Front Office
Management
for the
Veterinary Team

Front Office Management

for the

Veterinary Team

Heather Prendergast, BS, AS, RVT, CVPM
Certified Practice Manager
Jornada Veterinary Clinic
Las Cruces, New Mexico

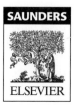

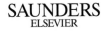

SAUNDERS
ELSEVIER

3251 Riverport Lane
St. Louis, Missouri 63043

Notice

Knowledge and best practice in this field are constantly changing. As new research and experience broaden our understanding, changes in research methods, professional practices, or medical treatment may become necessary.

Practitioners and researchers must always rely on their own experience and knowledge in evaluating and using any information, methods, compounds, or experiments described herein. In using such information or methods they should be mindful of their own safety and the safety of others, including parties for whom they have a professional responsibility.

With respect to any drug or pharmaceutical products identified, readers are advised to check the most current information provided (i) on procedures featured or (ii) by the manufacturer of each product to be administered, to verify the recommended dose or formula, the method and duration of adminis-tration, and contraindications. It is the responsibility of practitioners, relying on their own experience and knowledge of their patients, to make diagnoses, to determine dosages and the best treatment for each individual patient, and to take all appropriate safety precautions.

To the fullest extent of the law, neither the Publisher nor the author assumes any liability for any injury and/or damage to persons or property as a matter of products liability, negligence or otherwise, or from any use or operation of any methods, products, instructions, or ideas contained in the material herein.

Library of Congress Cataloging-in-Publication Data

Prendergast, Heather.
  Front office management for the veterinary team / Heather Prendergast. -- 1st ed.
      p. ; cm.
  Includes bibliographical references and index.
  ISBN 978-1-4377-0446-4 (pbk. : alk. paper)
  1. Veterinary services--Administration. 2. Animal health technicians. 3. Office management. I. Title.
  [DNLM: 1. Veterinary Medicine--organization & administration--United States. 2. Animal Technicians--United States. 3. Office Management--organization & administration--United States. 4. Practice Management, Medical--organization & administration--United States. 5. Veterinarians--United States. SF 756.4 P926f 2011]
  SF756.4.P74 2011
  636.089068--dc22   2010004577

Vice President and Publisher: Linda Duncan
Publisher: Penny Rudolph
Senior Developmental Editor: Shelly Stringer
Publishing Services Manager: Patricia Tannian
Project Manager: Carrie Stetz
Design Direction: Margaret Reid

Printed in the United States of America

Last digit is the print number: 9 8 7 6 5 4 3 2

Dedication

To my mother *~the wind beneath my wings~* you have guided me and
given me inspiration, motivation, and empowerment.
You have been *a truly amazing woman.*
I miss you dearly.

Preface

Veterinary assistants and technicians are an essential component to every practice. Practice managers and hospital administrators help guide the team and continue the progression of excellent medicine and customer service. All team members fulfill an ever-expanding role in the veterinary practice, both clinically and administratively. These increased responsibilities require a greater need for professional knowledge and skill. This text has been designed to provide the basics of administrative skills as well as a guide for more advanced practice management philosophies. Many technicians step into the role of practice management and learn as they go; this book will aid the understanding and application that you will face as your professional career grows.

FEATURES IN THIS TEXTBOOK

Important Features Include the Following:

- **Learning objectives** and **key terms** at the beginning of each chapter guide you in your study and enable you to check your mastery of the content in each chapter.

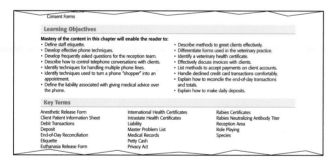

- **Veterinary Practice and the Law** boxes provide specific details regarding laws and regulations that pertain to each chapter.

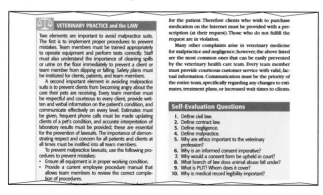

- **What Would You Do/Not Do?** boxes present real-life situations that occur in the veterinary practice and guide you through the appropriate responses.

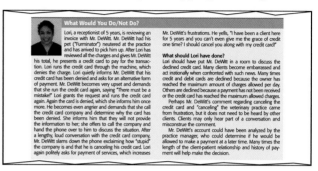

- **Practice Point** boxes spotlight important tips to running a successful practice.

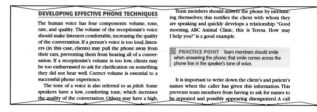

- **Self-evaluation questions** ensure that you have mastered complete comprehension of each chapter.
- An icon is placed next to the forms in this text that are available on the Evolve Web site as interactive working forms for student practice.
- **Recommended readings** provide additional sources of detailed information on important topics.

EVOLVE RESOURCES

The instructor Evolve site (for instructors only) includes:

- Chapter outlines, learning objectives, and key terms from the book.
- A test bank created in ExamView including 500 multiple-choice questions with rationales for the correct answers.
- An image collection containing all the images from the book (approximately 400 images).
- PowerPoint presentations for each chapter to assist with lecturing.

The student and instructor Evolve site includes:

- Interactive working forms to allow students to practice. These forms include sample checks and deposit slips, incident reports, history-taking forms, laboratory submission forms, and more!
- A quiz for each chapter taken from the book.
- A comprehensive glossary.

Acknowledgments

The completion of this text allows me to relay appreciation to the many individuals who contributed their time and effort. This book would not have been possible without any of them.

The photographs were taken by Clint Derk. I am indebted to him for his careful precision and patience in taking the photos, thus enhancing the value of this book. Clint has always said, "Life is too short not to enjoy what you do; make the best of everything you do!"

The team at Jornada Veterinary Clinic donated their time, skills, and smiles. Dr. Nancy Soules and Dr. Katie Larsen, my mentors and friends, have encouraged me and inspired me to take it to the next level. Without them, this hobby and career would not be as enjoyable as it has been.

Chris Delgado, Pam Dickens, Angela Winter, Melissa Supernor, and Elaine Anthony: thank you for your editing, ideas, and contributions. You guys are another amazing team that has taught me that dreams do come true! Penny and Shelly: you have made this endeavor an easy dream to accomplish. Others in the profession should strive to be as professional and positive as you.

To each of my students, past, present, and future: we know this career can be rewarding. Find a practice that allows you to shine and that will shine the light on you! Enjoy life while you can.

Heather Prendergast, BS, AS, RVT, CVPM

Table of Contents

Veterinary Practice as a Business

The veterinary health care team is what makes a veterinary practice a success. The team is made up of individuals with different qualities and intellectual levels. One team member may be great as an assistant but may lack the patience to work with clients in the reception area. A veterinarian may be a great surgeon but may have a less-than-desirable bedside manner. A great team is made of these different individuals who develop respect and rapport for one another. Each helps other team members at any time and is willing to help increase the knowledge of others.

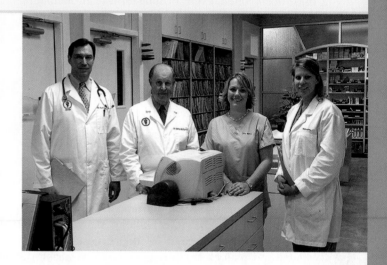

Kennel and veterinary assistants are critical to the team. Kennel assistants may be the first to notice abnormalities of hospitalized patients because they are in the kennels with the patients at all times. Assistants help restrain and aid in patient services. Excellent assistants are delegated certain responsibilities and duties, allowing the veterinarian to continue seeing patients and performing surgery. Credentialed technicians are excellent at providing education to clients and team members as well as performing diagnostic procedures for the veterinarian. Groomers may be the first to notice lumps or ear and anal gland infections and bring them to the attention of the owner and/or veterinarian. Receptionists are the front lines of the veterinary practice; they greet clients and accept criticism from clients, all with a smile on their faces. They make appointments, help organize appointments once clients have arrived, and maintain medical records. Office managers, practice managers, and hospital administrators help hold the practice together as a team. They problem solve, train, and develop procedures to maintain the team's efficiency. Veterinarians work hard to see patients, allowing them to examine, diagnose, prescribe medications, and perform surgery on the patients. With every team member's duties and responsibilities, all must work together to effectively and efficiently provide outstanding medicine and client service.

Team leadership requires a highly motivated and patient individual who is willing to learn about each team member. Some employees learn and retain information differently than others, and different teaching techniques must be used to have a successful team. Leaders must be effective at communication; team communication is essential in a successful practice. Once all team members understand and perform procedures in an efficient manner, tasks can be delegated to them, creating an empowering environment. Delegation and empowerment contribute to high employee retention rates. High retention rates signal a highly satisfied team.

Every team member lives by a code of ethics. Ethics are developed by society and are generally considered the cultural norm. Veterinary ethics are developed by the profession, and each team member must adhere to them. The American Veterinary Medical Association (AVMA), Veterinary Hospital Managers Association, and the National Association of Veterinary Technicians in the United States have developed a Code of Ethics for each member to follow. The AVMA's code of ethics has been adopted by many state veterinary boards and is the basis for many practice acts. Practice acts are the laws that have been established in each state to which veterinarians and veterinary technicians must adhere. If these laws are not followed, team members may be in violation, which allows for the removal of licenses.

Many laws have been established for the protection of employers as well as employees. Practice managers and owners must be familiar with federal and state laws, as penalties can be high for those in violation. Employee manuals should be developed both for the protection of the practice as well as the employees. A manual allows team members to understand what is expected of them once they are hired as well as policies of the practice and termination procedures if they are needed. Procedural manuals outline all of the procedures the practice follows; a simple guideline allows new team members to excel at their positions while providing a refresher for those long-term employees who do not practice the procedure often.

Team training is essential to the success of a team; it must occur often, even for long-term team members. Continuing education (CE) revitalizes everyone, creating excitement among the team. CE can be brought into the clinic; team members can attend local or state meetings without traveling far or attend national conferences that are out of state.

For new team members, the creation of a structured training plan is a must. Training in phases prevents the new team member(s) from becoming overwhelmed, as many procedures and tasks are learned in one day. It also prevents the skipping of procedures and tasks and allows the task to be mastered before moving on to the next skill level. Training in phases and regulation of employee hours can prevent stress and burnout that is so highly associated with veterinary technology. Many assistants and technicians work extended hours, ensuring quality client and patient care is achieved. However, those under high levels of stress may turn to drugs or alcohol to relieve stress or leave the profession all together. It is imperative for all team members to prevent career burnout—for oneself as well as the rest of the team.

Practice design is essential to the efficiency of the practice. Items needed for a task should be placed as close together as possible to decrease the time to complete tasks. Team members must use correct posture and lifting movements to prevent injury while on the job. Overuse and inappropriate lifting can injure the back over time; measures must be taken to prevent injuries before they happen. Placing computers in specific areas of the practice can increase the efficiency of the team, as can choosing appropriate veterinary software to help manage client accounts. Software can allow a practice to be completely paperless, which increases efficiency and decreases wastage. If a practice wishes to continue utilizing paper records, software can enhance inventory management, accounts receivable, and client communications.

Marketing techniques are used by every practice on a daily basis. Marketing to clients takes place without the team being aware of the activities occurring. Client education is a form of marketing, as are reminders and recalls. Web sites are developed to inform existing and potential clients of the services the practice offers as well as provide educational materials and links to recommended organizations or companies. Indirect marketing includes the cleanliness of the practice as well as the genuineness of the team members. Practice managers may develop marketing programs to drive clients into the practice for particular services, but a positive and energetic team spirit will retain clients and keep them returning for services. Practices must seize the opportunity to provide clients with exceptional service, education, and high-quality medicine.

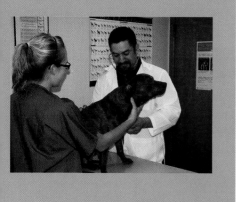

Veterinary Health Care Team Members

Learning Objectives

Mastery of the content in this chapter will enable the reader to:
• Define various positions within a veterinary practice.
• Identify courses of study to enhance the education of each
  position.

Key Terms

American Veterinary Medical
   Association (AVMA)
Groomer
Kennel Assistant
National Association of Veterinary
   Technicians in America (NAVTA)

Office Manager
Practice Manager
Receptionist
Veterinarian
Veterinary Assistant
Veterinary Practice Act

Veterinary Support Personnel
   Network (VSPN)
Veterinary Technician
Veterinary Technician National
   Examination Committee (VTNE)

The veterinary practice can be a highly structured environment that provides an excellent career for all team members. The goal of every practice should be to provide excellent medical care to patients and outstanding customer service to clients while providing a workplace that is friendly, efficient, and safe. Each team member contributes to the success of the practice. Veterinarians are responsible for providing the guidelines of medical care, and assistants and technicians are responsible for following these guidelines to provide excellent care.

In-hospital patients receive care from all team members—from kennel assistants to veterinarians—and all team members are responsible for ensuring patient safety and comfort. Patients can never be left in feces and urine; they must always have access to water and food when allowed and be hospitalized in a warm, comfortable environment. Team members share responsibilities for these hospitalized patients, and all must take initiative to provide the best care, whatever their positions are in

the practice (Figure 1-1). Any team member who sees a patient in a dirty cage must clean it immediately.

Outpatients include those that visit the practice for examinations, vaccinations, lab work, or services that do not require hospitalization. In general, one technician and one veterinarian provide service to these clients, and it is their responsibility to ensure the client receives the necessary services in a timely and professional manner. Medications, client instructions, and handouts should be supplied to the client when needed. Clients are often overwhelmed with information they obtain while at a veterinary hospital; therefore client handouts are pertinent for excellent customer service.

Clients are turning to the Internet more than ever to educate themselves about veterinary disease, products, and procedures. The Internet has a vast amount of information, but not all of it is correct. Veterinary practices must provide accurate and supplemental information to clients who have questions. The Internet should not

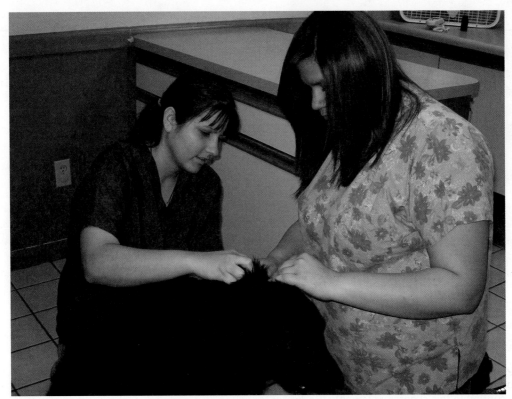

FIGURE 1-1 Two assistants discuss a case.

be looked at negatively, but incorporated appropriately as a means to educate clients. Once clients find new information on products and procedures, they should be encouraged to contact the practice with questions. Team members can use this opportunity to strengthen the client-patient-practice relationship.

Clients expect excellent customer service from veterinary practices. It can take weeks to receive laboratory results in human medicine, and many times the physician never calls the patient with results. In veterinary medicine, clients expect veterinarians to call the following day with results and often are upset if the results are not available sooner. Many opinion polls conducted in the past have placed veterinarians higher than physicians when respondents were asked to rank professions and the value they place on each. Some individuals value their veterinarians more than their physicians because the level of care they receive from their veterinary practice far exceeds the care they receive from their own physicians.

Team members have rights and responsibilities in practices, including a safe work environment. Practices cannot be completely hazard free. Dogs and cats will bite, but practices can ensure that the proper equipment to prevent those hazards from occurring is available. Team members must use proper equipment when needed, and all should receive proper training on when and how to use personal protective equipment. A safe work environment can lead to a fun, interactive workplace that results in a satisfying career.

A key ingredient to teamwork is open and honest communication among employees, managers, and owners. The second ingredient to a successful team is developing and embracing respect for one another. When teamwork is evident, clients notice and recommend the friendly, honest, genuine service that a veterinary practice can provide.

The veterinary health care team involves all members of the staff. Each person plays a significant role in a successful practice. Roles and duties vary by practice and typically are defined in an employee manual. Team members working together as a group provide better patient and client care than those who work as individuals. Team members may include, but are not limited to, students, groomers, kennel assistants, veterinary assistants, credentialed veterinary technicians, veterinary technologists, receptionists, veterinarians, office managers, and practice managers. Many clinics also have specializations within each team member position. Having a team leader can significantly improve communication and accountability.

Larger practices may have a structured hierarchy, with each team member having a specific role in the practice. Technicians may be limited to hospitalized patients, surgical recovery, or laboratory, whereas others may be assigned to outpatient visits only. Smaller practices have assistants and technicians assigned to all areas of the practice at the same time. Each area requires special knowledge and education and must not be overlooked when completing duties in various areas of the practice.

Each new team member must become familiar with a number of topics in each practice. Because many practices use different products and equipment or perform procedures with different methods, a list of questions has been developed that each team member should be familiar with when starting a new position (Box 1-1).

STUDENTS

Students may function as observers or hold paid positions within a hospital. Many students must complete externships as part of a program. High school students can earn grades while completing a required number of hours at the job site, and veterinary assistant and technician students may fulfill hours required for their coursework. Students may be assigned tasks by the school that must be done before course completion, which aids in the training process. Task lists can be used as a guide for both the practice and the student.

Many veterinary schools have in-clinic prerequisites that must be completed before application and/or admission. Veterinary students can also complete an externship in a private practice to obtain more experience before graduating from a professional program.

GROOMERS

Groomers perform technical skills that they have acquired in order to care for patients and satisfy clients. This takes patience. They must take precautions to prevent injury to animals as well as themselves. Animals can become scared and aggressive while being groomed. Clippers are loud and tables can scare pets, causing them to become more aggressive than usual.

Several courses are available to learn how to groom; on-the-job training is also available. The National Dog Groomers Association works with groomers throughout the country to promote and encourage professionalism and education to maintain the image of the pet grooming profession. Their goal is to unite groomers through membership, promote communication with colleagues, set recognized grooming standards, and offer those seeking a higher level of professional recognition the opportunity to have their grooming skills certified. In some states licensure or certification is required.

At times, groomers are the first to recognize abnormalities that should be further investigated by a veterinarian. Abnormal anal glands, skin tags, masses, and ear infections are often detected by groomers while they care for pets. Owners appreciate and respect groomers' opinions when these abnormalities are found and often follow up with a visit to a veterinary practice.

Groomers need to communicate clearly and professionally as a part of retaining clients. Many clients require extra time because they expect the best for their pets. Many times pets become uncooperative, producing a less than perfect cut; this can upset clients. Any grooming mistakes reflect on the groomers, who must be able to communicate well to handle dissatisfied clients.

Grooming can be an extremely satisfying career for many team members because results of an excellent job can be viewed immediately (Figure 1-2 and Box 1-2).

KENNEL ASSISTANTS

Kennel assistants are critical to the health care team. Kennel assistants keep the patients clean and alert the team of any changes in patient status. Most kennel assistants

Box 1-1	Common Questions for the New Team Member

- What are the common emergencies seen at the practice?
- What are the common diseases seen in the practice's geographic area?
- What are local vaccination protocols?
- What flea and tick preventive is recommended?
- What nutritional products and food are sold at the practice?
- What routine surgeries are performed in the practice?
- What specialty procedures are performed in the practice?
- Is the hospital accredited by the American Animal Hospital Association?
- Does the practice board animals?
- Are emergencies accepted after hours? If not, where are clients advised to go?
- At what age are pets recommended to be altered?

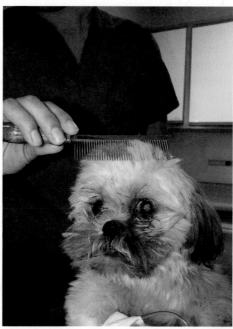

FIGURE 1-2 Groomers play an important role in the veterinary practice.

Box 1-2	Responsibilities of Groomers

Successful groomers must:
- Have patience
- Have excellent customer service skills
- Communicate clearly with clients
- Be flexible
- Know when new products are available
- Know about skin diseases and infections
- Be aware of communicable and zoonotic diseases
- Obtain continuing education to better serve their patients

receive on-the-job training, learning procedures and protocols while they gain proficiency.

Kennel assistants should become familiar with cleaning protocols as well as any harmful and potentially fatal cleaning products. Mixing cleaning chemicals should be against hospital policy because of the possibility of creating toxic fumes. Many team members are unfamiliar with chemical reactions that can cause harm to both employees and patients.

Kennel assistants should be trained to detect emergency situations that may occur while a patient is hospitalized, including anaphylactic shock and seizures. They must also receive education on the prevention of disease transmission. Many diseases can be transmitted by fomites (e.g., bowls, litter pans) that are not cleaned completely. Cages can also retain aerosolized droplets of disease organisms when not cleaned properly. Cages are considered to have seven sides: the front cage door (two sides) and the five sides of the interior of the cage. All sides should be cleaned with a safe disinfectant approved for killing viruses and fungi.

Kennel assistants must be able to interpret correct nutritional instructions, feed the correct diet and amount, and remove food from preoperative patients. Appropriate safety precautions should be taken when moving patients to another cage or when walking patients outdoors (Figure 1-3). This important team member reports any and all behavior and condition changes to the immediate patient supervisor (Box 1-3).

VETERINARY ASSISTANTS

Veterinary assistants are a strong asset to the team. Veterinary assistants may help a veterinary technician and/or veterinarian. They should excel at physical restraint, laboratory skills, patient care, and client relations (Box 1-4). Veterinary assistants often are key to clinics that excel in client satisfaction and patient care. Kennel assistants may report to a veterinary assistant, who in turn reports critical patient information to either a veterinary technician or veterinarian. Assistants can be trained on the job by veterinary technicians or practice managers or attend veterinary assistant classes. As the field of veterinary

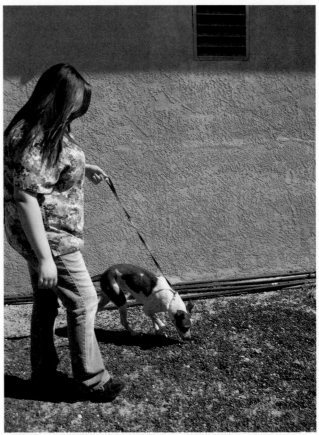

FIGURE 1-3 Kennel assistants use a leash and walk patients outdoors in safe, designated areas.

Box 1-3	Responsibilities of Kennel Assistants

Successful kennel assistants must:
- Have patience
- Communicate well with team members
- Accept tasks willingly
- Have knowledge of communicable diseases
- Understand the transmission potential of zoonotic diseases
- Understand nutrition and the importance of a proper diet
- Know when to report an emergency situation
- Safely use cleaning chemicals and procedures

medicine grows, education opportunities available to team members increase as well. Programs are available at every level to help educate each staff member (Box 1-5).

VETERINARY TECHNICIANS

Veterinary technicians are critical to the health care team. A credentialed technician is a graduate of a 2-year veterinary technology program approved by the American Veterinary Medical Association (AVMA). A technician must pass an examination given by the state and the Veterinary Technician National Examination Committee (VTNE) before receiving a license. Depending on the state, the

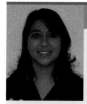

What Would You Do/Not Do?

Sabrina, a veterinary assistant of 5 years, is interested in furthering her career by attending a credentialed program to receive her license. She has seen the tasks and procedures credentialed technicians at other practices can complete and wonders if she would be able to perform them in her practice. Her practice currently does not employ a credentialed technician, so her scope of the level of activities is limited. She also wonders if she would receive a pay raise for her schooling as well as the potential added responsibilities. She cannot decide if she should attend a campus or distance program.

What Should Sabrina Do?

Sabrina should first address her enthusiasm for the profession with the owner of the practice. The veterinarian may be unaware of how much a credentialed technician could help the practice. Sabrina should mention the tasks and procedures other credentialed technicians complete and how these skills benefit their practices. Sabrina can make a comparison with how credentialing could benefit their practice.

Second, Sabrina could ask about the possibility of promotion and added responsibilities, along with a potential raise in the future, if she completes her degree. If Sabrina receives satisfactory answers, she can decide if a distance or campus program would be best for her. Finances, location, and the scope of the program should all be considered.

Box 1-4	**Responsibilities of Veterinary Assistants**

Successful veterinary assistants must:
- Accept tasks willingly
- Strive to provide the best service at all times
- Communicate clearly with team members and clients
- Excel at animal restraint
- Understand diseases and their prevention
- Understand nutrition and the importance of a proper diet
- Understand common procedures performed in the practice
- Have knowledge of common drugs used in the practice
- Have initiative to learn and raise the practice to the next level of care

---

Box 1-5	**Veterinary Assistant Programs**

- Animal Care Training in combination with Texas Veterinary Medical Association (distance education): www.4act.com
- National Collegiate Partners offers veterinary assistant programs at a variety of community colleges: 888-824-6667 or info@natcolpar.com
- VetMedTeam.com
- Veterinary assistant programs offered through local community colleges

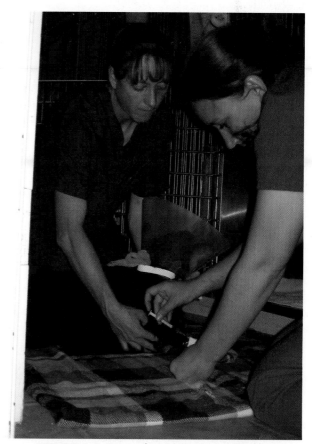

FIGURE 1-4 Two technicians treat a patient.

graduate may be considered registered, certified, or licensed or may be called an *animal health technologist.* Credentialed technicians are allowed to perform certain duties under the direct supervision of a veterinarian (Figure 1-4). Direct supervision is defined as having a licensed veterinarian on premises and readily available while a veterinary technician completes certain duties. These duties vary from state to state; therefore each state veterinary practice act must be evaluated individually. Credentialed technicians may be required to attend continuing education to maintain licensure; states vary regarding the minimal number of credits required (Boxes 1-6 and 1-7).

Box 1-6	Continuing Education Requirements for Technicians

STATE	REQUIREMENTS
Alaska	10 hours per 2 years
Alabama	8 hours per 1 year
Arkansas	4 hours per 1 year
Arizona	10 hours per 2 years
California	Not required
Colorado	16 hours per 2 years
Connecticut	Not required
Delaware	12 hours per 2 years
Florida	15 hours per 2 years
Georgia	10 hours per 2 years
Hawaii	Does not license
Idaho	14 hours per 2 years
Illinois	10 hours per 2 years
Indiana	16 hours per 2 years
Iowa	30 hours per 3 years
Kansas	Not required
Kentucky	6 hours per year
Louisiana	Not required
Maine	Not required
Maryland	24 hours per 3 years
Massachusetts	12 hours per year
Michigan	Not required
Minnesota	10 hours per 2 years
Mississippi	10 hours per year
Missouri	10 hours per year
Montana	Does not license
North Carolina	12 hours per 2 years
North Dakota	8 hours per 2 years
Nebraska	16 hours per 2 years
New Hampshire	12 hours per year
New Jersey	Does not license
New Mexico	8 hours per year
Nevada	5 hours per year
New York	Not required
Ohio	10 hours per 2 years
Oklahoma	10 hours per year
Oregon	15 hours per 2 years
Pennsylvania	16 hours per 2 years
Rhode Island	12 hours per year
South Carolina	10 hours per 2 years
South Dakota	12 hours per 2 years
Tennessee	12 hours per year
Texas	5 hours per year
Utah	Does not license
Virginia	6 hours per year
Vermont	6 hours per year
Washington	Not required
Washington, DC	Does not license
Wisconsin	15 hours per 2 years
West Virginia	8 hours per year
Wyoming	10 hours per 2 years

Each state has its own standards and requirements; review the specific state's veterinary board and practice act for more information.

Box 1-7	Responsibilities of Veterinary Technicians and Technologists

Successful veterinary technicians and technologists must:
- Have patience
- Accept tasks willingly
- Communicate well with team members and clients
- Educate team members and clients
- Listen to clients
- Understand, prevent, and teach the significance of diseases
- Understand and teach the importance of nutrition
- Develop safety protocols for assistants
- Perform common procedures and laboratory analyses
- Become proficient at obtaining samples for laboratory analysis
- Understand the mechanics, chemistry, and effects of the drugs used in the practice

PRACTICE POINT   Veterinary Technician Week is the third week in October, as designated by NAVTA.

Veterinary technicians are generally assigned a patient by the veterinarian. The technician follows all instructions for a treatment protocol, including medication, nutrition, laboratory tests, and exercise. Technicians must document all treatments given to the patient and include any observations, such as bowel movements or urination, in the record or on a hospital sheet (see Figure 14-12). This allows the veterinarian to follow the treatment progress of patients. Veterinary technicians are critical for client interaction as well. Clients should be updated daily regarding the progress of their pets by an informed staff member. Clients appreciate updates throughout the day as well as any education materials regarding their pets' disease or condition.

VETERINARY TECHNOLOGISTS

A veterinary technologist can be a graduate of a 4-year bachelor of science program in veterinary technology accredited by the AVMA (Box 1-8).

A veterinary technologist may also hold an associate's degree in veterinary technology along with a bachelor's degree in another program, such as business, management, or health science. Technologists tend to work in positions that require a higher level of education and may hold teaching positions within technology programs or veterinary schools.

The head veterinary technician or technologist is responsible for overseeing veterinary technicians, assistants, and kennel personnel. They are responsible for training employees, implementing new and/or updated protocols and procedures, as well as maintaining inventory and ordering products.

<table>
<tr><td>Box 1-8</td><td>Accredited Veterinary Technology Programs</td></tr>
</table>

- Total number of programs: 150
- Number offering 4-year degree: 16
- Number offering distance learning: 9

The following states do not have AVMA-accredited veterinary technology programs: Alaska, Arkansas, District of Columbia, Hawaii, Montana, and Rhode Island. For a complete, up-to-date listing of AVMA-accredited veterinary technician programs, visit www.avma.org.

VETERINARY TECHNICIAN SPECIALTIES

Veterinary technicians may decide to focus on a specific area of care, currently consisting of four specialty academies and one society. A *society* is defined as a group of individuals, veterinary technicians, hospital staff, and veterinarians interested in a specific discipline or area of veterinary medicine. An *academy* is the term selected by the National Association of Veterinary Technicians of America (NAVTA) to designate a group receiving recognition as a specialty (Box 1-9).

Technicians who choose to specialize must accumulate a specific number of hours within a particular specialty during a set number of years. For example, The Academy of Internal Medicine for Veterinary Technicians requires a minimum of 3 years' experience, with 6000 hours of experience as a credentialed veterinary technician in the field of internal medicine. All experience must be completed within 5 years before application. Candidates are also expected to have a minimum of 40 hours of continuing education on internal medicine before application submission.

Whether a veterinary assistant, veterinary technician, or technologist, every team member should be educated in basic laboratory work performed in a hospital. Veterinary technicians and technologists must be able to prepare and read blood smears, cytology preparations, urine samples, and fecal smears. Veterinary assistants may become proficient at running chemistry panels and complete blood cell counts on in-house laboratory equipment. All assistants and technicians should become proficient at radiology and learn the safety issues associated with all laboratory equipment, including the radiology machines. A veterinarian's productivity increases by delegating tasks associated with patient care to veterinary technicians and assistants. This allows the veterinarian to concentrate on diagnosing, prescribing medication, and performing surgeries.

RECEPTIONISTS

Receptionists are often the "face" of the veterinary practice (Box 1-10). They play a significant role in the success of a practice and must appear professional, polite, and

<table>
<tr><td>Box 1-9</td><td>Veterinary Technician Specialties</td></tr>
</table>

- Academy of Veterinary Emergency and Critical Care Technicians (AVECCT): www.avecct.org
- Academy of Veterinary Technician Anesthetists (AVTA): www.avta-vts.org
- Academy of Veterinary Dental Technicians (AVDT): www.avdt.us
- Academy of Internal Medicine for Veterinary Technicians (AIMVT): www.aimvt.com
- American Association of Equine Veterinary Technicians and Assistants (AAEVT): www.aaevt.org
- Society of Veterinary Behavior Technicians: www.svbt.org

<table>
<tr><td>Box 1-10</td><td>Responsibilities of Receptionists</td></tr>
</table>

Successful receptionists must:
- Have patience
- Communicate well with team members and clients
- Provide exceptional service to every client
- Determine wants and needs of every client and patient
- Have respect for others
- Educate clients on the phone
- Promote products and services provided by the practice
- Listen to clients

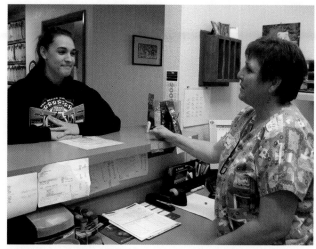

FIGURE 1-5 A receptionist greets a client with a smile, giving a positive first impression of the veterinary practice.

caring. They must listen to client stories, show empathy when needed, and be able to collect money from clients under difficult circumstances (Figure 1-5).

Receptionists greet clients, detail and clarify invoices, and receive money. They answer the phone and can turn an inquiring phone call into an appointment. Receptionists acknowledge clients when they walk in and out of the practice. They make the first impression on a client, whether on the phone or at the front desk.

OFFICE MANAGERS

The office manager is generally responsible for overseeing the front office staff as well as training receptionists to excel at customer service and public relations (Box 1-11). An office manager may allow a client to charge services and generally oversees accounts receivable. An office manager's realm of authority and decision making may be quite broad or limited depending on the administrative needs and criteria established by the practice. Many office managers are responsible for bank deposit preparation and performance. An office manager is courteous, friendly, and professional (Figure 1-6). His

Box 1-11	Responsibilities of Office Managers

Successful office managers must:
- Be a successful receptionist
- Educate team members
- Develop coping strategies to handle angry clients
- Handle accounts receivable with a smile
- Determine if and when clients may charge for services rendered

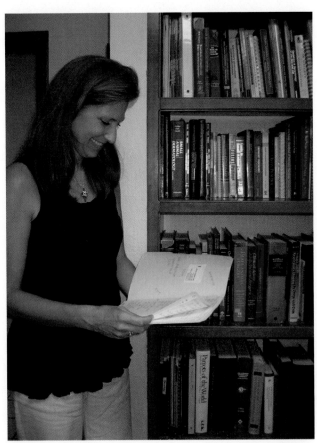

FIGURE 1-6 Office managers ensure that the front office is operating effectively. They must display a friendly attitude and a professional appearance.

or her demeanor, whether positive or negative, trickles down through the rest of the team.

VETERINARIANS

Veterinarians are the only members of the team allowed to diagnose, prescribe, and perform surgery on patients (Box 1-12). They have completed 4 years of a professional, AVMA-accredited school of veterinary medicine (Box 1-13). Veterinarians must be licensed in the state where they work and must pass both national and state examinations before receiving licensure. Veterinarians are required to complete a minimum number of hours in continuing education each year and must report their hours to the state veterinary board. These requirements ensure veterinarians offer the best medical care available to patients and clients (Figure 1-7).

PRACTICE MANAGERS

A practice manager helps keep the entire team working together and often reports to a hospital administrator. Practice managers generally handle client and personnel issues, supervise training sessions for team members, and hold team members accountable for their actions. Duties may also include reviewing records for completeness, observing for missed charges, and ensuring that policies are followed correctly. New strategies may be implemented by the practice manager to increase business as well as introduce new products to the clinic. Most practice managers hold a bachelor's degree in science or business administration; others hold an associate's degree in veterinary technology. Practice managers benefit from either type of degree, which allows them to excel at managing a veterinary hospital.

A practice manager may have to wear many hats while on the job: copier repair technician, computer technician, plumber, veterinary technician, kennel assistant, and/or counselor. Just as with the office manager, the practice manager must have a positive, friendly attitude with an open-door policy for all team members. Great attitudes encourage a professional and successful atmosphere (Box 1-14).

Box 1-12	Responsibilities of Veterinarians

Successful veterinarians must:
- Practice quality and current medicine
- Communicate well with clients and team members
- Educate clients and team members
- Attend continuing education seminars on a regular basis
- Have patience
- Have a positive attitude
- Delegate tasks
- Diagnose, prescribe medication, and perform surgery

Box 1-13	Veterinary Schools

- Auburn University College of Veterinary Medicine: www.vetmed.auburn.edu
- Colorado State University College of Veterinary Medicine and Biomedical Sciences: www.cvmbs.colostate.edu
- Cornell University College of Veterinary Medicine: www.vet.cornell.edu
- Cummings School of Veterinary Medicine at Tufts University: www.tufts.edu/vet
- Iowa State University College of Veterinary Medicine: www.vetmed.iastate.edu
- Kansas State University College of Veterinary Medicine: www.vet.ksu.edu
- Louisiana State University School of Veterinary Medicine: www.vetmed.lsu.edu
- Michigan State University College of Veterinary Medicine: cvm.msu.edu
- Mississippi State University College of Veterinary Medicine: www.cvm.msstate.edu
- North Carolina State University College of Veterinary Medicine: www.cvm.ncsu.edu
- Ohio State University College of Veterinary Medicine: www.vet.ohio-state.edu
- Oklahoma State University Center for Veterinary Health Sciences: www.cvm.okstate.edu
- Oregon State University College of Veterinary Medicine: oregonstate.edu/vetmed
- Purdue University School of Veterinary Medicine: www.vet.purdue.edu
- Texas A&M University College of Veterinary Medicine & Biomedical Sciences: www.cvm.tamu.edu
- Tuskegee University College of Veterinary Medicine, Nursing & Allied Health: www.tuskegee.edu/Global/category.asp?C=35019&nav=menu200_9
- University of California School of Veterinary Medicine: www.vetmed.ucdavis.edu
- University of Florida College of Veterinary Medicine: www.vetmed.ufl.edu
- University of Georgia College of Veterinary Medicine: www.vet.uga.edu
- University of Illinois College of Veterinary Medicine: www.cvm.uiuc.edu
- University of Minnesota College of Veterinary Medicine: www.cvm.umn.edu
- University of Missouri College of Veterinary Medicine: www.cvm.missouri.edu
- University of Pennsylvania School of Veterinary Medicine: www.vet.upenn.edu
- University of Tennessee College of Veterinary Medicine: www.vet.utk.edu
- University of Wisconsin-Madison School of Veterinary Medicine: www.vetmed.wisc.edu
- Virginia Tech Virginia-Maryland Regional College of Veterinary Medicine: www.vetmed.vt.edu
- Western University of Health Sciences College of Veterinary Medicine: www.westernu.edu/xp/edu/veterinary/about.xml

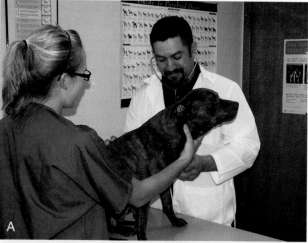
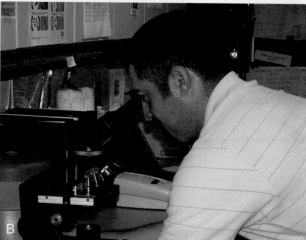

FIGURE 1-7 Veterinarians diagnose, prescribe, and perform surgery.

Box 1-14	Responsibilities of Practice Managers

Successful practice managers must:
- Have patience
- Lead the team in a positive manner
- Address conflict immediately
- Develop training protocols for the entire team
- Develop communication pieces for clients
- Develop sales strategies to increase revenue
- Hire, fire, and train in a legal manner
- Determine efficient methods for completion of tasks and procedures

HOSPITAL ADMINISTRATORS

A hospital administrator may be a veterinarian, technician, or a business manager. He or she generally has complete authority over the operation of the business and practice. This position is responsible for setting budgets, paying bills, creating organizational structure, and planning events (Box 1-15). A typical administrator is responsible for all the duties of the office manager and practice manager. Although a hospital administrator may not be a veterinarian, this person should have general knowledge of quality assurance and performance in veterinary medicine and may act in an advisory role in helping establish and supervise protocols of the practice. A hospital administrator may report to the owner or shareholders if the practice is owned by multiple members. Hospital administrators often make the final purchasing decisions.

TEAM

All roles on a veterinary team are important. All members contribute significantly (Figure 1-8). As is commonly said, there is no "I" in "team." Each team member must help others complete tasks in the most efficient manner (Box 1-16). Kennel assistants may need to help a technician restrain a patient for laboratory work, and a technician may need to clean kennels; a veterinarian may need to answer the phone when all receptionists are working actively with clients. This is why cross-training employees

Box 1-15	Responsibilities of Hospital Administrators

Successful hospital administrators must:
- Have patience
- Lead the team in a positive manner
- Oversee each department
- Develop, implement, and enforce budgets
- Develop and implement sales strategies to increase revenue
- Scrutinize medical records for completeness and quality medicine
- Ensure practice policies and procedures are being followed by each team member
- Attend continuing education seminars to improve the quality of the practice

Box 1-16	Characteristics of Successful Team Environments

- Team members understand one another's priorities and difficulties and offer help when the opportunity arises.
- Open communication exists among all employees, managers, and owners.
- Problem solving occurs as a team.
- The team is recognized for outstanding results, as are individuals for personal contributions.
- Team members are encouraged to make suggestions and test their abilities to improve the quality and quantity of work.

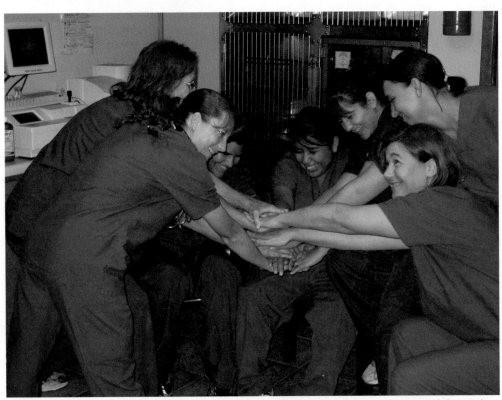

FIGURE 1-8 All team players need to be knowledgeable in several areas of responsibility and should work together to keep the practice running smoothly.

in all areas of the practice is crucial. Information and communication can be accessed and shared easier when team members are knowledgeable in several areas of the practice. When a team environment is created, any role in the veterinary health care team is rewarding. Patients receive better care, clients receive better communication, and employees enjoy coming to work. When employees enjoy their jobs, they work harder and more efficiently and strive to achieve higher goals. Every practice can benefit from a team attitude.

PROGRAMS TO ENHANCE STAFF EDUCATION

Several programs are available online and at community colleges across the United States to enhance staff education. Veterinary assistant courses are available to help teach the basics of animal restraint, disease development, and client communication. Veterinary technician courses are available on campus and through distance learning. Distance programs give students the advantage of working in a practice while attending classes in the evening or on weekends via the Internet. Students can practice techniques learned in class under the direct supervision of their employing veterinarians. Distance education technology schools must be accredited by the AVMA in order for the students to take the licensing examination upon graduation from the program.

Students physically attending veterinary technology programs participate in clinics that are either on campus or organized through local veterinary hospitals, allowing students to obtain the direct experience needed to graduate from the program. Once students graduate, state and national technician organizations offer continuing education opportunities (Boxes 1-17 and 1-18).

The Veterinary Support Personnel Network (VSPN) is a group for veterinary technicians and assistants, receptionists, office managers, and other support staff who work with, for, or in the field of veterinary medicine. To access all VSPN's features (message boards, chat forums,

Box 1-17	National Veterinary Technician Organizations

National Association of Veterinary Technicians in America (NAVTA)
50 S. Pickett, #110
Alexandria, VA 22304
703-740-8737
www.navta.net

Canadian Association of Animal Health Technologists and Technicians (CAAHTT)
339 Rue Booth Street
Ottawa, ON K1R 7K1
CANADA
800-567-2162, ext. 121

Box 1-18	State Veterinary Technician Organizations

STATE	ASSOCIATION
Alabama	www.alabamavettech.com
Alaska	Not active
Arizona	www.vhctaz.org
Arkansas	www.arkvetmed.org
California	www.carvta.org
Colorado	www.cacvt.com
Connecticut	Not active
Delaware	www.delvettech.com
Florida	www.fvta.net
Georgia	www.gvtaa.org
Hawaii	Not active
Idaho	Not active
Illinois	Not active
Indiana	www.invta.org
Iowa	www.civta.com
Kansas	www.kvta.net
Kentucky	www.kyvta.org
Louisiana	Not active
Maine	www.mevta.org
Maryland	No organization
Massachusetts	www.massvta.org
Michigan	www.mavt.us
Minnesota	www.mavt.net
Mississippi	No organization
Missouri	www.mvma.us/MOVMAWEB.nsf
Montana	www.mtbsvta.org
Nebraska	Not active
New Hampshire	www.nhvta.org
New Jersey	Not active
New Mexico	Not active
Nevada	No organization
New York	www.nysavt.org
North Carolina	www.ncavt.com
North Dakota	www.ndvta.org
Ohio	www.ohiorvt.org
Oklahoma	www.okvta.org
Oregon	www.ovtaa.org
Pennsylvania	pvta.affiniscape.com
Rhode Island	www.rivta.org
South Carolina	www.scavt.org
South Dakota	No organization
Tennessee	www.tnvta.org
Texas	www.tarvt.org
Utah	No organization
Vermont	No organization
Virginia	www.valvt.org
Washington	www.wsavt.info
Washington, DC	No organization
West Virginia	www.wvavt.com
Wisconsin	www.wvta.com
Wyoming	www.wyvta.org

Current as of November 2009.

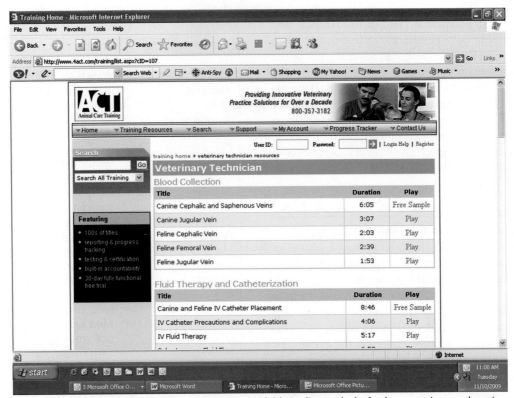

FIGURE 1-9 Animal Care Training videos are available online to help further veterinary education. (Courtesy Animal Care Technologies, Denton, Texas.)

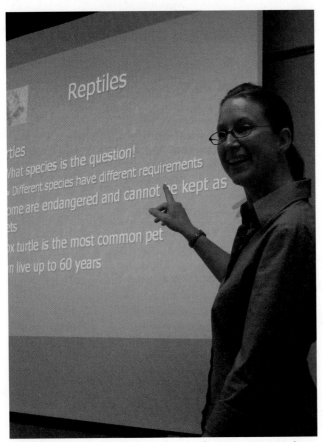

FIGURE 1-10 A veterinary technician lectures at a veterinary assistant program.

continuing education, etc.), team members can register at www.vspn.org. Membership to VSPN is free. The VSPN community brings together members from all over the world to interact, teach, and learn. Members of VSPN have access to thousands of colleagues worldwide who want to help each other become a success.

Animal Care Training offers exceptional educational videos that can be viewed online. These training videos cover all aspects of veterinary health care, including receptionist, veterinary assistant, and technician job functions. Sample videos can be viewed at www.4act.com (Figure 1-9).

Local specialty and emergency centers may offer continuing education for staff members of surrounding veterinary clinics. These seminars are generally free and cover a broad range of topics, including law and liability, emergency care, and practice management issues. In addition, local and regional veterinary technician organizations often offer continuing education at reasonable prices (Figure 1-10).

Manufacturer and distributor representatives are other excellent resources for continuing education for staff members. They have educational information available and are always willing to give presentations to staff.

VETERINARY PRACTICE and the LAW

Veterinary assistants are not licensed, and in most states their role is not clearly defined. State veterinary practice acts may allow veterinarians to delegate clinical tasks to qualified veterinary assistants under their supervision. Some states define the roles and regulations of veterinary assistants; therefore legal status should be determined on a state-by-state basis.

Credentialed veterinary technicians are licensed in some states. However, state practice acts may not clearly define the roles or procedures that technicians are allowed to perform. Just as with assistants, many state practice acts allow veterinarians to delegate duties to qualified technicians as long as they are under the direct supervision of the veterinarian.

Licensed technicians are responsible for maintaining a professional image and must renew their license annually or biannually. Licenses can be revoked for lack of continuing education, misconduct, or drug abuse.

Self-Evaluation Questions

1. What are the main duties associated with a groomer?
2. What are the main duties associated with a kennel assistant?
3. What are the main duties associated with a veterinary assistant?
4. What are the main duties associated with a veterinary technician?
5. What is a technician specialty?
6. What is the purpose of continuing education?
7. Where do you see yourself in 5 years? 10 years?
8. What qualities will you bring to the practice?

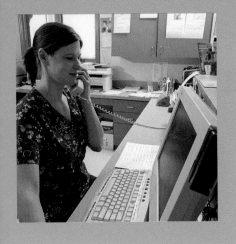

The Receptionist Team

Chapter Outline

Learning Objectives

Mastery of the content in this chapter will enable the reader to:

- Define staff etiquette.
- Develop effective phone techniques.
- Develop frequently asked questions for the reception team.
- Describe how to control telephone conversations with clients.
- Identify techniques for handling multiple phone lines.
- Identify techniques used to turn a phone "shopper" into an appointment.
- Define the liability associated with giving medical advice over the phone.
- Describe methods to greet clients effectively.
- Differentiate forms used in the veterinary practice.
- Identify a veterinary health certificate.
- Effectively discuss invoices with clients.
- List methods to accept payments on client accounts.
- Handle declined credit card transactions comfortably.
- Explain how to reconcile the end-of-day transactions and totals.
- Explain how to make daily deposits.

Key Terms

Anesthetic Release Form
Client Patient Information Sheet
Debit Transactions
Deposit
End-of-Day Reconciliation
Etiquette
Euthanasia Release Form

International Health Certificates
Intrastate Health Certificates
Liability
Master Problem List
Medical Records
Petty Cash
Privacy Act

Rabies Certificates
Rabies Neutralizing Antibody Titer
Reception Area
Role-Playing
Species

The ultimate goal of the receptionist team is to provide immediate, consistent, dependable, and courteous service to the client. The receptionist is the front line of any veterinary health care team. This person is responsible for clients' first impressions and should therefore greet them in a friendly manner when they call the practice or walk in the door. Receptionists offer helpful information and explain any charges for which the client is responsible. They are also the last member of the team to take care of clients; therefore the need to make a lasting positive impression is a must. Receptionists should have a professional demeanor and appearance. They monitor the reception area for any dirt or hair pets leave behind. The reception area should project a clean, warm atmosphere (Figure 2-1).

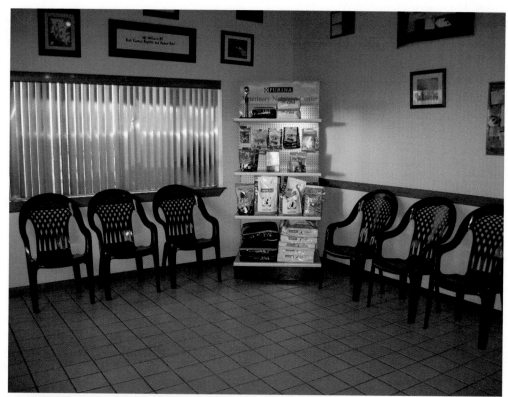

FIGURE 2-1 A clean reception area creates a warm, welcoming atmosphere for clients.

A second crucial goal is to support quality client and patient care through effective communication with team members. Clients often call throughout the day requesting updates on their pets. The receptionist team is responsible for either relaying the information to the owner or transferring the call to a knowledgeable team member. Clients may also call for suggestions or advice relating to their pets. It should be the goal of the receptionist to provide the most current, correct information available on the subject. If a receptionist does not know the answer, he or she is responsible for finding it.

MANAGING THE RECEPTION AREA

Many activities occur in the reception area; clients engage in conversation, pets may interact, and children may be in danger. The reception team monitors this area and must be able to control situations that may arise.

Clients often attempt to share knowledge with each other; however, on occasion the information is not accurate or appropriate. Receptionists should try to monitor conversations and may need to move a client into a room sooner than anticipated because of the topic being addressed. "Toxic" topics include a poor experience the client is having at the practice or has had in the past, incorrect information regarding diseases or treatments, and offensive topics and language. It can be easier to isolate the offender and apologize to the victim than to remove the victim and let the offender

repeat the conversation with another client arriving at the practice.

Pets may interact in smaller reception areas, which may result in tragedy. Dogs may try to attack each other, and cats may escape if they are not in a carrier. Receptionists should ensure every dog is on a leash and provide them when necessary. If cats are not in a carrier, the receptionist may offer to place the cat in a cage until a room is ready.

Children occasionally attempt to pet the other animals in the waiting room. This can be dangerous to the child and encourages the spread of contagious disease. Receptionists may need to remind parents to control their children while in the waiting room because not all pets are fond of children.

A receptionist may also need to triage patients as they arrive. Triage is prioritizing patients according to the severity of their conditions. If a patient arrives with symptoms of any contagious disease, such as the parvovirus, the patient should be immediately placed in isolation or kept in the car away from other animals in the reception area.

Basic animal instinct is just as important with the receptionist team as it is with technicians. Team members must not place their faces in the immediate face of an animal or behave aggressively with trained police or narcotics dogs. Receptionists must realize that not every animal is friendly and fearless. New smells, other animals, and unfamiliar people may place animals on alert and make them fearful.

TEAM ETIQUETTE

Etiquette is defined as the rules that society has set for the proper way to behave around other people. The most obvious facet of etiquette is being kind and polite to others; therefore every team member must appear professional and treat both clients and other team members with respect.

> **PRACTICE POINT**   Do unto others as you would have done unto you.

Actions of team members are observed by clients, patients, visitors, and fellow employees. The potential for veterinary practice growth, client acceptance, and compliance is based on team member etiquette. The failure to use etiquette among team members can be detrimental. Clients perceive the stress associated with poor etiquette, ultimately leading to decreased communication, client noncompliance, and poor profits (Box 2-1).

Etiquette must also be recognized when a client's pet is being euthanized. This is an extremely difficult time for clients, and the receptionist can make the experience less painful. The receptionist should notify all team members that a euthanasia is planned so everyone can be sensitive to the atmosphere of the clinic (e.g., no laughing or giggling in the halls). A sign can also be posted on the door to the room where the euthanasia is occurring so that team members are aware of the event.

Team members should always wear nametags to identify themselves to the clients. Clients appreciate knowing who is caring for their pets. If a technician is credentialed, the appropriate abbreviation should be on the badge as well. Veterinarians should also have name badges. Clients may assume a technician is still treating their pet when, in fact, the veterinarian has entered the room. Identification can be in the form of a pin, a magnet, or an embroidered name on the team member's scrubs.

DEVELOPING EFFECTIVE PHONE TECHNIQUES

The human voice has four components: volume, tone, rate, and quality. The volume of the receptionist's voice should make listeners comfortable, increasing the quality of the conversation. If a person's voice is too loud, listeners (in this case, clients) may pull the phone away from their ears, preventing them from hearing all of a conversation. If a receptionist's volume is too low, clients may be too embarrassed to ask for clarification on something they did not hear well. Correct volume is essential to a successful phone experience.

The tone of a voice is also referred to as *pitch*. Some speakers have a low, comforting tone, which increases the quality of the conversation. Others may have a high, squeaky pitch. Some clients may be unable to understand

| Box 2-1 | Ideas to Encourage Staff Etiquette |

- Greet team members with a smile every morning. Happiness is contagious.
- Introduce team members when they are not acquainted with visitors, clients, or new employees.
- Greet clients with a smile when they arrive.
- Always say goodbye to both clients and team members as they leave the practice—and mean it.
- Be a team player.
- Dress and act professionally.
- Do not criticize. Take the opportunity to educate employees instead of reprimanding.
- Have respect for each team member and client.
- Do not gossip.

a squeaky voice and become irritated. The tone of voice a receptionist uses to answer the phone can give a client a lasting impression. Team members should have a pleasant, confident, and understandable voice. Tones can indicate "I am too busy to take your call right now" or "I am at your service today; how may I help you?" Team members should smile as they answer the phone; the tone of that smile will come across the phone line (Figure 2-2).

The rate of speaking can greatly affect a conversation. Speaking too quickly can leave the listener confused and unable to follow instructions. People who naturally speak quickly should often remind themselves to slow their speaking rate. The receptionist must be efficient and knowledgeable and speak slowly and clearly. Many older clients cannot hear well and may not be able to understand a team member who is speaking rapidly. This can also imply that the practice is busy and that the receptionist does not have time for the client.

The quality of voice is a combination of clarity, volume, rate, and tone. All four factors are interrelated and have compounding effects on each other. Tape recording telephone conversations can help team members realize what they sound like on a phone and help improve skills and telephone etiquette.

Team members should answer the phone by introducing themselves; this notifies the client with whom they are speaking and quickly develops a relationship. "Good morning, ABC Animal Clinic, this is Teresa. How may I help you?" is a good example.

> **PRACTICE POINT**   Team members should smile when answering the phone; that smile comes across the phone line in the speaker's tone of voice.

It is important to write down the client's and patient's names when the caller has given this information. This prevents team members from having to ask for names to be repeated and possibly appearing disorganized. A call that has been placed on hold allows the team member to

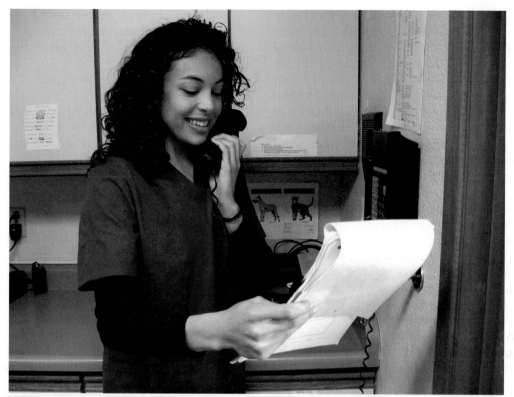

FIGURE 2-2 Answering the phone with a smile projects a friendly attitude that can be detected by the listener.

address the client personally when resuming the conversation. "Thank you for holding, Mrs. Jones. Sparky's record indicates that he is due for vaccines…"

Guidelines should be developed covering what to say and what not to say on the telephone. Many times, the same topic said with different words can have a very different meaning to the caller. For example, a client may call the hospital to request an appointment, believing that Fluffy's ear infection is a sudden emergency. The receptionist may respond, "There are no appointments available until next week; however, you can come in as a walk-in and wait to be seen." A better response, however, would be, "We don't have any appointments available today, but we are happy to accept you as a walk-in. We can work Fluffy in between our appointments if you don't mind waiting." Office managers may also develop a list of frequently asked questions and appropriate responses for topics such as:

- Setting up appointments
- Clients wanting to talk with the veterinarian immediately
- Clients asking for an update on a hospitalized pet
- A client asking questions regarding a statement or invoice
- Price shopping
- Angry and abusive caller
- Placing callers on hold
- Creating estimates

- Refill requests for food and medications
- Emergency calls
- Confirming upcoming surgeries and general appointments

> **PRACTICE POINT** Controlling client telephone conversations is imperative when handling multiple lines.

Role playing can facilitate correct responses to these potentially difficult situations.

Team members must learn not to say certain phrases. Expressions such as "I don't know" can imply the team member is not knowledgeable or does not care to get the correct information for the client. Instead of saying "I don't know," team members should reply, "that is a great question, let me find out." Rather than saying a hurried "just a second," a team member might say "give me just a moment to get that [information or product]." The combination of words and tone can have a powerful effect on clients. Words and phrases such as "absolutely!", "I know how much you care," and "I understand" are powerful in creating empathy with clients (Box 2-2).

Some clients enjoy casual phone conversations with the staff. Clients enjoy talking about their pets, and veterinary professionals are ideal listeners. However, the receptionist must control the conversation. Team members want to let clients know they are listening, caring, and compassionate, but another phone line may be ringing or another client may be waiting to pick up a pet (Figure 2-3). A few options exist to help control this conversation. It is acceptable to let the client know that there is another client waiting and that someone will call the client back with more information in approximately 10 minutes (then follow the general rule and call back in 5 minutes). Otherwise, ask closed-ended (yes or no) questions only, such as "Is Fluffy vomiting?" or "Does Fluffy have diarrhea?" Some clients may still attempt to prolong the conversation, but team members usually can get an appointment scheduled and end the conversation. It can be difficult to end a conversation without making the client perceive that the team member does not care. However, with practice and role playing team members can learn to convey sincerity.

Receptionists often hear the same questions repeatedly when answering phones at a veterinary practice. Frequently asked questions (FAQs) can be compiled to enhance the knowledge of the receptionist team, allowing questions to be answered immediately. Technicians and veterinarians may be unable to take a phone call to answer simple questions if they are with a client or patient. The receptionist team can enhance the client's experience by being able to answer simple questions such as:
- Vaccine protocols
  - How old do puppies and kittens have to be to start vaccinations?
  - What vaccinations are recommended?

Box 2-2 Powerful Words and Phrases

- "I understand."
- "I know you love your pet."
- "Unconditionally"
- "Extremely"
- "Absolutely"
- "Enormously"
- "Unquestionably"

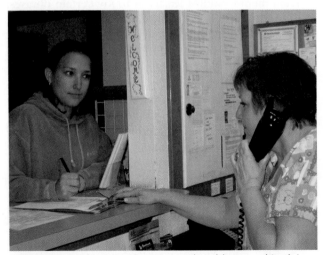

FIGURE 2-3 The receptionist must be able to multitask in a friendly and polite manner.

- What vaccinations are included?
- How often are vaccinations given?
- What is included in the initial puppy or kitten examination?
- How much do vaccinations cost?
- Spaying and neutering pets
  - How old do pets have to be to be altered?
  - Do vaccinations have to be current?
  - What does the surgical procedure entail?
  - Is pain medication included?
  - When do pets need to arrive at the practice?
  - When are they usually ready to go home?
  - Do they need to be held off food and water?
  - How much does the procedure cost?
  - What lab work is required? Are IV fluids required?
- Sick pets
  - Is the pet vomiting? If yes, for how long?
  - Does the pet have diarrhea? If yes, for how long?
  - Does the pet have an appetite?
  - Is the pet current on vaccinations?
- Heartworm preventive
  - What is it?
  - What tests are required to start the pet on preventive?
  - What products does the practice carry?
  - How is it administered?
  - How often is it administered?
  - How much does it cost?
- Flea and tick preventive
  - What diseases are carried by fleas and ticks?
  - Can people catch these diseases?
  - What products does the practice carry?
  - How are these products administered?
  - How often are these products administered?
  - How much do they cost?
- Diets
  - What special diets does the practice carry?
  - What maintenance diets does the practice carry?

New team members may be overwhelmed with new information. FAQ sheets can help new team members answer questions almost as well as those with experience.

MANAGING MULTIPLE PHONE LINES

Many practices have multiple phone lines to answer, clients to greet as they walk in and out of the practice, and invoices or charges to enter (Figure 2-4). As a general rule, phones should not ring more than three times before being answered. If a receptionist is with another client or on another line, it is acceptable to ask the client to hold momentarily because another phone line is ringing. For example, "Good morning, ABC Animal Clinic, this is Teresa. I am on the other line [or with another client], are you able to hold one moment?" Once the client answers yes, the team member should say thank you. This allows the receptionist to finish with the first client.

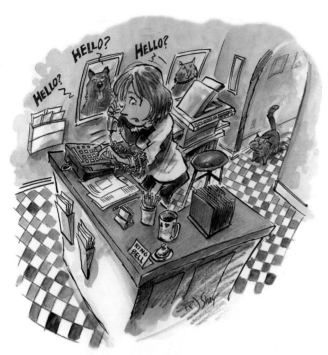

FIGURE 2-4 Receptionists are responsible for many duties, including managing multiple telephone lines and greeting incoming clients.

Asking a client "Are you able to hold one moment?" does exactly that; it *asks* the client politely. A short "can you hold?" becomes a demand rather than a question. "Thank you for holding, how may I help you?" can then resume the conversation. If multiple lines continue ringing, a receptionist may also ask clients if a return call is possible instead of waiting on hold. "Thank you for holding, this is Teresa. I have a client waiting for me, do you mind if I call you back in 10 minutes so you do not have to continue to hold?" Once again, the client should be called back within 5 minutes.

It is important not to leave callers on hold for more than 1 minute. Most current phone systems sound an alert after 1 minute; at this time clients should be told that the team member helping them will return momentarily. If the client will be on hold more than 1 or 2 minutes, the client should be asked if a team member can return the call as soon as the requested information is available. One minute on hold seems like 5 minutes to a client.

The time a client is on hold can be a valuable marketing resource time. Special on-hold systems can generate specific messages about the veterinary practice or specific diseases that may be a concern to the area. Clients can be educated on a variety of topics while they are on hold. This information can include practice hours, history of the veterinarians, or specialties or products that the practice offers. (See Chapter 10 for more information regarding marketing for the veterinary practice.) If the caller has something to listen to, the wait time does not seem as long. Recordings can also assure the client that the phone line has not been disconnected. It can be difficult to determine if a call has been disconnected if the line is silent.

Receptionists should also be able to call on cross-trained team members to help assist when the phone lines continue to ring. Team members should also realize that if a phone line has rung more than three times, the receptionist team needs help. This is an ideal time for cross-trained employees to make a difference. Telephone calls are one of the first impressions made to a client, whether new or existing. If a client believes he or she was rushed through a conversation or that a call was never answered, the client may go to another practice.

Veterinary practices should never have an answering machine on during the day to catch an overflow of phone calls. The majority of new clients will not leave a message and will call another practice. If a receptionist is too busy to check the messages, return phone calls may not be made until much later in the shift. Every phone call must be answered during business hours. Current trends indicate clients dislike answering machines and automated phone services and want to talk to a live person. Prevent this potential irritant by having several team members available to answer the phone.

> **PRACTICE POINT** Cross-training team members to work the reception desk can improve the efficiency of the practice during busy times.

An ideal scenario is to have a call center located separately from the reception area (Figure 2-5). This allows the receptionist to give clients full attention as they enter and leave the practice. Mistakes are decreased when team members can concentrate on one client at a time. The call center can concentrate on answering calls promptly and can review patient histories without other clients overhearing conversations. Some practice owners may argue that this will increase labor costs; however, if a receptionist can increase an average transaction by $10 either by catching a missed charge or by selling a client an extra $10 of service, then one receptionist has covered the cost of the labor and increased the profits at the end of the day (Box 2-3). Ultimately, clients are satisfied and will return because they experienced superior customer service within the veterinary practice.

> **PRACTICE POINT** A call center located away from the reception area allows team members to concentrate on clients visiting the practice without interruptions.

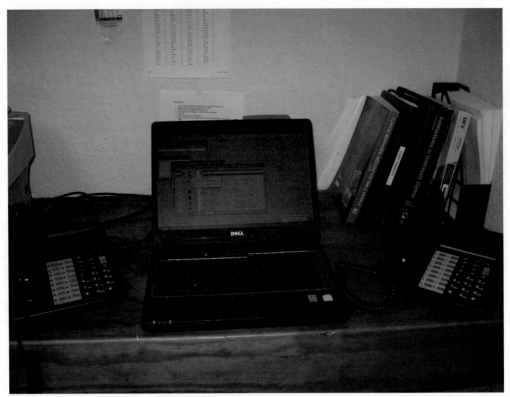

FIGURE 2-5 Some practices have a call center separate from the reception area.

Box 2-3   Labor Versus Service

- If 20 clients are seen in one day and a receptionist increased the average transaction of each client by $10, the receptionist has added $200 to the gross profits for the day (20 × $10 = $200).
- If the employee is paid $9 per hour and works an 8-hour day, she would be paid $72 per day. The labor formula of 20% is added for tax purposes ($72 × 20%) = $14.40. $72 + $14.40 = $86.40. The employee costs the employer $86.40.
- $200−$86.40=$113.60 gross profit per day. $113.60 × 5 days = $568 gross profit per week!

TURNING PHONE CALLS INTO APPOINTMENTS

A receptionist has the potential to turn every inquiring phone call into a client. A friendly and genuine voice makes a potential client feel comfortable and encourages the caller to ask questions. When the receptionist can answer questions in a polite, educated, and unhurried manner, the caller is inclined to make an appointment with the veterinary practice. The receptionist can ask open-ended questions to generate conversation. Open-ended questions do not require a "yes or no" answer; they open the door for discussion. The more education a team member can provide a potential client, the more likely the practice will gain a new patient. Receptionists should always ask if they can make an appointment for a client at the end of a phone conversation and end the discussion with "Mr. Jones, have I answered all of your questions today? Please call back anytime with any other questions you may have."

> **PRACTICE POINT**   Giving phone "shoppers" details regarding available services can gain a new client for the practice.

TAKING MESSAGES FOR VETERINARIANS AND TECHNICIANS

Clients often call and want to speak to a doctor as soon as possible. The receptionist should be able to determine if a technician would be able to answer a client's questions. Technicians know many answers and can verify any additional information with the veterinarian. This allows veterinarians to continue providing service for clients and patients currently on the premises. Receptionists should always pull the applicable medical records for either the technician or veterinarian taking the call; this allows the team member to review the case before answering questions. Once the team member has answered the client's question, comments regarding the telephone conversation must be documented in the medical record. This allows the next team member to be able to follow the case if the client comes to the veterinary practice for

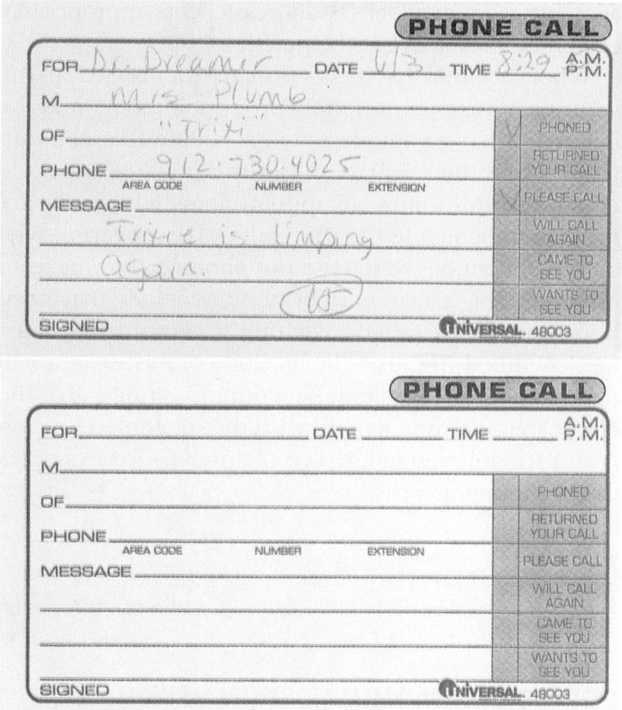

PHONE CALL

FOR _Dr. Dreamer_ DATE _6/3_ TIME _8:29_ A.M. P.M.

M _Mrs. Plumb_

OF _"Trixi"_

PHONE _912-730-4025_
AREA CODE NUMBER EXTENSION

MESSAGE _Trixie is limping again._

☐ PHONED
☒ RETURNED YOUR CALL
☒ PLEASE CALL
☒ WILL CALL AGAIN
☐ CAME TO SEE YOU
☐ WANTS TO SEE YOU

SIGNED _(5)_   UNIVERSAL. 48003

PHONE CALL

FOR _____ DATE _____ TIME _____ A.M. P.M.

M _____

OF _____

PHONE _____
AREA CODE NUMBER EXTENSION

MESSAGE _____

☐ PHONED
☐ RETURNED YOUR CALL
☐ PLEASE CALL
☐ WILL CALL AGAIN
☐ CAME TO SEE YOU
☐ WANTS TO SEE YOU

SIGNED _____   UNIVERSAL. 48003

FIGURE 2-6 Duplicate message pads prevent lost messages.

an appointment or follow up with another phone call. It is important that every conversation with clients be documented in the medical record. Every case should be treated as if it will go to court. Simply speaking, if something is not documented in the record, legally it never happened. (See Chapter 4 for more information on documentation and the law.)

Messages need to be legible and contain accurate information. Team members should ask for a current phone number and repeat the number back to the client. Veterinarians and team members lose valuable time when information is incorrect or has been transcribed incorrectly. Messages can be written on a duplicate message pad; if a message is lost or misplaced, a copy is available for referral (Figure 2-6).

> ◉ **PRACTICE POINT** Duplicate message pads prevent the loss of important messages.

LIABILITY OF TELEPHONE CALLS

Team members can be held accountable for incorrect verbal communication. Misunderstood conversations can be held against the veterinary practice. Every telephone call must be documented in the patient's record, with details regarding the conversation. No one but the veterinarian should give health care advice over the phone. Advice from another staff member is inappropriate and can be

considered malpractice. Phrases such as "you may want to wait and watch," "this does not sound like an emergency," or "you can just give some Pepto-Bismol if your pet is vomiting" **must never be said.** If the pet happens to die overnight, have complications, or be seen at an emergency clinic, the veterinary practice can be held liable. Always advise clients that if they are concerned about their pet's health, they should bring the animal in for an examination. Then document this call in the medical record. They have called for a service; offer to solve it with an appointment.

Veterinarians can also be held liable for giving medical advice over the phone if something happens to the patient. Malpractice lawsuits may have fewer consequences if the veterinarian gives advice compared with staff giving advice; however, the potential still exists. Veterinarians must also remember to document the conversation immediately; many veterinarians rush into the next room and forget to write in the medical record.

PERSONAL PHONE CALLS

Business lines must be available for business use at all times. The employee manual must clearly state that personal phone calls are limited to emergencies only. If a personal call occurs, it must be kept short and to the point to keep lines available for clients. Potential clients who cannot reach the office may dial the next clinic in the phone book, or clients with emergencies may panic if they cannot reach the practice immediately.

MANAGING AND PROCESSING MAIL

Veterinary practices receive many pieces of literature on a daily basis. Some is junk, but the majority consists of statements, laboratory reports, information on upcoming continuing education opportunities, or ads for the release of new products and books. All mail must be given to the person to whom it is addressed. Some veterinarians and technicians may like their mail to be opened, allowing greater efficiency in sorting, but others may prefer to keep their privacy. Statements and invoices should be given to the manager in charge of paying bills; all statements must be reviewed for correct charges. All laboratory reports should be placed within the clients' records and placed on the veterinarian's desk for review. Magazines and journals must be given to the subscriber. Continuing education brochures should be posted, allowing the entire team to note the opportunities available to further their knowledge.

CLIENT RELATIONS

Clients draw preliminary conclusions about a practice within the first 2 to 5 minutes of entering the building. This conclusion (especially if it is negative) can continue through the rest of the visit. Team members should always greet clients as they enter the facility, regardless of what other tasks they may be doing. If a receptionist is on the phone, acknowledging clients with a smile and a wave is acceptable. If a receptionist is helping another client, greet the entering client with a smile and say "Hello, I will be with you in a moment." If the receptionist is working with another team member, that task should be put aside and the client should receive the full attention of both team members.

> **PRACTICE POINT**   Clients must be acknowledged when they enter the practice.

Greeting clients by their names and addressing their pets create a positive first impression (Figure 2-7). This can be difficult with first-time clients; however, if team members can find something to compliment the owner or patient about, this can be overcome. Conversation starters such as "Fluffy is such a beautiful girl," or "Your necklace is beautiful, Mrs. Jones," make clients feel acknowledged. Small comments help provide exceptional service. Many clients prefer to be addressed as Mr., Mrs., or Dr. Once the initial appointment has began, team members may ask the new client how they wish to be addressed. A notation can be made in the record, allowing team members to address clients appropriately each time they arrive at the practice.

When a client has been provided a service at the veterinary hospital, a follow-up appointment may be needed. It is very important to schedule that appointment while the client is still in the practice. Most clients return for follow-up appointments when they are previously scheduled. If the patient is recovering well and the client has to initiate the phone call to make an appointment, it may not get done. Vaccines that need boosters and to be given within a certain time must be scheduled because clients "forget" and do not call to make an appointment. Receptionist should give the client an appointment card with the scheduled time on it as a friendly reminder. (See Chapter 13 for examples of appointment cards.)

> **PRACTICE POINT**   Follow-up appointments should be scheduled for clients before they leave the practice.

FORMS COMMONLY USED IN VETERINARY PRACTICE

Clients may be asked to fill out various forms regarding their personal contact information, their pet's information and history, or a variety of release forms (Figure 2-8).

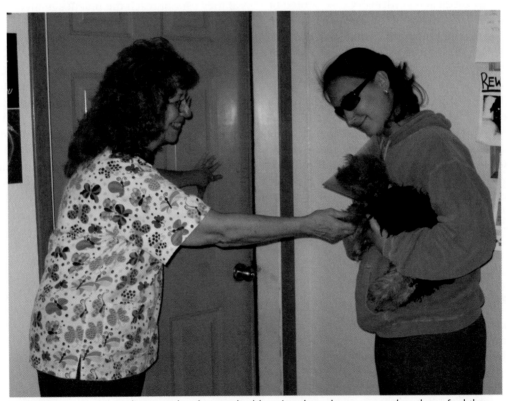

FIGURE 2-7 Greeting clients at the door and addressing them by name makes them feel they are getting personalized attention.

Receptionists need to be sure all forms are filled out completely when a new client enters information. Obviously, contact information is vital in order to call the owner with updates regarding his or her pet's health. Address information must be current so that reminders may be mailed for vaccines, tests, and medication refills. Anytime a client returns to the clinic, the receptionist must verify that the contact information in the record is still current. It is also important that the client sign the bottom of the form, which should state that he or she (the client) is responsible for any charges regarding the listed patients.

The pet's information is an essential portion of the record. Details should include species, gender, date of birth, breed, color, and alteration status. *Species* refers to the classification: dog, cat, bird, rabbit, reptile, and so forth. Team members must learn about breeds within a species; owners can be easily offended when team members are unfamiliar with their pet's breed. Purebred animals are generally easy to classify; mixed breeds can be referred to by the breed they most resemble. Mixed-breed cats can be difficult to classify and are generally described by their hair coat (Box 2-4). Domestic

shorthair (DSH) refers to a short-haired cat, domestic mediumhair (DMH) refers to a cat with medium-length hair, and domestic longhair (DLH) refers to a long-haired cat.

The Medical Record

Each animal should have its own medical record as part of the overall record (Figure 2-9). The medical record should be dated each time an entry is made, listing the presenting problems and the author's initials. Some clinics choose a card-filing system to conserve space and costs. In this system the medical records are kept on 5 × 8 inch cards stored in plastic folders that also hold lab results, radiology reports, and financial information. These plastic folders are then stored in a file drawer. As society becomes more litigious, practices are switching to full paper or paperless records. Clinics that are paperless must still document everything in the medical record. Paperless clinics have the benefit of being able to access client records, laboratory results, and radiographs at any computer station. Paperless records increase clinic space that was once consumed by file cabinets; they also result in decreased numbers of lost files and results.

ABC Animal Clinic
555 Uptown Circle
Anytown, MN 89000
314-134-4431

Please print clearly

Date: _____

Name _____

Mailing address _____ Zip code _____

Street address _____ Zip code _____

Home phone _____ Work phone _____

Drivers license # _____ State _____

Animals:

Name	Date of birth	Species	Breed	Color	Gender	Spayed or neutered?
_____	_____	_____	_____	_____	_____	_____
_____	_____	_____	_____	_____	_____	_____
_____	_____	_____	_____	_____	_____	_____

I understand that payment is required in full on the same date that services are rendered.

_____
Signature

A

FIGURE 2-8 A and **B,** Examples of client patient information sheets.

A disadvantage of paperless records is that some software companies allow record alteration after a record has been completed (See Chapter 14).

> ◎ **PRACTICE POINT**   Medical records are not complete without the initials of the team member making the notes.

Consent Forms

Clients may be asked to sign a variety of consent forms before various treatments and procedures can be performed on their pets (Figure 2-10). Every member of the team must be able to explain the meaning of any form a client is asked to sign. The forms are self-explanatory, but team members must read the consent forms aloud to the client to ensure the client understands what he or she is

---

Arroyo Vista Animal Clinic
2303 Inspiration Lane

Owner's name _____   Spouse _____

Address _____

Home telephone _____   Work telephone _____

Employer's name and address _____

Spouse's employer and address _____

Best time to call regarding your pet _____   Phone number _____

In case of emergency, please call _____

WRITTEN ESTIMATES ARE AVAILABLE UPON REQUEST. Please ask the receptionist if an estimate is needed. **ALL FEES ARE DUE AT THE TIME SERVICES ARE RENDERED.** If you plan to pay with a check or credit card, please complete the following:

MC ___   Visa ___   Exp Date _____   Driver's License Number _____   State _____   Expires _____

How did you hear of Arroyo Vista Animal Clinic? Yellow Pages ___ Referral (Name) _____ Other _____

Number and type of pets in your household? _____

Pet's origin: Humane Society ____   Pet Shop ____   Kennel ____   Breeder ____   Friend ____   Stray ____   Other ____

	Pet #1	Pet #2	Pet #3
Name			
Species (dog, cat)			
Breed			
Color			
Age			
Date of birth			
Sex			
Length of time owned			
Spayed or neutered			
Vitamins? (type)			
Diet (kind of food)			
Type of grooming products			
Inside or outside?			
Last rabies vaccine?			
Last DHLP vaccine? (Dog)			
Last parvo vaccine? (Dog)			
Last FVRCP vaccine? (Cat)			
Last FeLV vaccine? (Cat)			
Last leukemia test? (Cat)			
Last heartworm test? (Dog)			
Heartworm prevention?			
Last fecal exam?			
Last dental?			
Prior illness?			
Prior surgery?			

B

FIGURE 2-8, cont'd Example of a client patient information sheet.

signing. Release forms are not required by law; their purpose is to protect the veterinary health care team. If the form is documented in the record, it can be submitted if a court case arises. If it is not documented, the assumption is that it was never discussed. All releases should contain the owner's and patient's names along with the date and the initials of the team member helping the client sign the forms.

> **PRACTICE POINT**   Consent forms must be verbally explained to the owner. Once they understand, they must sign and date the form.

Information included on consent forms should include known risks, alternatives, prognosis, and possible complications. Anesthetic release forms clearly indicate that anesthesia could result in death. Vaccination release forms (see Figure 2-10, *G*) state the risks and benefits of vaccinating pets along with the possibility of anaphylactic reaction, which may result in death. Euthanasia release forms (see Figure 2-10, *H* and *I*) state that the owner is presenting the pet for a painless, humane death (and should state that *euthanasia results in death*). Owners declining treatment or recommended diagnostic tests may also need to sign a release based on practice policies. Owners can

Box 2-4	Species Identification	
SPECIES	**COMMONLY REFERRED TO AS**	**ABBREVIATION**
Canine	Dog	K-9
Feline	Cat	Fe
Avian	Bird	Av
Iguanas, snakes, etc.	Reptiles	Re
Lagomorph	Rabbit	Ra
Equine	Horse	Eq
Bovine	Cow	Bo

Patient Medical Record

Client Name _____   Telephone Number _____

Address _____   Client Number _____

Pet Name _____ Breed _____ Color _____

Sex _____ Altered _____ DOB _____ Age _____ Species _____

Date		Charges

A

FIGURE 2-9 A, Sample medical record sheet.

refuse to vaccinate their pets, prevent heartworm disease, or test for heartworm disease. For the best interests of the practice, the owner should sign a release indicating that he or she, the client, does not hold the hospital, veterinarian, or any team member liable for any disease the client's pet may encounter when not accepting preventive measures recommended by the veterinarian and/or practice.

Patient History

Comprehensive patient medical history forms are essential when collecting information about new patients. Clients should fill out a form answering questions regarding the pet's health history. This helps the veterinary team diagnostically if any problems arise. History forms can also include an area for the owner to sign that allows the practice to treat the patient and acknowledges that the owner agrees to pay for services rendered.

Rabies certificates are often printed by veterinary software systems. The team member enters the rabies tag number, lot number, and manufacturer of the vaccine (Figure 2-11). If a rabies vaccine book is used, the correct owner and patient information must be legible. The date and the owner's name, address, and phone numbers are required. The patient's name, age, breed,

FIGURE 2-9, cont'd B, Sample medical record sheet.

and gender are also required. The rabies tag number and lot number are then entered, along with the veterinarian's signature and license number. Lost animals are often identified by their rabies tag number. Therefore it is important to ensure the information has been added correctly and legibly.

Spay and neuter certificates are generated once a pet has been altered. This provides the owner with proof that the pet was altered if such proof is ever needed. This certificate may also be required when ordinances require pets to be registered with a city or county. Many city and county agencies require pets to be licensed, capping the number of pets allowed per household. All pets may be required to be licensed, including dogs, cats, rabbits, and ferrets, as well as some exotic species. Practices should be familiar with local laws regarding pet licensing. Local chapters of the Humane Society of the United States and animal shelters are excellent sources of information regarding laws and ordinances pertaining to pets.

PRACTICE POINT Dogs and cats are required by each state to have a current rabies vaccine.

Arroyo Vista Animal Clinic
2303 Inspiration Lane

Owner's name_____ Patient's name_____

Breed _____ Color _____ Sex _____ Species _____

Date	SOAP	

C

FIGURE 2-9, cont'd C, Sample medical record sheet.

ABC Veterinary Clinic

Surgery/Anesthesia Consent Form

Client Name _____ Date _____

Pet's Name _____

Your pet has been scheduled for a procedure requiring sedation or anesthesia. By signing this form, you authorize ABC Veterinary Clinic and its agents to administer tranquilizers, anesthetics, and/or analgesics that are deemed appropriate for your pet. Please be aware that all drugs have the potential for adverse side effects in any particular animal. The chances of such occurrence are extremely low.

I am aware that staff is not on premises after hours, and I agree to indemnify ABC Veterinary Clinic and its agents harmless from and against any and all liability arising from the care that is provided.

In an effort to ensure your pet's safety and to anticipate any problems before they may occur, we have available preanesthetic electrocardiogram and blood testing capabilities to detect hidden heart, liver, kidney, or other problems that may increase the risk to your pet. This testing is available for an additional charge. If abnormalities are detected, we will attempt to notify you, and the anesthetic procedure may be delayed or modified. Please verify the procedures being performed and indicate your wishes concerning the option of preanesthetic testing. If you have any questions, please ask BEFORE signing this form.

Procedures scheduled: _____

Routine surgical procedures are painful. We recommend postoperative pain medication for each procedure. Pain medication is automatically dispensed for each patient. If you **decline postoperative pain medication, please sign here:** _____

How may we contact you **today?** _____

Home phone _____ Work phone _____

Cell phone/pager _____ Client signature _____

A

FIGURE 2-10 **A** through **K,** Examples of various release forms. **A,** Surgery/anesthesia consent form.

A master problem list is a summary of the patient's health status (Figure 2-12). Vaccinations, laboratory tests, acute and chronic diseases, and current medications can be listed on one sheet. Master lists can increase efficiency when team members do not have to search through the entire record to find medication refill information. The list can clearly indicate when a patient is overdue for an examination, vaccinations, or laboratory work. Master problem lists should also include any vaccine, medication, or anesthetic reaction the pet may have had in the past.

Health Certificates

Health certificates are required by airlines, as well as some state and federal agencies, when traveling with pets. Airlines want to ensure the pet is in healthy condition before accepting it for transport, and states want to ensure the pet is not importing any diseases. Both federal and state agencies are responsible for the prevention of disease and have different regulations regarding the entry of animals. Interstate health certificates are generally good for 10 days before shipment (Figure 2-13).

◎ **PRACTICE POINT** A master problem list can increase the efficiency of the veterinary health care team.

◎ **PRACTICE POINT** Health certificates are required by airlines to ensure that pets are healthy enough for travel.

Arroyo Vista Animal Clinic
2303 Inspiration Lane, Anywhere, USA
Dr. Larsen, Dr. Cooke, and Dr. Thompson
Hospitalization/Surgical Consent Form

Owner's Name _____

Pet's Name _____ Breed _____ Sex _____ Age _____ Color _____

I certify that I own the above described animal and do hereby consent and authorize Dr. Larsen or her associates to hospitalize and/or administer vaccinations, medication, tests, surgical procedures, or treatments the doctor and her associates deem necessary for the health, safety, or well-being of the above animal while it is under their care and supervision.

If the pet should injure itself in an escape attempt, refuse food, urinate or defecate on itself, become ill or die while in the hospital, I will hold Dr. Larsen and her associates, along with the staff of Arroyo Vista Animal Clinic, free of any responsibility and/or liability in the absence of gross negligence.

I realize that my pet will only be discharged during regular office hours and when the doctor or her associates are present, and the fee due for its care will be paid in full at that time. If I neglect to pick up my pet within five (5) days of written notice, you may assume the animal is abandoned and you are thereby authorized to dispose of it as you see fit. I further realize that should I not pay the amount due at the time of pickup, I will be responsible for reasonable costs of collection, including court costs and reasonable attorney's fees.

In the event that I become ill, move, or change my address, it shall be my duty to inform the hospital of such changes.

I hereby acknowledge that I have read the foregoing and fully understand the terms and conditions set forth.

Signed _____ Dated _____

Staff Member Signature _____ Dated _____

B

FIGURE 2-10, cont'd B, Hospitalization/surgical consent form.

The pet must be fully examined by a veterinarian before the certificate is issued. Most states require submission of a copy of the health certificate. International health certificates are generally good for 30 days and require the signature of the state veterinarian. These certificates are for shipment of pets out of the United States. Both forms of health certificates require the owner's name, address, and phone number along with the name, address, and phone number of the person who will be accepting and taking responsibility of the pet. All the animal's identifying information must be included, including age, breed, gender, and microchip or tattoo number. the animal's vaccines must be current and the vaccination information clearly stated. Small animal and large animal health certificates differ; large animal certificates should indicate tests that were required and completed, with the results stated. Before shipment to any state or country, regulations should be verified. Some countries have strict regulations regarding the importation of animals, mostly to limit disease transmission.

Many countries require a series of rabies vaccines and a rabies titer to import animals. The rabies neutralizing antibody titer test (RNATT) is a general term for the methods that measure rabies virus neutralizing antibody (RVNA) titers. Other countries may require a microchip before importation, along with deworming and the application of flea and tick preventive immediately before shipment. Visit the U.S. Department of Agriculture at www.aphis.usda.gov/regulations/vs/iregs/animals/for the most current information regarding animal importation procedures.

Release Forms

A signed consent form to release medical records may be required by some states. It is important to understand the Privacy Act and not release any records without the

{CLINICNAME}
{CLINICADDRESS1}
{CLINICADDRESS2}
{CLINICCITY} , {CLINICSTATE} {CLINICPOSTALCODE}
{CLINICPHONE}

Standard Consent Form
{CURRENTDATE[SHORT]}

Client ID:	{ID}	Patient ID:	{PATIENTID}
Client Name:	{FULLNAME}	Name:	{NAME}
Address:	{ADDRESS1}	Species:	{SPECIES}
	{ADDRESS2}	Breed:	{BREED}
	{CITY} , {STATE} {POSTALCODE}	Sex:	{SEX}
Telephone:	{PHONENUMBER}	Color:	{COLOR}
		Markings:	{MARKINGS}
		Birth Date:	{BIRTHDATE[SHORT]}

I hereby certify that I am the owner of the above-named animal or am responsible for it and have the authority to execute this consent.

I hereby authorize the performance of the following procedure(s):

_____

_____

I hereby also authorize the use of such anesthetics as you deem advisable and performance of such surgical or therapeutic procedures as you determine to be indicated. I understand that conditions not known may make it advisable that other surgical/treatments be done. {CLINICNAME} will try to contact me before doing added treatments, should they not be able to contact me, I authorize such treatments/anesthetics/surgeries, etc. when and if they are deemed necessary.

I agree to indemnify and hold {CLINICNAME} harmless from and against any and all liability arising out of the performance of any of the procedures referred to above.

All charges including boarding costs will be paid when the pet is released from the hospital. If the pet is not called for within 10 (ten) days after the specified time for return and if the doctor/clinic is not notified of an alternate date within this ten day period, the pet will be considered ABANDONED. {CLINICNAME} is given the right to dispose of the animal as the doctor/clinic sees fit -- including giving the animal away or euthanasia. It is understood that abandonment does not relieve me of my responsibility for all costs of services, medication, and boarding.

_____
(Signature of legal owner or responsible person)

AT WHAT NUMBER CAN YOU BE CONTACTED TODAY?

C

FIGURE 2-10, cont'd C, Standard consent form.

client's authorization. The Privacy Act of 1974 states, in part:

> No agency shall disclose any record which is contained in a system of records by any means of communication to any person, or to another agency, except pursuant to a written request by, or with the prior written consent of, the individual to whom the record pertains.

Many practices have owners fill out medical release forms and return them to the clinic either by mail or fax (Figure 2-14). Medical records release forms should also give an estimated time of when records will be available for pickup or fax so the client will know when to expect them. Some practices charge a fee for copying records; this price should be included on the release.

Boarding

Boarding consent forms may list services offered by veterinarians that clients might need to be reminded of (Figure 2-15). It is important to document the names and dosages of medication(s) the pet receives as well as what kind of food the animal eats at what frequency and times. It must also contain emergency contact information in case of an emergency as well as an authorization to treat the pet according to veterinary recommendations. Figure 2-15, *C,* shows an example of a boarding form available

Pre-Surgery Questionnaire

	Yes	No
1. Has your pet eaten within the last twelve hours?	____	____
2. Has your pet had anything to drink within the last four hours?	____	____
3. Has your pet vomited or had any diarrhea within the last week?	____	____
4. Have you noticed any rashes or itching?	____	____
5. Any history of trauma in the last week?	____	____
6. Any previous problems with anesthesia?	____	____
7. Is your pet current on all vaccinations?	____	____
8. Has your dog been tested for heartworms in the last twelve months?	____	____
9. Is your dog currently on heartworm prevention?	____	____
10. Is your cat feline leukemia negative?	____	____
11. Is your pet currently on medication?	____	____

If so, please list: _____

_____

12. Does your pet have any other medical problems or conditions?	____	____

If so, please explain:_____

13. Would you like your pet's nails trimmed at no additional cost?	____	____

14. Purebred cats may require an alternate anesthesia protocol to lessen the anesthetic risk. Please initial the line to the right that you understand there will be additional charges. _____

15. Would you like an Elizabethan collar to take home? (If the patient starts licking while in our care, we will automatically send home a collar.)	____	____
16. Is your pet microchipped?	____	____

Signature: _____ Date: _____

If you are not certain about the questions above, please consult a veterinary assistant prior to admission for advice.

D

FIGURE 2-10, cont'd **D,** Pre-surgery questionnaire.

from veterinary software. Once the client and form are selected, the software automatically populates the information. Figure 2-15, *D,* shows a form that the client fills in regarding medications, belongings, or any other important information that the practice should be aware of at the time of the pet's admission.

HANDLING SPECIAL SITUATIONS WITH CLIENTS

Clients can be pleasant or difficult depending on the kind of person they are, the type of day they have had, or the type of situation presented to them once they arrive at the practice. If a client has had a bad day, the team may take the brunt of the person's frustration. Team members should remember not to take the comments of these clients personally and instead try to make it a better day for the client.

Receptionists must effectively handle hostile clients on the phone. Although clients may call and be angry with the practice for some reason, the receptionist handling the conversation can turn the call into a positive experience. First, the receptionist should listen to the client. Once the client has finished his or her portion of the conversation, the receptionist should review the facts, ensuring that a miscommunication does not occur. If a manager is available to take the telephone call, the manager and client can discuss the case. If a supervisor is not available, the receptionist can politely state that the manager who can handle the situation is not available at the moment but he or she will return the call as soon as possible. A delay in the conversation may allow the client to calm down before a manager returns the call, allowing an easier resolution to the issue.

Angry clients at the practice should be taken into an exam room and allowed to vent in private. A team member who simply listens to the client often diffuses the situation. The team member can try to offer a solution that is satisfactory to the client to resolve the problem. If the fault lies with the practice, the mistake must be admitted and apologized for. Many times this repairs the situation immediately. (See Chapter 11 for more resolution techniques for angry clients.)

Grieving clients can be difficult because they have just suffered an emotional loss, sometimes similar to that experienced when losing a family member. Depending

Arroyo Vista Animal Clinic
Dr. Larsen, Dr. Cooke, and Dr. Thompson

Owner's Name _____ Patient's Name _____

Phone Number to Contact Today _____

All patients undergoing a dental procedure may receive the following:
- Pre-surgical exam
- Bloodwork
- IV catheter and fluids
- Induction anesthesia
- General anesthesia
- Anesthetic monitoring
- Ultrasonic cleaning/scaling and polishing
- Fluoride treatment
- Extractions
- Digital radiographs
- Doxirobe gel
- Antibiotics

After all of the tartar and plaque have been removed, our dental technician uses special equipment to determine if there is advanced gum disease. If deep pockets or an infection is found, dental radiographs and/or extractions may be necessary. Additional anesthesia may be needed due to the extended length of the procedure.

I authorize dental radiographs to be taken _____ Yes _____ No
I authorize extractions if needed _____ Yes _____ No
I wish to be contacted before any further procedure _____ Yes _____ No
If I cannot be reached I: Do not OK any further procedures _____
                          OK all procedures needed for my pet's health _____

It is our clinic policy to administer and dispense pain medication to every animal receiving extractions.

I authorize the veterinarians and their designated technicians to administer treatment as needed: perform surgical procedures as deemed necessary, perform diagnostics as indicated during the course of the procedure, as well as administer anesthetics. I have read and fully understand the above authorization for medical and/or surgical treatment. I also understand that no guarantee has been made of the results that may be obtained. I agree to pay the agreed upon estimate for surgery, with a ±15% range on the given estimate.

Signature of Owner or Representative _____ Date _____

E

FIGURE 2-10, cont'd E, Dental consent form.

on the situation, clients may be in shock and disbelief; others have accepted the situation and are sad. Clients in shock and disbelief may be angry. The pet may have just been hit by a car, and they are angry at the driver as well as at the practice for not doing more to save their pet. On occasion a poor prognosis has been given for a patient, but the client believes that more could be done to save the pet. The client may leave quickly, ask for a copy of the animal's records, and go to another veterinarian for a second opinion.

In all of these situations, clients must be taken to an isolated area to discuss their pet's condition; the reception area is not appropriate for providing sensitive information. The clients must be allowed to vent their anger (only verbally, *not* physically) before they leave the practice. Once they have been able to discuss the situation with a team member, the situation will likely calm down. Chapter 12 discusses the stages of grief in detail and provides more information on how team members can help clients cope with a traumatic situation.

Arroyo Vista Animal Clinic
Dr. Larsen, Dr. Cooke, and Dr. Thompson

Owner's Name _____   Patient's Name _____
Phone Number to Contact Today _____

Pre-Anesthesia Bloodwork

Under 2 Years of Age	**2-7 Years of Age**	**Above 7 Years of Age**
ALT, BUN, CREA, ALK Phos, Glucose, TP	ALT, BUN, CREA, ALK Phos, Glucose, TP, Electrolytes	Comprehensive bloodwork: ALT, ALB, AMY, BUN, Ca, CREA, ALK Phos, Glob, Bili, Glucose, TP, Electrolytes, CBC
Total: $39.91	**Total: $55.67**	**Total: $117.35**

I choose the appropriate bloodwork for my pet's age. _____ (initial)
I decline the recommended bloodwork and assume anesthetic risk. _____ (initial)

Your pet's health is our primary concern. Our most effective and safest anesthetic drugs require the use of an intravenous catheter (IV) placed on the forearm of you pet's leg. This requires a small area to be shaved and disinfectant applied. Your pet will receive IV fluids during and after the anesthetic period, which provides for safer anesthesia, a quicker recovery, and better pain management. An IV also gives the ability to provide emergency drugs if needed. An additional $39.11 will be applied to your account.

I give permission for my pet to receive IV fluids. _____ (initial)
I do not give permission for my pet to receive IV fluids. _____ (initial)

It is our belief that pain control is necessary for patients that have surgery. Not only is it humane to prevent pain, it has been scientifically proven that pets recover faster with pain medication. Additional pain medication ranges from $15.00 to $30.00 based on the size of your pet.
I request that my pet receive pain medication. _____ (initial)
I decline pain medication for my pet. _____ (initial)

I am the owner or caretaker of the pet, and I assume all responsibility of care after surgery. I understand that all anesthesia and surgical procedures involve a degree of risk and realize results cannot be guaranteed. While performing the surgery, should the veterinarian find the procedure to involve more than originally estimated, I will be contacted prior to continuation. If I cannot be contacted, I authorize the veterinarian to continue with the procedure deemed appropriate for my pet. I understand that I will be responsible for full payment upon patient discharge.

Signature of owner/caretaker _____
Contact phone number _____
Signature of staff member _____

F

FIGURE 2-10, cont'd F, Anesthesia consent form.

> **⊙ PRACTICE POINT** Grieving clients may be temporarily upset with team members, believing the team should have provided better treatment to save their pet in an emergency situation.

Clients who arrive at the practice under the influence of drugs or alcohol can be dangerous to team members and clients. Impaired individuals cannot reason because their ability to comprehend information is decreased. Drugs and alcohol distort thought processes; trying to hold a rational conversation can be dangerous. The client should be asked to leave, and the practice manager or veterinarian can call the client at a later time. If the client refuses to leave, the police should be called. The situation should not be allowed to progress, and the team should not make an effort to satisfy the client. Satisfaction will not occur when drugs have influenced the person's mental state.

Pet Immunization Information/Consent
ABC Veterinary Clinic

Immunizing your pet is an important procedure that in most cases will provide protection against an illness that may be life threatening. In past years, veterinarians have followed the vaccine manufacturer's guidelines and recommended annual revaccination for diseases that were believed to be a threat to our patients. Recent studies have shown that annual revaccination may not be necessary for some diseases because many pets are protected for three years or longer when vaccinated. Although most pets do not react adversely to vaccination, some have had allergic or other systemic reactions after receiving a vaccine. Rarely, the allergic reaction can be so profound that it may be life threatening. Certain immune-mediated diseases such as hemolytic anemia (anemia caused by red blood cell destruction), thrombocytopenia (low blood platelet numbers), and polyarthritis (joint inflammation and pain) in dogs may be triggered by the body's immune response to a vaccine. A serious additional concern has been a lump forming at the site of the vaccination. Why this occurs in cats is controversial at best, but it is considered extremely rare. In some cats, if these lumps persist, a tumor known as a fibrosarcoma may form that may have grave consequences if ignored. If your cat develops a lump under the skin after a vaccination that persists for longer than four weeks, you should have it examined as soon as possible.

Vaccinating your pet should not be taken lightly. Failure to vaccinate could result in your pet contracting a serious preventable disease. However, unnecessary vaccinations should be avoided. A decision to vaccinate should only come after you and your veterinarian consider your pet's age and the risk of exposure to disease. Vaccinations given at the appropriate age and at the appropriate intervals will greatly benefit your pet and protect it against some life-threatening diseases.

I understand the risks and benefits associated with vaccinating my pet. I hereby release ABC Veterinary Clinic of all liabilities associated with vaccinating my pet.

Owner _____ Date _____

G

Euthanasia Release

I, the undersigned, do hereby certify that I am the owner of the animal, and hereby give ABC Veterinary Clinic full and complete authority to euthanize the animal in whatever manner the doctor shall deem fit. I hereby release the doctors and staff from any and all liabilities for euthanizing said animal. I understand that euthanasia results in death.

I do also certify that the said animal has not bitten any person or animal during the last 15 days and to the best of my knowledge has not been exposed to rabies.

Owner _____ Date _____

H

FIGURE 2-10, cont'd G, Immunization information and consent form. **H,** Euthanasia release form.

Clients may slip and fall in the practice, presenting a significant liability. Signs must be posted when the floor is wet, and a team member should be available to direct clients around the wet area until it is dry. Clients may trip on rugs, shelving units, or any other object that sits on the floor. Wall-to-wall carpets should not curl up at the seams, and area rugs should have anti-skid material on the back to prevent tripping and slipping. Objects such as scales should have large warning barriers at the corners to prevent tripping (Figure 2-16). Team members should rush to the side of any client who has fallen in the practice. Many times team members are in shock when a client falls, and they stop and stare. The client should be asked if he or she feels any pain and where it is coming from. If needed, stabilize the patient in the same location until an ambulance arrives. Once the client feels stable enough to leave independently or the ambulance leaves for the hospital, pictures of the area should be taken. All team members who witnessed the accident should immediately write down the facts of the accident. If time passes before members write out the events, details will be forgotten. It may be advised to call the liability insurance company to inform

```
                        {CLINICNAME}
                       {CLINICADDRESS1}
                       {CLINICADDRESS2}
         {CLINICCITY}, {CLINICSTATE} {CLINICPOSTALCODE}
                       {CLINICPHONE}

                   Euthanasia Authorization
                     {CURRENTDATE[SHORT]}

Client ID:     {ID}              Patient ID:   {PATIENTID}
Client Name:   {FULLNAME}        Name:         {NAME}
Address:       {ADDRESS1}        Species:      {SPECIES}
               {ADDRESS2}        Breed:        {BREED}
               {CITY}, {STATE}   Sex:          {SEX}
               {POSTALCODE}
Telephone:     {PHONENUMBER}     Color:        {COLOR}
                                 Markings:     {MARKINGS}
                                 Birth Date:   {BIRTHDATE[SHORT]}

I, the undersigned, do hereby certify that I am the owner (duly authorized agent for the owner) of the animal
described above, that I do hereby give the doctors of {CLINICNAME} permission to euthanize and dispose of said
animal in whatever manner the said doctors of {CLINICNAME}, their agents, servants or representatives deem fit. I
also release the doctors, {CLINICNAME}, their agents, servants and representatives for any and all liability for so
euthanizing and disposing of said animal. I do also certify that to the best of my knowlege the said animal has not
bitten any person or animal during the last ten (10) days and has not been exposed to rabies.

                          SIGNED _____
```

FIGURE 2-10, cont'd **I,** Euthanasia authorization form.

it of the accident in case a lawsuit is brought against the practice. Chapter 21 discusses a variety of safety issues within the practice that should be addressed.

REVIEWING INVOICES WITH OWNERS

A team member should always review invoices with owners before collecting money. Services that have been provided should be detailed, and the receptionist should be knowledgeable enough to answer questions easily (cross-training helps in this area) (Figure 2-17). An invoice of the services should be detailed to include every facet of the service. The client should be able to review the invoice while the team member explains the charges (Figure 2-18). Following is a detailed example.

> **PRACTICE POINT** Client invoices should be reviewed in detail before presenting the total due from the client.

Scruffy had surgery at ABC Animal Clinic, and the client has arrived to pick her up. The receptionist greets the client, "Hello, Mrs. Rogers, are you here to pick up Scruffy? I have her invoice ready for you. Today she had a preoperative exam at no charge; preoperative bloodwork for $45.99; a preoperative ECG for $49.99; and IV fluids for $54.85, which includes the IV catheter, IV administrative set, and the fluids. Her ovariohysterectomy was $97.89, which includes anesthesia, surgery pack, and suture material as well as her postoperative

pain medication for $24.99. Scruffy's total is $398.34. Do you have any questions for me?"

This detailed presentation allows the client to read and understand the services provided. The value of the service has increased to the client once all procedures that have been provided are explained. An alternative conversation would be, "Hello, Mrs. Rogers. I have Scruffy's invoice ready. The total is $398.34. How would you like to pay for that today?" In this situation, the client does not know what she is paying for and may have a sense of sticker shock at the cost of a "simple spay." She will not perceive the value of the services her pet was provided and may respond, "Wow, that is expensive!" She may look for a cheaper clinic for her next veterinary visit.

PAYMENT FOR SERVICES

The most common forms of payment are by cash (including debit card), check, or credit card. The practice manager may choose which credit cards to accept. Practices pay a percentage of the total credit card transaction to the bank issuing the card. Most machines are very simple to operate; a team member slides the card and enters the expiration date and charge amount, and the machine connects to a designated terminal and either approves or declines the transaction (Figures 2-19 and 2-20). Debit transactions are quite similar, except the client enters a personal identification number (PIN) code before the transaction is approved. The signature on the credit card must match the signature on the slip. If any questions arise, the signature on a driver's license should be verified.

AAHA AMERICAN ANIMAL HOSPITAL ASSOCIATION	Comprehensive Patient Medical History Form	

	Yes	No
Are your address and phone still correct?		
Do you have pet health insurance?		
Are your pet's vaccinations up to date?		
Is your pet spayed or neutered?		
Was there a heartworm test in the last year?		
Is your pet taking heartworm prevention Rx?		
Has your pet been tested for worms in the last year?		
Have you seen your pet passing any worms?		
Has your pet had any illness/injury in the last year?		
Has your pet ever had a seizure?		
Does your pet get table scraps?		
Did your pet eat in the last four hours?		
Does your pet ever strain to urinate?		
Has there been any recent vomiting?		
Has your pet been coughing?		
Has your pet been sneezing?		
Has your pet been gagging?		
Any listlessness?		
Any weakness?		
Any lameness? Circle leg: RF LF RR LR		
Shaking of the head?		
Scratching? Where?		
Significant hair loss?		
Scooting of rear?		
Unusual lumps or bumps?		
Bad breath?		
Unusual discharge?		
Diarrhea?		
Constipation?		
Stiffness?		
Behavior changes?		

	Increased	Decreased
Drinking?		
Appetite?		
Urination?		
Defecation?		
Weight?		

Reason for visit today?

_____
_____
_____

Has your pet been examined elsewhere for the same condition?   Yes   No

If so, where?_____

What medication is your pet now taking?

_____
_____

Is your pet allergic to any food or Rx?   Y   N

If yes, please describe _____

What flea control is used?

Anything else we need to know?

_____
_____
_____
_____
_____

I hereby authorize the hospital to prescribe for and treat the conditions presented on this form for the pet presented by me. The hospital and staff will not be held liable for any problems that develop provided that reasonable care is provided. Furthermore, I agree to pay fees in full for services rendered when pet is discharged from the hospital's care unless other prior arrangements have been agreed upon by both parties.

_____   _____
        Signature   Date

FIGURE 2-10, cont'd J, Comprehensive patient medical history form. (Courtesy American Animal Hospital Association, Lakewood, Colo.)

PRACTICE POINT   A majority of transactions are paid by debit or credit cards.

Care Credit is a credit card used exclusively for veterinary medicine. Other divisions of Care Credit are available for human medical care. Clients can apply either online or while at the practice. A receptionist can enter the information online or through a telephone operator, and approval can be received in as little as 10 minutes. Care Credit generally runs specials with the first-time use of the card. Visit www.carecredit.com for current information. Many veterinary clinics in the United States accept Care Credit, allowing clients to charge veterinary care costs if their pet has an emergency while traveling.

Accepting cash has associated risks. Cash can be counterfeit. A local bank should be consulted regarding tips to recognize counterfeit money. Counterfeit money has no value, and detecting the passer can be difficult. Ask the local police department if it alerts local businesses to the passing of counterfeit money.

PRACTICE POINT   Counterfeit money is a loss to the practice because it cannot be deposited. Team members must learn how to identify counterfeit bills.

Large amounts of cash should be kept in a separate, locked safe, out of the sight of clients. It only takes a second for a client or person off the street to reach over the counter and grab money from the drawer. Cash

Pre-Anesthetic Bloodwork Options

Please initial all options you are accepting.

_____   Heartworm/Ehrlichia/Lymes test...$45.52
If not on prevention or tested recently

_____   Feline Leukemia/FIV test...$44.87
If never tested and/or unknown history

_____   CBC (Complete Blood Count)...$34.26
To check for anemia, clotting abilities, and infection
Recommended for all ages and all surgeries

_____   Chemistry Profile Prep II..$48.76
To check liver and kidney function
Recommended for animals 6 years and younger for all anesthesia

_____   Chemistry Profile Complete..$66.95
Full 12 chemistry profile
Recommended for animals 6 years and older for all anesthesia

_____   CBC and Chemistry Profile Prep II...$73.51

_____   CBC and Chemistry Profile Complete..$92.75

_____   IV Catheter...$40.91
Open line for emergency medications and/or fluids
Recommended for all geriatric animals or patients with ongoing health risks

_____   IV Catheter + Fluids..$63.68
To maintain blood pressure and hydration and for rapid recovery
Recommended for all geriatric animals or patients with ongoing health risks

_____   HomeAgain Microchip...$38.81

_____   E-Collar...$7 to $30

_____   I have been advised of the importance of these options and have declined all bloodwork.

Ear Crops:

_____   Required to have a CBC, IV catheter, and fluids (included in ear crop price).

_____   I have been advised that an additional pain medication will be administered to my pet if
needed at an additional charge of $13 to $20 per injection.

Signature _____ Date _____

K

FIGURE 2-10, cont'd   K, Pre-anesthetic bloodwork form.

drawers should have a lock and be locked immediately after it has been closed. Drawers should never be left unattended, especially if left unlocked. One moment of inattention can result in the loss of hundreds of dollars.

Many clinics also use check machines. Once checks are swiped through the terminal and the transaction has been approved, the money is automatically withdrawn from the customer's account and deposited into the clinic's bank account. If the client has insufficient funds in the account, the transaction will be declined and the client will need to use another source of payment.

When accepting checks, the receptionist must always make sure the check is signed, dated, and written

OWNER'S COPY	**RABIES VACCINATION CERTIFICATE**	Rabies Tag Number

NASPHV Form #51
Owner's Name and Address **Print - use ball point pen or type**

PRINT - Last	First	M.I.	Telephone

No.	Street	City	State	Zip

Species:	Sex:	Age:	Size:	Predominant Breed:	Colors:
Dog ☐	Male ☐	3 mo to 12 mo ☐	Under 20 lbs. ☐	_____	_____
Cat ☐	Female ☐	12 mo or older ☐	20 - 50 lbs. ☐		_____
Other: ☐ (Specify)	Neutered ☐	Actual Age_____	Over 50 lbs. ☐ Actual_____lbs.	Name:	_____

DATE VACCINATED:

Producer: [ ][ ][ ]
(First 3 letters)

Veterinarian's: # _____ (License No.)

_____ _____ _____
Month Day Year

☐ 1 yr. Lic./Vacc.
☐ 3 yr. Lic./Vacc.
_____ Other

(Signature)
Address:

VACCINATION EXPIRED:

_____ _____ _____
Month Day Year

Vacc. Serial (lot) no. _____

FIGURE 2-11 Rabies certificate. (Courtesy National Association of State Public Health Veterinarians.)

Master Problem List

Client name_____ Telephone number_____
Address _____ Client number _____
Pet name_____ Breed _____ Color _____
Sex _____ Altered _____ DOB _____ Age _____

	Date received	Date received	Date received	Date recieved
DHLPP				
FVRCP				
FeLV				
Rabies				
HWT				
FeLV/FIV				

Chronic diseases/date of onset:_____
_____
_____
_____

Current medications and directions:_____
_____
_____
_____

A

FIGURE 2-12 **A, B,** and **C,** Examples of master problem lists.

AVAC
Master Problem List

Client Name _____ Patient Name _____

Breed _____ Species _____

Allergies _____ Color _____ Sex _____ DOB _____

Rabies																
FVRCP																
FeLV																
FIP																
FeLV Test																
FIP Test																
HW Test																

MAJOR PROBLEMS

Date	Description	Treatment

MINOR PROBLEMS

Date	Description	Treatment

See reverse side for laboratory analysis.

B

FIGURE 2-12, cont'd (Courtesy AVAC Ltd., Calgary, Alberta, Canada.)

for the correct amount. Second, always make sure the check is in the team member's hand or the cash drawer, not still in the client's checkbook. A cashier's check is a check from the bank itself and represents guaranteed funds. Traveler's checks are similar to cashier's checks but must be signed and completed in front of a team member. The signature must match the person's identification and the previous signature on the face of the traveler's check. Cashier's and traveler's checks are much less risky than personal checks (for practices that do not use a check authorization service).

Receptionists should always verify identification when processing payments. Team members must protect the clinic against consumer fraud and stolen checks or credit cards. Most check reader terminals require a driver's license number to be entered into the machine before accepting the transaction.

Date									
WBC									
NEUTRO									
LYMPH									
MONO									
EOS									
BASO									
RBC									
Hb									
HCT									
PLT									
Date									
GLU									
BUN									
CREA									
Na									
P									
Cl									
CO2									
Ca									
Phos									
Trig									
CHOL									
ALK PHOS									
TP									
ALB									
GLOB									
T BILI									
SGPT (ALT)									
SGOT (AST)									
LDH									
GGT									
CPK									
Date									
Thyroid									
Phenobarb									

C

FIGURE 2-12, cont'd Reverse side of AVAC master problem list.

PRACTICE POINT Every credit card and check transaction should be verified by client identification to prevent fraud.

Pet health insurance is also an option for owners. Many companies now offer veterinary health care for pets. Owners pay the practice for services their pet receives and are then reimbursed by the insurance company. See Chapter 19 for more information.

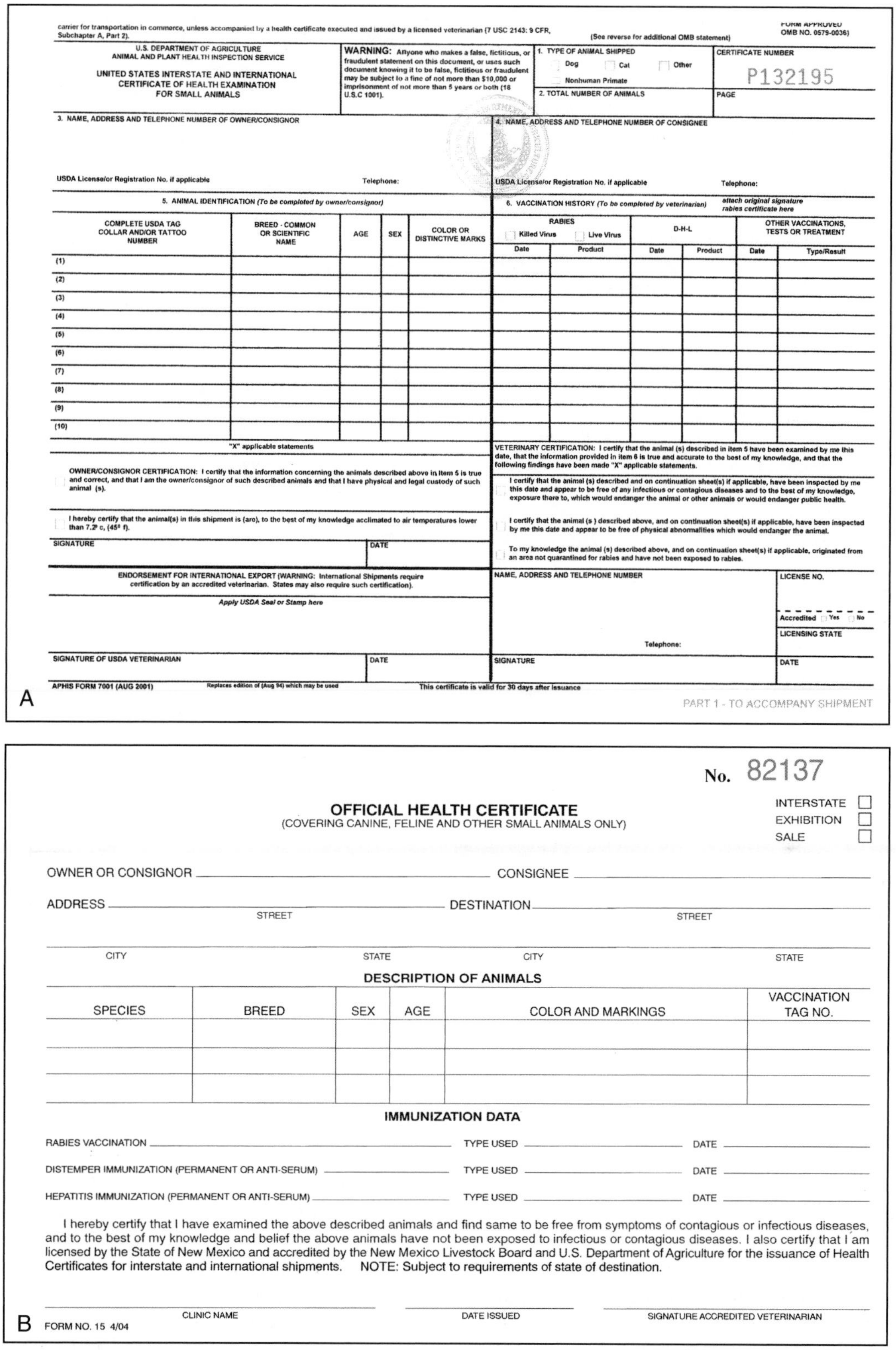

carrier for transportation in commerce, unless accompanied by a health certificate executed and issued by a licensed veterinarian (7 USC 2143: 9 CFR, Subchapter A, Part 2).

(See reverse for additional OMB statement)

FORM APPROVED OMB NO. 0579-0036)

U.S. DEPARTMENT OF AGRICULTURE
ANIMAL AND PLANT HEALTH INSPECTION SERVICE

UNITED STATES INTERSTATE AND INTERNATIONAL CERTIFICATE OF HEALTH EXAMINATION FOR SMALL ANIMALS

WARNING: Anyone who makes a false, fictitious, or fraudulent statement on this document, or uses such document knowing it to be false, fictitious or fraudulent may be subject to a fine of not more than $10,000 or imprisonment of not more than 5 years or both (18 U.S.C 1001).

1. TYPE OF ANIMAL SHIPPED ☐ Dog ☐ Cat ☐ Other ☐ Nonhuman Primate

2. TOTAL NUMBER OF ANIMALS

CERTIFICATE NUMBER P132195

PAGE

3. NAME, ADDRESS AND TELEPHONE NUMBER OF OWNER/CONSIGNOR

USDA License/or Registration No. if applicable Telephone:

4. NAME, ADDRESS AND TELEPHONE NUMBER OF CONSIGNEE

USDA License/or Registration No. if applicable Telephone:

5. ANIMAL IDENTIFICATION *(To be completed by owner/consignor)*

COMPLETE USDA TAG COLLAR AND/OR TATTOO NUMBER	BREED - COMMON OR SCIENTIFIC NAME	AGE	SEX	COLOR OR DISTINCTIVE MARKS
(1)				
(2)				
(3)				
(4)				
(5)				
(6)				
(7)				
(8)				
(9)				
(10)				

6. VACCINATION HISTORY *(To be completed by veterinarian)* *attach original signature rabies certificate here*

RABIES ☐ Killed Virus ☐ Live Virus		D-H-L		OTHER VACCINATIONS, TESTS OR TREATMENT	
Date	Product	Date	Product	Date	Type/Result

"X" applicable statements

☐ OWNER/CONSIGNOR CERTIFICATION: I certify that the information concerning the animals described above in Item 5 is true and correct, and that I am the owner/consignor of such described animals and that I have physical and legal custody of such animal (s).

☐ I hereby certify that the animal(s) in this shipment is (are), to the best of my knowledge acclimated to air temperatures lower than 7.2° c, (45° f).

SIGNATURE DATE

ENDORSEMENT FOR INTERNATIONAL EXPORT (WARNING: International Shipments require certification by an accredited veterinarian. States may also require such certification).

Apply USDA Seal or Stamp here

SIGNATURE OF USDA VETERINARIAN DATE

VETERINARY CERTIFICATION: I certify that the animal (s) described in item 5 have been examined by me this date, that the information provided in item 6 is true and accurate to the best of my knowledge, and that the following findings have been made "X" applicable statements.

☐ I certify that the animal (s) described and on continuation sheet(s) if applicable, have been inspected by me this date and appear to be free of any infectious or contagious diseases and to the best of my knowledge, exposure there to, which would endanger the animal or other animals or would endanger public health.

☐ I certify that the animal (s) described above, and on continuation sheet(s) if applicable, have been inspected by me this date and appear to be free of physical abnormalities which would endanger the animal.

☐ To my knowledge the animal (s) described above, and on continuation sheet(s) if applicable, originated from an area not quarantined for rabies and have not been exposed to rabies.

NAME, ADDRESS AND TELEPHONE NUMBER Telephone:

LICENSE NO.

Accredited ☐ Yes ☐ No

LICENSING STATE

SIGNATURE DATE

APHIS FORM 7001 (AUG 2001) Replaces edition of (Aug 94) which may be used This certificate is valid for 30 days after issuance

PART 1 - TO ACCOMPANY SHIPMENT

A

No. 82137

OFFICIAL HEALTH CERTIFICATE
(COVERING CANINE, FELINE AND OTHER SMALL ANIMALS ONLY)

INTERSTATE ☐
EXHIBITION ☐
SALE ☐

OWNER OR CONSIGNOR ____ CONSIGNEE ____

ADDRESS ____ STREET ____ DESTINATION ____ STREET ____

CITY STATE CITY STATE

DESCRIPTION OF ANIMALS

SPECIES	BREED	SEX	AGE	COLOR AND MARKINGS	VACCINATION TAG NO.

IMMUNIZATION DATA

RABIES VACCINATION ____ TYPE USED ____ DATE ____

DISTEMPER IMMUNIZATION (PERMANENT OR ANTI-SERUM) ____ TYPE USED ____ DATE ____

HEPATITIS IMMUNIZATION (PERMANENT OR ANTI-SERUM) ____ TYPE USED ____ DATE ____

I hereby certify that I have examined the above described animals and find same to be free from symptoms of contagious or infectious diseases, and to the best of my knowledge and belief the above animals have not been exposed to infectious or contagious diseases. I also certify that I am licensed by the State of New Mexico and accredited by the New Mexico Livestock Board and U.S. Department of Agriculture for the issuance of Health Certificates for interstate and international shipments. NOTE: Subject to requirements of state of destination.

CLINIC NAME DATE ISSUED SIGNATURE ACCREDITED VETERINARIAN

B FORM NO. 15 4/04

FIGURE 2-13 **A,** International health certificate. (Courtesy U.S. Department of Agriculture.) **B,** Interstate health certificate.

Declined Transactions

If a client's credit card, check, or debit card has been declined, politely and discreetly inform the client of the decline. Ask for an alternate method of payment. Some credit card and debit cards have a maximum charge amount per day, so the overdraft may be unintentional. Do not assume that a client has bad credit because of a refusal; there may be an innocent reason behind the decline.

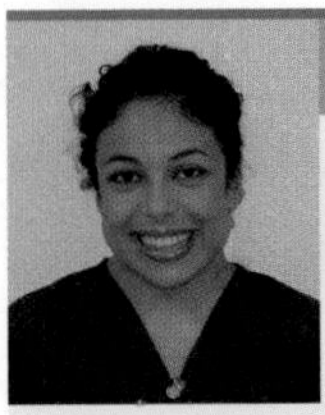

What Would You Do/Not Do?

Lori, a receptionist of 5 years, is reviewing an invoice with Mr. DeWitt. Mr. DeWitt had his pet ("Furminator") neutered at the practice and has arrived to pick him up. After Lori has reviewed all the charges and gives Mr. DeWitt his total, he presents a credit card to pay for the transaction. Lori runs the credit card through the machine, which denies the charge. Lori quietly informs Mr. DeWitt that his credit card has been denied and asks for an alternative form of payment. Mr. DeWitt becomes very upset and demands that she run the credit card again, saying "There must be a mistake!" Lori grants the request and runs the credit card again. Again the card is denied, which she informs him once more. He becomes even angrier and demands that she call the credit card company and determine why the card has been denied. She informs him that they will not provide the information to her; she offers to call the company and hand the phone over to him to discuss the situation. After a lengthy, loud conversation with the credit card company, Mr. DeWitt slams down the phone exclaiming how "stupid" the company is and that he is canceling his credit card. Lori again politely asks for payment of services, which increases

Mr. DeWitt's frustrations. He yells, "I have been a client here for 5 years and you can't even give me the grace of credit one time? I should cancel you along with my credit card!"

What should Lori have done?

Lori should have put Mr. DeWitt in a room to discuss the declined credit card. Many clients become embarrassed and act irrationally when confronted with such news. Many times credit and debit cards are declined because the owner has reached the maximum amount of charges allowed per day. Others are declined because a payment has not been received or the credit card has reached the maximum allowed charges.

Perhaps Mr. DeWitt's comment regarding canceling the credit card and "canceling" the veterinary practice came from frustration, but it does not need to be heard by other clients. Clients may only hear part of a conversation and misconstrue the comment.

Mr. DeWitt's account could have been analyzed by the practice manager, who could determine if he would be allowed to make a payment at a later time. Many times the length of the client-patient relationship and history of payment will help make the decision.

Request to Release Medical Records

I request that copies of the medical records for my pet(s) named:

_____

be released to the following new practice name:

_____

New practice street address, city, state, and zip:

_____

Printed name of owner _____

Signature and date of owner _____

Records will be available for pickup or available by fax within 24 hours after receipt of the signed release form.

FIGURE 2-14 Request to release medical records.

Hospital policy regarding declined charges should be developed and instituted so that consistency runs throughout the practice. Some clinics allow a client to return to pay on the account; others may keep medication that was to be dispensed until a client can return with payment. Never keep a client's pet because of a declined payment. Practices are then responsible for the upkeep and care of the pet until the owner returns. If it is a sick and debilitated pet, the owner may not return! It is against the law in many states to hold a pet for ransom. Each state has different lien laws regarding holding pets; practice owners and managers should check with the their state board of veterinary medicine for clarification.

The practice owner is responsible for determining if the clinic will allow clients to charge for services rendered. Every member of the team must be familiar with the policy, including the veterinarians. Practice owners, practice managers, and/or office managers should be the only team members allowed to approve this type of transaction. Often, veterinarians and technicians empathize with the client and wish to extend credit; unfortunately, many clients will not return to make a payment. Care Credit should always be offered to clients wishing to charge services. This allows the clinic to give clients an option when they may not be able to pay for services rendered (the practice will receive immediate payment, and the client can make payments to Care Credit).

Arroyo Vista Animal Clinic
2303 Inspiration Lane, Anywhere, USA
Dr. Larsen, Dr. Cooke, and Dr. Thompson
Boarding Admission Form

Owner's Name _____ Date _____
Address _____ Phone _____
City _____ In case of emergency, please call _____

Pet's Name _____ Breed _____ Sex ___ Age ___ Color _____
Date of last vaccine _____ Please circle which vaccine: DHPP   FVRCP   FeLV
Date of last rabies vaccine _____ Date of last Bordetella vaccine _____
Medications while boarding _____
Belongings _____
Pet's Name _____ Breed _____ Sex ___ Age ___ Color _____
Date of last vaccine _____ Please circle which vaccine: DHPP   FVRCP   FeLV
Date of last rabies vaccine _____ Date of last Bordetella vaccine _____
Medications while boarding _____
Belongings _____
Pet's Name _____ Breed _____ Sex ___ Age ___ Color _____
Date of last vaccine _____ Please circle which vaccine: DHPP   FVRCP   FeLV
Date of last rabies vaccine _____ Date of last Bordetella vaccine _____
Medications while boarding _____
Belongings _____
While boarding, please perform the following procedures:
Physical exam _____ Vaccinations _____
Heartworm test _____ Bath _____ Dip _____ Nail trim _____
Other: _____
_____
_____
_____

All animals entering the hospital must be up to date on vaccinations and free of external parasites (fleas, ticks) or they will be treated upon admission at the owner's expense.
I authorize Arroyo Vista Animal Clinic to treat my pet(s) in case an emergency situation should arise.
Pets are released only during the regular office hours. It is my responsibility to inform the hospital if I will be delayed in picking up my pets; I will assume all costs associated with an extended stay.

Owner's signature _____ Date _____

A

FIGURE 2-15 **A,** Sample boarding admission form.

Not all clients can afford the most expensive services, so several payment options should be available. Clients may elect conservative treatment because of the cost of services and should not be judged for their decisions. On the other hand, do not assume clients cannot afford necessary services.

PRACTICE POINT Care Credit is a credit card used exclusively for veterinary services.

Daily Reconciliation

Balancing the accounts at the end of the day is a crucial task. Incomplete transactions, errors, and missing money, credit card receipts, or checks can all be found when balancing. It is much easier to find errors at the end of the day than searching for them the next day or following week (Figures 2-21 and 2-22).

PRACTICE POINT Reconciliation must occur on a daily basis.

Boarding Admission Form

Please read the following statements and sign below.

All animals entering the hospital for boarding must be current on vaccinations and free of parasites. If not, they will be treated upon entering at the owner's expense.

All dogs that have boarded five days or more will be bathed prior to discharge unless the animal's health or temperament makes it hazardous to the animal or handlers. If tranquilizers are necessary for treatment/handling, permission is granted.

Pets are released only during regular clinic hours.

I expect to pick up my pet(s) on _____ (date).

If I neglect to contact/pick up my pet(s) within 7 days of said date, Arroyo Veterinary Clinic may assume my pet has been abandoned and is hereby authorized to dispose of the pet(s) as it deems best (including euthanasia).

I authorize Arroyo Veterinary Clinic to treat as needed _____

OR

I request Arroyo Veterinary Clinic to treat, but not to exceed $ _____

Signed _____

Dated _____ Emergency # _____

I request Arroyo Veterinary Clinic to walk my pet daily for exercise. I understand that Arroyo Veterinary Clinic and its staff will do all that is possible to prevent the escape of my pet. But if my pet slips out of its collar/leash and is NOT retrievable (runs off), I will not hold Arroyo Veterinary Clinic responsible for negligence or punitive damages.

Signed _____

Belongings: _____

Medications: _____

Feeding schedule: _____

B

FIGURE 2-15, cont'd B, Sample boarding admission form.

Reconciliation is the process of matching and comparing figures from a transaction totals sheet with the actual receipts and funds accepted as payments. The balance of the transaction totals sheet must match the funds. Reconciliation compares account records to uncover any possible discrepancies. Practices may have different methods of ensuring reconciliation but the goal is the same; the computer daily total transactions must equal the daily flow sheet.

The cash drawer or register will contain an opening amount of cash predetermined by the practice owner. It should be the same amount every day, comprised of a variety of bills to give change when needed. A recommendation may be $200, broken into one $20 bill, four $10 bills, eight $5 bills, 50 $1 bills, and $50 in quarters, dimes, nickels, and pennies. At the end of the day, the total amount in the cash drawer should be $200 plus any cash payments made by clients (Figure 2-23). This cash amount must equal the cash payments on the computer daily total transaction sheet. If the remaining cash does not equal $200, the error must be found. Once the cash balances, the cash from the clients should be removed from the cash drawer and placed in a bank bag and set aside in preparation for a deposit.

Guest: {PATIENTID} - {NAME}   Breed: {BREED}
Owner: {ID} - {FULLNAME}   Age: {AGE}
Cage: {CAGETYPE} {CAGENUMBER}   Sex: {SEX}
Date in: {ARRIVALDATE[SHORT]}   Weight: {CURRENTWEIGHT} {CURRENTWEIGHTUNIT}
Date/time out: {DEPARTUREDATE[SHORT]} {DEPARTURETIME}

Diet: _____   Amount: _____ cups _____ times a day

DATE:					Medication:			
MONDAY	AM	AFT	PM	Other	___ AM ___ PM _____			
Feeding								
Confirmed					___ AM ___ PM _____			
Water								
Potty Break					___ AM ___ PM _____			
Urination								
Defecation					Comments:			
20 Min Exercise								
Brush					_____			
Medication								
Bath					_____			
Daycare					_____			
Nighttime Treat					_____			
Grooming					_____			

DATE:					DATE:			
TUESDAY	AM	AFT	PM	Other	FRIDAY	AM	AFT	PM	Other
Feeding					Feeding			
Confirmed					Confirmed			
Water					Water			
Potty Break					Potty Break			
Urination					Urination			
Defecation					Defecation			
20 Min Exercise					20 Min Exercise			
Brush					Brush			
Medication					Medication			
Bath					Bath			
Daycare					Daycare			
Nighttime Treat					Nighttime Treat			
Grooming					Grooming			

DATE:					DATE:			
WEDNESDAY	AM	AFT	PM	Other	SATURDAY	AM	AFT	PM	Other
Feeding					Feeding			
Confirmed					Confirmed			
Water					Water			
Potty Break					Potty Break			
Urination					Urination			
Defecation					Defecation			
20 Min Exercise					20 Min Exercise			
Brush					Brush			
Medication					Medication			
Bath					Bath			
Daycare					Daycare			
Nighttime Treat					Nighttime Treat			
Grooming					Grooming			

DATE:					DATE:			
THURSDAY	AM	AFT	PM	Other	SUNDAY	AM	AFT	PM	Other
Feeding					Feeding			
Confirmed					Confirmed			
Water					Water			
Potty Break					Potty Break			
Urination					Urination			
Defecation					Defecation			
20 Min Exercise					20 Min Exercise			
Activity Toy					Activity Toy			
Brush					Brush			
Medication					Medication			
Bath					Bath			
Daycare					Daycare			
Nighttime Treat					Nighttime Treat			
Grooming					Grooming			

C

FIGURE 2-15, cont'd C, Sample boarding admission form.

The checks must also be reconciled and compared against the check totals on the computer daily total transaction sheet (Figure 2-23, *B*). If a check machine is used, the machine will require team members to "batch out" at the end of the day. The total on the check batch sheet must match the total of the checks themselves as well as the transaction daily total sheet. If they do not match, the error must be found.

The credit card slips must also be totaled and matched against the transaction daily total sheet (Figure 2-23, *C*). If there are any missing credit card slips or transactions, the error must be identified. Credit card machines will also need to be "batched out" at the end of the day; the total on the batch sheet must match the totals of the credit card slips and the transaction sheet. Finally, the cash, checks, and credit cards must equal the total on the daily

Boarding Client Information Sheet

In case of an emergency, please contact

Name _____

Number _____

My animal has medications to be given: Yes   No

If yes, please list medications and instructions:

_____

_____

_____

_____

Belongings: _____

_____

_____

_____

Any other important information we should know?

_____

_____

_____

_____

D

FIGURE 2-15, cont'd D, Sample boarding admission form.

transaction total sheet (Figure 2-23, *D*). If they do not match, the error must be found.

> **PRACTICE POINT**   Cash, checks, and credit cards must be counted and matched against the end-of-day reconciliation sheet.

Credit card slips and checks deposited through an automatic check machine need to be stored in a safe and locked place. It is important that these documents be kept for 7 years in case a client chooses to dispute a transaction.

As a last check (see Figure 2-23):
- A + B + C = D, and E + F + G = H.
- B = F and C = G.
- Finally, D = H − $200 (the starting cash balance)

Deposits

Deposits to the bank must be recorded on a deposit slip. Cash is entered on the cash line and checks typically are entered individually. If a check machine is used, the checks do not need to be deposited at the end of the day. For practices without check machines, checks should be stamped "for deposit only, ABC Veterinary Clinic" on the

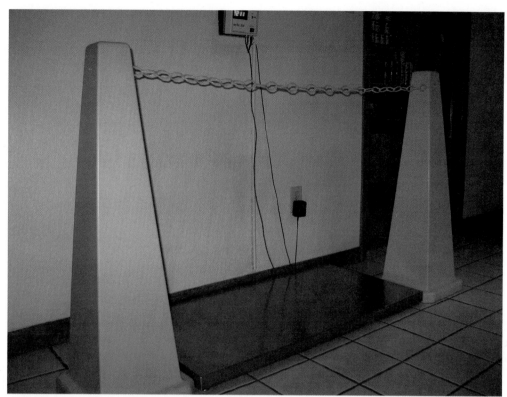

FIGURE 2-16 Bright yellow barriers around the weight scale prevent clients and team members from tripping.

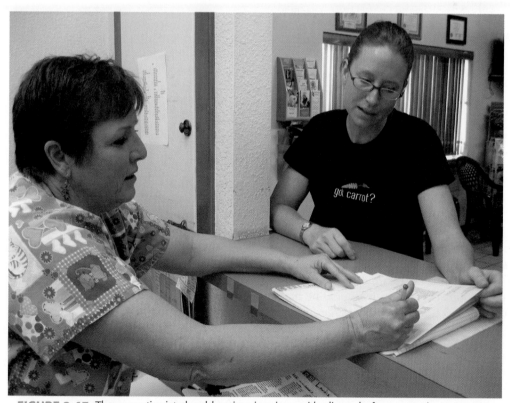

FIGURE 2-17 The receptionist should review invoices with clients before accepting payment.

ABC Animal Clinic
134 Uptown Circle
Anytown, MN 89000
800-555-5555

Maria Rogers
6454 Downtown Circle
Anytown, MN 89001   Account # 21312

"Scruffy" Rogers
Age: 9 years
Weight: 45#
Reminders: DHPP due 5/10/10
             Rabies due 5/10/11
             Heartworm Test due 5/10/09

Invoice Number: 10090
Date: 04/28/08
Dr. Nancy Dreamer

Date	Service	Unit	Extended Cost
04/28/09	Pre-Anesthetic Exam	1	0.00
04/28/09	Pre-Anesthetic Bloodwork	1	$45.99
04/28/09	CBC/Chemistry	1	
04/28/09	Electrolytes	1	
04/28/09	Pre-Anesthetic ECG	1	$49.99
04/28/09	IV Fluids – Surgery	1	$54.85
04/28/09	IV Catheter	1	
04/28/09	IV Administration Set	1	
04/28/09	Normosol 1 Liter	1	
04/28/09	General Anesthesia	1	$101.20
04/28/09	Pre-Anesthetic	1	
04/28/09	Sevoflurane	1	
04/28/09	K-9 OVH under 50#	1	$97.89
04/28/09	OVH Pack	1	
04/28/09	Suture Material	2	
04/28/09	Biohazard Fee	1	
04/28/09	Surgical Monitoring	1	
04/28/09	Post-Operative Pain Medication	1	$24.99

	Subtotal	$374.91
	Tax 6.25%	23.43
	Invoice Total	$398.34

A

FIGURE 2-18 A, Sample invoice.

back, including an account number. The cash and checks are totaled and entered at the bottom of the deposit slip (Figure 2-24). This total must match the cash and check total on the transaction sheet. Deposits should be made on a daily basis because it is unsafe to leave large amounts of cash in the office.

It is important to have a checks and balance system in place. All totals should match and must be double checked. It is very important to eliminate errors as much as possible; double checking a team member's work helps. Each transaction total should be initialed by the person checking and double checking the transactions.

Loving Care Animal Clinic

#5 Sugar Creek Road
Piedmont, MO 63957

800-555-5555

"Our Goal Is To Make
Your Pet Happy"

For: Mrs. Jessica Albert
     P.O. Box 16
     Piedmont, MO 63957

Printed: 02-18-09 at 11:11a
Date: 02-18-09
Account: 474
Invoice: 169740

Date	For	Qty	Description	Price
12-19-09	Alvin	1	Canine DA2PP 1st	18.50
12-19-09		1	Fecal examination, <8 weeks	19.00
12-19-09		1	Eukanuba puppy 8 lbs	13.70
12-19-09		1	Nylon collar 5/8"	4.49
12-19-09		1	Rawhide bone - 6" curl	2.10

Total charges, this invoice	57.79
Tax	4.33
Total, this invoice	62.12
Your previous balance	0.00
Total payment(s) received	62.12
02-18-09 Check payment #512	62.12
Your new balance	0.00

Reminders for: Alvin (Weight: 7.0 lbs - 17w)   Last done

10-17-10	Annual examination
04-07-10	Dental cleaning first
02-06-10	Canine rabies vaccination
01-09-10	Canine DA2PP 2nd

Doctor's instructions

Eukanuba puppy 8 lbs
To assure that we provide your pet with the freshest food available, effective July 2010, we are changing our pet food distribution policies. We will rotate to an order system for food refills. In the past, food was ordered and stocked. There were times that we would run out of stock and therefore did not have the food your pet needed. On the other hand, we might have a bag sitting on the shelf for many months before it was needed. We would like to eliminate both of these possibilities and provide you with an increased level of service.

B

FIGURE 2-18, cont'd B, Sample invoice.

Adding machine tape should be banded around receipts from checks and credit cards in case any questions arise regarding reconciliation. Deposit totals can be recorded in the practice checkbook or in a daily log book maintained by the practice manager. The practice manager should always compare deposits from the bank statement to the log entry.

PRACTICE POINT Practices using check machines do not need to deposit checks at the bank.

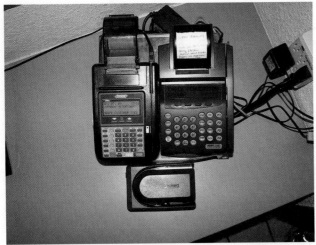

FIGURE 2-19 Credit card and check machine.

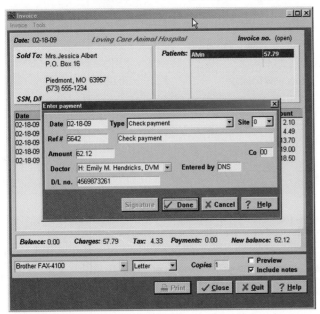

FIGURE 2-20 Sample payment screen from Avimark, a veterinary software program. (Courtesy McAllister Software Systems, Piedmont, Mo.)

Petty Cash

Petty cash is a term used to describe cash set aside in the practice to purchase items needed for the business when a check is not available. For example, the veterinarian may need some turkey meat for a special patient that will not eat regular dog food. In this situation, a team member can take some money from the petty cash bag and purchase the meat. A receipt must be returned and placed in the bag for balancing and reconciliation purposes. The money should be counted at the end of every shift to ensure that money is not missing and that receipts account for any money spent.

VETERINARY PRACTICE and the LAW

When a telephone call concerns an emergency, the team member answering it becomes responsible for providing immediate assistance. The most desirable response from a team member is to transfer the call to a veterinarian or a team member who can provide assistance. If no one is available, the receptionist may need to provide comfort and ask questions to determine the extent of the emergency.

Treatment procedures cannot be given over the phone without direct consultation with the veterinarian. If a client has a concern, team members must advise owners to immediately bring the pet in for an examination. Any advice given over the phone can be misconstrued, leading to a poor resolution that may place the practice in jeopardy of a malpractice lawsuit.

Each receptionist team should keep an emergency procedural manual in the front office. This manual should list specific questions to ask and appropriate answers to provide. The name of the client, patient, and a phone number should be written down as documentation and used for a follow-up call if the client never arrives at the practice.

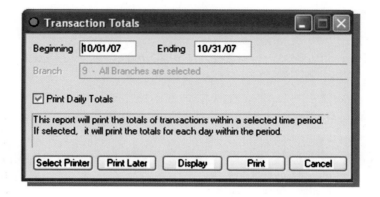

Total Invoices	*(add)*	199108.23
Total Discount	*(subtract)*	0.00
Total (Invoice-Discount)		199108.23
Total Tax	*(add)*	854.94
Total Net Invoices		199963.17
Total Returns	*(subtract)*	253.83
Total Returned Tax	*(subtract)*	0.86
Total Credit Adj	*(subtract)*	1315.24
Total Debit Adj	*(add)*	1111.79
Total Net Services		**199505.03**

Total Cash	*(add)*	5611.15
Total Cash Change	*(subtract)*	441.64
Total Cash Refund	*(subtract)*	0.00
Total Net Cash		5169.51
Total Check	*(add)*	38012.36
Total Card	*(add)*	154590.42
Total Payment		197772.29
Total Check Refund	*(subtract)*	0.00
Total Card Refund	*(subtract)*	674.26
Total Net Payments		**197098.03**

Debit Transactions (Adjustments)	
NSF Check Fee	60.00
Returned Check	1051.79
Furry Friends Fund	0.00
Balance write off	0.00
Beginning Balance	0.00
Refund Adj	0.00
Monthy Interest	0.00
Billing Fee	0.00
No Transaction Type	0.00
Total:	**1111.79**

Credit Transactions (Adjustments)	
Dr. Approved Credit	958.81
Furry Friends Fund	0.00
Col Agency Writeoff	0.00
Balance write off	0.00
Beginning Balance	0.00
Return Adj	356.43
No Transaction Type	0.00
Total:	**1315.24**

Transaction Totals INTRAVET VETERINARY CARE

10/01/2007 - 10/31/2007

CALCULATION METHOD:

Total Invoices	= (Total Item Amounts) before tax and discount applied
Tax	= (Tax) - (Returned Tax)
Net Services	= (Total Invoice) + (Tax) - (Discount) - (Returns) - (Credit Adj) + (Debit Adj)
Total Payment	= (Cash) + (Check) + (Card) - (Change) - (Refund)

Date	Invoices	Disc.	Tax	Returns	Deb Adj	Cre Adj	Services	Cash	Check	Card	Refund	Payment
10/01/2007	7968.74		31.63				8000.37	239.18	846.78	6996.60		8082.56
10/02/2007	5938.20		31.93	53.35			5916.78	214.31	1928.26	3889.15		6031.72
10/03/2007	6665.07		29.92				6694.99	263.20	480.44	6092.60		6836.24
10/04/2007	4347.51		10.52				4358.03	14.67	1746.91	2596.44		4358.02
10/05/2007	5269.28		26.45				5295.73	45.01	836.79	4016.91		4898.71
10/06/2007	4665.07		30.71				4695.78	348.61	262.11	3979.04		4589.76
10/07/2007	2679.07		9.32				2688.39	238.27	472.06	2187.87		2898.20
10/08/2007	8125.15		40.98				8166.13	195.72	703.62	6476.92		7376.26
10/09/2007	9290.25		7.39				9297.64	132.93	1516.38	8079.38		9728.69
10/10/2007	7369.77		43.64	111.90			7301.51	222.88	1633.25	6892.93		8749.06
10/11/2007	8006.12		13.69				8019.81	10.93	1069.69	6939.03		8019.54

FIGURE 2-21 A transaction totals screen. (Courtesy IntraVet, Effingham, Ill.)

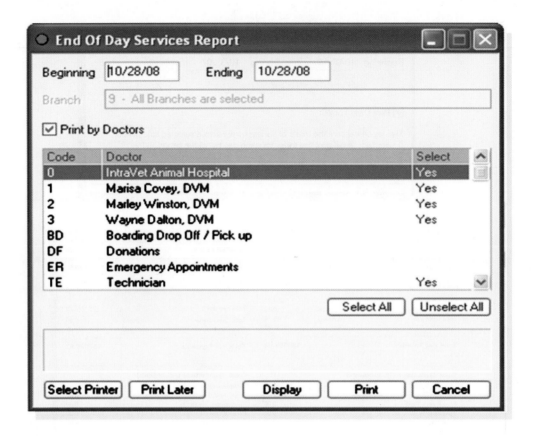

FIGURE 2-22 End-of-day services report. (Courtesy IntraVet, Effingham, Ill.)

Transaction Totals		6/1/09			ABC Animal Clinic	
Total Invoices	$ 5,497.69					
Total Cash	$ 1,409.65	(A)	Cash Counted	$ 1,209.65	(E)
Total Checks	$ 382.96	(B)	Checks Counted	$ 382.96	(F)
Total Credit Card	$ 4,105.08	(C)	Credit Card Slips Counted	$ 4,105.08	(G)
Total Payment	$ 5,497.69	(D)	Total Counted	$ 5,697.69	(H)

A = E + $200.00
B = F
C = G
D = H - $200.00 (starting cash balance)

FIGURE 2-23 Transaction totals sheet.

ABC Veterinary Clinic
1234 Street
Anywhere, US 10001

Date _____

_____
SIGN HERE IF CASH RECEIVED

32112   321   34890491   01

CASH		
List Checks:		
TOTAL		
LESS CASH RECEIVED:		
NET DEPOSIT		

FIGURE 2-24 Deposit slip.

Self-Evaluation Questions

1. Record a phone conversation between two students. One should act as a receptionist team member; the other should be a client. Have the team member use the following techniques while talking with the "client."
   - Speak loudly
   - Speak softly
   - Speak rapidly
   - Do not smile when answering the phone
   - Smile while answering the phone

   Analyze the recording. What were the differences? Is the call confusing? What changes could improve each call?

2. Identify mistakes and incompleteness on the following client form.

ABC Animal Clinic
555 Uptown Circle
Anytown, MN 89000
314-134-4431

Please print clearly

Date: _____4/30/09_____

Name _____Santiago Garcia_____

Mailing address __1645 Horse Lane, Mesa, AZ__   Zip code ___06070___

Street address _____   Zip code _____

Home phone ___576-895-8576___   Work phone __867-869-8695__

Drivers license # _____   State _____

Animals:

Name	Date of birth	Species	Breed	Color	Gender	Spayed or neutered?
Chuck	12/15/06	Canine	Chih	Black		N

I understand that payment is required in full on the same date that services are rendered.

_____
Signature

Self-Evaluation Questions—cont'd

3. Reconcile the end-of-day report for the veterinary practice below and develop a deposit for your cash and checks.

Total Invoices:	$6579.08
Total Cash:	$568.90
Total Checks:	$2567.78
Total Credit Cards:	$3442.40

   Your opening cash drawer was $200.00

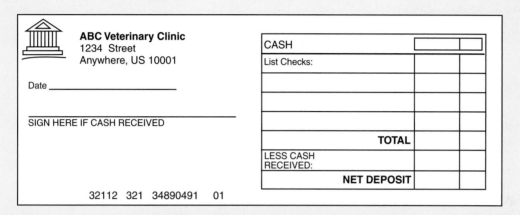

4. Determine mistakes on the following end-of-day reconciliation:

Total invoices:	**$6798.34**
Total cash:	$235.68
Total cash counted:	*$435.68*
Total checks:	$564.67
Total checks counted:	*$480.98*
Total credit card transactions:	$5977.99
Total credit card slips counted:	*$4478.67*
Total payments:	$6798.34

   Total counts: _____

5. Why are health certificates required?
6. What makes the first impression on clients?
7. What information should not be given to clients over the phone?
8. How can a phone shopper be turned into a client?
9. How should a declined credit card be handled?
10. Why should invoices be reviewed with clients, not just given to them?

Recommended Reading

Finch L: *Telephone courtesy and client service,* Los Altos, CA, 1994, Crisp Publications.

Gearson RF: *Beyond customer service. Keeping clients for life,* Schaumburg, IL, 2001, Crisp Publications.

Heinke MM: *Practice made perfect: a guide to veterinary practice management,* Lakewood, CO, 2001, AAHA Press.

McCurnin D: *Veterinary practice management,* Philadelphia, PA, 1988, JB Lippincott.

Wilson JF, Lacroix LA: *Legal consent forms for the veterinary practice,* ed 3, Yardley, PA, 2001, Priority Press.

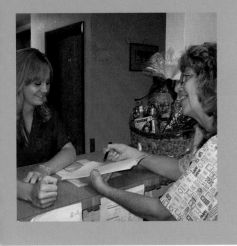

Team Management

Chapter Outline

Learning Objectives

Mastery of the content in this chapter will enable the reader to:
- List methods to become an effective leader.
- Describe and understand various management styles.
- Discuss the empowerment of team members.
- Discuss effective delegation.
- Clarify methods to increase team communication.
- List methods to resolve conflict.
- Discuss methods to increase team efficiency.
- Identify methods to decrease loss in the practice.

Key Terms

Accountability
Conceptual Skill
Conflict Management
Delegation

Directive Management
Effective Communication
Empowerment
Evaluation

Human Skill
Supportive Management
Technical Skill
Travel Sheet

Successful management of the veterinary health care team is essential to practice survival. The team attracts new clients, retains clients, educates clients, and satisfies clients. The team includes every member of the veterinary hospital, from the kennel assistants to the veterinarians. Each person contributes significant time and energy to each client and patient. Practice managers and hospital administrators may not have direct contact with clients, but they support the team by developing and providing staff training, client education materials, and excellent managerial structure to help the organizational run smoothly.

In a veterinary practice there are many benefits to employees acting as a team rather than a set of individuals. Team members recognize and understand their interdependence, allowing personal and team goals to be accomplished with mutual support. They feel a sense of pride and ownership in the practice and are committed to reaching goals that they have helped establish. All team members contribute to the success of the practice by applying their unique skills and talents to obtain those goals and by always being willing to accept new challenges. New ideas and challenges can stimulate team members to become strong performers and encourage others to follow. Team members continually work together to improve their service to clients, patients, and each other, and all of these team qualities make participation in a veterinary practice an excellent and rewarding

---

Box 3-1	Suggestions for Creating Positive Team Interactions

- Help others be right, not wrong.
- Have fun.
- Smile!
- Be enthusiastic.
- Seek ways for new ideas to work, not reasons why they won't.
- Be courageous.
- Maintain a positive attitude.
- Maintain confidentiality.
- Verify information given to you; do not gossip.
- Speak positively of others at all times.
- Say "thank you" for kind gestures.
- If you don't have something positive to say, don't say anything.

---

career. A dedicated and proficient team that understands basic practice management is likely to achieve extraordinary goals and boost the practice's compliance rate. Team building is a continuous process that never ends; the trial and error that are a part of this process allow each team member to learn and grow from the mistakes made along the way (Box 3-1).

Successful leadership comes with practice, education, and time. Many managers have learned success through trial and error and by finding what works best in their particular practices. What works in one practice may not work in another, and continuing education can help with developing ideas to help take a veterinary hospital to the next level.

LEADERSHIP

Leadership is vital to the success and growth of a practice. Leadership is influence; a leader is one who influences others, motivating them into action and inspiring them to become the best they can be. Leaders in veterinary practice must guide effective communication and create an environment that facilitates teamwork. Through good leadership, team members can appreciate how they contribute to the big picture of exceptional patient and client care.

PRACTICE POINT Strong leadership facilitates a well-organized and profitable practice.

In modern society, leaders must strive to achieve short- and long-term goals; create effective, efficient methods to complete tasks; and be proactive instead of reactive to situations. A leader's personal effectiveness can directly influence a hospital's success. Leaders must determine the most effective method to manage team members and be able to recognize their own strengths and weaknesses

as well as those of others. A motivating leader generates enthusiasm and excitement and an organized leader provides the path to achieve goals; the best kind of leader does both. A leader sets the practice's vision and goals, communicating the vision to the staff so they may help accomplish those goals.

Leaders must hold themselves to a higher standard of patient care, customer service, performance, and personal behavior. Leading by example has a much more profound effect on team members than leading by directive. Examples show team members what is expected of them when it comes to patient and client care. All team members should be held accountable for providing the best care possible, and leaders can set the stage for this to occur. Leadership that promotes a poor standard of care and professionalism will also affect the team, as team members realize that they do not need to perform their best or maintain themselves in a professional manner. Leaders of this type should be terminated because they will cause the team to disintegrate and the practice to fail.

Leadership skills are not developed overnight; they come with patience, education, and trial and error. Managing a practice has both wonderful and terrible days. A leader is sometimes viewed as a "good guy," sometimes as a "bad guy," and sometimes as uncaring and lacking compassion. However, the success of a business can depend on the quality of the leader. Someone who is capable of being either a good guy or bad guy when necessary will keep the team focused so they provide excellent quality of care.

PRACTICE POINT A leader makes mistakes; a successful leader admits the mistakes and learns from them.

Excellent leaders use human, technical, and conceptual skills to succeed in that role. *Human skill* is the ability to understand people and what motivates them and to be able to direct their behavior through effective leadership. Not all team members respond to leadership, training, or education in the same manner. Characteristics such as shyness, lack of confidence, and poor communication skills make it hard to train some team members. Domineering, independent, and strong-willed individuals may also have a hard time accepting training. Effective leaders can determine what motivates these various personality types and have a positive influence on each (Box 3-2).

Technical skill is the ability to apply leadership, skill, and knowledge of equipment, procedures, and hospital policies to team members in an effective, ambitious manner. Leaders must be able to train or provide training to team members on all equipment, maintenance of equipment, functions, and supplies needed to maintain that piece of equipment. Team members need training on policies and procedures that have been developed to have a successful implementation. Policy training

Box 3-2	Fundamentals That Build Effective Leadership

- **Trust:** Development of a trusting relationship with each employee facilitates open communication.
- **Accept change:** Effective leaders understand that disruptions occur and are willing to make and accept change to succeed.
- **Focus:** Leaders have the ability to achieve and direct their time and energy to achieve goals.
- **Commitment:** Effective leaders work continually to find new ideas to help make policies and procedures succeed. Accepting change helps promote commitment.
- **Compassion:** Leaders care about and desire to understand team members and their families.
- **Integrity:** Integrity demands that leaders seek to create quality assurance for their clients, patients, and team members and facilitate a positive relationship with all.
- **Endurance:** Leaders demonstrate courage, perseverance, and strength when situations, people, or the environment becomes chaotic or difficult.

Box 3-3	Characteristics of Effective Leaders

- Self-confident
- Sincere
- Enthusiastic
- Effective listener
- Effective communicator
- Accepting of diverse cultures
- Team player
- Problem solver
- Innovator and renovator
- Will admit mistakes

can be difficult for some employees, especially long-term employees, because they may be resistant to policy change or implementation.

Conceptual skill is the ability to sense how the leadership style affects the practice and to make change in a positive way. Not all leadership styles have a positive effect on team members. An effective leader can determine when changes are needed and try various leadership styles until success has been attained.

> **PRACTICE POINT** Effective leaders are able to change leadership styles as needed to lead different team members.

Leaders must possess several qualities to be successful. Self-confidence, sincerity, and enthusiasm for the job are essential. Leaders are effective listeners and accept diverse cultures. To have an effective team, a leader must be a team player and work to solve problems, innovate, and renovate existing policies, procedures, and environments. Leaders explain how to accomplish a task and give a challenge to the team. This allows the team members to think for themselves creatively, which can develop leaders for the future (Box 3-3).

Effective leaders possess **self-confidence.** They believe they have the ability to complete tasks efficiently and effectively. Leaders accentuate positive personal attributes and do not dwell on negative weaknesses. Self-confident leaders take risks and are able to make recommendations and changes without delay.

Genuineness and **sincerity** come from within and promote trust and communication. Team members know the suggestions and changes made by sincere leaders enhance the skills of all involved.

Enthusiasm shows that leaders are interested in their practices and the steps needed to make it successful. Enthusiasm is contagious to fellow team members and should be a part of practice culture. Enthusiastic team members are excited to come to work, enjoy sharing experiences with others, appreciate humor, and enjoy the team work environment.

Listening effectively has become a lost skill in today's world; talking has overtaken listening. Listening is the ability to receive, attend to, interpret, and respond to words and body language. Poor listening skills can result in misinterpretation of information, leading to malpractice in the medical field. Poor listening and interpretation can cause a communication breakdown when a leader is trying to manage a practice effectively and lead team members in a positive style.

One of the most important skills for effective leadership is to be an **effective communicator.** Communications must be done in a clear and pleasant manner. Effective communicators think clearly, talk sparingly, and listen intently. It is imperative to think topics through before jumping to a conclusion. All issues must be understood and interpreted before an action can be taken. Rash decisions should not be made, or devastating results may occur. Time should be taken to interpret the facts and prevent immediate judgments. Talking too much can be a problem itself and greatly inhibits listening. Tone is as important as talking; positive, enthusiastic tones are much more effective than negative, authoritarian tones.

Cultures have different means of communication, and an effective leader must be able to determine the best method of communication for each culture. Morals and ethics vary among cultures, ultimately affecting the learning and training abilities of different team members. Leaders must be **accepting of diverse cultures,** welcoming the different qualities each possesses, and work with them to provide the best leadership possible.

Veterinary practice is a team business. A team is a simple concept: a group of individuals with different skills and attributes. Effective leaders **build teams** that allow the business to succeed at all levels, including providing excellent patient and client care and maintaining a

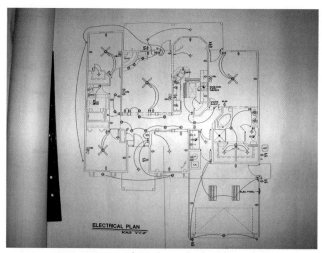

FIGURE 3-1 Blueprints of a building plan.

friendly and cohesive work environment while being able to create and maintain a profit for the practice.

Leaders must possess **skills to solve problems** before they arise—to be proactive instead of reactive. Leaders determine the problem; collect, listen, and interpret the facts; and present a variety of solutions to the team. Team members should be asked how they would resolve a situation; their point of view is also important in problem resolution.

> **PRACTICE POINT** An effective leader is a team player with excellent problem-solving skills.

Managing a practice requires attention to both internal and external forces (Figure 3-1). Change is required to keep up with modern technology and medicine. Leaders must be **aware of innovations** available and how they can improve the practice. Pharmacology, equipment, computer technology, and medicine reveal new science every year; flexibility is a must. If one innovation does not work within the practice, another should be tried. Trial and error produce the best results. Practice policies and procedures must undergo refinement on a yearly basis. Review policies that need updating, make a plan, set goals, and implement the change needed.

All people make mistakes. An effective manager must be able to **admit mistakes** that have been made and correct them. Team philosophy allows mistakes to be made while creating an environment for employees to learn from those mistakes. When environments are created in which team members are not afraid to take on new responsibilities and skills, mistakes are bound to be made. However, effective leaders can help all team members learn from those errors and prevent the mistake from occurring again (allowing mistakes does not allow the team member to complete tasks carelessly; mistakes should be accounted for and learned from).

Four Steps of Management

The four steps of management philosophy include *planning, organization, directing,* and *evaluating.* All four stages are of equal importance, and each is present in all applications of management. If one topic is ignored, the others will suffer. Many organizations fail to plan, thereby eliminating the need to evaluate because the goal is never achieved. It is imperative to master each step; this results in success in every aspect of management and leadership.

> **PRACTICE POINT** The four steps of management must be fully addressed to maintain a successful practice.

Sound **planning** before beginning a project or task may eliminate the need for crisis management, or the experience of handling one catastrophe after another. Planning identifies what needs to be accomplished in the future. Planning determines the goals of the practice and develops strategies to accomplish these goals. At times, planning is overlooked and managers try to implement a procedure without proper planning. This sets the stage for failure.

Planning can be divided into three categories: strategic planning, tactical planning, and operational planning. *Strategic planning* is long-range planning, approximately 5 to 10 years in the future. It can involve the practice's long-term goals, equipment purchases, and the type of medicine the practice wants to offer in the future.

Tactical planning evolves from strategic planning, beginning 1 to 3 years in advance of proposed changes, and includes the steps required to achieve the long-range goals (Box 3-4). Tactical goals might include a current equipment purchase along with continuing education for staff to become efficient with that particular piece of equipment. Ultrasound machines, for example, cost a significant amount of money and have a long learning curve. A practice must purchase the equipment and attend a significant amount of continuing education classes to become proficient at making a diagnosis with the machine. Dates should be set when developing a tactical plan; this helps facilitate and keep the strategic plan on schedule.

Third, *operational planning* evolves from tactical planning and is used for immediate planning. Operational planning sets the budget and develops the resources needed to achieve the tactical and strategic plans.

A strategic plan includes creating a budget to purchase the equipment and researching needed information to find the equipment that fits the needs of the practice. A date should be set to accomplish the strategic plan. A tactical plan includes the purchase of the ultrasound machine and attendance at multiple seminars to become

Box 3-4	Four Steps of Effective Management

- Planning
- Organizing
- Leading
- Evaluating

proficient in the use of it. A date should also be set at which time the machine will be of optimal use to the practice. Operational planning then comes into play by developing actions needed to make the ultrasound profitable to the practice. This may include marketing (both internal and external), staff continuing education, and the capacity to create a flexible appointment schedule to fit in emergency referrals from other local practices.

Organizing determines how the work will be divided and accomplished by the team. Organizing involves communication with the team to plan and develop the framework and resources required to implement the plan. A team may discuss the positive and negative aspects of purchasing an ultrasound machine and methods to accommodate the equipment. Teams may organize a special room or develop marketing themes to successfully implement the new procedures.

Leading is directing, guiding, and supervising the staff in performance of their duties and responsibilities while implementing the plan. Directing uses management skills to motivate team members to accomplish various steps of the plan through appropriate resources.

> **PRACTICE POINT**   Leading is not micromanaging; it is guiding team members to make correct decisions while they complete their responsibilities.

Management includes **evaluating** whether plans are being achieved and making decisions to modify them if needed. Every policy and procedure needs to be evaluated for effectiveness on a yearly basis. In the example above, once an ultrasound machine has been purchased, it must be used frequently to maintain the staff's efficiency and skills at using it. If the ultrasound machine is not being used, it is not paying for itself and the policies and procedures must be reevaluated. Questions should be asked to identify issues: Why is the machine not being used? Does the veterinarian feel inadequate at using the machine? Do clients decline the service because of cost? Is the procedure not being recommended by staff? Evaluation must occur, allowing a positive change to take place. A clear distinction cannot always be made among these four steps. At times they overlap each other, and they do not always occur in numeric order. Goals and activities can be modified on a daily basis depending on the success and achievement of goals.

Leadership Styles

Leadership and communication styles are essential in the management of people and business. Leadership depends on and results from the behavior of the manager; therefore the most effective form is to lead by example. A solid leader understands what motivates each individual and how he or she will respond, and can direct the employee's behavior to have a desired outcome. Ultimately, leaders must accept the task and responsibility of influencing the behavior of others.

Two theories of effective management are *directive* and *supportive*. Directive management is task oriented, whereas supportive behavior is people oriented. Some managers are task oriented and others are supportive; some leaders may use a combination of the two styles. Effective managers can determine which style will work best with each situation that rises. Directive managers are task oriented and are more interested in achieving results than in discussing how a task will be completed. Supportive managers listen to employees and encourage them to express their thoughts and opinions. Tasks may be discussed in detail to be completed.

Supportive managers provide feedback and recognition as well as an open level of communication. The best managers are flexible and adapt to the differing needs of different employees. Some employees may need a directive style of management; others may require a supportive environment. A combination may yield the best results. Assigning tasks in a directive fashion allows team members to complete them in their own fashion, developing self-confidence and leadership abilities that will benefit the practice in the future. By offering some supportive management, leaders can provide positive feedback on a project and invite the team members to discuss problems that may arise during the project.

> **PRACTICE POINT**   Team members respond to leadership styles differently; a leader must be able to adapt to the different techniques needed for each team member.

The style of leadership in a practice can make or break the practice by severely affecting team member performance. Five main leadership styles include the absolute dictator, the benevolent leader, the unpredictable leader, the responsibility avoider, and the democratic leader. Each of these styles is well described by its title.

The **absolute dictator** has strong opinions, makes all decisions, and rarely delegates. This leader criticizes in public, never offers positive reinforcement, and gives orders. Employees are simply that: employees. No team exists, and employees feel unworthy and, on occasion, stupid. Eventually employees burn out and leave the practice.

The **benevolent leader** is dominated by the need to be loved and labeled as the nice guy. This leader publicly recognizes work well done and caters to all the needs of the team. Benevolent leaders end up doing the work because they do not want to burden someone else with the responsibility. This nice guy attitude prevents the practice from taking the next step to success.

The **unpredictable leader** is moody and unstable and may be a dictator one day and a benevolent leader the next. Team members spend much of their time trying to figure out which leader they have for the day.

The **responsibility avoider** lacks self-confidence and/or ambition. The practice drifts without direction and is unable to take the next step to success.

The **democratic leader** listens to team members and involves them in decision making. Open-door communication is the key, and leaders welcome suggestions for improvement by staff members. Democratic leaders build a great team with members who are loyal to the practice and consistently perform their best while on the job.

Leadership Commitment

Effective leaders are committed to their jobs, their team members, and themselves. It is imperative that leaders keep commitments that they have made to their team; again, the best leadership style is to lead by example. Commitments are made to others, and others depend on that person to complete them. Leaders who do not uphold commitments cannot expect team members to follow through either. If commitments cannot be followed through, they should not be made in the first place.

> **PRACTICE POINT** Leaders should pledge themselves to a higher level of commitment, thereby creating an example that others want to follow.

Become an Effective Leader

The preceding suggestions will help every leader become more efficient at managing team members. Ideas listed below will help enhance the skills already developed.

- *Learn something new every day.* Often, managers feel they have mastered the skills to be effective leaders. This may be true, but something can be learned from every situation. Make it a point at the beginning of each day to look for at least one new thing that can enhance the team. Once the new idea or topic has been mastered, share it with the team.
- *Strive for excellence every day.* It is unrealistic to expect perfection on every task and skill, but all team members should perform their best at all times; this includes all leaders, managers, and owners.
- *Take charge of team morale.* Negative environments are difficult to work in, and clients pick up on negative interactions. Improving team morale improves employee performance, enhances client relationships, and creates a wonderful working environment.

- *Smile every day.* Smiling is contagious.
- *Inspire trust.* Keep commitments, tell the truth, and say, "I am sorry" when needed.
- *Accept and embrace suggestions.* Some ideas may not be the best, but do not reject ideas given by team workers. Embrace an idea and build on it.
- *Do not spread gossip or foster rumors.* Curtail gossip to improve the quality of the workplace environment. Effective teams are built on trust and respect. Determine the facts and kill the gossip.
- *Provide motivation.* Not all team members are motivated by the same technique. Learn what motivates each individual and foster an environment that will create and maintain motivation for everyone.
- *Remember that actions speak louder than words.* Lead by example and the team will follow (Boxes 3-5 and 3-6).

THE POSITIVE EFFECTS OF A TEAM

Realistic and achievable goals can be established by a team. Because each team member contributes to the establishment of goals, members will work hard to ensure they are achieved. This contributes to a sense of pride and ownership of the practice. Because of this pride, team members recognize the importance of disciplined work habits and ensure their behavior meets team standards. This prevents behaviors such as calling in and leaving the rest of the team short staffed. If team members need time off, they do everything in their power to have their shift covered or provide coverage for the team member who needs time off.

Box 3-5 Applying Leadership

- Define a mission in 50 words or less.
- Set goals for 1 year, 5 years, and 10 years.
- Facilitate open-door communication.
- Share information.
- Build trust.
- Delegate.
- Recognize the value of diversity.
- Develop a reward system.
- Generously praise; carefully criticize.

Box 3-6 Ideas to Improve Employee Morale

- Share cartoons.
- Hold team lunches, dinners, and outings.
- Celebrate every birthday.
- Congratulate team members on personal or professional achievements.
- Create a "star" chart. Each time team members do something that deserves recognition, award a star and share a summary of what the person accomplished.

> **PRACTICE POINT** Practices that use teams instead of individuals have higher employee retention rates, increased morale, and decreased stress among the staff.

Team members often understand one another's priorities and offer help or support when difficulties arise. This may occur in both the practice and in personal life. Offering a supportive work environment can ease the burden of personal issues; views and opinions from co-workers can help solve personal problems.

A leader of a team is one who guides the group. A leader does not run a group or dictate a group; a leader simply guides. Teams may discuss topics, problems, and solutions and develop and plan to implement a new policies or procedures. An effective leader will help guide the team through the appropriate steps to achieve the goal(s).

THE FOUR R'S OF TEAM MANAGEMENT

*R*esponsibility, *r*espect, *r*apport, and *r*ecognition contribute to managing a successful team. Responsibility denotes a duty or obligation that a team member is expected to uphold. Team members should be delegated responsibilities that they are expected to complete and follow through. Completion should be expected within a set time and may need some guidance; however, team members should be given space to complete the project and not be micromanaged. If a team member cannot be given responsibility, cannot complete a project, or must be micromanaged, it may be questioned why the team member is an employee. A successful manager establishes a team that can accept delegated tasks and complete those tasks responsibly without the need for micromanaging. Micromanaging decreases the leader's time and efficiency; a leader who chooses to micromanage should complete the project herself.

Respect is consideration or esteem given to another person. Each member of the team must respect other team members' education, skills, and values. Without respect for each other, team members' morale and self-esteem drop, producing a negative attitude for the entire team. Team members must learn that not all employees have the same thoughts and philosophies, and many people complete tasks differently based on education or previous skill sets. This can be accepted as long as the same ultimate goal is reached in a timely manner and all team members understand this accepted philosophy. Each member possesses expert skills and credentials that warrant respect.

> **PRACTICE POINT** Team members must respect one another to have a productive environment.

Rapport is a mutual trust or emotional relationship that exists among team members. Great rapport starts at the top with owners and managers. Magnificent rapport is effused to clients who recognize how well the team works together during busy and stressful times and how they enjoy each other's company. Team members with great rapport have respect for each other and are delegated responsibilities on a daily basis. They complete tasks as a team and seek others' opinions while completing those tasks.

Recognition is achievement. Team members should be recognized for a job well done as soon as it is warranted. Many team members only hear of mistakes they have made and the necessary corrections and never hear about the excellent quality of work they produce. Positive situations need to be recognized and brought to the attention of all team members so they can all benefit.

EMPOWERING EMPLOYEES

Employee empowerment is essential to the success of a veterinary practice. *Empower* means to give power or authority to; to authorize; to enable or permit. This entails giving team members the ability and permission to complete tasks and objectives. Empowering is the concept of encouraging and authorizing workers to take initiative to improve operations, reduce costs, and improve the quality and quantity of service. Client education is an essential task that all team members should be allowed to complete. By empowering team members to educate clients with the information the practice has implemented, the staff will work above and beyond its usual level. Team members should be allowed to complete laboratory analysis, answer client questions, and treat patients (as directed by the veterinarian). All tasks require extensive training, which should be provided to obtain the best team possible. Once team members have achieved these skills, they must be allowed to use them in the best way possible. Empowering team members to use their skills brings satisfaction to the employee, veterinarian, and client. The goal is to have team members who can manage themselves individually as well as their own projects. Teams that are engaged in daily operations are proactive and strive for the highest quality of care for patients and clients while striving to improve profits for the business.

> **PRACTICE POINT** Empowerment means to give [someone] the power or authority to do something.

Empowered employees are only as good as their expertise, and expertise comes from training. It is imperative to train team members on a continual basis. The strongest employees accept training as a way to improve themselves and the practice. When employees have pride for their workplace and are empowered to improve the daily operations, they will exceed expectations. Emotional ownership of a practice (vs. financial ownership) yields high returns. Team members can never receive enough training. Training motivates team members on a continual basis and also helps retain the strongest employees.

DELEGATION

Independent and strong-willed employees find it hard to delegate tasks to others, often feeling that other team members will not complete the tasks as well as they can. Delegation and empowerment are critical tasks that must be learned and used by all members of management (Figure 3-2). One person cannot possibly manage all

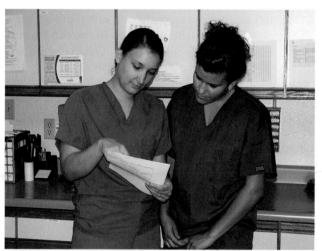

FIGURE 3-2 Delegating tasks appropriately is the key to an efficient veterinary practice.

aspects of a veterinary practice. A veterinarian or manager cannot see and discharge patients, receive payments, and manage accounts receivable, inventory, and accounts payable while continuing to provide the best treatment possible for hospitalized patients. Delegation and empowerment are the keys to a successful veterinary practice. Delegation frees time, reduces stress, and shows team members they are capable of completing their assigned tasks.

> **PRACTICE POINT** Delegation means to give an assignment or task to someone to complete.

Team members who are a "10" can be easily trained to manage tasks delegated by a manager. It takes more time to learn to delegate than it takes employees to complete the tasks delegated to them. Some managers fear that by delegating tasks, they are admitting failure and the inability to complete all tasks. This is not the case. Delegation increases the efficiency of a manager.

It is important to take small steps when learning to delegate. One task should be delegated and completed, then the next. Often leaders delegate many projects and then receive negative results from a portion of them. The leader then feels that he or she cannot delegate successfully and stops the delegation process. It is also essential, when delegating large tasks, that the team member is involved in the developing of an action plan. This will help motivate the delegating team member and ensure success of the project.

When choosing to delegate duties, choose an employee who has interest in the task, and the ability to accomplish

---

What Would You Do/Not Do?

Frances, the practice manager of ABC Veterinary Clinic, has been asked to oversee the construction of the new boarding facilities. On top of the new duty, she is also responsible for the account receivables, reminders, and recall systems. She also must place orders for products and supplies and monitor and improve sales during a specified period. Frances becomes overwhelmed trying to complete all her assigned tasks; she therefore sends out reminders late and does not complete recalls or callbacks. Also, statements were completed incorrectly and did not get recorded in the client accounts. When Frances was confronted by the owner of the practice about the ineffective management strategies, Frances became extremely defensive and stated it was the owner's fault for expecting too much of her.

What Should Frances Have Done?

Frances should have delegated tasks to other employees. An office manager can be trained to maintain the account receivables, and a receptionist can be taught to print reminders on a regular basis. A head veterinary technician who works on the floor can oversee inventory and inventory management, potentially improving the management of the products. Inventory can be scrutinized more easily by someone who uses the supplies and dispenses products on a daily basis.

By delegating, Frances would still be able to oversee all the tasks; the person that the tasks were assigned to could provide feedback and ask any questions that may arise. Changes could be made with the involvement of both Frances and the other team member, ensuring maximum efficiency and task completion. By delegating, Frances could have provided maximum attention to the new project and used the team to improve the client services.

When Frances was confronted by the owner, instead of becoming defensive she should have admitted that she had become overwhelmed and was sorry that she did not admit her mistake earlier. The qualities of a great leader are to admit mistakes, delegate effectively, and train others to follow in a leadership position. A great team aids in making delegation easier and more efficient.

it. Explain the details of the task and how it should be completed, then turn the task over to the team member. Set a date for completion and check in frequently, making sure the team member has no problems or questions. Positive reinforcement should be provided during the project while avoiding micromanaging. Rewarding team members at the end encourages pride and innovation.

> **PRACTICE POINT** Delegation increases the efficiency of a leader.

To become efficient and understand delegation and empowerment, one must accept error. When empowering and delegating tasks to team members, they will make mistakes. Team members will learn will learn from their mistakes through trial and error. Mistakes offer a learning opportunity for all when they are shared with the entire team. Effective leadership, delegation, and empowerment help create and motivate other team members to become individual team leaders through personal development, improved self-confidence, and lessons on how to solve problems.

Along with delegation skills, it is imperative that leaders learn to accept help graciously. Again, many leaders will not accept help from others because they believe it makes them appear ineffective or weak. In reality, accepting help when needed is a part of teamwork culture. Not accepting help and having to make excuses for not finishing tasks or completing them in an unsatisfactory manner carries a greater stigma than accepting help. Asking for help or delegating work to team members shows commitment to the team and leads members to ask for help when needed.

METHODS OF COMMUNICATION

Communication between and among team members is just as critical as communication with clients. Team members should fully understand policies and procedures as well as any changes that may occur. Communication is the key to the success of any change. Many times changes in policies and procedures fail because of a lack of communication among team members. Team members may not understand the change, the reason for the change, and what benefit is likely to result. The manager should hold staff meetings when wishing to implement changes. When team members discuss a change and give their opinions on how a policy or procedure ought to be changed, they are more likely to accept and implement the change. Team members may have ideas or methods to better implement the change and may have positive or negative thoughts on the process that management had not considered. Employee concerns must be addressed when making changes or the transition will not occur. If it does, it may not occur smoothly.

Box 3-7	Ideas to Increase Communication in a Practice

- Meetings
- Newsletters
- Team member evaluations

Poor communication can be caused by several barriers, including poor listening, preoccupation, impatience, and/or resistance to change or new ideas. Poor listening, preoccupation, and impatience can be on the part of either the leader or team member. It is imperative that a manager not show these qualities and that he or she is always mindful of them to prevent them from occurring. Office and practice managers have many duties, tasks, and responsibilities to complete, but employee communication should be the top priority. If team members feel they have not been heard or that the manager was preoccupied, they will follow the example that was set for them. Good listeners are good problem solvers. It should be a priority for everyone on the team to be a good listener. Listening to clients and team members improves the level of communication at all stages (Box 3-7).

> **PRACTICE POINT** Listening to clients and team members is a task at which every manager must become proficient.

Because of the aforementioned barriers, the information being communicated may not be received the way it was intended. Practice managers should be aware of misinterpretations, work to overcome barriers, and improve channels of communication with team members. Additional channels may be used to ensure complete understanding. Changes to policies and procedures may be announced at a meeting (channel 1); a summary of the notes should then be given to all team members (channel 2); a discussion regarding the success of the change should be on the agenda for the following meeting (channel 3); and a newsletter addressing the new change may be circulated 1 month after the change (channel 4). Other channels may be developed by practices to make sure all team members are on board. Managers should periodically evaluate channels and make sure they are understood by all team members.

Teams that practice open and honest communication encourage ideas and opinions and are open to disagreements and discussions. Each team member is more likely to accept and understand others thoughts and opinions, and accept them with an open mind. With open communication, members are more likely to resolve conflicts quickly and constructively and will not need the help of management. Open communication is a major component of a successful practice.

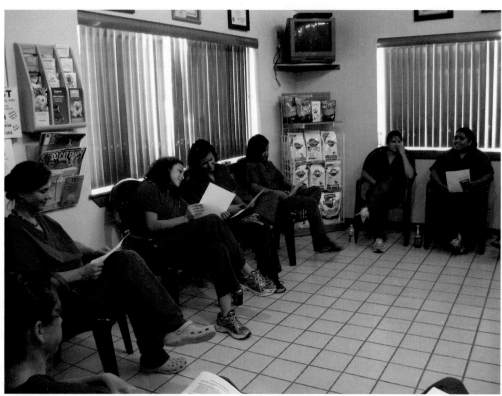

FIGURE 3-3 Team meetings are critical to clear and open communication among all employees.

Box 3-8	Meeting Rules

- Start and end on time.
- Set a maximum length of 1.5 hours.
- Create an agenda.
- Facilitate topic movement.

Meetings

Regular team meetings should become routine in the veterinary practice. Meetings allow the communication channels to remain open and persuade team members to discuss problems and create solutions as a team (Figure 3-3). They allow goals for the practice to be developed and reviewed on a regular basis. They can also raise practice benchmarks, thereby providing for total quality management, increased profits, and improved compliance with staff recommendations and client acceptance (Box 3-8).

Meetings cost money and therefore must be useful and beneficial to the practice. Employees must be paid for their time, and food may be provided. An hour-long meeting with 13 staff members and two veterinarians costs an average of $462 in wages; this does not account for the cost of food or lost profits from closed doors.

A meeting facilitator has a difficult but important job. The facilitator is responsible for starting and ending the meetings on time, controlling the topics, and preventing negativity from overcoming the team. Facilitating meetings does not come naturally; acquired skills may be needed to run meetings efficiently and with a minimum of stress. Community colleges offer facilitator classes that may benefit those leading meetings, making the job easier and more pleasant.

Some practices allow a lunch meeting one day per week; others close for half a day and incorporate training sessions into the meeting. Others may have short daily breakfast meetings at which they discuss the plan for the day and the clients and/or cases that are expected. If meetings are held at lunchtime, team members should be allowed to eat first and decompress from the morning activities. Once a majority of the team has finished eating, the meeting can begin.

> **PRACTICE POINT**   To be most effective, meetings should contain both educational material and policy or safety review.

Whatever method works best for a given hospital, it is very important to begin and end meetings on time. Employees resent attending meetings that start late and run late. Meetings should begin when they are scheduled, regardless of who is present. Team members who arrive late must take responsibility to find out at a later time what they missed. The meeting should not be stopped and repeated for latecomers; this devalues the meeting for those who were on time. Meetings should

| Box 3-9 | Sample Meeting Agenda |

1. Task list
2. Doctors' schedules for the holidays
3. Dry food for Petunia and Jesse at all times
4. Dispensing Buprinorphine
5. Christmas party...*after Christmas!*
6. No meeting December 24
7. Happy holidays!

also end on time. Reviews of topics should be avoided at the end of the meeting; these can be typed into a summary and given to team members after the meeting. If tasks were assigned to fellow team members, those assignments should be quickly reviewed before the meeting breaks up.

The value of the meeting is lost when team members lose interest and watch the clock instead of the speaker. Meetings should not last for more than 1 to 1½ hours. Those that last longer are less productive because of lost interest, and active participation in the meeting begins to drop. Larger groups may require longer meeting times so that each member can participate. If longer meetings are needed, breaks should be factored in to allow the team to reenergize so they can fully focus and participate in the discussions.

Agendas may be created for meetings, which can expedite the meeting process (Box 3-9). Team members know what topics are on the list and when to address concerns they have. This helps keep the meeting running on time and prevents getting off topic and further delaying the meeting. Suggestions for meeting topics can be asked of team members. A note board can be placed in a central location of the practice, and team members can add topics that they want to discussed. Topics may include further education on a specific procedure, policy clarification, or education regarding a disease. The meeting facilitator can take the topics and prioritize them. This ensures that the most important topics are addressed first, allowing ample time for discussion. Other topics must also be addressed, if only briefly. If a topic is left off the agenda, team members may feel that their input was not important, and they may be reluctant to volunteer topics in the future.

> **PRACTICE POINT** Meeting facilitators must run meetings in a positive manner.

Once the agenda has been created, the meeting should adhere to those items. It is vital that the meeting stay on track and on time. If one person dominates the discussions and rambles, employees will soon lose interest in the meeting and it will be a waste of everyone's time. The meeting leader is responsible for not letting this happen and must use tact when guiding the discussion

back to the agenda. If a heated discussion begins and emotions run high, it may be suggested that the topic be researched and readdressed at the next meeting. This allows emotions to settle before the next meeting and gives time to find resolution to the problem. The next topic can then be addressed. The same applies to topics that are taking an extensive amount of time to decide or solve. The team members can then be assigned homework; their job would be to provide a solution at the next meeting as well as develop a list of pros and cons regarding the subject. The topic can then be at added to the top of the agenda for the next meeting and the remainder of the current agenda can be addressed.

Meetings should not be allowed to become a gripe session, and it is important that the meeting facilitator prevent this from happening. If team members begin to gripe, the leader can ask how that team member would recommend fixing the problem. The problem can then be opened for discussion to all team members so that a solution can be found as a team. The leader can guide the discussion into a positive frame by using encouraging and exciting words. Positive energy trickles from the top down, with the remaining team members taking nonverbal cues from the management team. This can turn a gripe session into a positive problem-solving meeting. The end result is a team that works better together in a happy and friendly environment.

> **PRACTICE POINT** Any accomplishment a team member has made, either professional or personal, should be celebrated at a weekly meeting.

Always review accomplishments and successes before ending a meeting. Client compliments, employees' personal accomplishments, and successful changes should all be addressed. Meetings ending on a positive note leave team members feeling important, empowered, and willing to continue to work above and beyond the call of duty to make the practice a success.

A summary of the meeting should be provided to team members after the meeting. Many topics are often forgotten about because many ideas and/or changes may be discussed in meetings. Other team members may have been absent or were tardy for the meeting. Notes should be detailed and summarized in a positive fashion (Box 3-10). They should not incorporate an authoritarian tone; absent team members may unconsciously reject the information. The notes should be a friendly reminder for those who were in attendance. Meeting notes also serve as a proof of discussion for all team members when they forget a topic has been addressed. Notes from previous meetings can be pulled from the file and handed to employees who need a friendly reminder.

Successful teams discuss problems and use a method of decision making called *consensus*. This means that all team members discuss possible solutions, all voices and

Box 3-10	Sample Summary of Notes

- Afternoon and evening duties must be completed **before anyone leaves at night.** This includes Friday afternoons. Tasks that are being left incomplete:
  - Putting the clinic cats away
  - Taking the trash outside (Fridays)
  - Washing the tub table
  - Breaking down boxes
- The tech responsible for treatments is now responsible for **all** cleaning and duties that must be completed. This does not mean that only that person is to complete those duties; they are simply making sure everything is complete before **anyone** leaves. **Sabrina, Alex, Reese,** and **Sarah** are responsible for treatments and duties until the schedule changes. If you work with one of these techs, **do not get offended** if they delegate duties to you; everything must be done before you leave!
- Please check the doctors' schedules before making appointments for the holidays. Schedules have changed.
- Please make sure Jesse and Petunia have dry food at all times now. They are fed canned food in the morning and evening; they like both forms of food. They are thin, old, and want more choices! ☺
- Buprinorphine will always be dispensed in red top tubes and pill vials from now on. Please show the owners how much they will need to administer when discharging patients. This allows the medication to be in a child-proof container and the client does not have the perception that they are giving an injection (many think they are giving injections when it is drawn up in syringes).
- CHRISTMAS PARTY: Saturday, January 3, 2010, 6 PM (Remember: Bring a White Elephant gift!)
- No meeting next week on Wednesday, December 24. We close at 12 PM and reopen Monday, December 29!

HAPPY HOLIDAYS!

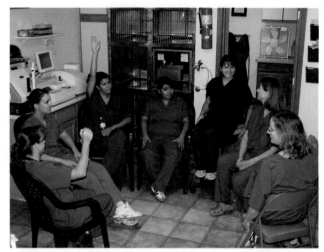

FIGURE 3-4 Allowing team members to participate in decision making improves their acceptance of changes in the practice.

opinions are heard, and the entire team works toward a group decision (Figure 3-4). This does not mean that every decision is going to satisfy each team member; however, employees will realize that compromises are necessary. Consensus ensures that every member of the team has agreed to support the decision, and no resentment should be left on the table. Each team member understands that the best decision was made based on the presenting circumstances. If everyone takes responsibility for reaching a consensus, the problem will be solved, the task will be completed, and the team will have a much higher chance of avoiding each individual's need to be right.

PRACTICE POINT Consensus means an opinion or position reached by a group as a whole.

Team members should be asked to participate in meetings and should be held responsible for paying attention and actively listening. To help engage participation, team members can be asked to present topics. This will help create accountability and develop a sense of pride among the staff, along with developing self-confidence and independence. Learning games, videos, brochures, and team handouts can all be used by staff to enhance the education they provide.

Team Newsletter

Team newsletters are an effective form of communication for large veterinary hospitals. Monthly newsletters can inform the teams of birthdays, special anniversaries (employment anniversaries, marriage, stop-smoking, etc.), and special events that will occur in the coming months. Changes to procedures and policies can be discussed, as well in-house continuing education topics. Smaller hospitals can use the same newsletter format; it may only be a two-page newsletter, but it opens the communication channels with employees. It shows respect for one another, adds rapport, and highlights the accomplishments of the team. Fun photos can be included, as well as fun facts and catchy phrases. The goal is team member communication; making it fun for employees adds to the success of the project (Figure 3-5).

Evaluations

Employee evaluations are an excellent time to address concerns and issues and to open the door for communication between team members and management. Concerns can be addressed and documented. Managers can be of assistance to help solve personal issues and personnel issues and/or address concerns regarding policies or procedures. Some team members may not feel comfortable addressing their concerns in front of other team members and may use evaluation time to do so. Managers should readdress and follow up with concerns throughout the year to ensure problems have been resolved. This time can also be used to encourage team members to discuss issues year-round because the practice should have an open-door communications policy. Team members will feel comfort in knowing that their concerns are not going to be publicly addressed and that they will not receive harassment for doing so.

> **◎ PRACTICE POINT**   Team member evaluations should be completed on a yearly basis to address competencies of that team member as well as address future goals and methods to accomplish those goals.

Team member accomplishments should also be addressed during evaluations. Many team members complete projects, receive certifications, and obtain licensure and must be commended for their achievements.

Team members may be encouraged to fill out an employee survey (Box 3-11). This can help management address issues or topics that may not have surfaced. Management can then be proactive at preventing and solving problems before they arise. Practices can develop their own employee surveys, highlighting policies and procedures within the hospital. Receptionists may answer different questions than technicians because their goals may be slightly different (Figure 3-6).

Employee evaluations should be task specific and listed in detail. Restraint, client education, and work ethic are a few examples that can be used in a veterinary technician's evaluation. Customer service, phone skills, and client-oriented personality may be examples for a receptionist's evaluation.

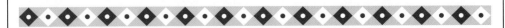

Inside the Paw Print - A Newsletter for the Team!

ABC Veterinary Clinic

Rabies Awareness Month

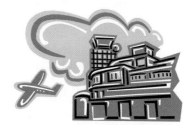

January is Rabies Awareness Month for Anytown, USA! For the month of January, rabies vaccines will be discounted to our clients for $10.00. According to Dr. Dreamer, the purpose of this deeply discounted vaccine is for the promotion of rabies awareness, and to protect the community from this potentially fatal virus.

Rabies awareness draws clients that would not normally come into the practice for yearly exams and vaccines. Clients must be advised that rabies can be fatal to both them and their pets should either of them be exposed. "The more animals that we can vaccinate, the safer our community is," stated Dr. Love, a longtime veterinarian.

Along with discounted rabies vaccines, clients can also receive a discounted DHPP for their dogs or an RCP for their cats. Clients must have their pets vaccinated by January 31 to receive the discount.

Volume 3, Issue 2
January 15, 2009

Special points of interest:

- *Rabies Awareness month*
- *Birthdays*
- *HG Promo*
- *We will be closed Monday January 19th in observation of Martin Luther King Day*
- *Parvo*

Inside this issue:

Inside Story	2
Inside Story	2
Inside Story	2
Inside Story	3
Inside Story	4
Inside Story	5
Inside Story	6

Parvo Virus is Among us Again

Springtime is arriving, along with our beautiful temperatures! With these beautiful temperatures comes the potentially fatal Parvo virus.

If any clients call with a puppy with symptoms that include vomiting or diarrhea, we must advise them to leave the puppy in the vehicle (with them) until we have an available room. We must try and prevent

the transmission of the disease as much as possible. When puppies arrive for vaccinations, we must advise owners not to take their puppy for walks in

continued page 2

FIGURE 3-5 A team newsletter is an effective form of communication for the veterinary hospital.

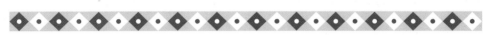

Parvo... continued from Page 1

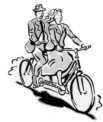

in public places until the vaccination series is complete. Pets that are fully vaccinated at 12 weeks of age are guaranteed to be protected from the virus by the vaccination manufacturer. Should a puppy contract the virus after we have fully vaccinated them, then the manufacturer will pay for the treatment itself.

We give one of the finest vaccines available that utilizes one of the best technologies available to produce vaccinations. Vaccine reactions are rare with this vaccine; however, all owners must be warned that any pet may have a vaccine reaction at any time. If a pet has immediate vomiting or diarrhea or within 45 minutes of vaccine administration, then we should recheck the pet.

Vaccinate all puppies and kittens!

Puppies should be vaccinated for DHPP every 3 weeks until they are 12 weeks of age; they must receive at least 2 vaccines, the second vaccine being after 12 weeks to be considered fully vaccinated.

Dr. Larsen Heads to Western Veterinary Conference

Dr. Larsen and Brooke held down the fort while many team members and Dr. Jay were able to attend the Southwest Veterinary Conference in September. "The staff had such a great time and learned so much information," stated Dr. Jay. "Many team members picked up information that they have been able to pass onto the clients. The clients love the information they have received!"

In order to continue providing continuing education, Dr. Larsen and Brooke will be attending the Western Veterinary Conference in February. According to Dr. Larsen, "WVC offers a wide variety of topics to choose from, ranging from small to large animal medicine. It should be a great conference!" The two will leave on Sunday February 15th, returning the evening of Thursday February 19th.

"Continuing Education is an excellent opportunity for the entire staff."

Heartgard Promotion through February 13!

Thanks to our wonderful Merial Representative, we will be giving away a Valentines Day gift certificate on February 13th! Any client that purchases a one-year supply of Heartgard will be entered into a drawing to receive a $50.00 gift certificate to Roadhouse for dinner on the big V-Day!

In addition to being entered into the drawing, clients will receive $5.00 cash back on their purchase, ALONG WITH one month free of HEARTGARD!

SAVE THE DATE!

Merial will sponsor lunch for the entire staff on Wednesday February 18th! Heartworm and Heartworm Prevention will be discussed. Bring your questions and your appetite!

FIGURE 3-5, cont'd

Performance feedback is more meaningful with teams because they understand what is expected of them and can monitor their performance against expectations. Many times, team members will judge their own actions harder than management and critique themselves severely. Any correction needed is merely a suggestion that the employee takes to the next level. When a team environment such as this has been created and is successful, managing employees becomes a rewarding opportunity.

CONFLICT MANAGEMENT

Conflicts are normal between team members and occur whenever two or more people work together. Some team members can manage the conflict by themselves, but others need a leader to intervene and confront the conflict. Conflict should be viewed as an opportunity to solve problems. Confidential, open discussions can resolve issues before they become destructive. When conflict is properly handled, it can stimulate new thinking, progress, and growth. Unmanaged conflicts divide team members and should be dealt with as soon as possible.

PRACTICE POINT Conflicts must be dealt with as soon as they arise.

Practices without conflict can be just as harmful as those with conflict. Employees may be afraid to speak their opinions, or they have learned to work in a culture

Box 3-11	Guidelines for Creating Employee Surveys

- Make them task oriented.
- Make them position oriented.
- Ask specific questions that relate to the practice's visions and goals.
- Provide an area for questions, comments, and suggestions.
- Ask team members to state goals for the following 12 months.

where they survive best by simply completing orders given to them. A culture of this sort can be detrimental; it prevents creative thinking, innovation, and change. It can also encourage passive resistance because opinions are not permitted. Employees are simply employees in environments such as this, not team members. They may become disgruntled and leave the practice for a more positive, creative environment.

The top three reasons that cause conflict in the workplace environment are gossip, lack of training, and lack of communication. Conflicts should be identified and confirmed with all parties involved. A leader does not need to stir the nest when there is no conflict or spread gossip about a possible conflict. Once the problem has been confirmed, leaders should ensure they fully understand the problem. Leaders may repeat the problem to the presenting team member(s) and express empathy on both parts. Understanding and explaining the other team member's opinion and view of the problem may solve the problem immediately if a simple misunderstanding has occurred. Both team members should be aware that the problem is understood and that their concerns are valid. Once problems and opinions have been stated and are open for discussion, the emotions are released from the problem and the tension decreases. Team members should not be told how to act or what to think, which does not solve the problem. A caring and empathetic environment makes it easier for honesty and open communication to be a normal part of practice culture, allowing conflicts to be resolved relatively easily.

When determining the extent of conflict, questions such as those listed in Box 3-12 can be asked. Open-ended questions stimulate discussion. Who, what, when, where, why, and how introduce open-ended questions. To help correct conflict, specific examples can be used when discussing the problem (see Box 3-12). As an example, "Patients did not receive 12 PM treatments today because of a personality conflict between two technicians." In this example patient care has been compromised; this must not occur because of a simple personality issue! Team members may be encouraged to discuss the personality conflict together. Clear expectations can be set regarding how a problem can be solved and a solution created based on the compromises.

PRACTICE POINT   Conflicts may be the result of more than one topic; all issues must be explored and handled in a professional manner.

Occasionally, team members may need to be addressed regarding poor work ethic and performance. Leaders may first ask why the poor performance has begun. Perhaps the employee is having medical issues that had not been revealed, or resentment of "lazy" team members may be to blame. The source of the problem should be identified. Once the problem is identified, the employee should be shown what impact his or her poor performance has on other team members, clients, and patients. When poor performers see the impact they have on others, they may make suggestions for change and be willing to implement their own changes. If suggested changes do not occur, a written warning may be needed (Box 3-13).

Some conflicts may involve managers, who can become defensive when confronted with a complaint. Just as with other team members, some will take complaints personally. Opinions need to be listened to, internalized, and thought through. Some points may be valid; team members often try to help the leader just as the leader has helped team members in the past. If numerous complaints arise against one team member, a serious problem may exist. Regardless of the nature of the complaint, the details should be reviewed and a resolution should be developed. Unmanaged conflicts can lead to unprofessional behavior.

INCREASING STAFF EFFICIENCY

Productivity is not enhanced by overbooking appointments and surgeries. It is about increasing client compliance and education and following up with clients. Increasing staff efficiency can increase the doctor's productivity and satisfy clients; satisfied clients increase client compliance and the average client transaction.

A fine balance often exists between increasing efficiency and not compromising quality of care. Quality of patient and client care can actually improve with increased team efficiency. Veterinarians only have so many hours in a day; by delegating tasks, veterinarians can see more patients. However, team members must be fully trained to accept the delegated tasks and accomplish them in an efficient manner while maintaining a high quality of care. Therefore protocols and standards of care should be written out and easily accessible to all team members. New team members may need a reminder of the correct procedure to follow; older team members may need a reminder if they have not performed a procedure in several months. See Chapter 5 for more information on employee procedural manuals.

Leveraging teams increases the profitability and productivity of all team members. Once team members have been trained, they should be used appropriately.

Employee Survey

Please give your honest, most objective assessment of your performance over the past 12 months of your employment. Please return survey no later than _____ .

Please rate the following from 1 (poor) to 5 (outstanding). Assign NA if not applicable.

1. Accomplishes tasks _____

2. Enthusiastic and positive attitude _____

3. Leadership abilities _____

4. Honest and trustworthy _____

5. Team player _____

6. Work ethic _____

7. Client education and communication skills _____

8. Provides timely service to clients _____

9. Attentiveness and response to client needs _____

10. Observance of practice policies _____

11. Participation in staff meetings _____

12. On time for shift _____

13. Provides innovative ideas for practice improvement _____

What are your goals for the next 12 months? _____
_____
_____

What can you do to help increase client satisfaction and compliance? _____
_____
_____
_____

What can you do to help your team members improve themselves over the next 12 months?
_____
_____
_____

List any suggestions, comments, or improvements that you feel would help benefit the practice.
_____
_____
_____

FIGURE 3-6 Employee surveys alert management to possible problems in the practice.

PRACTICE POINT To help increase team efficiency, task lists may be created; team members must complete tasks by the end of each shift.

Underused team members often leave a practice in search of one that will use their skills.

To help improve team efficiency and decrease client wait time, several recommendations can be made. The veterinarian is responsible for providing care, diagnostics, prescriptions, and surgery to patients. The receptionist and office manager are responsible for entering charges and collecting money for services rendered. The veterinarian should not have any part of collecting funds or enforcing no-charge policies. This decreases the efficiency of the team and affects clients waiting to be seen. Second, travel sheets can eliminate any discrepancy in charge amounts and decrease lost charges. The team schedule

---

Box 3-12   Determining the Extent of Conflicts

- Is this an individual problem?
- Who is involved?
- Does this problem relate to job satisfaction? Why?
- Is patient or client care compromised? How?
- Is poor service the issue? How?
- Does the team need more training? What kind of additional training is needed?
- Is the practice short staffed? Why?

Box 3-13   Guidelines for Conflict Resolution

- Discuss the problem as soon as possible. A delay in discussion may result in additional conflict or may be interpreted to mean that management is not interested in the problem.
- Listen to all the issues and keep an open mind. Encourage team members to talk.
- Determine the real issue. Frequently, a complaint is made about a superficial problem when, in reality, a deeper problem exists. For example, a team member may have a workload complaint when a personality conflict is the real problem.
- Exercise control and avoid arguments. Everyone has opinions; let them be stated. Emotional outbursts lead nowhere.
- Avoid a delay in decision making. Unresolved problems spread like wildfire and can add undue stress to the entire team.
- Maintain records of the problem. Document the conflict in case the same problem arises in the future. Recalling details at a later date usually is impossible.

---

should be evaluated next, eliminating any overstaffing or understaffing with the client schedule. Additional team members may be needed during a busy time of the day. For example, at 5 PM, when clients arrive to pick up animals that were dropped off earlier in the day, pick up medications, or arrive for appointments, extra team members may be added to assist in these areas. Fewer team members may be needed when surgery is the only activity occurring in the practice. The team member schedule should be analyzed to match the client schedule.

Common areas of waste include time, money, energy, products, and supplies. Team members must use time efficiently to continue to provide excellent customer service and prevent clients from having to wait. Laboratory analysis should be performed efficiently and without mistakes. Team members may need to learn to multitask and perform several analyses at the same time to increase efficiency. By multitasking, team members can save energy as well. Products and supplies used to provide services to clients are often overlooked. Waste in these areas is generally high in most practices; teams should brainstorm ways to become more efficient, with an ultimate goal of decreasing waste.

PRACTICE POINT   Multitasking saves time and energy and increases the pace at which tasks or treatments are completed.

Task lists can also be developed for each area of the practice to ensure that all tasks are completed before the end of the shift. Many times, team members are excellent at taking care of clients and patients but forget the "small stuff" that must be completed to keep the practice running smoothly. For example, microscopes should be cleaned on a daily basis at the end of each shift. Ear cones must be cleaned and disinfected, and paper towel dispensers must be refilled. These tasks are essential for the efficiency of the team for the following day and must be completed before leaving the practice. Task lists can help ensure these and other tasks are completed.

Teams should try to maximize team members, schedules, and equipment. Maximizing the client schedule can help increase the profits of the practice (see Chapter 13). Nail trims and suture removal appointments can be made for technicians, and yearly exams or ear infection

appointments can be made for a veterinarian. An example of maximizing equipment comes in the form of dental machines. Routine dental prophylaxis can be scheduled for veterinary technicians throughout the day, allowing the veterinarian to see more patients. If a technician needs the assistance of a veterinarian, one can help as needed. The dental machine will not produce profits sitting alone and should be used to its maximum potential.

TIME MANAGEMENT OF LEADERS

It is essential to work efficiently, especially in a veterinary practice. There is never enough time in the day or week to complete all tasks needed. Leaders need to know how to perform a task, how to prioritize tasks, and how long each task will take. Understanding the relation of time to production is essential. Planning and scheduling of work decrease wasted time.

The behaviors that result in wasted time include failure to plan and budget time, interruptions, failure to follow through and complete tasks, slowness in making decisions, unnecessary work, and failure to delegate. Other time wasters include lack of privacy and desk clutter. When items are needed and cannot be found, time is wasted looking for them. Efficient time management requires that staff organize tasks, maintain a daily schedule, establish deadlines, and organize work flow.

PRACTICE POINT   Efficient time management requires organizing tasks, maintaining a daily schedule, establishing deadlines, and organizing work flow.

To help maintain a daily work flow, a manager may create a to-do list and determine priorities that need to be accomplished. Many people make a list when tasks become overwhelming but do not create a list for everyday tasks. A to-do list helps prioritize tasks and can ensure they are completed on a daily basis. If a task does not get completed on the day stated, it can roll over to the following day, especially if the priorities of the listed tasks change. Long-term lists can also be developed to keep long-range goals in mind. Often, managers become overwhelmed with short-term goals and lose sight of long-term tasks. Leaders must set standards high and set an example for other team members. If a manager cannot complete tasks early or on time, the rest of the team cannot be expected to complete their tasks on time either. A calendar or planner can also help keep personal and work appointments organized. Each person responds to organization differently, and different methods should be tried as long as the ultimate goal is reached: completion of all tasks created and assigned.

> **PRACTICE POINT** To help implement time management, create daily to-do lists.

DECREASING LOSS

An essential task of a manager is to develop practices and policies to increase profits and decrease loss. Loss can come in a variety of avenues. Employee theft tops the list, followed by missed charges, excess use of products and supplies in the hospital, and undercharging for services provided. It is unfortunate to think that the great team that has been developed is at risk for employee theft. However, employee theft can account for a high percentage of loss each year. Internal controls must be implemented to prevent the temptation. The cost adds up if each employee takes one box of heartworm preventive home (Box 3-14).

Missed charges account for a majority of lost money. Fecal smears, heartworm tests, and nail trims are often forgotten. Practices should review 10 records per day and look for lost charges. Almost every record will have at least one item that was not charged. It is imperative to implement procedures to help control loss through missed charges.

Travel Sheet

Many practices have found that travel sheets are an excellent way to decrease lost charges (Figure 3-7). A travel sheet lists the most common procedures provided

and products carried in the practice. The travel sheet is attached to the medical record and travels with it throughout the day. When a service is performed, the procedure is then circled or highlighted on the sheet. In multiple-doctor practices, it is advised to use a specific colored highlighter for each veterinarian. The receptionist can then be sure to add charges under that specific doctor (this is imperative when veterinarians are paid on production). When the medical record is complete, the receptionist can enter the charges and double check the record against the travel sheet, looking for any missed charges (Figure 3-8).

For those who wish to save paper, travel sheets can be laminated and reused. Simply place them in a pile and clean them at the end of the day.

Inpatient charges are missed more often than outpatient charges. Team members may only miss one charge for an outpatient; that number is at least doubled, if not tripled, for hospitalized patients. Outpatients are considered those that did not stay in the hospital. Exams, vaccines, fecal checks, and so forth are all outpatient services. Inpatient services include IV catheters, injections, bloodwork, and radiographs. Medications are often forgotten, as are individual lab tests that may have been added after the initial diagnosis. It may be useful for practices to develop a travel sheet for hospitalized patients. Each time a test or treatment is completed, it should be circled on the sheet with the specific colored highlighter of the veterinarian who ordered the treatment or test.

Each hospital may create individualized hospital travel sheets that can include the most common hospitalized procedures performed in that particular practice. Each patient will have one hospital travel sheet per day, allowing charges to be entered at the end of each day. Team members are less likely to forget charges for patients when the case is fresh in their mind versus entering charges before patient discharge (Figure 3-9).

Box 3-14	Ways to Decrease Loss

- Implement internal controls to prevent employee theft.
- Use travel sheets to decrease missed charges.
- Have team members be accountable for all supplies used.
- Set appropriate fees.

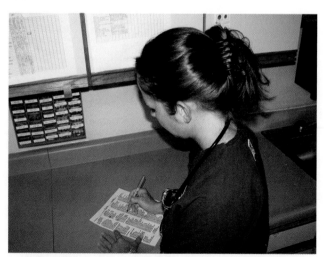

FIGURE 3-7 Travel sheets can decrease lost charges.

Accountability

Team members should be held accountable for the amount of materials used in clinic to provide services for clients. For example, a sloppy surgeon who drops suture material on a daily basis can cost the practice a significant amount. Technicians who must retake radiographs because of positioning errors cost the practice money. Not every employee contributes to loss, but if each is held accountable the lost dollars will decrease. Meetings are a great place to discuss loss and brainstorm ideas to reduce it as well as bring awareness to product loss.

Inventory Management

Inventory management is discussed in detail in Chapter 15. It is important to realize that inventory control is a large factor in controlling loss within the practice. A good

> **PRACTICE POINT** Accountability means a form of trustworthiness—the trait of being answerable to someone for something or being responsible for one's conduct.

inventory system ensures that product will be available for use while maintaining inventory at a cost-effective level. Reorder points and reorder quantities are vital to a successful inventory system. Inventory levels should be decreased so that excess levels do not tempt employee theft. Excess products can be kept in a central supply location, allowing the inventory manager to monitor supply use closely. See Chapter 15 for other ideas of effective inventory management.

Client Number _____ Client Name _____ Pet _____ Doctor _____

DISCOUNTS
0107 Monthly Special
0108 Senior Wellness
Senior Citizen

OFFICE CALL
0214 Brief Office Call
0216 Regular Office Call
0219 Well K-9/Fe Exam
0222 Exotics Exam-Reg
0220 Exotics Exam-Brief
226 Exam w/ vaccines
0228 Pre-Op Exam
0232 Recheck N/C
0234 Recheck
0109 Health Certificate
0106 Int'l Health Certificate
0104 Duplicate Rabies Tag

FELINE VACCINES
0608 FVRCP Booster
0612 FVRCP 1 year
0609 FVRCP 3 year
0613 FELV Booster
0610 FELV 1 year
0611 FVRCP/FELV
0607 Rabies Only Fe -1 yr
0618 Rabies Feline 1 year
0605 Feline Yearly Exam
0621 Feline Sr Wellness

PET WEIGHT_____

CANINE VACCINES
0603 Parvo
0615 Bordetella
0616 DHPP Booster
0602 DHPP 1 year
0617 DHPP 3 year
0604 Rabies Canine 1 year
0601 Rabies 3 year
0690 Canine Yearly Exam
0620 Canine Sr Wellness
0606 Rattlesnake Vaccine
0619 Lepto

ANESTHESIA
0302 Anesthesia
0304 Extended
0306 Short
0308 Local
0310 Tranquilization
0316 Geriatric Anesthesia

GROOMING
0506 Beak Trim- Small
0508 Beak Trim- Large
0510 Nail Trim
0512 Nail Trim- Exotic
0514 Wing Trim- Small
0516 Wing Trim- Large
0520 Trim Teeth
0518 Pluck ears
0502 Medicated Bath
0501 Shave Cat

DENTAL
0702 Sm Normal Prophy
0704 Lg Normal Prophy
0701 Feline Normal Prophy
0706 Severe Periodontal Dz
0710 Follow-Up
0714 Tooth Ext. Minimum
0716 Tooth Ext. Moderate
0718 Tooth Ext. Extensive
0712 Dental Sutures

HOSPITALIZATION
0902 Board-Canine
0904 Board-Feline
0903 Overnight Board, Sx
0906 Day Board/Obsvtn
907 Hospital Day
0908 Hospital Overnight
909 Hospital Day w/ IV
0910 Hospital Weekend
0912 Hospital Exotic
911 O2 Therepy Half Day
0914 O2 Therepy Full Day
0916 IV Care Daily
0918 IV Care Intensive
0920 IV Catheter
0922 IV Catheter, 2nd
0924 IV Fluids per Liter
0926 IV Fluids One time
0928 Fluid Additives
0925 IV Fluids Hetastarch
0930 SQ Fluids Once
0932 SQ Fluids Per Day
0934 SQ Fluids Exotic
0936 SQ Fluids Disp.
938 SQ Fluids No Tech/Dr.

RADIOLOGY
4125 Radiographs
4126 Radiographs-dental

LAB SERVICES
3505 ACTH Stim
3515 Automimmune Profile
3520 Avian Comp Profile
3526 Avian Post Purchase
3535 Bile Acids
3611 BIPS
3621 Blood Pressure
3560 CBC/Diff
3580 Coagulation Profile
3770 Chemistry #1
3775 Chemistry >2
3590 Culture and Sensitivity
3605 Cytology In house
3593 Cytology-Lab
3610 DTM
3615 Ear Mite Check
3620 Ear Smear
3631 Electrolytes
3603 EKG
3626 EKG >1 per day
3628 EKG Senior Wellness
3630 EKG Repeat
3641 Ehrlichia Canis PCR
3655 Fecal-Direct
3660 Fecal Flotation/Smear
3665 Fecal- Recheck
3675 FELV Snap Test
3685 FELV/FIV Snap Test
4081 Fine Needle Aspirate
3695 Fungal Serology
3815 General Health Profile
3710 Heartworm SNAP
3715 Heartworm Difil
3705 HCT/TP
3720 Histopath
3725 Histopath Additional
3730 Histopath Derm
3731 Histopath-Bone Decal
3527 Mammalian Comp Prof
0438 Necropsy In house
0436 Necropsy NMDL
0441 Necropsy Avian-NMDL
3745 Parvovirus Snap Test
3750 Phenobarb Levels
3749 Platelet Count
3601 Pre-Op EKG
3755 Pre-Op Profile
3785 Reptile Std. Profile
3786 Reptile Comp Profile
3795 Schirmer Tear Test
3805 Skin Scrape

LAB SERVICES
3821 T-4 Equilibrum Dialysis
3820 T-4 Dogs
3822 T-4 Cats
3830 Tick Born Dz Panel
4141 Tonopen
3850 Urinalysis- In house
3855 Urinalysis-Lab
3880 Urinalysis-SG
3854 Urinalysis Sediment
3853 Urinalysis-Stick
3852 Urinalysis- Yearly Exam
3860 Vaginal Smear

CLINICAL PROCEDURES
4005 Abdominocentesis
4010 Anal Sac Expression
4015 Anal Sac recheck
4020 Artifical Insemination
4025 Bandage Wound Sm
4030 Bandage Wound Med
4035 Bandage Wound Lg
3085 Cast
4050 Clean Ears
4055 Clip/Clean Wound Sm
4060 Clip/Clean Wound Med
4065 Clip/Clean Wound Lg
4070 Corneal Stain (1)
4071 Corneal Stain (2)
4080 Enema
4083 Flush Anal Glands
4085 Flush ears (1)
4090 Flush ears (2)
4095 Flush Nasal Duct
4105 Home Again Implant
4110 Pass Stomach Tube
4130 Semen Collection/Eval
7002 Splint-Small
5126 Re-Splint Small
7001 Splint-Medium
5131 Re-Splint Medium
7000 Splint-Large
5136 Re-Splint-Large
4140 Thoracocentesis
4145 Transtracheal Wash
4150 Urinary Catheter

EUTHANASIA
WT_____
Dog _____ Cat _____
Mass Cremation
Private Cremation
402 Exotic

FIGURE 3-8 Sample travel sheet.

SURGICAL PROCEDURES		CONSULTS	INJECTIONS
4205 Abcess Debride	4405 Feline Neuter	202 Cardiology	
4210 Amputate Limb Sm	4410 Feline Neuter/Declaw	213 Repeat EKG	# of ML _____
4215 Amputate Limb Lg	4420 Feline OVH	204 Internal Medicine	
4220 Amputate Digit	4425 Feline OVH In heat	206 Miscellaneous	1220 Amiglyde #1
4225 Amputate Tail	4430 Feline OVH Pregnant	208 OFA 1225 Amiglyde >1	
4235 Ant. Cruc. Repair	4435 Feline OVH Declaw	210 Radiology	1256 Baytril 100mg/ml
4240 Aural Hematoma-K-9	4441 FHO Feline	212 Shipping	1255 Baytril 22.7mg/ml
4341 Aural Hematome-Fe	4442 FHO Canine		1265 Cephazolin
4245 Biopsy - Wedge	4455 Growth Removal SM	**HEARTWORM MEDICATION**	1270 Cephazolin >1
4250 Biopsy - Punch	4460 Growth Removal MED	HG Small # _____	1281 Cortrosyn
4246 Biopsy - Bone	4465 Growth Removal LG	HG Medium # _____	1289 Dexameth 2mg/ml
4260 C-Section	4470 Growth Removal >1	HG Large # _____	1290 Dexameth 4mg/ml
4265 C-Section w/ OVH	4480 Hernia Repair Inguinal	HG Feline 0-5# #6	1305 Diphenhydramine
4270 Canine Neuter <50	4485 Hernia Repair Abdom	HG Feline 5-15# #6	Ivomec
4275 Canine Neuter >50	4490 Hernia Repair Diaphm.		1335 Immiticide
4285 Canine OVH <50	4495 Hernia Repair Umbil.		1390 Methyl Pred Acetate
4290 Canine OVH 50-99	4505 Patellar Luxation #1	Revolution Feline	1410 Pred Acetate
4272 Canine OVH >100	4510 Patellar Luxation #2	Revolution Canine	1417 Solu-delta Cortef 100mg
4295 Canine OVH/Heat	4511 Prostatic Wash		1418 Solu-delta Cortef 500mg
4305 Canine OVH/Preg	4515 Puppy Dewclaws Each	Frontline Feline	1430 Torbugesic
4236 Cranial Cruc. SM (1)	4520 Puppy Tail Docks Each	Frontline Canine	
4238 Cranial Cruc. LG (1)	4525 Pyometra w/ OVH	Frontline In Hosp Use	**E-COLLAR**
4237 Cranial Cruc. SM (2)	4530 Rabbit Neuter		
4239 Cranial Cruc. LG (2)	4535 Rabbit OVH	**POST OP PAIN MEDS**	**N/C ITEMS**
4315 Cherry Eye Repair 1	4540 Staple Wound per staple	Rimadyl 25mg	818 HG SM
4320 Cherry Eye Repair 2	4545 Stenotic Nares Repair	Rimadyl 75mg	822 HG M
4325 Cryptorchid Fe-Flank	4550 Suture Wound SM	Rimadyl 100mg	826 HG LG
4330 Cryptorchid Fe-Abdm	4555 Suture Wound MED	Metacam	2790 Strongid
4345 Cryptorchid K-9 Abdm	4560 Suture Wound LG	Buprinex	510 Nail Trim
4340 Cryptorchid K-9 Flank	4575 Third Eyelid Flap	Tramadol	
4350 Cystotomy			
4355 Debride wound			
4360 Declaw/Tendonectomy			
4365 Dewclaw Unjointed #1			
4370 Declaw Jointed #1			
4375 Drain Placement			
4385 Entropion per lid			
4390 Exploratory			
4395 Eye Enucleation			

FIGURE 3-8, cont'd

Appropriate Fee Setting

Many practices do not charge appropriately for the services provided. Veterinarians often believe the costs are too high and that clients cannot afford to pay those fees. In reality, the veterinary practice has a large overhead cost that is, for the most part, hidden. Payroll taxes, team member benefits, and credit card fees are just a few of the hidden costs veterinary practices must absorb. Obvious costs include product purchases, utilities, and mortgages that must be paid monthly regardless of the profit the practice produces. See Chapter 20 for more information on budgeting and financial planning in a veterinary hospital.

> **PRACTICE POINT** Fees must be charged appropriately for services provided to cover overhead expenses the practice has incurred.

If clients complain of the fees they are charged, they may not fully understand the value associated with those fees. Client education should be reviewed to ensure clients are being fully educated by the team when they visit the practice. Clients value honesty, compassion, and timeliness. They want to understand the information being presented to them. Without this knowledge, they will feel that they cannot pay the fees practices charge.

When developing a pricing structure, fees should be divided into two categories: shopped services and in-hospital fees. Shopped fees include vaccinations, heartworm tests, and routine procedures. These fees can be competitively priced with other practices in the community. The fees should cover the cost of the product, the cost of the items needed to complete that service, and the time of the technician or veterinarian to complete the service. For example, a heartworm test should include the cost of the test itself, the syringe and needle needed to draw the blood for the test, and the technician's time to draw the blood and run the test. A percentage needs to be added on top to contribute to the hidden overhead costs of the practice. Many times, practices forget to add the cost of the items needed to complete the service as well as the technician's time.

Once shopped service fees have been set, in-hospital fees can be determined. A simple formula provided by Mark Opperman works well.

Overhead costs/min + Direct costs + Return on time to Dr.

Overhead costs can be determined from the previous year's financial statements and include every cost except veterinarian compensation and drug and supply costs. Most overhead costs range from $1.50 to $2 per minute. Direct costs include all materials used for any given procedure. Once all direct costs have been calculated, double it to include the costs of ordering, shipping, and unpacking the products. If practices only charge the true direct costs, income will be lost.

Return on veterinarian time covers how much it costs to pay doctors for their skills. The average small-animal veterinarian return is $180 per hour for in-house medical procedures, $2 to $3 per minute for soft tissue surgery, and $3 to $4 per minute for orthopedic surgery. These figures can be used to create a baseline fee for any in-hospital procedure. This formula is essential to setting fair, profitable fees and helps the staff understand how and why charges are set.

PRACTICE POINT Fair fees must be set for a practice to be profitable and be able to reinvest money into the practice.

Pharmaceuticals must also be charged appropriately and include the cost for the label, the pill vial, and the time to count the pills to be dispensed. The average markup on the true product is two times for shopped products and two and half times for others. The computer should have an automatic default dispensing fee per medication dispensed. The average dispensing fee is generally $6 to $12 each time a prescription is dispensed. A minimum prescription fee should be charged when the total cost does not equal the minimum charge.

Outside laboratory fees are generally doubled, adding $5 to $10 to cover the cost of supplies used to obtain the sample, plus labeling, packaging, and filling out the form.

CLIENT'S LAST NAME _____ WORKING DIAGNOSIS _____

PET'S NAME _____ PRIMARY DOCTOR _____

DATE:	8AM	9	10	11	12	1	2	3	4	5	6	7	8
FEED													
WATER													
WALK/LITTER													
TEMPERATURE													
WEIGHT													
APPETITE?													
ATTITUDE?													
URINE?													
BM OR DIARRHEA													
VOMIT?													

OFFICE CALL
0214 Brief Office Call
0216 Regular Office Call
0222 Exotics Exam-Reg
0220 Exotics Exam-Brief
0232 Recheck N/C
0234 Recheck
FELINE VACCINES
0608 FVRCP Booster
0612 FVRCP 1 year
0609 FVRCP 3 year
0613 FELV Booster
0610 FELV 1 year
0611 FVRCP/FELV
0618 Rabies Feline 1 year
0605 Feline Yearly Exam
0621 Feline Sr Wellness
CANINE VACCINES
0603 Parvo
0615 Bordetella
0616 DHPP Booster
0602 DHPP 1 year
0617 DHPP 3 year
0604 Rabies Canine 1 year
0601 Rabies 3 year
0690 Canine Yearly Exam
0620 Canine Sr Wellness
0606 Rattlesnake Vaccine
0619 Lepto

HOSPITALIZATION
0902 Board-Canine
0904 Board-Feline
0903 Overnight Board, Sx
0906 Day Board/Obsvtn
907 Hospital Day
0908 Hospital Overnight
909 Hospital Day w/ IV
0910 Hospital Weekend
0912 Hospital Exotic
911 Oxygen Therepy Half Day
0914 Oxygen Therepy Full Day
0916 IV Care Daily
0918 IV Care Intensive
0920 IV Catheter
0922 IV Catheter, 2nd
0924 IV Fluids per Liter
0926 IV Fluids One time
0928 Fluid Additives
0925 IV Fluids Hetastarch
0930 SQ Fluids Once
0932 SQ Fluids Per Day
0934 SQ Fluids Exotic
0936 SQ Fluids Disp.
RADIOLOGY
4125 Radiographs
CONSULTS
202 Cardiology
213 Repeat EKG
204 Internal Medicine
210 Radiology

LAB SERVICES
3611 BIPS
3621 Blood Pressure
3560 CBC/Diff
3770 Chemistry #1
3775 Chemistry >2
3590 Culture and Sensitivity
3605 Cytology In house
3610 DTM
3615 Ear Mite Check
3620 Ear Smear
3631 Electrolytes
3603 EKG
3626 EKG >1 per day
3655 Fecal-Direct
3660 Fecal Flotation/Smear
3675 FELV Snap Test
3685 FELV/FIV Snap Test
4081 Fine Needle Aspirate
3815 General Health Profile
3710 Heartworm SNAP
3705 HCT/TP
3745 Parvovirus Snap Test
3750 Phenobarb Levels
3601 Pre-Op EKG
3755 Pre-Op Profile
3795 Schirmer Tear Test
3805 Skin Scrape
0000 T-4

LAB SERVICES
0000 Urinalysis
3860 Vaginal Smear
CLINICAL PROCEDURES
4005 Abdominocentesis
4010 Anal Sac Expression
0000 Bandage Wound
3085 Cast
4050 Clean Ears
4055 Clip/Clean Wound Sm
4060 Clip/Clean Wound Med
4065 Clip/Clean Wound Lg
4070 Corneal Stain (1)
4071 Corneal Stain (2)
4080 Enema
4083 Flush Anal Glands
4085 Flush ears (1)
4090 Flush ears (2)
4110 Pass Stomach Tube
7002 Splint-Small
5126 Re-Splint Small
7001 Splint-Medium
5131 Re-Splint Medium
7000 Splint-Large
5136 Re-Splint-Large
4140 Thoracocentesis
4145 Transtracheal Wash
4150 Urinary Catheter
E-COLLAR

FIGURE 3-9 Sample hospital travel sheet.

SELECTING, MOTIVATING, AND RETAINING TEAM MEMBERS

Chapter 5 covers the selection of employees and retaining current team members. The selection process of team members is important. It is critical to choose the best employee possible, not just fill a position with anyone available.

People who work well together understand the importance of positive reinforcement. It is essential for maintaining the team's enthusiasm and motivation. The simplest form of positive reinforcement comes in words and phrases that recognize an individual's hard work and dedication to the practice. Positive reinforcement is

Box 3-15	Ideas for Motivating Team Members

- Setting goals together
- Thinking "career"
- Humor
- Benefits
- Lifelong learning
- Time off
- Generational preferences
- Praise
- Coupons
- Gift cards
- Celebrating victories
- "Firing" bad clients

a tremendous incentive for strengthening teams. Lack of recognition and appreciation is a top reason for employee dissatisfaction. Seize the moment to show each team member the recognition he or she deserves (Box 3-15).

> **PRACTICE POINT** Positive reinforcement is a tool that many managers do not use to its maximum potential.

Positive reinforcement should be given on an individual basis. A team member who has gone above and beyond expectations should be rewarded immediately with something that is useful for that particular person. For example, if an employee has just purchased a new home and has previously discussed the need to buy new kitchen utensils, then a simple reward of new pots and pans may be warranted. If a team member is remodeling a home, a gift certificate to a local hardware store may be appropriate. However, a gift certificate to the local roller rink for a team member who is 50 years old would devalue the positive reinforcement. Take the time to reward appropriately, and the positive reinforcement will double in value.

Job enrichment is also important for retaining team members. For example, the main job of kennel attendants is to clean the kennels on a daily basis, but this position can be enriched by allowing them to assist technicians (Figure 3-10). They can hold animals for treatments or

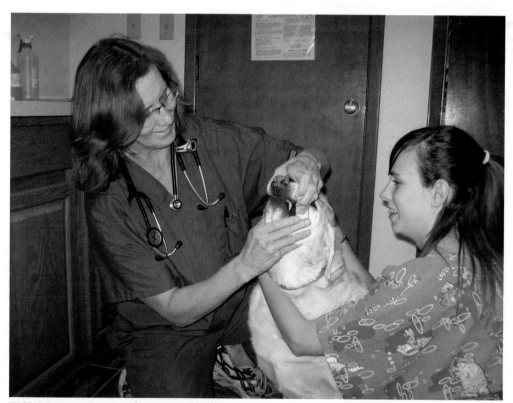

FIGURE 3-10 Encouraging team members to assist with tasks outside their regular responsibilities keeps them motivated.

help position patients for radiographs. Individuals can get bored with their daily duties. By allowing them to do something other than clean kennels, their job can be exciting and interesting and give them incentive to take the next step up the ladder within the veterinary hospital.

VETERINARY PRACTICE and the LAW

Effective team management includes training team members in proper oral communication. It is imperative to add to job descriptions that team members must be able to communicate effectively with clients. Team members with thick accents or those who talk too fast may be hard for some clients to understand. Keep in mind, however, that employers cannot discriminate against team members because of a foreign accent; both state and federal laws protect against national origin discrimination, including discrimination based on foreign accent, fluency, and cultural traits (e.g., clothing).

If an excellent team member has difficulty communicating with clients, it may be worth advising the person to seek the assistance of a speech therapist. Employers may want to contribute to the therapy assistance if the team member is a potential long-term and dedicated employee.

Self-Evaluation Questions

1. What are some characteristics of effective leaders?
2. What are four steps of management?
3. Why are these four steps critical to the management of a veterinary practice?
4. What are two theories of effective management? Define each.
5. How can you become a better leader?
6. Why are respect and rapport imperative when managing a team?
7. What are some methods that can be used to empower team members?
8. How long should a meeting last?
9. What is a consensus?
10. Why should conflicts be resolved immediately?

Recommended Reading

Belaso JA, Stayer RC: *Flight of the buffalo: soaring to excellence, learning to let employees lead*, New York, 1993, Warner.

Hersey P, Blanchard K: *Management of organized behavior*, ed 9, Englewood Cliffs, NJ, 2008, Prentice Hall.

Nelson R: *1001 ways to reward employees*, New York, 2005, Workman.

Tropman J: *Making meetings work: achieving high quality group decisions*, ed 2, New York, 2003, Sage Press.

Ackerman L, Stowe JD: *Blackwell's five minute veterinary practice management consult*, section 6.11, Ames, IA, 2007, Blackwell.

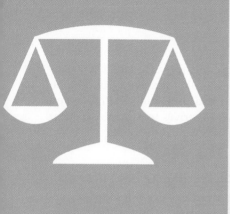

CHAPTER 4

Veterinary Ethics and Legal Issues

Chapter Outline

Code of Ethics
Veterinary Ethics
Legal Issues
    Veterinary Practice Act
    Definitions of Law
    Consent
    Emergency Care

Malpractice
Abandoned Animals
Impending Laws
Medical Records
Most Common Complaints to the Board of Veterinary
    Medicine

Learning Objectives

Mastery of the content in this chapter will enable the reader to:
- Differentiate ethics and law.
- Define the branches of ethics.
- Identify a veterinary practice act.
- Differentiate criminal and civil law.
- Describe informed consent.

- Develop an informed consent form.
- Clarify methods used to prevent malpractice and negligence.
- Manage abandoned animals.
- List the most common complaints in veterinary medicine.

Key Terms

Administrative Ethics
Civil Law
Code of Ethics
Consent
Contract Law
Criminal Law

Informed Consent
Law
Malpractice
Negligence
Normative Ethics
Personal Ethics

Professional Ethics
Social Ethics
Standard of Care
Tort
Veterinary Ethics
Veterinary Practice Act

Three areas of ethics exist and affect each team member on every level. Social, personal, and professional ethics are interrelated, yet they affect each person differently. Social ethics are the consensus principles adopted or accepted by society at large and codified into laws and regulations. Laws include those against murder, rape, and stealing along with ordinances such as those that regulate pets on leashes. Personal ethics define what is right or wrong on an individual basis. This can include religious beliefs and values as they relate to relationships and marriages. Professional ethics, as stated, are developed by the professionals of a particular discipline, developing rules, codes, and conduct for the profession to follow.

> **PRACTICE POINT** Professional veterinary ethics are developed by veterinarians to cultivate rules, codes, and conducts for the profession.

CODE OF ETHICS

Ethics is a branch of philosophy and a systematic, intellectual approach to the standards of behavior. The purpose of a professional code of ethics is to help members of a profession achieve high levels of behavior through moral consciousness, decision making, and practice. A sense of ethics in daily practice challenges veterinarians to determine right from wrong. Each organization within the profession also has a code of ethics for its members and is based on moral principles that reflect concern and care for the client and patient.

Historically, ethics relate to standards of conduct promoted by and demanded of members of veterinary associations. The American Veterinary Medical Association (AVMA) *Principles of Veterinary Medical Ethics* is a document on ethical issues in veterinary practice focusing more on the relationships one has with colleagues than on the broader range of moral and ethical issues relating to animals (Box 4-1).

The Veterinary Hospital Managers Association (VHMA) holds a strong code of ethics for the profession, practice, and patient. Practice and hospital managers must protect the interest and integrity of the practice itself while providing a professional image for the profession (Figure 4-1).

The National Association of Veterinary Technicians in America (NAVTA) code of ethics for veterinary technicians is a combination of professional ethics that focus both on the practice of medicine and protecting the profession as a whole (Box 4-2). NAVTA strives to provide excellent guidelines for its members as well as the public.

VETERINARY ETHICS

Four branches of veterinary ethics exist: descriptive, official, administrative, and normative ethics. *Descriptive ethics* refers to the study of ethical views of veterinarians and veterinary professionals regarding their behavior and

---

Box 4-1   AVMA Principles of Veterinary Medical Ethics

Introduction

Veterinarians are members of a scholarly profession who have earned academic degrees from comprehensive universities or similar educational institutions. Veterinarians practice the profession of veterinary medicine in a variety of situations and circumstances.

Exemplary professional conduct upholds the dignity of the veterinary profession. All veterinarians are expected to adhere to a progressive code of ethical conduct known as the Principles of Veterinary Medical Ethics (the Principles). The basis of the Principles is the Golden Rule. Veterinarians should accept this rule as a guide to their general conduct, and abide by the Principles. They should conduct their professional and personal affairs in an ethical manner. Professional veterinary associations should adopt the Principles or a similar code as a guide for their activities.

Professional organizations may establish ethics, grievance, or peer review committees to address ethical issues. Local and state veterinary associations should also include discussions of ethical issues in their continuing education programs.

Complaints about behavior that may violate the Principles should be addressed in an appropriate and timely manner. Such questions should be considered initially by ethics, grievance, or peer review committees of local or state veterinary associations, when they exist, and/or when appropriate, state veterinary medical boards. Members of local and state committees are familiar with local customs and circumstances, and those committees are in the best position to confer with all parties involved.

The Judicial Council may address complaints, prior to, concurrent with, or subsequent to review at the state or local level, as it deems appropriate.

All veterinarians in local or state associations and jurisdictions have a responsibility to regulate and guide the professional conduct of their members.

Colleges of veterinary medicine should stress the teaching of ethical and value issues as part of the professional veterinary curriculum for all veterinary students.

The National Board of Veterinary Medical Examiners is encouraged to prepare and include questions regarding professional ethics in the National Board Examination.

The AVMA Judicial Council is charged to advise on all questions relating to interpretation of the Bylaws, all questions of veterinary medical ethics, and other rules of the Association. The Judicial Council should review the Principles periodically to ensure that they remain complete and up to date.

Professional Behavior

Veterinarians should first consider the needs of the patient: to relieve disease, suffering, or disability while minimizing pain or fear.

Veterinarians should obey all laws of the jurisdictions in which they reside and practice veterinary medicine. Veterinarians should be honest and fair in their relations with others, and they should not engage in fraud, misrepresentation, or deceit.

Veterinarians should report illegal practices and activities to the proper authorities.

The AVMA Judicial Council may choose to report alleged infractions by nonmembers of the AVMA to the appropriate agencies.

Veterinarians should use only the title of the professional degree that was awarded by the school of veterinary medicine where the degree was earned. All veterinarians may use the courtesy titles *Doctor* or *Veterinarian*. Veterinarians who were awarded a degree other than DVM or VMD should refer to the *AVMA Directory* for information on the appropriate titles and degrees.

It is unethical for veterinarians to identify themselves as members of an AVMA recognized specialty organization if such certification has not been awarded.

It is unethical to place professional knowledge, credentials, or services at the disposal of any nonprofessional organization, group, or individual to promote or lend credibility to the illegal practice of veterinary medicine.

Veterinarians may choose whom they will serve. Both the veterinarians and the client have the right to establish or decline a Veterinarian-Client-Patient Relationship (see Section III) and to decide on treatment. The decision to accept or decline treatment and related cost should be based on adequate discussion of clinical findings, diagnostic techniques, treatment, likely outcome, estimated cost, and reasonable assurance of

Box 4-1 AVMA Principles of Veterinary Medical Ethics—cont'd

payment. Once the veterinarians and the client have agreed, and the veterinarians have begun patient care, they may not neglect their patient and must continue to provide professional services related to that injury or illness within the previously agreed limits. As subsequent needs and costs for patient care are identified, the veterinarians and client must confer and reach agreement on the continued care and responsibility for fees. If the informed client declines further care or declines to assume responsibility for the fees, the VCPR may be terminated by either party.

In emergencies, veterinarians have an ethical responsibility to provide essential services for animals when necessary to save life or relieve suffering, subsequent to client agreement. Such emergency care may be limited to euthanasia to relieve suffering, or to stabilization of the patient for transport to another source of animal care.

When veterinarians cannot be available to provide services, they should arrange with their colleagues to assure that emergency services are available, consistent with the needs of the locality.

Veterinarians who believe that they haven't the experience or equipment to manage and treat certain emergencies in the best manner, should advise the client that more qualified or specialized services are available elsewhere and offer to expedite referral to those services.

Regardless of practice ownership, the interests of the patient, client, and public require that all decisions that affect diagnosis, care, and treatment of patients are made by veterinarians.

Veterinarians should strive to enhance their image with respect to their colleagues, clients, other health professionals, and the general public. Veterinarians should be honest, fair, courteous, considerate, and compassionate. Veterinarians should present a professional appearance and follow acceptable professional procedures using current professional and scientific knowledge.

Veterinarians should not slander, or injure the professional standing or reputation of other veterinarians in a false or misleading manner.

Veterinarians should strive to improve their veterinary knowledge and skills, and they are encouraged to collaborate with other professionals in the quest for knowledge and professional development.

The responsibilities of the veterinary profession extend beyond individual patients and clients to society in general. Veterinarians are encouraged to make their knowledge available to their communities and to provide their services for activities that protect public health.

Veterinarians and their associates should protect the personal privacy of patients and clients. Veterinarians should not reveal confidences unless required to by law or unless it becomes necessary to protect the health and welfare of other individuals or animals.

Veterinarians who are impaired by alcohol or other substances should seek assistance from qualified organizations or individuals. Colleagues of impaired veterinarians should encourage those individuals to seek assistance and to overcome their disabilities.

The Veterinarian-Client-Patient Relationship

The veterinarian-client-patient relationship (VCPR) is the basis for interaction among veterinarians, their clients, and their patients. A VCPR exists when all of the following conditions have been met:

The veterinarian has assumed responsibility for making clinical judgements regarding the health of the animal(s) and the need for medical treatment, and the client has agreed to follow the veterinarian's instructions.

The veterinarian has sufficient knowledge of the animal(s) to initiate at least a general or preliminary diagnosis of the medical condition of the animal(s). This means that the veterinarian has recently seen and is personally acquainted with the keeping and care of the animal(s) by virtue of an examination of the animal(s), or by medically appropriate and timely visits to the premises where the animal(s) are kept.

The veterinarian is readily available, or has arranged for emergency coverage, for follow-up evaluation in the event of adverse reactions or the failure of the treatment regimen.

When a VCPR exists, veterinarians must maintain medical records (See Section VII).

Dispensing or prescribing a prescription product requires a VCPR.

Veterinarians should honor a client's request for a prescription in lieu of dispensing.

Without a VCPR, veterinarians merchandising or use of veterinary prescription drugs or their extra-label use of any pharmaceutical is unethical and is illegal under federal law.

Veterinarians may terminate a VCPR under certain conditions, and they have an ethical obligation to use courtesy and tact in doing so.

If there is no ongoing medical condition, veterinarians may terminate a VCPR by notifying the client that they no longer wish to serve that patient and client.

If there is an ongoing medical or surgical condition, the patient should be referred to another veterinarian for diagnosis, care, and treatment. The former attending veterinarian should continue to provide care, as needed, during the transition.

Clients may terminate the VCPR at any time.

Attending, Consulting and Referring

An *attending veterinarian* is a veterinarian (or a group of veterinarians) who assumes responsibility for primary care of a patient. A VCPR is established.

Attending veterinarians are entitled to charge a fee for their professional services.

When appropriate, attending veterinarians are encouraged to seek assistance in the form of consultations and referrals. A decision to consult or refer is made jointly by the attending veterinarian and the client.

When a consultation occurs, the attending veterinarian continues to be primarily responsible for the case.

A *consulting veterinarian* is a veterinarian (or group of veterinarians) who agrees to advise an attending veterinarian on the care and management of a case.

Continued

Box 4-1   AVMA Principles of Veterinary Medical Ethics—cont'd

The VCPR remains the responsibility of the attending veterinarian.

Consulting veterinarians may or may not charge fees for service.

Consulting veterinarians should communicate their findings and opinions directly to the attending veterinarians.

Consulting veterinarians should revisit the patients or communicate with the clients in collaboration with the attending veterinarians.

Consultations usually involve the exchange of information or interpretation of test results. However, it may be appropriate or necessary for consultants to examine patients. When advanced or invasive techniques are required to gather information or substantiate diagnoses, attending veterinarians may refer the patients. A new VCPR is established with the veterinarian to whom a case is referred.

The *referral veterinarian or receiving veterinarian* is a veterinarian (or group of veterinarians) who agrees to provide requested veterinary services. A new VCPR is established. The referring and referral veterinarians must communicate.

Attending veterinarians should honor clients' requests for referral.

Referral veterinarians may choose to accept or decline clients and patients from attending veterinarians.

Patients are usually referred because of specific medical problems or services. Referral veterinarians should provide services or treatments relative to the referred conditions, and they should communicate with the referring veterinarians and clients if other services or treatments are required.

When a client seeks professional services or opinions from a different veterinarian without a referral, a new VCPR is established with the new attending veterinarian. When contacted, the veterinarian who was formerly involved in the diagnosis, care, and treatment of the patient should communicate with the new attending veterinarian as if the patient and client had been referred.

With the client's consent, the new attending veterinarian should contact the former veterinarian to learn the original diagnosis, care, and treatment and clarify any issues before proceeding with a new treatment plan.

If there is evidence that the actions of the former attending veterinarian have clearly and significantly endangered the health or safety of the patient, the new attending veterinarian has a responsibility to report the matter to the appropriate authorities of the local and state association or professional regulatory agency.

Influences on Judgment

The choice of treatments or animal care should not be influenced by considerations other than the needs of the patient, the welfare of the client, and the safety of the public.

Veterinarians should not allow their medical judgement to be influenced by agreements by which they stand to profit through referring clients to other providers of services or products.

The medical judgements of veterinarians should not be influenced by contracts or agreements made by their associations or societies.

When conferences, meetings, or lectures are sponsored by outside entities, the organization that presents the program, not the funding sponsor, shall have control of the contents and speakers.

Therapies

Attending veterinarians are responsible for choosing the treatment regimens for their patients. It is the attending veterinarian's responsibility to inform the client of the expected results and costs, and the related risks of each treatment regimen.

It is unethical for veterinarians to prescribe or dispense prescription products in the absence of a VCPR.

It is unethical for veterinarians to promote, sell, prescribe, dispense, or use secret remedies or any other product for which they do not know the ingredient formula.

It is unethical for veterinarians to use or permit the use of their names, signatures, or professional status in connection with the resale of ethical products in a manner which violates those directions or conditions specified by the manufacturer to ensure the safe and efficacious use of the product.

Genetic Defects

Performance of surgical or other procedures in all species for the purpose of concealing genetic defects in animals to be shown, raced, bred, or sold, as breeding animals is unethical. However, should the health or welfare of the individual patient require correction of such genetic defects, it is recommended that the patient be rendered incapable of reproduction.

Medical Records

Veterinary medical records are an integral part of veterinary care. The records must comply with the standards established by state and federal law.

Medical Records are the property of the practice and the practice owner. The original records must be retained by the practice for the period required by statute.

Ethically, the information within veterinary medical records is considered privileged and confidential. It must not be released except by court order or consent of the owner of the patient.

Veterinarians are obligated to provide copies or summaries of medical records when requested by the client. Veterinarians should secure a written release to document that request.

Without the express permission of the practice owner, it is unethical for a veterinarian to remove, copy, or use the medical records or any part of any record.

Fees and Remuneration

Veterinarians are entitled to charge fees for their professional services.

In connection with consultations or referrals, it is unethical for veterinarians to enter into financial arrangements, such as fee splitting, which involve payment of a portion of a fee to a recommending veterinarian who has not

Continued

Box 4-1   AVMA Principles of Veterinary Medical Ethics—cont'd

rendered the professional services for which the fee was paid by the client.

Regardless of the fees that are charged or received, the quality of service must be maintained at the usual professional standard.

It is unethical for a group or association of veterinarians to take any action which coerces, pressures, or achieves agreement among veterinarians to conform to a fee schedule or fixed fees.

Advertising

Without written permission from the AVMA Executive Board, no member or employee of the American Veterinary Medical Association (AVMA) shall use the AVMA name or logo in connection with the promotion or advertising of any commercial product or service.

Advertising by veterinarians is ethical when there are no false, deceptive, or misleading statements or claims. A false, deceptive, or misleading statement or claim is one which communicates false information or is intended, through a material omission, to leave a false impression.

Testimonials or endorsements are advertising, and they should comply with the guidelines for advertising. In addition, testimonials and endorsements of professional products or services by veterinarians are considered unethical unless they comply with the following:

The endorser must be a bona fide user of the product or service.

There must be adequate substantiation that the results obtained by the endorser are representative of what veterinarians may expect in actual conditions of use.

Any financial, business, or other relationship between the endorser and the seller of a product or service must be fully disclosed.

When reprints of scientific articles are used with advertising, the reprints must remain unchanged, and be presented in their entirety.

The principles that apply to advertising, testimonials, and endorsements also apply to veterinarians' communications with their clients.

Veterinarians may permit the use of their names by commercial enterprises (e.g. pet shops, kennels, farms, feedlots) so that the enterprises can advertise under veterinary supervision, only if they provide such supervision.

Euthanasia

Humane euthanasia of animals is an ethical veterinary procedure.

Glossary

Pharmaceutical Products

Several of the following terms are used to describe veterinary pharmaceutical products. Some have legal status, others do not. Although not all of the terms are used in the Principles, we have listed them here for clarification of meaning and to avoid confusion.

Ethical Product: A product for which the manufacturer has voluntarily limited the sale to veterinarians as a marketing decision. Such products are often given a different product name and are packaged differently than products that are sold directly to consumers. "Ethical products" are sold only to veterinarians as a condition of sale that is specified in a sales agreement or on the product label.

Legend Drug: A synonymous term for a veterinary prescription drug. The name refers to the statement (legend) that is required on the label (see *veterinary prescription drug* below).

Over the Counter (OTC) Drug: Any drug that can be labeled with adequate direction to enable it to be used safely and properly by a consumer who is not a medical professional.

Prescription Drug: A drug that cannot be labeled with adequate direction to enable its safe and proper use by non-professionals.

Veterinary Prescription Drug: A drug that is restricted by federal law to use by or on the order of a licensed veterinarian, according to section 503(f) of the federal Food, Drug, and Cosmetic Act. The law requires that such drugs be labeled with the statement: "Caution, federal law restricts this drug to use by or on the order of a licensed veterinarian."

Dispensing, Prescribing, Marketing, and Merchandising

Dispensing is the direct distribution of products by veterinarians to clients for use on their animals.

Prescribing is the transmitting of an order authorizing a licensed pharmacist or equivalent to prepare and dispense specified pharmaceuticals to be used in or on animals in the dosage and in the manner directed by a veterinarian.

Marketing is promoting and encouraging animal owners to improve animal health and welfare by using veterinary care, services, and products.

Merchandising is the buying and selling of products or services.

Advertising and Testimonials

Advertising is defined as communication that is designed to inform the public about the availability, nature, or price of products or services or to influence clients to use certain products or services.

Testimonials or *endorsements* are statements that are intended to influence attitudes regarding the purchase or use of products or services.

Fee Splitting

The dividing of a professional fee for veterinary services with the recommending veterinarian (see Section VIII B).

Bold print states the principles, and standard print explains or clarifies the principle to which it applies. Revised by the Council in October 2006. Approved by the Ethics Board in November 2006.
Courtesy American Veterinary Medical Association, Schaumburg, Ill.

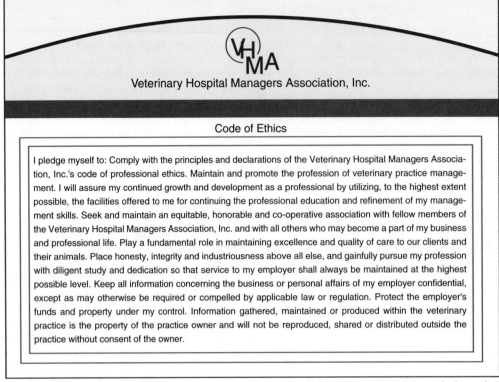

FIGURE 4-1 VHMA code of ethics. (Courtesy Veterinary Hospital Managers Association, Alachua, Fla.)

Box 4-2   NAVTA Code of Ethics
1. Aid society and animals through providing excellent care and service for animals.
2. Prevent and relieve the suffering of animals.
3. Promote public health by assisting with the control of zoonotic disease and informing the public about these diseases.
4. Assume accountability for individual professional actions and judgments.
5. Protect confidential information provided by clients.
6. Safeguard the public and profession against individuals deficient in professional competencies or ethics.
7. Assist with efforts to ensure conditions of employment are consistent with the excellent care for animals.
8. Remain competent in veterinary technology through commitment and lifelong learning.
9. Collaborate with members of the veterinary medical profession in efforts to ensure quality health care services for all animals.

Courtesy National Association of Veterinary Technicians in America, Alexandria, Va.

attitudes. This relates to what members of the profession think is right and wrong and does not involve making value judgments about what is moral or immoral in a professional's behavior. *Official veterinary ethics* involve the creation of the official ethical standards adopted by organizations of professionals and imposed on their members. *Administrative veterinary ethics* involve actions by administrative government bodies that regulate veterinary practice and activities in which veterinarians engage. Many organizations incorporate the AVMA's principles of ethics into their statutes or regulations. License revocation can result if any civil or criminal violation of these regulations occurs. *Normative ethics* refer to the search for correct principles of good and bad, right and wrong, justice or injustice. The difference between ethics and law lies in enforcement; laws are enforced by the government, whereas ethics are enforced by the professional associations that developed them.

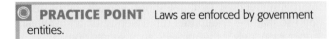

PRACTICE POINT   Laws are enforced by government entities.

LEGAL ISSUES

Laws are bodies of rules developed and enforced by government to regulate people's conduct. Veterinarians are faced with legal obligations on a daily basis. Many laws stem from society's moral and ethical concerns for life, death, and how people should conduct themselves. The veterinary practice act of each state defines the requirements necessary to practice veterinary medicine within that state. Standards of care rise from both the practice act and statutory law and must be followed. Principles of ethics also govern veterinary medicine and are implemented for the protection of the profession and society itself.

Veterinary Practice Act

The veterinary practice act emphasizes that the right to practice veterinary medicine is a privilege granted by state law and is thus subject to regulation to protect and promote public health, safety, and welfare. This statute is enacted as an exercise of the powers of the state to promote public health, safety, and welfare by ensuring the delivery of competent veterinary medical care. Therefore veterinary medicine must be practiced by individuals who posses the personal and professional qualifications specified in this act.

PRACTICE POINT Each state grants the right to practice veterinary medicine.

AVMA has created a model practice act that most states have followed while developing their state veterinary practice acts. Each state varies by laws and regulations; therefore each practice should be familiar with its own state's veterinary practice act (Box 4-3).

Because veterinary practice acts are umbrella laws that govern the practice of veterinary medicine, changes cannot be made easily. Changes must be submitted to the House and Senate, and then ultimately signed into law by the governor. State associations and boards can circulate proposed changes among members of the veterinary and veterinary technician communities, soliciting opinions and changes that members may recommend. Once the board and associations agree, a lobbyist may be hired to find state senators and representatives to support the bill. It may be introduced into the legislative process, amended, and updated various times before the final product is presented to the governor for acceptance. The governor can than accept or deny it but cannot make changes to the bill.

Practice acts are then regulated and enforced by the state veterinary medical board, which oversees both veterinarians and veterinary technicians. This group is responsible for testing and licensure, collection of renewal fees, and the evaluation of complaints presented by the public. With adequate evidence of wrongdoing, boards can revoke any professional veterinary license. The most common complaints are listed later in this chapter.

Definitions of Law

A law generally consists of established rules, statutes, and administrative agency rules that can be enforced to establish limits of conduct for governments and individuals in society. Law is divided into two categories: civil and criminal law. Civil law relates to the duties between people and the government. A contract dispute between a veterinarian and an employee is an example of a case that falls under civil law. Criminal law prosecutes crimes

Box 4-3	AVMA Model Veterinary Practice Act
	PREAMBLE
SECTION 1	Title
SECTION 2	Definitions
SECTION 3	Board of Veterinary Medicine
SECTION 4	License Requirement
SECTION 5	Veterinarian-Client-Patient Relationship Requirement
SECTION 6	Exemptions
SECTION 7	Veterinary Technicians and Technologists
SECTION 8	Status of Persons Previously Licensed
SECTION 9	Application for License: Qualifications
SECTION 10	Examinations
SECTION 11	License by Endorsement
SECTION 12	Temporary Permit
SECTION 13	License Renewal
SECTION 14	Discipline of Licensees
SECTION 15	Impaired Veterinarian
SECTION 16	Hearing Procedure
SECTION 17	Appeal
SECTION 18	Reinstatement
SECTION 19	Veterinarian-Client Confidentiality
SECTION 20	Immunity from Liability
SECTION 21	Cruelty to Animals—Immunity for Reporting
SECTION 22	Abandoned Animals
SECTION 23	Enforcement
SECTION 24	Severability
SECTION 25	Effective Date

Courtesy American Veterinary Medical Association, Schaumburg, Ill.

committed against the public as a whole. Most criminal laws focus on acts that injure people or pets or offend public morality. Violation of civil law generally results in fines paid to the opposing party, whereas violation of criminal law results in jail time and/or fines.

PRACTICE POINT A noncompete agreement falls under the division of civil law.

Civil law can be further broken down into tort and contract law. A tort is a civil offense to an opposing party in which harm has occurred. Standards of care exist for the protection of one's body, business interests, personal property, and reputation. Tort law permits people to sue for relief of an injury that occurred as a result of damages inflicted on their bodies, to their families, or to their property. Furthermore, tort law can be determined to be intentional or unintentional and must be proved to the court. An *intentional tort* is defined just as that: an intentional action that has taken place in which harm has occurred to another member of society. Examples of intentional torts include assault and battery, defamation of character, invasion of privacy, immoral conduct, and fraud. An example of an unintentional tort claim would be the failure to practice the standard of care. If a veterinarian did not practice the standard of care that has been developed by veterinary professionals and an animal suffered injury because of neglect, the veterinarian could be guilty of an unintentional tort of negligence. Torts are generally resolved with a civil trial and a monetary settlement is made.

Contract law deals with duties established by individuals as a result of contractual agreement. This area of law was developed to ensure that promises made by people would be fulfilled; if they are not fulfilled, a breach of duty is established.

A crime is an unlawful activity against a member of the public and is prosecuted by a public official, normally the district attorney or the attorney general's office. A crime is further classified as a misdemeanor or a felony. A misdemeanor charge is less serious than that of a felony and generally results in less jail time

> **PRACTICE POINT** Animal abuse cases fall under criminal law.

Negligence is the performance of an act that a reasonable person under the same circumstances would not perform. Malpractice can be considered a form of negligence and can be considered intentional or unintentional. Overall, malpractice can refer to any unprofessional, illegal, or immoral conduct. Malpractice is the dereliction of duty, resulting in injury to the patient. Box 4-4 lists the most common errors in veterinary practice that can result in malpractice claims.

Consent

By definition, consent is the voluntary acceptance or agreement to what is planned or is done by another person. Informed consent is when a veterinary practice has given information to a client regarding the proposed treatment, allowing the client to make an informed decision regarding whether to proceed with a treatment. Courts have established several elements that must be fully addressed to have complete informed consent. The consent must be given freely, and the treatment and diagnosis must be given in understandable terms. The risks, benefits, and prognosis of the defined procedure must be stated as well as the prognosis if no treatment is elected. The practice must provide a statement of alternative treatments or procedures along with the risks, benefits, and cost of each. The client must be given the right to ask questions and have them answered. See Figure 2-10, *A* through *K,* for a variety of sample consent forms. Figure 4-2 is an example of an informed consent form; the pet owner and technician sign each section together after the risks and benefits have been discussed with the owner.

If an informed consent is challenged in a court of law and these conditions have not been met, the court may conclude that the client did not consent to the procedure and the veterinarian may be held liable. Documentation of the discussion must be in the record. If a record does not indicate that risks were discussed, the court may assume the discussion did not occur. A signed consent form does not indicate that an informed consent occurred because many people sign consent forms without reading them. Therefore a verbal discussion must occur. Practices should never rely on clients who state "do what is best" because this is not an informed consent; they have not been educated on the risks and benefits of the procedure. The average client does not possess the skill or knowledge to make informed decisions without all the available information.

Information should be given to clients in a manner that they can understand. Each client should be evaluated for the level of education, skill, and knowledge that he or she possesses with which to comprehend the information. It may be questioned of minors or those whose reasoning or judgment is impaired (by mental illness, intoxication, mental retardation, etc.) whether their understanding of the information is valid; acceptance of consent should be made with caution in these cases.

The best consent form available is one that is tailored to specific clients and procedure being recommended. If anesthesia is advised to complete a procedure, the consent form should clearly indicate that death is a risk. A blank should be placed next to that statement for both the client and the team member reviewing the consent form to sign. All risks, benefits, and prognoses should be listed as such and initialed by both individuals. This will help the court determine that each topic was fully addressed and that the client was fully informed before signing the form.

Box 4-4   Acts of Malpractice
• Incorrect drug administration • Incorrect strength of drug administration • Failure to clean animals that have defecated and/or urinated on themselves • Abandonment • Leaving foreign objects in patient after surgery • Failure to exercise good judgment • Failure to communicate • Loss or damage to patients personal property • Disease transmission • One patient attacking another while in the veterinary practice • Use of defective equipment or medication

> **PRACTICE POINT** Informed consent forms should be required by every practice.

Emergency Care

Veterinary practices often face the dilemma when a good samaritan brings in a pet that has been hit by a car. Can the practice treat this emergency? Who is the owner? Can the owner be contacted? Is the good samaritan going to be responsible for the bill? The first thought that most practices experience is that there is no consent to treat the animal. However, if the owners are found, they may hold the practice liable for not performing lifesaving techniques. The law of unjust enrichment allows protection for the practice if critical factors are met. If there is value to the pet, the courts may allow a recovery of cost. The more valuable the pet appears, the greater the chance of recovery. Value can be based on either economic or emotional attachment with respect to the human-animal bond. The severity of the injuries must be proven. Photographs documenting injuries and supportive treatment will help assure the client and the court that unnecessary procedures were not completed. Attempts to reach the owner must be documented in the record with the name of the person trying to make contact, phone numbers, time of the calls, as well as the number of attempts made. Once the patient is stable, only supportive care should be rendered. Plating a fracture would not be considered supportive care of a trauma patient unless it was a lifesaving technique.

ABC Veterinary Clinic
Surgery, Anesthesia, and Treatment Consent Form

Client Name _____   Patient Name _____

Date _____ Procedure _____   Male/Female

Your pet has been scheduled for a procedure requiring sedation or anesthesia. By signing this form, you authorize ABC Veterinary Clinic and its agents to administer tranquilizers, anesthetics, and analgesics that are deemed appropriate. Please be aware that all drugs have a potential for adverse side effects in any particular animal. The chances of such occurrence are extremely low; however, death can result in any anesthetized patient.

Owner initials _____ Tech initials _____

In an effort to ensure your pet's safety and to anticipate any problems before they occur, we advise pre-anesthetic bloodwork and electrocardiogram prior to anesthesia. Bloodwork will determine the kidney and liver functions, which participate in the metabolism of anesthesia. An electrocardiogram can detect abnormal arrhythmias, heart rate, and conductivity.

I accept/decline bloodwork   I accept/decline an electrocardiogram

Owner initials _____ Tech initials _____

IV fluids are advised for all patients undergoing anesthesia. IV fluids help maintain blood pressure of the patient while offering support for the kidneys to metabolize the medications. Pets may take longer to recover without IV fluids.

I accept/decline IV fluids

Owner initials _____ Tech initials _____

Heartworm tests are recommended for dogs over 6 months of age. Heartworm disease can cause anesthetic complications. We advise FeLV/FIV testing for cats. FeLV or FIV infection can delay healing of any surgical site.

I accept/decline heartworm test   I accept/decline FeLV/FIV test

Owner initials _____ Tech initials _____

Vaccinations are important for disease prevention in your pet. We advise that pets be current on vaccines. Rabies vaccination is required by law; every pet must receive a rabies vaccine.

Vaccines due (booster?): DHPP FVRCP FeLV   Rabies

Owner Initials _____ Tech Initials _____

FIGURE 4-2 Sample informed consent form.

Did pet eat this morning?	Yes	No
Has pet had any allergies or vaccine reactions in the past?	Yes	No
Are we declawing the pet?	Yes	No
Are we removing dewclaws?	Yes	No
Does the pet have 2 testicles?	Yes	No
If the pet is pregnant, can we continue with surgery?	Yes	No
Does the pet have an umbilical hernia?	Yes	No
May we repair?	Yes	No
Does the pet have retained teeth?	Yes	No
May we remove?	Yes	No
Does the pet need an Elizabethan collar?	Yes	No
Dental: OK to extract teeth?	Yes	No
OK to take dental radiographs if indicated?	Yes	No
OK to apply Doxirobe gel if indicated?	Yes	No
Is pet currently on antibiotics?	Yes	No
When was last dose? _____		
How many pills are left? _____		
Growth Removal: Histopath?	Yes	No
Location of growths: _____		

You may contact me **today** at: _____

Alternative contact phone number: _____

I understand that anesthesia is a risk and authorize the above procedures. I understand that I will be contacted first if any changes in the discussed protocol occur.

Client signature _____ Date _____

FIGURE 4-2, cont'd

Many times, the only way for a practice to recover the costs associated with emergency care is to take the client to court (if the owner was identified). This has led to many practices refusing to treat animals without owners. There is no law that states that practices must treat; in fact, duty to treat is only initiated once a valid client-patient relationship has been established. Once a valid client-patient relationship has been established, a practice must continue the treatment until the animal recovers, the veterinarian has completed all the treatments agreed upon, the patient dies, or the client terminates the client-patient relationship.

Treatment can be declined by the practice because of the client's inability to pay; however, once treatment has begun, it is extremely difficult to terminate treatment if the result would be neglect or harm to the animal. If treatment by the veterinarian must be terminated for any reason, including nonpayment of services, the veterinarian should make a good faith effort to find a veterinarian that will continue the treatment.

Veterinary practices are ethically obligated to provide emergency services to their clients after hours (as stated in the AVMA Code of Ethics); if they do not provide services themselves, they must refer their clients to a location that accepts emergencies after hours.

Malpractice

Lawsuits against veterinarians and veterinary technicians are almost always based on neglect versus breach of contract, defamation, or breach of warranty.

Negligence is defined as performing an act that a person of ordinary prudence would not have done under similar circumstances (or failure to perform an act that a person of ordinary prudence would have done). If a veterinarian or technician is sued for negligence, four basic elements must be proven in the court of law. The first is the establishment of a valid client-patient relationship. This is rarely an issue because most client-patient relationships were established when the patient was presented to the practice by the owner. Second, breach of duty must be proven. *Breach of duty* is the failure of the veterinarian or technician to act in accordance with the standard of care. This breach can occur by either performing an act that should not have been performed or not performing an act that should have been performed. Third, *proximate cause* must be established. Proximate cause is the connection between the negligent act of the veterinarian and/or technician and the harm to the patient caused by the act. Fourth, damages or harm incurred by the patient as a result of the negligent act must be displayed.

> **PRACTICE POINT** Technicians who do not show up for weekend treatments can be held liable for negligence.

The *standard of care* can be defined as the duty to exercise the care and diligence that is ordinarily exercised by a reasonably competent veterinarian under normal circumstances. With the availability of specialists in many metropolitan and suburban areas around the United States, the standard of care will be held to the specialist level. This means that veterinarians should refer or recommend referrals to a specialty center when a case is complex and requires the intervention of a specialist. Veterinarians may be held liable if they do not make the recommendation and/or not document the referral recommendation in the record. If the client declines the referral, the declined treatment should be documented clearly.

> **PRACTICE POINT** If a client declines a referral to a specialist, the refusal must be documented in the record.

To help avoid a malpractice lawsuit against a veterinarian or practice, several topics can be addressed with team members. Medical records must be complete, with every detail of the case. "If it is not in the record, it did not happen," is a common statement in the court of law. Every treatment and recommendation must be clearly documented along with any refusals the client has made. Clients must be informed when making decisions, and proof of informed consent must be included in the record. If a patient is in need of a higher level of care, the veterinarian must advise referral of the case. Should the client decline, it should be clearly documented in the record.

Most veterinarians purchase liability insurance through AVMA, which is supported by Professional Liability Insurance Trust (PLIT). This insurance provides coverage for veterinarians, veterinary technicians, and support staff who are engaged in activities involved in the practice. Each veterinarian in the practice must carry his or her own liability insurance.

Abandoned Animals

Many animals are left at practices unclaimed, especially puppies with parvovirus or other incurable or expensive ailment. Practices may make repeated attempts to contact the owner, to which no replies are made. Because a valid client-patient relationship was developed when the owner dropped off the pet, the practice is responsible for providing treatment that will prevent harm or neglect to the patient. The practice is not required to perform lifesaving techniques; however, the pet cannot receive injury by withholding treatment. After repeated attempts to contact the owner, a certified letter should be sent to the owner indicating the confirmation of abandonment of the pet. Local and state laws should be reviewed indicating the length of time the practice is required to hold the pet to confirm abandonment. A second certified letter may be required by some localities. If there is no response from the owner within the stated time, the pet can be considered abandoned and the practice can make the pet available for adoption or euthanize it, whichever provides the best outcome for the practice.

> **PRACTICE POINT** Repeated attempts must be made to contact the owner of an abandoned animal.

Impending Laws

Local laws have been amended in several cities that animals may no longer be considered to be owned, but rather to be cared for by guardians. This can affect the veterinarian-client relationship in many ways. In human cases, a guardian is generally given that authority or designation to care for a person who is a minor, incapacitated, or disabled. A *guardian ad litem* is a person appointed to protect the interests of a minor or legally incompetent person in a lawsuit or, in this case, an animal.

Change in the status of owner to guardian can present many issues. Who will determine what is best for the animal—the guardian or veterinarian? Could the veterinarian be sued for wrongful death on behalf of the pet? Other questions will certainly be raised as well as concerns for animal abuse or neglect by veterinarians. If a veterinarian does not immediately provide pain relief for an animal or send home postoperative pain medication, the practice may be held liable for neglect.

Many have questioned the validity of this change, and many questions remain unanswered. Practices must stay abreast of both city and state laws and the amendments made in them to ensure that the veterinarian is protected while administering professional care.

Medical Records

The laws concerning the legal ownership of records vary from state to state; however, in general, medical records are owned by the practice, not the pet owner. The owner can request a copy of the medical record at anytime. In fact, most clients request copies of records when they are changing veterinary hospitals.

> **PRACTICE POINT** The veterinary practice, not the client, owns the medical record.

Clients should sign a medical record release for medical records to be copied and released to someone other than the client. This includes faxing records to other hospitals, boarding facilities, or new owners. The only time medical records should be released without a consent is if the patient has a reportable disease that must be reported to the state or U.S. Department of Agriculture.

It should be kept in mind that medical records are legal documents. Therefore they must be legible at all times. Medical records are generated to ensure consistent and accurate care as well as protect the veterinarian in the event of a malpractice suit. Inaccurate, illegible medical records could be interpreted as professional incompetence with substandard care. It must also be remembered: if it was not written down, it did not occur.

If mistakes are written in a record, a single line should be drawn though the mistake, initialed, and corrected. Correction fluid or scratch-outs should not be permitted because this could be interpreted as altering of records, rendering them inadmissible in the court of law (see Chapter 14 for more information on medical records).

MOST COMMON COMPLAINTS TO THE BOARD OF VETERINARY MEDICINE

A complaint is a formal action noting dissatisfaction with the services of a licensed veterinarian or credentialed veterinary technician. A complaint is filed with the state veterinary board office, which then sends a letter to the veterinarian and/or technician. An investigator is assigned to the case and completes all needed interviews and record reviews. The complaint is reviewed by the review committee, who then submits it to the board. The board takes ultimate action against the veterinarian or technician and can dismiss the case or settle the case without a hearing (continuing education and fines may be imposed). If the complaint is found to be severe, a Notice of Contemplated Action is sent requesting a

hearing. The result of the hearing may impose continuing education, fines, license suspension, or revocation. All decisions can be appealed.

Owners tend to file complaints because of dissatisfaction resulting from experiences at the practice. Dissatisfaction may come from service that displeased them or did not fulfill their expectations. Many times, clients are unsatisfied with a treatment that their pets received. For example, a cast or splint may have been too tight, resulting in cast or bandaging sores. A common complaint is that a pet chewed a cast off and removed the sutures or staples without the veterinary team having warned the owner to keep the pet from chewing. Many times, the wrong medication is dispensed, infuriating owners.

Occasionally, a patient incurs severe trauma, necessitating the team to become dedicated to taking care of the patient's immediate needs. The aftercare and prognosis of the pet are the last items communicated to the owner and are often forgotten. Many clients become upset that they spent so much money saving a pet. They feel that if they had only known the prognosis and the amount of aftercare required, they may have chosen to euthanize the pet instead. The entire treatment process, from the immediate care to the year after the trauma, must be communicated to the owner and documented in the record to prevent this complaint from arising.

Clients are often unhappy with the results of a surgery or treatment. Many fractures do not heal properly, and the client believes the veterinarian is responsible. The team must recommend the best procedure available to repair fractures, regardless of whether the practice provides that procedure. If possible, the patient should be referred to a practice that is able to provide the best possible procedure. If the client declines the referral and opts for the lesser treatment, it must be noted in the record. The recommendation should also be written on a release sheet that the owner signs when the patient is discharged; this provides proof that the owner was made aware of the recommendation.

The unexpected death of a patient is also a common complaint. If a client brings a pet to the practice for treatment, regardless of the use of anesthesia, a treatment authorization form must be signed by the owner. As stated above, an informed consent **must** be discussed with the owner, listing the risks and benefits of treatments or procedures. The client must be fully informed that death may result. A simple blood draw on an unhealthy cat can induce a sudden, unexpected death. It is imperative that risks be discussed with the owner.

Team members treating clients disrespectfully loses clients for the practice and can result in formal complaints. Disrespect may include being rude to a client, not listening to client wishes, or not returning a client's phone calls.

Many clients are unsatisfied with the invoice at the end of the procedure. Estimates must be provided to owners at all times, regardless of whether the information is given over the phone or in the examination room. The estimate copy must remain in the medical record for future referencing. If the estimate should change in any way, the client must be notified immediately of the impending change. If services were not approved by the owner, a formal complaint may be filed.

Poor communication is the top complaint. Communication is integral to most aspects of the veterinary practice, from the receptionist to the veterinarian. Many times, veterinary technicians relay too much information and overstep their professional boundaries. Veterinary technicians cannot diagnose a disease; only veterinarians are permitted to do so. In the process of providing information to the client before the veterinarian has seen the case, the technician may give incorrect or invalid information. The different information provided by the veterinarian and veterinary technician can confuse the client, resulting in a complaint

When patients are discharged from the hospital, a signed copy of the information provided must remain with the record; this covers the practice if clients state they did not receive the information. When the patient is discharged, the team member must ensure that the client fully understands the instructions and can medicate the patient as advised.

Conduct, record keeping, premises, and pharmaceutical violations are four common violations given in veterinary medicine. Correct conduct is defined as

> Veterinarians shall exercise the same degree of care, skill, and diligence in treating patients as are ordinarily used in the same or similar circumstances by reasonably prudent members of the veterinary medical profession in good standing. A veterinarian shall not use or participate in any form of representation or advertising or solicitation which contains false, deceptive, or misleading statements or claims.
>
> Record keeping is a difficult challenge for many practices; however, records must be fully completed to avoid a violation [see Chapter 14].

The most common premises violation is that a surgery room must be a room separate and distinct from all other rooms that is reserved for aseptic surgical procedures requiring aseptic preparation. Only items used for surgical procedures may be kept in the surgical room. Dental machines cannot be stored in the surgical room because they are not part of an aseptic procedure.

Veterinarians should honor a client's request to dispense or provide a written prescription for a drug that has been determined by the veterinarian to be appropriate

What Would You Do/Not Do?

Fluffy was admitted to the hospital for lab work because she "was not feeling right." Teresa, the technician admitting the case, was advised by Dr. Mortinger to perform a complete blood count and chemistry panel, radiographs, and a urinalysis. Teresa reviewed the medical record as she placed the test results in the folder. She did not see an estimate for the services that were recommended and asked Dr. Mortinger if an estimate had been provided, because it is practice policy. Dr. Mortinger said the clients advised her that they did not need an estimate. "Do whatever is needed," was their reply. Since the bloodwork returned normal results, with slight abnormalities in the radiographs and urinalysis, the veterinarian advised an ultrasound of the abdomen. The owners agreed and said "Do whatever is needed" yet again. The ultrasound revealed a tumor in the bladder, with high suspicion of a transitional cell carcinoma. The veterinarian called the owners to deliver the news, who were devastated that their dog had cancer. "She was just in to see you last month for her yearly exam! How could you have missed this on her exam, Dr. Mortinger?" The owners were on their way to the practice to pick up Fluffy.

Once the owners arrived, Lori, the receptionist, reviewed the invoice with the owners before the pet was released. The owners were enraged at the price of the invoice and refused to pay for the services. "We did not authorize those services! You just wait," exclaimed Mrs. Smith. "Not only did Dr. Mortinger miss cancer in my dog last month, she ran tests I did not know about! I WILL file a complaint, and I am going to sue her!"

What Should the Team Members Have Done?

First, since it was practice policy, an estimate should have been created initially, regardless of whether the owners believed that they did not need one. An estimate lists all the advised services along with a cost. Second, when Teresa noticed that an estimate had not been provided, she should have made one and called the owner with an updated estimate when the ultrasound was approved. Third, if Lori had placed the owner in a room, other clients would not have heard the outburst of Mrs. Smith.

An estimate may have prevented the shock regarding costs and would have clearly listed the services. The owners may have responded differently had communication been clearer. At this point in the conversation, it would be wise to place the Smith family into a room and have a veterinarian explain the history of bladder tumors and provide written information regarding treatment options. This may defuse the anger, allowing the client to understand that this type of tumor is not usually diagnosed on a yearly exam.

If the client wants to file a complaint with the state board of veterinary medicine and continue with a suit of malpractice or negligence, the professional liability company must be contacted for further information. The case should no longer be discussed with the client.

VETERINARY PRACTICE and the LAW

Two elements are important to avoid malpractice suits. The first is to implement proper procedures to prevent mistakes. Team members must be trained appropriately to operate equipment and perform tests correctly. Staff must also understand the importance of cleaning spills or urine on the floor immediately to prevent a client or team member from slipping or falling. Safety plans must be instituted for clients, patients, and team members.

A second important element in avoiding malpractice suits is to prevent clients from becoming angry about the care their pets are receiving. Every team member must be respectful and courteous to every client, provide written and verbal information on the patient's condition, and communicate effectively on every level. Estimates must be given, frequent phone calls must be made updating clients of a pet's condition, and accurate interpretation of laboratory results must be provided; these are essential for the prevention of lawsuits. The importance of demonstrating respect and concern for all patients and clients at all times must be instilled into all team members.

To prevent malpractice lawsuits, use the following procedures to prevent mistakes:

- Ensure all equipment is in proper working condition.
- Provide a current employee procedure manual that allows team members to review the correct completion of procedures.
- Use informed consents; ensure clients fully understand the risks and benefits of all procedures to be completed on the patient.
- Document conversations, procedures, and recommendations completely and clearly in the record.
- **Protect patients from injury.**
- Label all specimen samples correctly.
- Post signs indicating a wet floor.
- Never guarantee an outcome.
- Follow up on all patients after surgery or procedures.

for the patient. Therefore clients who wish to purchase medication on the Internet must be provided with a prescription (at their request). Those who do not fulfill the request are in violation.

Many other complaints arise in veterinary medicine for malpractice and negligence; however, the above listed are the most common ones that can be easily prevented by the veterinary health care team. Every team member must provide courteous customer service with valid, factual information. Communication must be the priority of the entire team, specifically regarding any changes to estimates, treatment plans, or increased wait times to clients.

Self-Evaluation Questions

1. Define civil law.
2. Define contract law.
3. Define negligence.
4. Define malpractice.
5. Why are ethics important to the veterinary profession?
6. Why is an informed consent imperative?
7. Why would a consent form be upheld in court?
8. What branch of law does animal abuse fall under?
9. What is PLIT? Whom does it cover?
10. Why is medical record legibility important?

Recommended Reading

Pratt PW, Rollin BE, Picut CA: *Principles and practice of veterinary technology,* Chapter 3, St Louis, 1998, Mosby.

Wilson JF: *Laws and ethics for the veterinary profession,* Yardley, PA, 1990, Priority Press.

Wilson JF, Fishman AJ, Nemder JD: *Contracts, benefits, and practice management for the veterinary profession,* Yardley, PA, 2002, Priority Press.

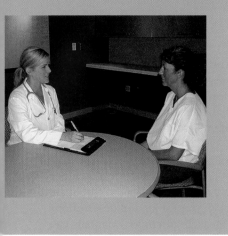

CHAPTER 5

Human Resources

Chapter Outline

Organizational Behavior
Hiring the Perfect Team
  Reviewing Resumes
  Reviewing Letters of Reference
  Asking the Right Questions
  Questions Not to Ask
  Pre-employment Screening
  References
  The First Day With a Number 10
Laws That Require Familiarity
  Fair Labor and Standards Act
  Family and Medical Leave Act
  Uniformed Services Employment and Reemployment Rights Act
  Immigration Reform and Control Act
  Employee Polygraph Protection Act
Equal Employment Opportunity
  Occupational Safety and Health Administration
  Pregnancy and Maternity Leave
  Required Posters
Employee Manual
  Developing an Employee Manual

Employee Procedure Manual
  Developing an Employee Procedure Manual
  Implementing an Employee Procedure Manual
  Updating the Employee Procedure Manual
Payroll
  Determining Staff Wages
  Determining Raises
  Managing Payroll
  Payroll Taxes
Personnel Files
Contract Employee Versus Employee
Team Training
  Developing a Training Protocol
  Providing All Levels of Continuing Education
  Role-Playing
  Methods to Retain Employees
Workers' Compensation Insurance
Theft and Embezzlement
Termination
Troubleshooting and Problem-Solving Skills

Learning Objectives

Mastery of the content in this chapter will enable the reader to:
- Compare and review resumes.
- Discuss methods used to interview candidates effectively.
- Describe questions that can legally be asked of candidates.
- Clarify specific laws associated with human resources.
- Identify required posters.
- Develop an employee personnel manual.
- Develop an employee procedure manual.

- Calculate staff wages when hiring new employees.
- Calculate raises.
- Efficiently manage payroll and calculate taxes.
- Explain how to maintain payroll files.
- Develop team training protocols.
- List methods used to effectively terminate team members.

Key Terms

401(k)
Benefits
COBRA
Contract Employee
Direct Deposit
Employee Manual
Employee Polygraph Protection Act
Employee Procedure Manual
Equal Employment Opportunity
ERISA

Fair Credit and Reporting Act
FLSA
FMLA
FUTA
IRCA
MISC-1099
Mission Statement
Noncompete Agreement
Organizational Behavior
OSHA

References
Resume
SEPS
sIRA
USERRA
W-2
W-4
Workers' Compensation Insurance

ORGANIZATIONAL BEHAVIOR

Basic management of a veterinary practice includes organizational development and employee development. Organizational development is the development, improvement, and effectiveness of an organization and includes the culture, values, system, and behaviors of such practice. Employee development helps improve the vision, empowerment, learning, and problem-solving abilities of employees.

The vision of such practice is built by a team and shared by a team. All team members should know what the vision of the practice is and live it on a daily basis. The vision can be reevaluated by the team each year, making changes if necessary. With vision comes structure, practice culture, norms, codes of conduct, and core values. The culture created should be positive and happy and provide an open communication policy for all employees. A code of conduct can be established and written in the employee manual, allowing all employees to know what is expected of them.

Team development is essential to the success of a practice. Creating the perfect team takes time and begins with correct hiring procedures. Job descriptions must be correct and job duties should be clear, allowing potential and current employees to know what is expected of them. Retaining the perfect team is of upmost importance and must be a top priority for the practice. Encouraging teamwork and motivation will help ensure a high retention rate, as do positive feedback and evaluations for all team members. Effective organizations have teams, not individuals.

Team members should be encouraged to communicate with practice management, clients, and other team members. Team meetings can help facilitate communication among employees and allow discussion of protocols and procedures. Meetings should run on time and be as effective as possible in the short time allotted. Communication with clients is essential because this is where most client dissatisfaction occurs. Exceptional client communication increases client compliance because they can accept the recommendations made by the team more easily.

Development of employee and procedure manuals may take time, but they greatly increase the efficiency and communication of a practice. By allowing the team to help create the manuals, fewer duties and descriptions are forgotten and more ideas are included. Manuals can help hold the team together and allow greater leadership in all areas of the practice. When a team creates manuals together, implementing and using them is achieved with greater success.

HIRING THE PERFECT TEAM

Hiring a team of "10s" can make a practice successful and take it to the next level. An employee who is a 1 can break a practice. An 8 or a 9 can be molded into a 10, but a 7 or lower can be difficult to manage. If a practice is going to achieve the goals and dreams that it has set as its mission, then a team of 10s must be hired. Practices can hire for personality and work ethic and train for the skill that is needed. One cannot hire for skill and train personality or work ethic. Team members have it or they do not, and it is useless to hire an unmotivated person. Unmotivated and irritable staff members affect all team members and create a negative environment. This can be detrimental to a practice and should be avoided at all costs.

PRACTICE POINT A "10" employee is the most efficient and effective employee a practice can have.

What Would You Do/Not Do?

It has been brought to the attention of a practice manager that inappropriate behavior may have occurred between team members at a recent continuing education seminar held out of town. Rumor has it that a male veterinarian and a female veterinary technician had a couple of alcoholic beverages and shared a room together. Other team members who attended the seminar with the pair felt that this gave the technician an advantage over them and that favoritism may occur from this point on.

What Should a Practice Manager Do?

First, the employee manual must be consulted to see if any reference is made to sexual relations between employees. If no reference is made, nothing can be done. If the manual covers this topic, then both team members should be interviewed individually to verify the rumor. The interview may reveal that the rumor was false; however, if the rumor is true, both team members must be sanctioned as outlined in the employee manual. Third, a team meeting should be held outlining the employee manual and communicating the expectations of all team members. Open communication must be a top priority to prevent events such as this from occurring.

Leaders are only as good as their weakest player. If a team member is only rated as a 1 or a 2 on a 10-point scale, the leadership may only be as good as a 1 or a 2. What happens when the problem is not fixed? The 9s and 10s begin to resent the fact and become less effective, doubt the leader's abilities, and break down the team. Any 5s or 6s should be eliminated and replaced with 8s or 9s.

Reviewing Resumes

Applicants may provide a resume for review when applying for a position within the hospital. Resumes should be short and to the point, with applicants clearly stating what they are looking for in a position. Do not make notes on resumes because they remain part of the personnel file if the applicant is hired. Notes should be made on a separate piece of paper. Also remember that the threat involving claims of discrimination in the hiring process is real, so good defensive tactics must be practiced throughout the entire hiring process.

Reviewing Letters of Reference

It is important to follow up on any letter of reference. Some letters are written to ease a difficult termination; others may have been unwilling to express any reservations that were held at the time of the employee resignation or termination. An outstanding letter of reference is not always that. Phone calls are advised on all applicants; one candidate cannot be treated differently from another.

Asking the Right Questions

With a team of 10s in mind, it is essential to ask the right questions when interviewing potential candidates (Figure 5-1). Questions such as "Tell me about yourself," "What do you know about our practice?" and "What is

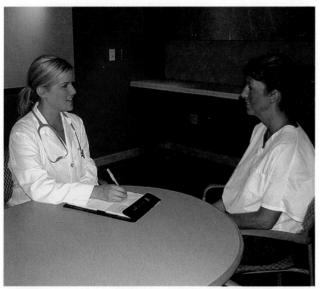

FIGURE 5-1 Specific questions must be asked in an interview to determine if a candidate is right for the practice.

your single greatest achievement?" stimulate discussion instead of elicit a yes or no answer. "Describe a typical day in your last job," promotes discussion regarding work ethic. Questions should prompt the candidate to show his or her skill and potential. Open-ended questions allow the applicant to discuss the question asked. *What, when, where, why,* and *how* are excellent words to use when asking an open-ended question. Every person believes he or she has an excellent work ethic and a great personality; the interviewer must be able to distinguish whether this is true. Closed-ended questions allow only a yes or no answer (Box 5-1).

> **PRACTICE POINT** Many questions are considered illegal and may not be asked during an interview.

A working interview can also help determine an individual's work ethic and skill. Many applicants may state they are qualified for the position, and a working interview will help determine whether certain skills are met. It is important to remember what questions cannot be asked during this working interview (see below).

One may also ask candidates if previous employers can be called; answers may provide a clue to the past employment history. Once employers are called, an important question to ask is, "Would you rehire this person?" The response can provide valuable information regarding the candidate.

Questions Not to Ask

The hiring process is highly regulated by federal and state laws. These laws exist for the protection of potential employees. Many questions cannot be asked in an interview. Any questions related to marriage, age, gender, religion, and military status are strictly prohibited. The interviewer cannot ask female applicants different questions than male applicants and cannot ask if they have any children. See Box 5-2 for a list of questions that cannot be asked.

Box 5-1	Asking the Right Questions

- Are you currently employed? Why or why not?
- How long have you been employed at your current job?
- Why would you want to leave your current position?
- Describe a typical day at your last job.
- What did you enjoy about your past job?
- What position do you expect to fill?
- If you joined our team, what abilities would you bring?
- Describe your summer employment.
- What do you feel are your outstanding qualities?
- What was the least enjoyable aspect of your last job?
- What are some areas you feel you need improvement on?
- Are you able to work a weekend schedule?
- When would you be available to begin work?
- What is your salary requirement?

Box 5-2	Questions NOT to Ask

- Do you have any children?
- What is your national origin?
- Where are your parents from?
- What is your maiden name?
- Have you ever been arrested?
- Do you have any physical disabilities?
- Have your wages ever been garnished?
- What type of military service have you been involved with?
- What is your native language?
- What clubs and societies do you belong to?
- Have you ever filed for Workers' Compensation?
- What is your religion?
- What holidays do you observe?
- Do you prefer to be addressed as Ms., Miss, or Mrs.?
- When did you graduate from high school?

Pre-employment Screening

The Fair Credit Reporting Act is a federal law that regulates prescreening reports issued to employers by outside agencies called *credit reporting agencies*. Employers may use these consumer reports to help screen employees. These can also be referred to as part of a background check. Background checks are a matter of public record; however, employers must have the consent of the applicant.

> **PRACTICE POINT**   Candidates must give consent to a potential employer before a background check can be completed.

Practices can also administer a grammar and/or spelling test, perhaps including some medical terminology. A typing test may also be appropriate if the position includes a large amount of typing or transcription services.

References

It is imperative to call all references listed. If a candidate has not provided a list of references with the resume and/or application, one should be asked for at the time of the interview. It can be difficult to obtain useful information when calling references. Because of the increase in defamation lawsuits, past employers are reluctant to provide any information, either positive or negative. Information that is permissible must be factual and documented in written evidence. All references on all candidates should be checked, and the same questions should be asked. One applicant cannot be treated differently from another. Calling references can also reveal discrepancies with the applicant's resume and/or interview.

The First Day With a Number 10

A new team member's first day can be intimidating, overwhelming, and daunting. The employee should be introduced to the rest of the staff, given a tour of the practice, and then taken to a quiet area to review practice policy and procedures. The new employee should fill out new-hire forms, including a W-4 (federal income tax withholding form), state tax forms (if required), I-9 (employment eligibility verification form), forms for accepting or declining any employee benefit plans, and emergency contact information. Copies of any credentials should be made at this time. The employee should receive his or her own copy of the employee personnel manual, review it verbally with a manager, and sign a document stating he or she has received, read, and understands the manual.

> **PRACTICE POINT**   The first day for a new team member should be comfortable and rewarding.

The new team member should be given a copy of the procedure manual and reassured that he or she is not expected to know all the information within the manual on the first day. The phase training program that the hospital has implemented should be explained, along with the expected dates of completion. The new employee should be allowed to observe the whole team for the rest of the day and encouraged to ask questions. Hands-on training can begin the following day. Taking the new employee to lunch adds a personal touch to the day. Team members can ask questions and learn about each other out of the office.

LAWS THAT REQUIRE FAMILIARITY

Many laws and regulations apply to veterinary medicine. Laws and regulations change on a regular basis at both the federal and state levels. Every practice manager and office manager should be familiar with changes that occur, update the team with changes, and add or modify the personnel manual as needed (Box 5-3).

Fair Labor and Standards Act

The Fair Labor and Standards Act (FLSA) was created to establish minimum wage and overtime pay standards as well as regulate the employment of minors. State minimum wage may be more or less than the federal minimum wage; whichever is higher supersedes the other. Minimum wage changes periodically and managers

Box 5-3	Laws With Which to Be Familiar

- Family and Medical Leave Act
- Uniformed Services Employment and Reemployment Rights Act
- Fair Labor and Standards Act
- Equal Employment Opportunity
- Occupational Safety and Health Administration
- Immigration Reform and Control Act
- Employee Polygraph Protection Act

should be aware of changes. Any employee working more than 40 hours within 1 work week must be paid overtime at 1.5 times the regular rate of pay. The FLSA makes reference to a work week as 7 consecutive, regularly recurring, 24-hour periods totaling 168 hours. For the first 40 hours worked in any given work week, each employee must be paid at least minimum wage. Overtime pay must be paid for any hours worked above 40 in a given week at the stated hourly wage.

An exemption to overtime pay applies to any individual involved in executive, administrative, or professional duties. In the case of a professional employee, at least 80% of the duties must require knowledge of an advanced type of science or learning, artistic work, or teaching. Veterinarians and some practice managers are exempt from overtime. It is imperative to monitor team member hours because staff in veterinary medicine often work longer and harder than allowed. Excess hours lead to burnout. Prevention of burnout is imperative or the employee retention rate will drop dramatically. Technicians who work on a salary basis must also receive overtime pay for any hours accumulated after 40 hours. Technicians are not exempt from overtime regardless of salary status. Practices can receive large fines from the Department of Labor for not paying team members overtime.

Another exemption to FLSA is full-time students (who may be paid at 85% of minimum wage), apprentices, or handicapped workers. The Wage and Hour Division of the U.S. Department of Labor issues certificates of exemptions, which must be applied for by the employer, to pay wages less than minimum wage.

Employees must be at least 16 years of age to work in non–farm-related jobs; youths who are 14 or 15 may be allowed to work outside school hours with a work permit. They are allowed to work only 3 hours per day during school days and 8 hours per day on non-school days. Work cannot begin before 7 AM and cannot end after 7 PM. During the summer, hours are extended until 9 PM. Work permits can generally be obtained from the school district that the child is enrolled in.

Employers are required to keep records on wages and hours for a minimum of 3 years.

Family and Medical Leave Act

The Family and Medical Leave Act (FMLA) was established in 1993 to protect and preserve the integrity of the family. It was designed to benefit employees without adversely affecting employers. It allows employees to take up to 12 weeks of unpaid leave for the birth and care of a newborn child of the employee; for placement with the employee of a son or daughter for adoption or foster care; to care for an immediate family member (spouse, child, or parent) with a serious health condition; or to take medical leave when the employee is unable to work because of a serious health condition. The employee is guaranteed his or her job, or an equivalent one, upon return to work.

Employees must have worked for the organization for at least 12 months, with at least 1250 hours acquired during those 12 months. The employee must give the employer at least 30 days notice before leaving regarding when the period will begin and end. If these requirements are not met, the employer can deny the leave. FMLA applies to organizations with more than 50 employees; an organization with fewer employees is exempt from the act.

Uniformed Services Employment and Reemployment Rights Act

The Uniformed Services Employment and Reemployment Rights Act (USERRA) was created to protect individuals who are enrolled in any branch of the military service. USERRA protects the rights of employees who voluntarily or involuntarily leave an employment position to undertake any military service. Employers cannot discriminate against past, present, and potential employees who are uniformed service members. Employees have the right to return to the employment position they had before leaving as well as any benefits that are or were available at that time.

> **PRACTICE POINT** Team members who are in the military cannot be discriminated against and must be able to retain their positions upon returning from a tour of duty.

Immigration Reform and Control Act

The Immigration Reform and Control Act (IRCA) prohibits employer discrimination against any employee or potential employee because of national origin. I-9 forms should be filled out by new hires to confirm that they can legally work in the United States. The I-9 form is required to be completed by employers and states that the employer has examined the required documents verifying employment eligibility (Figure 5-2) (see the Evolve site accompanying this text for the complete form). Documents to verify include a birth or naturalization certificate, a U.S. passport, a valid foreign exchange passport authorizing employment in the United States, a resident alien card (green card), Social Security card, and driver's license or state identification card. The documents should be photocopied and kept in the personnel file. The I-9 form must be kept for 3 years from the date of hire, or 1 year after termination, whichever is longer.

Employee Polygraph Protection Act

The Employee Polygraph Protection Act prohibits most employers from using lie detector tests for either pre-employment screening or during the course of employment. Employers cannot discriminate against employees who refuse to take a lie detector test. An exemption does apply to a practice that prescribes and dispenses controlled substances. It is advised to review this law further

OMB No. 1615-0047; Expires 06/30/09

Department of Homeland Security
U.S. Citizenship and Immigration Services

Form I-9, Employment Eligibility Verification

Instructions

Please read all instructions carefully before completing this form.

Anti-Discrimination Notice. It is illegal to discriminate against any individual (other than an alien not authorized to work in the U.S.) in hiring, discharging, or recruiting or referring for a fee because of that individual's national origin or citizenship status. It is illegal to discriminate against work eligible individuals. Employers **CANNOT** specify which document(s) they will accept from an employee. The refusal to hire an individual because the documents presented have a future expiration date may also constitute illegal discrimination.

What Is the Purpose of This Form?

The purpose of this form is to document that each new employee (both citizen and non-citizen) hired after November 6, 1986 is authorized to work in the United States.

When Should the Form I-9 Be Used?

All employees, citizens and noncitizens, hired after November 6, 1986 and working in the United States must complete a Form I-9.

Filling Out the Form I-9

Section 1, Employee: This part of the form must be completed at the time of hire, which is the actual beginning of employment. Providing the Social Security number is voluntary, except for employees hired by employers participating in the USCIS Electronic Employment Eligibility Verification Program (E-Verify). **The employer is responsible for ensuring that Section 1 is timely and properly completed.**

Preparer/Translator Certification. The Preparer/Translator Certification must be completed if **Section 1** is prepared by a person other than the employee. A preparer/translator may be used only when the employee is unable to complete **Section 1** on his/her own. However, the employee must still sign **Section 1** personally.

Section 2, Employer: For the purpose of completing this form, the term "employer" means all employers including those recruiters and referrers for a fee who are agricultural associations, agricultural employers or farm labor contractors.

Employers must complete **Section 2** by examining evidence of identity and employment eligibility within three (3) business days of the date employment begins. If employees are authorized to work, but are unable to present the required document(s) within three business days, they must present a receipt for the application of the document(s) within three business days and the actual document(s) within ninety (90) days. However, if employers hire individuals for a duration of less than three business days, **Section 2** must be completed at the time employment begins. **Employers must record:**

1. Document title;
2. Issuing authority;
3. Document number;
4. Expiration date, if any; and
5. The date employment begins.

Employers must sign and date the certification. Employees must present original documents. Employers may, but are not required to, photocopy the document(s) presented. These photocopies may only be used for the verification process and must be retained with the Form I-9. **However, employers are still responsible for completing and retaining the Form I-9.**

Section 3, Updating and Reverification: Employers must complete **Section 3** when updating and/or reverifying the Form I-9. Employers must reverify employment eligibility of their employees on or before the expiration date recorded in **Section 1**. Employers **CANNOT** specify which document(s) they will accept from an employee.

A. If an employee's name has changed at the time this form is being updated/reverified, complete Block A.

B. If an employee is rehired within three (3) years of the date this form was originally completed and the employee is still eligible to be employed on the same basis as previously indicated on this form (updating), complete Block B and the signature block.

C. If an employee is rehired within three (3) years of the date this form was originally completed and the employee's work authorization has expired **or** if a current employee's work authorization is about to expire (reverification), complete Block B and:

1. Examine any document that reflects that the employee is authorized to work in the U.S. (see List A **or** C);
2. Record the document title, document number and expiration date (if any) in Block C, and
3. Complete the signature block.

Form I-9 (Rev. 06/05/07) N

FIGURE 5-2 I-9 form.

for additional information as it applies to veterinary medicine.

Equal Employment Opportunity

An Equal Employment Opportunity policy prohibits discrimination against employees on the basis of race, color, sex, religion, or national origin. Employers cannot deny a promotion, terminate, or not hire a potential employee for any of those reasons. Equal Employment Opportunity also prevents discrimination of those with disabilities who can perform the job as described in the job duties. The law also requires that organizations provide to qualified applicants and employees with disabilities reasonable accommodation that does not impose undue hardship on the employer. The Age Discrimination in Employment Act of 1967 protects applicants and current employees over the age of 40 years from discrimination on the basis of age in hiring, promotion, discharge, and compensation. The Civil Rights Act of 1964, Title VII, prohibits sex discrimination in payment of wages to men and women performing substantially equal work in the same establishment.

Occupational Safety and Health Administration

The Occupational Safety and Health Administration (OSHA) has set safety standards to protect employees. Employers must provide a safe work environment and comply with safety standards set forth by OSHA (see Chapter 21 for more information). OSHA has the authority to inspect workplace environments without advance notice to the employer. Safety hazard plans should be in place to help protect employees from dangers, and they must be enforced by the employer on a daily basis.

> **PRACTICE POINT**   OSHA rules and regulations must be enforced by employers.

Pregnancy and Maternity Leave

State labor boards or commissions should be contacted to determine the most recent regulations regarding the required length of pregnancy and maternity leave. Employers cannot prohibit pregnant employees from working once risks associated with their position have been discussed. It is unlawful to exclude employees from job duties unless the claim is supported by objective, scientific evidence. If employees insist on continuing to work in a potentially harmful environment, they should sign a statement releasing the employer from liability.

Required Posters

Posters informing employees of their rights are required and must be posted in a location visible by all employees. Posters can be picked up at any local or state labor department free of charge and do not have to be purchased from solicitors. Posters required include OSHA: It's the Law, Equal Employment Opportunity, Family and Medical Leave Act of 1993, Employee Polygraph Protection Act, Immigration Reform and Control Act, the Uniformed Services Employment and Reemployment Rights Act, and the Fair Labor Act (Box 5-4; Figures 5-3 through 5-7).

Box 5-4	Posters That Must Be Displayed in a Highly Visible Area

- Occupational Safety and Health
- Equal Employment Opportunity
- Family and Medical Leave Act
- Employee Polygraph Protection Act
- Immigration Reform and Control Act
- Uniformed Services Employment and Reemployment Rights Act
- Fair Labor and Standards Act

EMPLOYEE MANUAL

An employee manual provides a guide for employees as well as a quick resource when a personnel issue arises (Figure 5-8). (See the Evolve site accompanying this text for the complete form.) A manual can solve workplace problems quickly and fairly because topics and policies have already been determined. If an employee manual has not been developed, it is important to take the time to establish one. It may be a good idea to have the practice attorney review the manual before distribution to ensure the practice is legally protected in every way possible. A court may find the employee manual to be a contract although a signed contract has not been established. Violations of the terms of the manual can be seen as a breach of contract; therefore it is important to state in the front of the manual that it is not a contract, and that the manual can be changed and updated at any time. New employees should read the manual, sign a document stating that they have received it, and understand that it is not a contract—simply a guide to employee policy. If any changes have been made, employees should read them and sign a document indicating that they have received the update (see Figure 5-7).

Each state has different laws regarding employee manuals and laws that must be covered within them. It is advisable to contact an attorney for review. Employment and labor laws change frequently, and policies and manuals must be updated to reflect these changes. Practices should reserve the right to update and modify employee manuals at any time. It is important to remain flexible, and employees should be made aware of changes as they occur; once again, it is important that they sign a form acknowledging any updates.

Developing an Employee Manual

Employee manuals should maintain a positive tone, avoiding any authoritarian manner. Their purpose is to create a positive work environment, prevent problems before they arise, and allow communication to occur freely. Many problems can be prevented by creating an atmosphere of open communication between team members and management.

> **PRACTICE POINT**   Employee personnel manuals should have a positive tone and provide guidance to the team members.

Many topics are addressed in employee manuals, including the philosophy of the practice. Every practice should have a goal that can be measured and obtained. Job descriptions and duties are essential and must be in written form so that both current and potential employees clearly understand the responsibilities associated with a given position. Benefits are generally offered by all practices, but the extent of benefits offered varies. Benefits packages can play a large role in attracting and

text continued on p. 107

U.S. DEPARTMENT OF LABOR

EMPLOYMENT STANDARDS ADMINISTRATION

Wage and Hour Division
Washington, D.C. 20210

NOTICE

EMPLOYEE POLYGRAPH PROTECTION ACT

The Employee Polygraph Protection Act prohibits most private employers from using lie detector tests either for pre-employment screening or during the course of employment.

PROHIBITIONS

Employers are generally prohibited from requiring or requesting any employee or job applicant to take a lie detector test, and from discharging, disciplining, or discriminating against an employee or prospective employee for refusing to take a test or for exercising other rights under the Act.

EXEMPTIONS*

Federal, State and local governments are not affected by the law. Also, the law does not apply to tests given by the Federal Government to certain private individuals engaged in national security-related activities.

The Act permits *polygraph* (a kind of lie detector) tests to be administered in the private sector, subject to restrictions, to certain prospective employees of security service firms (armored car, alarm, and guard), and of pharmaceutical manufacturers, distributors and dispensers.

The Act also permits polygraph testing, subject to restrictions, of certain employees of private firms who are reasonably suspected of involvement in a workplace incident (theft, embezzlement, etc.) that resulted in economic loss to the employer.

EXAMINEE RIGHTS

Where polygraph tests are permitted, they are subject to numerous strict standards concerning the conduct and length of the test. Examinees have a number of specific rights, including the right to a written notice before testing, the right to refuse or discontinue a test, and the right not to have test results disclosed to unauthorized persons.

ENFORCEMENT

The Secretary of Labor may bring court actions to restrain violations and assess civil penalties up to $10,000 against violators. Employees or job applicants may also bring their own court actions.

ADDITIONAL INFORMATION

Additional information may be obtained, and complaints of violations may be filed, at local offices of the Wage and Hour Division, which are listed in the telephone directory under U.S. Government, Department of Labor, Employment Standards Administration.

THE LAW REQUIRES EMPLOYERS TO DISPLAY THIS POSTER WHERE EMPLOYEES AND JOB APPLICANTS CAN READILY SEE IT.

*The law does not preempt any provision of any State or local law or any collective bargaining agreement which is more restrictive with respect to lie detector tests.

U.S. DEPARTMENT OF LABOR

EMPLOYMENT STANDARDS ADMINISTRATION

Wage and Hour Division
Washington, D.C. 20210

WH Publication 1462
September 1988

FIGURE 5-3 Employee Polygraph Protection Act poster.

Your Rights
under the
Family and Medical Leave Act of 1993

FMLA requires covered employers to provide up to 12 weeks of unpaid, job-protected leave to "eligible" employees for certain family and medical reasons. Employees are eligible if they have worked for their employer for at least one year, and for 1,250 hours over the previous 12 months, and if there are at least 50 employees within 75 miles. The FMLA permits employees to take leave on an intermittent basis or to work a reduced schedule under certain circumstances.

Reasons for Taking Leave:

Unpaid leave must be granted for *any* of the following reasons:

- to care for the employee's child after birth, or placement for adoption or foster care;
- to care for the employee's spouse, son or daughter, or parent who has a serious health condition; or
- for a serious health condition that makes the employee unable to perform the employee's job.

At the employee's or employer's option, certain kinds of *paid* leave may be substituted for unpaid leave.

Advance Notice and Medical Certification:

The employee may be required to provide advance leave notice and medical certification. Taking of leave may be denied if requirements are not met.

- The employee ordinarily must provide 30 days advance notice when the leave is "foreseeable."
- An employer may require medical certification to support a request for leave because of a serious health condition, and may require second or third opinions (at the employer's expense) and a fitness for duty report to return to work.

Job Benefits and Protection:

- For the duration of FMLA leave, the employer must maintain the employee's health coverage under any "group health plan."

- Upon return from FMLA leave, most employees must be restored to their original or equivalent positions with equivalent pay, benefits, and other employment terms.
- The use of FMLA leave cannot result in the loss of any employment benefit that accrued prior to the start of an employee's leave.

Unlawful Acts by Employers:

FMLA makes it unlawful for any employer to:

- interfere with, restrain, or deny the exercise of any right provided under FMLA:
- discharge or discriminate against any person for opposing any practice made unlawful by FMLA or for involvement in any proceeding under or relating to FMLA.

Enforcement:

- The U.S. Department of Labor is authorized to investigate and resolve complaints of violations.
- An eligible employee may bring a civil action against an employer for violations.

FMLA does not affect any Federal or State law prohibiting discrimination, or supersede any State or local law or collective bargaining agreement which provides greater family or medical leave rights.

For Additional Information:

If you have access to the Internet visit our FMLA website: **http://www.dol.gov/esa/whd/fmla.** To locate your nearest Wage-Hour Office, telephone our Wage-Hour toll-free information and help line at 1-866-4USWAGE (1-866-487-9243): a customer service representative is available to assist you with referral information from 8am to 5pm **in your time zone;** or log onto our Home Page at **http://www.wagehour.dol.gov**.

U.S. Department of Labor
Employment Standards Administration
Wage and Hour Division
Washington, D.C. 20210

WH Publication 1420
Revised August 2001

*U.S. GOVERNMENT PRINTING OFFICE 2001-476-344/49051

FIGURE 5-4 Family and Medical Leave Act poster.

Your Rights Under the Fair Labor Standards Act

Federal Minimum Wage

$4.75 per hour
beginning October 1, 1996

$5.15 per hour
beginning September 1, 1997

Employees under 20 years of age may be paid $4.25 per hour during their first 90 consecutive calendar days of employment with an employer.

Certain full-time students, student learners, apprentices, and workers with disabilities may be paid less than the minimum wage under special certificates issued by the Department of Labor.

<u>Tip Credit</u> – Employers of "tipped employees" must pay a cash wage of at least $2.13 per hour if they claim a tip credit against their minimum wage obligation. If an employee's tips combined with the employer's cash wage of at least $2.13 per hour do not equal the minimum hourly wage, the employer must make up the difference. Certain other conditions must also be met.

Overtime Pay

At least $1\frac{1}{2}$ times your regular rate of pay for all hours worked over 40 in a workweek.

Child Labor

An employee must be at least **16** years old to work in most non-farm jobs and at least **18** to work in non-farm jobs declared hazardous by the Secretary of Labor. Youths **14** and **15** years old may work outside school hours in various non-manufacturing, non-mining, non-hazardous jobs under the following conditions:

No more than –

- **3** hours on a school day or **18** hours in a school week;
- **8** hours on a non-school day or **40** hours in a non-school week.

Also, work may not begin before **7 a.m.** or end after **7 p.m.**, except from **June 1** through **Labor Day**, when evening hours are extended to **9 p.m.** Different rules apply in agricultural employment.

Enforcement

The Department of Labor may recover back wages either administratively or through court action, for the employees that have been underpaid in violation of the law. Violations may result in civil or criminal action.

Fines of up to $10,000 per violation may be assessed against employers who violate the child labor provisions of the law and up to $1,000 per violation against employers who willfully or repeatedly violate the minimum wage or overtime pay provisions. This law <u>prohibits</u> discriminating against or discharging workers who file a complaint or participate in any proceedings under the Act.

Note:
- Certain occupations and establishments are exempt from the minimum wage and/or overtime pay provisions.
- Special provisions apply to workers in American Samoa.
- Where state law requires a higher minimum wage, the higher standard applies.

For Additional Information, Contact the Wage and Hour Division office nearest you – listed in your telephone directory under United States Government, Labor Department.

This poster may be viewed on the Internet at this address: http://www.dol.gov/esa/regs/compliance/posters/flsa.htm

The law requires employers to display this poster where employees can readily see it.

U.S. Department of Labor
Employment Standards Administration
Wage and Hour Division
Washington, D.C. 20210

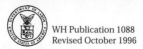

WH Publication 1088
Revised October 1996

FIGURE 5-5 Minimum wage poster.

You Have a Right to a Safe and Healthful Workplace.

IT'S THE LAW!

- You have the right to notify your employer or OSHA about workplace hazards. You may ask OSHA to keep your name confidential.

- You have the right to request an OSHA inspection if you believe that there are unsafe and unhealthful conditions in your workplace. You or your representative may participate in the inspection.

- You can file a complaint with OSHA within 30 days of discrimination by your employer for making safety and health complaints or for exercising your rights under the *OSH Act*.

- You have a right to see OSHA citations issued to your employer. Your employer must post the citations at or near the place of the alleged violation.

- Your employer must correct workplace hazards by the date indicated on the citation and must certify that these hazards have been reduced or eliminated.

- You have the right to copies of your medical records or records of your exposure to toxic and harmful substances or conditions.

- Your employer must post this notice in your workplace.

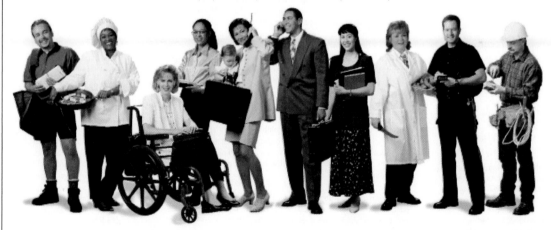

The *Occupational Safety and Health Act of 1970 (OSH Act)*, P.L. 91-596, assures safe and healthful working conditions for working men and women throughout the Nation. The Occupational Safety and Health Administration, in the U.S. Department of Labor, has the primary responsibility for administering the *OSH Act*. The rights listed here may vary depending on the particular circumstances. To file a complaint, report an emergency, or seek OSHA advice, assistance, or products, call 1-800-321-OSHA or your nearest OSHA office: • Atlanta (404) 562-2300 • Boston (617) 565-9860 • Chicago (312) 353-2220 • Dallas (214) 767-4731 • Denver (303) 844-1600 • Kansas City (816) 426-5861 • New York (212) 337-2378 • Philadelphia (215) 861-4900 • San Francisco (415) 975-4310 • Seattle (206) 553-5930. Teletypewriter (TTY) number is 1-877-889-5627. To file a complaint online or obtain more information on OSHA federal and state programs, visit OSHA's website at **www.osha.gov**. If your workplace is in a state operating under an OSHA-approved plan, your employer must post the required state equivalent of this poster.

1-800-321-OSHA
www.osha.gov

U.S. Department of Labor • Occupational Safety and Health Administration • OSHA 3165

FIGURE 5-6 Occupational Health and Safety Administration 3165 poster.

Equal Employment Opportunity is

THE LAW

Employers Holding Federal Contracts or Subcontracts

Applicants to and employees of companies with a Federal government contract or subcontract are protected under the following Federal authorities:

RACE, COLOR, RELIGION, SEX, NATIONAL ORIGIN

Executive Order 11246, as amended, prohibits job discrimination on the basis of race, color, religion, sex or national origin, and requires affirmative action to ensure equality of opportunity in all aspects of employment.

INDIVIDUALS WITH DISABILITIES

Section 503 of the Rehabilitation Act of 1973, as amended, prohibits job discrimination because of disability and requires affirmative action to employ and advance in employment qualified individuals with disabilities who, with reasonable accommodation, can perform the essential functions of a job.

VIETNAM ERA, SPECIAL DISABLED, RECENTLY SEPARATED, AND OTHER PROTECTED VETERANS

38 U.S.C. 4212 of the Vietnam Era Veterans' Readjustment Assistance Act of 1974, as amended, prohibits job discrimination and requires affirmative action to employ and advance in employment qualified Vietnam era veterans, qualified special disabled veterans, recently separarted veterans, and other protected veterans.

Any person who believes a contractor has violated its nondiscrimination or affirmative action obligations under the authorities above should contact immediately:

The Office of Federal Contract Compliance Programs (OFCCP), Employment Standards Administration, U.S. Department of Labor, 200 Constitution Avenue, N.W., Washington, D.C. 20210 or call (202) 693-0101, or an OFCCP regional or district office, listed in most telephone directories under U.S. Government, Department of Labor.

Private Employment, State and Local Governments, Educational Institutions

Applicants to and employees of most private employers, state and local governments, educational institutions, employment agencies and labor organizations are protected under the following Federal laws:

RACE, COLOR, RELIGION, SEX, NATIONAL ORIGIN

Title VII of the Civil Rights Act of 1964, as amended, prohibits discrimination in hiring, promotion, discharge, pay, fringe benefits, job training, classification, referral, and other aspects of employment, on the basis of race, color, religion, sex or national origin.

DISABILITY

The Americans with Disabilities Act of 1990, as amended, protects qualified applicants and employees with disabilities from discrimination in hiring, promotion, discharge, pay, job training, fringe benefits, classification, referral, and other aspects of employment on the basis of disability. The law also requires that covered entities provide qualified applicants and employees with disabilities with reasonable accommodations that do not impose undue hardship.

AGE

The Age Discrimination in Employment Act of 1967, as amended, protects applicants and employees 40 years of age or older from discrimination on the basis of age in hiring, promotion, discharge, compensation, terms, conditions or privileges of employment.

SEX (WAGES)

In addition to sex discrimination prohibited by Title VII of the Civil Rights Act of 1964, as amended (see above), the Equal Pay Act of 1963, as amended, prohibits sex discrimination in payment of wages to women and men performing substantially equal work in the same establishment.

Retaliation against a person who files a charge of discrimination, participates in an investigation, or opposes an unlawful employment practice is prohibited by all of these Federal laws.

If you believe that you have been discriminated against under any of the above laws, you should contact immediately:

The U.S. Equal Employment Opportunity Commission (EEOC), 1801 L Street, N.W., Washington, D.C. 20507 or an EEOC field office by calling toll free (800) 669-4000. For individuals with hearing impairments, EEOC's toll free TDD number is (800) 669-6820.

Programs or Activities Receiving Federal Financial Assistance

RACE, COLOR, RELIGION, NATIONAL ORIGIN, SEX

In addition to the protection of Title VII of the Civil Rights Act of 1964, as amended, Title VI of the Civil Rights Act prohibits discrimination on the basis of race, color or national origin in programs or activities receiving Federal financial assistance. Employment discrimination is covered by Title VI if the primary objective of the financial assistance is provision of employment, or where employment discrimination causes or may cause discrimination in providing services under such programs. Title IX of the Education Amendments of 1972 prohibits employment discrimination on the basis of sex in educational programs or activities which receive Federal assistance.

INDIVIDUALS WITH DISABILITIES

Sections 501, 504 and 505 of the Rehabilitation Act of 1973, as amended, prohibits employment discrimination on the basis of disability in any program or activity which receives Federal financial assistance in the federal government. Discrimination is prohibited in all aspects of employment against persons with disabilities who, with reasonable accommodation, can perform the essential functions of a job.

If you believe you have been discriminated against in a program of any institution which receives Federal assistance, you should contact immediately the Federal agency providing such assistance.

FIGURE 5-7 Equal Employment Opportunity poster.

WHO WE ARE

ABC Veterinary Clinic is a full-service small animal, avian, and exotic veterinary hospital owned by Dr. Nancy Stover. Our mission is to provide high-quality, progressive veterinary care for people and their pets while at the same time providing an environment that is efficient, friendly, clean, and safe.

SERVICES AND CAPABILITIES

ABC Veterinary Clinic provides the following veterinary services to our clients:

- Preventative medicine for dogs, cats, birds, reptiles, and exotic pets
- Senior pet health care
- Surgical procedures
- Laboratory diagnostics
- Radiology
- Dental procedures
- Referrals to specialty practices

PERSONNEL POLICIES
Employee Rights and Responsibilities

ABC Veterinary Clinic strives to provide a safe, pleasant, and professionally rewarding atmosphere in which to work. Employees are expected to fulfill their designated tasks in a professional and productive manner. Should a negative relationship develop that hinders the workplace environment, it should be promptly brought to the attention of the immediate supervisor.

Security: The nature of our business requires that staff members have access to the facility after hours. Consequently, security becomes an individual matter. Each staff member has the responsibility to see that the clinic is secured if he or she is the last person to leave. This includes turning off lights, air conditioners, and coffee maker and setting the alarm when leaving. Keys will be issued to employees based on the discretion of the practice manager. Keys must be returned at the end of employment or at the request of the practice manager.

Hiring/Discipline/Termination Procedures: New employees are subject to a 3-month trial period. At the end of 3 months, ABC Veterinary Clinic reserves the right to discontinue employment as a result of poor employee performance. Employees may be terminated at any time, with or without cause, at the discretion of the owner.

Facility: Facility care is the responsibility of all employees. Each staff member is expected to treat the facility, equipment, and lab instruments with due care and diligence.

FIGURE 5-8 Sample pages from an employee personnel manual.

retaining employees. Various benefits should be defined and clearly stated regarding which employees qualify for them. If seasonal team members are employed, length of employment, pay, and benefits should be stated. Noncompete agreements must be addressed in employee manuals, as well as work schedule policies, codes of conduct, and safety procedures (Box 5-5).

Philosophy and Mission Statements

Employee manuals should cover a variety of topics, including an overview of the practice philosophy and a vision or mission statement. The practice philosophy may be the same as a purpose statement: the fundamental reason for the organization to exist. It sets the ultimate standards for developing an outstanding organization. What is the purpose? What services are provided? Why are they important? These are just a few questions that can be answered when developing a practice philosophy.

A vision or mission statement may include goals the practice wishes to achieve and how they will be achieved. A positive and achievable goal must be established. The statement should be measurable and simple, and all employees should be able to participate in achieving the mission. Once it has been accomplished, a new mission can be developed. Missions can take two or three

Housekeeping: Each individual is responsible for leaving the work area in a clean and orderly condition. Although we have cleaning personnel, it is each individual's responsibility to clean up after themselves and after animals they have cared for.

Professionalism: Each employee is required to act and dress in a professional manner. Scrubs are provided for employees and should not be wrinkled or stained. Hair should be styled and colored in a professional manner. Body piercing should be kept to a minimum and must be eliminated from the facial area. Small, professional earrings are allowed.

Use of Telephone: ABC Veterinary Clinic depends on the phone lines for communication with our clients. It is very important to keep personal phone calls to a minimum. Please do not allow friends to call the clinic for personal matters; they can call once you are done with your shift. Long-distance personal calls are not allowed.

Confidential Information: All information pertaining to clients and employees is confidential. No staff member should reveal any information unless expressly authorized to do so. Clients must request a copy of the records themselves or have another veterinary clinic request them. Information regarding a client or employee is not to be given out over the phone. If an animal is lost, we cannot give out the owner's information. It is our responsibility to get in contact with the owner and convey the information on the lost pet.

Safety and Health: Safety is of paramount importance. Prevention of accidents is the responsibility of each staff member. Before undertaking any task, the hazards should be fully evaluated and appropriate precautions should be taken to avoid accidents and injury. Suggestions for improvement of working conditions and elimination of hazards are always welcome.

- Always wear lead gowns, thyroid collars, gloves, and radiation badges when taking radiographs.
- Wear exam gloves while debriding wounds or handling any case that has zoonotic potential.
- Do not lift animals over 50 pounds without assistance.
- Use your knees and legs to lift, not your back.
- Use muzzles when needed to prevent bites.
- In the event of a dog or cat bite, employees must report the injury immediately to the practice manager and owner. If the bite has penetrated the skin, you are required to visit a physician as soon as possible. Dog and cats bites are serious and must be treated accordingly.

FIGURE 5-8, cont'd

years to achieve and perfect, and developing an action plan will help achieve these goals (Box 5-6).

Job Descriptions and Duties

Another section to be included in an employee manual is list of job descriptions and duties for each position in a practice. Job descriptions must be detailed and include every aspect and expectation of that job. An employee may be asked to complete a task that is not listed as a description or duty; therefore it is important to add some flexibility into the description. The phrase "and any other task assigned by a supervisor" can be added to most job descriptions. If the practice is large and has several departments, a description may include a statement such as "Every employee works for ABC Veterinary Hospital as a whole, not for a particular supervisor or department." It is clearly defined that each team member is to help anyone who needs help, not just those within his or her own department.

> **PRACTICE POINT**   Job descriptions and duties must be clearly stated to allow potential and current team members to fully understand what is expected of them.

A kennel assistant can be defined as any person who assists a veterinarian, veterinary technician, or assistant in the care of animals. He or she may be expected to lift animals up to 50 pounds; clean up vomit, diarrhea, and urine; walk animals; provide correct food and water to patients or boarding animals; and wash dishes. If the duties are not clearly defined, the kennel assistant may not expect to, and/or may not be able to, complete the tasks. This rule is the same for each team member. All duties must be clearly defined, and team members must be able to complete those tasks. To help cover all duties, ask team members to write out all duties or tasks they complete on a daily and weekly basis. Once an informal list as been created, distribute the list to all team members and ask what has been forgotten. This will help

Box 5-5	Sample Table of Contents for Employee Personnel Manual

Statement or purpose of manual
Philosophy and/or mission statement
Job duties and descriptions
Laws of importance
   EOE
   Sexual harassment
   Pregnancy safety
Employment policies
   Code of conduct
   Appearance, dress code, uniforms
   Hours of operation
   Probationary period
   Attendance, work schedule policy
Termination procedures
Hours of operation
Holidays recognized
Benefits
Vacation
Sick leave
Holiday pay
Insurance
   Liability
   Health
   Disability
Continuing education
Dues and license fees
Full-time, part-time, and seasonal employment
Drug and alcohol abuse policy
Sexual harassment policy
Personal telephone calls
Noncompete agreement
Jury duty
Training procedures
Safety
OSHA/MSDS
   Reporting an accident
   Security
Probationary period

Each state has different laws regarding employee manuals and laws that must be covered. It is advised to contact an attorney for review. Employment and labor laws change frequently, and policies and manuals must be updated to reflect the changes. Practices should reserve the right to update and modify employee manuals at any time. It is important to remain flexible, and employees should be made aware of changes as they occur and sign a form acknowledging the update. *EOE,* Equal Opportunity Employment; *OSHA,* Occupational Safety and Health Administration; *MSDS,* Material Safety Data Sheets.

ensure that no duties or tasks have been missed (Boxes 5-7 and 5-8).

These examples of job duties and descriptions are in no way complete. They can be added to or deleted. Each practice varies, and duties and descriptions should be developed for each hospital. Each description should have the following fundamentals addressed:

- A position title. This helps give form to the position and may help create a hierarchy in larger hospitals.
- A summary.

Box 5-6	Examples of Mission Statements

- ABC mission: ABC Veterinary Clinic is a full-service small-animal, avian, and exotic veterinary hospital that is owned by Dr. Nancy Stover. Our mission is to provide high-quality progressive veterinary care for people and their pets, while at the same time providing an environment that is efficient, friendly, clean, and safe.
- To provide comprehensive high-quality veterinary care with emphasis on exceptional client service and patient care, while providing employees with desirable, fulfilling, and financially rewarding employment.

- Duties and responsibilities. Skilled, specialized, and basic duties must all be listed. Essential skills, such as lifting a 50-lb dog or providing client education, cannot be left out.
- Description of required skills and qualifications.
- Accountability. State the person to whom this person or position will report.

Job descriptions and duties should be given to each applicant during the interview process. Applicants must fully understand the entire job of a veterinary hospital. This will allow the interviewer and candidate to compare skills and abilities and determine whether the applicant is a match for the position.

Full-Time and Part-Time Employment

Full-time and part-time employment must be defined. Each practice can determine the number of hours per week required for a full-time position. Some practices may choose 40 hours per week, others may only require 34 hours. Overtime must be paid for any employee who works more than 40 hours per week. A week is defined by the Department of Labor as 7 consecutive days, with 24 hours within a day. For example, a work week may begin Monday at 12 AM through Sunday at 11:59 PM. The first 40 hours must be paid at a regular rate; any time accumulated after the initial 40 hours must be paid at time and a half. Those in violation of the act can be penalized severely.

PRACTICE POINT A week is defined by the Department of Labor as 7 consecutive days, with 24 hours within a day.

Seasonal Employees

Some practices are extremely busy during specific months and must hire seasonal employees to survive the busy time. Job descriptions, duties, and dates of employment should be established, preventing any miscommunication. Seasonal employees should also sign for the employee manual and personnel handbook. Benefits are generally not offered to seasonal employees; however, this is at the discretion of the practice.

Box 5-7	Sample Job Descriptions

KENNEL ASSISTANT

A kennel assistant will be expected to assist a veterinarian, veterinary technician, or assistant in the care of animals. This may include restraining, cleaning, and walking the patients. The kennel assistant will maintain the constant cleanliness of the kennels, cages, and ward area, including the care and feeding of all animals. Kennel assistants are expected to have knowledge of cleaning and disinfecting methods and use proper chemicals and equipment to complete the task safely and efficiently. The assistant should be able to patiently treat sick and debilitated patients as well as understand and carry out written and oral instructions. Kennel assistants must be able to lift and carry patients up to 50 lb as needed and required by team members. If any problems arise, kennel assistants should report them to the practice manager immediately.

VETERINARY ASSISTANT

A veterinary assistant will be expected to assist the veterinarian and veterinary technician in the care of animals. This may include restraining, cleaning, and walking the patients; providing medical care assigned by the veterinarian; as well as offering any communication to the client as specified by the veterinarian. The assistant will also perform laboratory analysis, take and develop radiographs, and assist the receptionist with answering the phone and providing customer service as needed. An assistant is expected to be pleasant, patient, courteous, and polite to clients and team members at all times and contribute to keeping the office flowing in an organized, efficient manner. Assistants must have knowledge of vaccination protocols, pharmacology, nutrition, animal husbandry and care and must be able to lift and carry patients up to 50 lb as needed and required by team members. If any problems arise, assistants should report them to the practice manager immediately.

VETERINARY TECHNICIAN

A veterinary technician will be expected to assist the veterinarian in the care of animals. This may include restraining, cleaning, and walking of the patients; providing medical care assigned by the veterinarian; as well as offering any communication to the client as specified by the veterinarian. The technician will also perform laboratory analysis, take and develop radiographs, and assist the receptionist with answering the phone and providing customer service as needed. The technician may oversee the kennel and veterinary assistants and provide continuing education for these staff members. The veterinary technician is held to the highest standard of care and must ensure all patients receive the appropriate treatments and nutrition and be kept in a safe and clean environment. A technician must be able to educate clients on the care and condition of their pets. Veterinary technicians are expected to be pleasant, patient, courteous, and polite to clients and team members at all times and contribute to keeping the office flowing in an organized, efficient manner. Technicians must have knowledge of vaccination protocols, pharmacology, nutrition, and animal husbandry and care. Veterinary technicians must be able to lift and carry patients up to 50 lb as needed by team members. If any problems arise, veterinary technicians should report them to the practice manager immediately.

RECEPTIONIST

A receptionist is expected to provide the highest level of customer service and care. This is to be done by answering phones, scheduling appointments, answering client questions, pulling patient charts, checking clients in and out, and accepting payments. A receptionist will maintain a professional appearance and behave in a professional manner at all times, speak clearly and slowly for clients to understand, and relay reliable information to clients as directed by the veterinarian and/or veterinary technicians. If any problems arise, the receptionist should report them to the office manager immediately.

OFFICE MANAGER

An office manager is expected to provide the highest level of customer service and care. This is to be done by answering phones, scheduling appointments, answering client questions, pulling patient charts, checking clients in and out, and accepting payments. Office managers will maintain a professional appearance and behave in a professional manner at all times, speak clearly and slowly for clients to understand, and relay reliable information to clients as directed by the veterinarian and/or veterinary technician. Managers are responsible for the training of receptionists and for overseeing all duties that are expected of them. The office manager is held to the highest standard and should ensure that all customers are satisfied and have received the value of service they have paid for. If any problems arise, office managers should report them to the practice manager immediately for guidance.

PRACTICE MANAGER

The practice manager oversees all the kennel assistant, veterinary assistant, veterinary technician, reception, and office management teams. The practice manager ensures that all team members receive proper training and that all standards of care are being met. The practice manager may oversee inventory management, scheduling, and maintenance of equipment. If problems arise, the practice manager should report them to the hospital administrator or owner for guidance.

VETERINARIAN

A veterinarian will see patients to diagnose and treat disease, perform surgery, and prescribe medications. A veterinarian will delegate duties of laboratory analysis and animal care to technicians and assistants, allowing more client/veterinarian interaction and education. Veterinarians are held to the highest standard of care; they are ultimately responsible for the care and treatment of patients and must advise clients of the best options available for their patients. Problems with training or with team members not completing their duties correctly should be discussed with the practice manager and hospital administrator.

HOSPITAL ADMINISTRATOR

A hospital administrator oversees the entire function of the veterinary hospital. The administrator is responsible for creating and maintaining budgets, finances, hospital protocols, and procedures. This position requires the use of accounting and financial tools, which must be used for the practice to be successful.

Box 5-8 Sample Job Duties

KENNEL ASSISTANT:
- Clean debris in cages as soon as it is present and record any bowel movements or urination
- Wash dishes, litter pans, and blankets
- Use cleaning chemicals in a safe manner
- Safely lift and move patients from one area to another
- Provide patient restraint assistance to team members when asked
- Provide humane treatment of patients
- Report any patient emergency to veterinary team members
- Provide food and water to patients at the request of team members and record patients' appetites and water consumption
- Walk patients in a safe environment
- Practice safety at all times
- Bathe animals if needed so that all patients will be clean at all times
- Recognize any unusual patient behavior or condition, record it, and report it to a veterinary technician or veterinarian
- Other duties as assigned or required

VETERINARY ASSISTANT
Be able to perform all the kennel assistant duties as well as:
- Perform laboratory analysis and provide results to the doctor in a timely manner
- Take and develop radiographs
- Treat patients with correct medications, whether by oral, subcutaneous, intramuscular, or intravenous route, as directed by the veterinarian
- Monitor hospitalized patients
- Check-in exam rooms and review recommendations with owners
- Review procedures and protocols with clients, including vaccinations, heartworm tests, and FELV/FIV tests
- Educate clients verbally and with written materials
- Provide estimates developed by the veterinarian to the owner and verbally review them
- Answer phones with a positive tone of voice
- Schedule appointments
- Assist clients to their cars with their animals and/or purchases
- Prepare, count, and properly label medications for owner
- Show owners how to administer medications
- Keep working area free of trash, hair, and other unneeded material
- Complete duties or tasks as needed and assigned by other team members or supervisors

VETERINARY TECHNICIAN:
Be able to perform all kennel and veterinary assistant duties as well as:
- Induce and maintain anesthesia
- Prepare animals for surgery; assist in surgery if needed by the veterinarian
- Monitor recovering surgical patients
- Prepare surgical packs before and after surgery
- Maintain surgical instruments (cleaning, lubricating, and sharpening if needed)
- Maintain autoclave and anesthetic machines
- Dental prophylaxis
- Provide medical treatment as directed by the veterinarian
- Assist, educate, and act as a mentor to kennel and veterinary assistants
- Complete any other duties or tasks assigned or required by other team members or supervisors

RECEPTIONIST:
- Answer phones with a smile
- Schedule appointments on the phone and as clients check out
- Provide superior customer service
- Accept payments for services rendered
- Check clients in; greet with a smile and address clients by name
- Update client files with each visit
- Help maintain proper and efficient client flow and organization within the practice on a daily basis
- Communicate delays with clients as they occur
- Prepare reminder cards
- File medical records in the appropriate location once each record has been completed
- Refill prescriptions in accordance with hospital policy
- Prepare end-of-day closing and reconciliation sheet along with a deposit sheet
- Ensure reception area stays clean
- Other related duties as assigned

OFFICE MANAGER
Be able to perform all receptionist duties, along with:
- Training and overseeing receptionists
- Accounts receivable

PRACTICE MANAGER
Be able to perform all duties previously listed for kennel and veterinary assistants, veterinary technicians, receptionist, and office manager, along with:
- Follow hiring and termination procedures
- Develop training programs and protocols
- Perform inventory management
- Perform employee scheduling
- Ensure proper maintenance and working order of equipment

VETERINARIAN
- Diagnose
- Prescribe medications
- Perform surgery
- Educate clients in a friendly, polite, and patient manner
- Educate team members when needed
- Help the practice flow in an organized and professional manner

HOSPITAL ADMINISTRATOR
Be able to perform all duties previously listed for kennel and veterinary assistants, veterinary technicians, receptionist, and office manager, along with:
- Provide a safe work environment for employees
- Ensure procedures and protocols are followed as developed

Continued

Box 5-8	Sample Job Duties—cont'd
• Oversee all departments and ensure compatibility • Offer solutions to problems • Create and manage budgets • Maintain and produce profit and loss statements, chart of accounts, and balance sheets • Conduct long-range financial planning	• Maintain accounts payable • Maintain payroll and taxes • Maintain knowledge of current developments in accounting theory and practice and in financial techniques for measurement, analysis, and planning

FEL/FIV, Feline leukemia/feline immunodeficiency virus.

Benefits

Once full-time and part-time employees have been established, the benefits each position receives should be defined. Many benefit plans are included in full-time employment; however, it is up to the practice to decide what to offer. No governing agency requires benefits to be offered, but they certainly help in recruiting and retaining employees. It is highly recommended to offer as many benefits as possible to all employees (Box 5-9).

Employee salary and benefits statements should be provided to employees on an annual basis. Employees generally only see the monetary compensation they have received, as shown on their year-end W-2 forms. Annual statements provide the overall picture because many employees do not know the value of the benefits they receive, and employers need to know that they are compensating their employees fairly.

> **PRACTICE POINT** Employee benefits statements are essential for ensuring that team members understand the full wage amount they receive for a given 1-year period.

Statements can be developed by each practice, but basic information should be included in each statement. Statements should run for the entire fiscal year, giving a clear picture to the employee of how much the employer has paid in the previous year. Pretax compensation should be listed, along with Medicare and Social Security contributions made by the employer. Many employees do not realize the practice contributes to these funds. Insurance, vacation, continuing education, uniforms, sick days, holidays, pet health care, and any other benefits should be listed individually because each employee's benefit summary will be different. It should not take an excessive amount of time to prepare the statements because all information should be easily retrievable through paid invoices of such benefits.

It is advised to discuss the statements with employees instead of handing them out without comment so that the employees will comprehend the full compensation and benefits plan. Historically, employees only consider their paycheck as compensation and forget that benefits are a real cost to the employer as well (Box 5-10).

Box 5-9	Examples of Employee Benefits
• Health insurance • Continuing education • Vacation • Sick leave • Holiday pay • Professional liability insurance • Retirement plans • Dues and licenses • Veterinary care Less frequently offered: • Disability insurance • Life insurance • Dental insurance	

Vacation

The amount of vacation that may be taken is determined by the practice and is generally built up over time. Vacation must be offered and employees should be encouraged to take it. Without a vacation, stress, fatigue, irritability, and decreased production can result. These can be detrimental to the practice.

Factors to consider when determining vacation for the practice include length of employment time required before vacation can be used, time allotment, eligibility, accrual, schedule approval, and whether unused vacation is paid at the time of termination or resignation. In general, practices allow 1 week per year for the first year, then increase 1 week per year to a maximum of 3 weeks. Practices often state that vacation should be used up within the fiscal year and should not be allowed to roll over to the following year, but this is the choice of a practice. No law states how vacation should be determined or used. Team members should be asked to give sufficient notice to use vacation time, allowing schedules to be adjusted accordingly. Overtime is not paid when vacation is used within the week.

> **PRACTICE POINT** It should be required that vacation be taken; it helps to prevent burnout and fatigue of team members.

Box 5-10 Example of Benefits Statement

Name of employee:	D.J. Stover
Period covered:	January 1, 2007, to December 31, 2007
Date of hire:	April 15, 1993
Salary or hourly wage:	$45,768.98 = $22/hour
Emergency compensation:	$0
Bonus:	$2500
Social Security and Medicare contribution:	$2837.68 + $663.63 = $3501.31
Health insurance:	$309.87/month (pay 100%) = $3718.44
Liability insurance:	$1200
Disability Insurance:	$102/month = $1224
Holiday pay:	8 paid days; $22/hour × 8 hours/day = $176 × 8 days = $1408
Vacation:	3 weeks, 40 hours/week; $22 × 40 = $880/week × 3 = $2640
Sick time:	1 week (40 hours) = $22 × 40 = $880
Retirement:	3% of matching contribution = $3042/year
Uniforms:	New uniforms twice yearly = $180
Continuing education:	$1500 to be used at your discretion
Dues:	City and state veterinary medical associations, American Veterinary Medical Association = $350
Licenses:	State, controlled substances = $325
Pet medical care:	Total discounted services this year = $1650.89
Miscellaneous:	Lunches, ice cream breaks = $67.89/employee
Total benefits:	**$20,187.53**
Total salary and benefits:	**$65,956.51**
Benefits as a percentage of salary:	**31%**

Vacation can also be accrued by the number of hours worked per week. A long-term employee may receive 8 hours of vacation for every 80 hours of work.

Sick Leave

Just as with vacation, the amount of sick leave is generally built up with the time of service, and its use should be encouraged. Allowing one person time off when sick is better than having four people sick at once. Trying to prevent the spread of a virus is more economically advantageous!

Factors to account for when determining the rules for sick leave include how long a person must be employed before receiving paid sick leave, accrual, whether the practice will allow it to accrue year to year, and whether it is paid on termination or resignation. Overtime is not paid when using sick leave.

Insurance

Liability Insurance is available in a variety of forms. Veterinarians must carry liability insurance, which is generally paid for by the practice. It is imperative that the liability insurance be high enough to cover any accident that may occur within the practice. This includes any animal-related injury, client injury, or accusation of malpractice. Managers should ensure these premiums are paid annually.

Health Health insurance can and should be available for team members. It is generally cheaper for a business to offer health insurance than for individuals to buy health insurance. Practices may offer to pay 100% of the monthly payment, or less if they so choose. The employee is then responsible for the remaining percentage if the employer does not cover the entire premium. Health insurance should be reviewed on an annual basis because premiums and coverage change frequently. When deciding which insurance plan to choose, team members should review both health maintenance organization (HMO) and preferred provider organization (PPO) plans because they can differ greatly in the doctors and laboratories covered as well as in copayments and annual deductibles. HMOs are usually well managed and generally cover all medical expenses if patients use the doctors and laboratories within the approved network. PPOs offer a network of physicians and laboratories and encourage patients to use them; this is not required, but subscribers receive lower amounts of coverage if they choose a doctor that is out of the network.

Disability Disability insurance is a benefit that some employers offer. Disability insurance is maintained to protect the employee against injury that results in the inability to perform tasks needed to complete the job. Back injuries, bite wounds that result in permanent damage, and carpal tunnel syndrome are just a few conditions that may prevent a team member from working. Three forms of disability insurance are available. *Own occupation* disability insurance covers any disability that does not allow a team member to return to that particular line of work. For example, if a veterinarian could no longer perform surgery because of a permanent hand injury but could see patients in a limited way, he would receive a small disability pension. *Any occupation* disability insurance covers any disability that does not allow the team member to return to any occupation. *Residual coverage* is important to professionals who become partially disabled and incur a loss of income from reduced duties. Residual benefits are based on the percentage of income lost. Team members need coverage in case they are permanently injured, especially if they are the main income producer of the family.

> **PRACTICE POINT** Disability insurance provides lifetime coverage if a team member becomes permanently injured and unable to work.

Workers' compensation insurance is not required in all states, but it is recommended. The Workers' Compensation Act was developed to protect the employer against any accident or injury that occurs on the job site. This type of compensation is detailed later in this chapter.

Insurance agents are excellent at helping small businesses find the right insurance plan at all levels. Ask clients and other local practices for referrals of reputable and reliable agents who provide courteous service. They can maximize the benefits for both the employer and employee while finding the most economically feasible policy.

Retirement Funds

A great benefit to offer employees is a retirement fund. Retirement funds are a growing trend in veterinary medicine and complement the benefits package well. The most common form of a retirement fund in general veterinary practice is a SIMPLE IRA (sIRA). SIMPLE is the abbreviation for Savings Incentive Match Plan for Employees, and IRA is short for Individual Retirement Account. sIRA plans are established by employers who want to allow eligible employees to set aside part of their pretax compensation as a part of their retirement savings plan. The employer must contribute either dollar for dollar or a percentage to all eligible employees. The employee can either contribute a set dollar amount per pay period or a percentage of the total pretax compensation. 401(k) plans are another common form of retirement fund in

which employers are not required to contribute to the employee's account but can do so if wished. Employees determine how much they wish to contribute on a monthly basis to their 401(k) plan.

> **PRACTICE POINT** Common retirement plans include sIRA, 401(k), profit-sharing, and SEP plans.

Practices may also create a profit-sharing plan for employees in which they receive an annual share of the practice's profits. Profit-sharing gives employees a sense of ownership in the company. This plan generally requires a plan administrator, and the percentage of profits is determined by management. Simplified Employee Pension plans (SEPs) are similar to profit-sharing plans and are appropriate for small organizations. They are funded by tax-deductible employer contributions, and employees are not allowed to contribute.

Retirement funds are highly regulated by the government through the Employee Retirement Income Security Act (ERISA) because of past negligence and abuse in the management of pension plans. Professional guidance from a broker is advised to determine which plan is best for the practice.

Retirement funds encourage team members to stay with the practice for the long term and reward employees for their dedication and hard work. The employer's match is tax deductible, making contributions a benefit for the practice.

Continuing Education

Continuing education (CE) should be a benefit available to all team members required to hold a license as well as those expected to continue to improve their job description and duties and those wanting to better themselves and the practice. Hospitals may determine a specific amount and give that dollar amount to each individual on a yearly basis, allowing team members to attend whatever form of CE they prefer. The set amount should include travel expenses, hotel, CE registration fees, and money to cover the cost of meals. If the practice chooses to cover those costs individually, team members should bring receipts back to the practice for reimbursement. These receipts should be kept for year-end taxes.

Allowing a set dollar amount per team member can prevent overspending and holds team members accountable for their spending. They may choose CE on a local or state level, which ultimately saves money for the practice. CE can average $895 to $1850 per person for national or regional conferences.

Many local and state veterinary medical associations, along with manufacturers, hold continuing education events throughout the year covering a variety of topics. Lunches or dinners are often offered at these free lectures, defraying some costs of attending. Technicians and veterinarians alike are normally invited to attend.

Holiday Pay

Practices may elect whether to pay employees for holidays and for which ones. Holidays may include New Year's Eve, New Year's Day, Martin Luther King, Jr. Day, Presidents' Day, Easter, Memorial Day, Independence Day, Labor Day, Veterans Day, Thanksgiving, Christmas Eve, and Christmas Day. Some practices only observe the major holidays; others prefer to observe a day that is meaningful to the practice. Holiday pay is usually paid to an employee who would normally work those hours on days when the practice has chosen to close. Holiday pay is generally only 8 hours of pay, and overtime is not paid when holiday pay has been accumulated.

Uniforms

If team members are required to wear scrubs, the practice should provide them or compensate individuals for their purchase. The benefit to the practice in providing scrubs is the ability to control the clothing appearance of team members. If scrubs do not appear professional, they can be replaced without harassment. The negative side of providing uniforms is the cost. Employees should be held accountable for maintaining their uniforms in the best condition possible. Requiring all team members to wear the same color uniform on specific days adds to the professional appearance of the staff. Ask the team to pick the best colors and assign days to those colors. When having input, the team will comply much easier with the request. Many companies offer discounts when large orders are placed. Inquire with several companies to find the best price that fits the budget of the practice.

Membership Fees

Both veterinarians and credentialed technicians pay a variety of membership fees each year. State veterinary medical associations, national organizations, and specialty boards are just a few. Practices may offer to cover the dues, especially if the organization or association helps the practice in some way. Many state and national organizations have a voice in government affairs, and political action committees watch and defend veterinary interests. Practices should analyze all potential dues and set a guideline to follow when choosing to cover such expenses.

Licenses

Licenses held by veterinarians and technicians are renewed each year or biannually with a fee. Practices may wish to cover this expense, including the controlled substance license, state license, and any other license required to practice veterinary medicine.

The total cost of licensure fees and dues to organizations for one veterinarian averages $1200 per year. Practices should remember that these fees can be considered a write-off at the end of the year when taxes are being completed.

Employee Discounts

The practice has the discretion to determine employee discounts and how much they should be. Many practices allow team members to purchase items at cost and take advantage of a percentage discount available on services rendered. Many veterinarians will perform services at no charge to team members as long as items used are paid for. It is a great benefit to allow employee discounts on services and products. Some team members may not be able to afford all the services that are recommended on a daily basis to clients. This, in turn, makes recommending the product and services to clients difficult for these team members because they cannot follow the protocol themselves. If these team members are allowed to use and believe in the medicine, they can make better recommendations to clients, which will in turn allow higher average transactions per client.

Some practices have found that some employees take advantage of this benefit and that they must place a cap on either the dollar amount or the number of pets covered. Practices may also purchase pet insurance in lieu of discounts. Most pet care insurance carriers provide discounts as well to practices and practice employees, making pet health insurance a reasonable benefit for employees.

Code of Conduct

Employees are expected to maintain professionalism while on the premises. The code of conduct section of the employee manual should define each area in which there are specific expectations of team members. Appearance, confidentiality, quality of patient care, equipment care, and accountability for supplies and equipment are some topics that should be addressed.

Appearance is more than just looks. Clients respect and trust team members who appear professional. Body piercings, hair color, and tattoos should be addressed. Cleanliness, body odor, and wrinkle-free uniforms may be discussed as well as the appropriate application of makeup.

Although it seems impossible that team members will misunderstand that client and patient confidentiality is of utmost importance, it must be addressed in the employee manual. Team members must also understand that employee information and phone numbers are confidential and must never be given out. Information can never be given out without employee or client consent.

PRACTICE POINT   Client, patient, and employee information must be kept confidential.

If a pet is lost and an unknown person calls the practice indicating that he or she has found a pet, the phone number and information should be written down, informing the unknown person that the client will be calling. The client should then be called and the information passed on to him or her. Never give the client's name and phone number to an unknown person. The practice does not know if the unknown person really has the pet, or if the person has criminal intentions. The practice can be held liable for giving out confidential information if this scenario ever occurs.

Work Schedule Policy

All team members need to be aware of the work schedule policy. Veterinarians are expected to be available during set appointment hours, and vacation or personal time must be scheduled in advance to accommodate the request. All other team members are expected to cover the shifts that have been assigned to them and must schedule vacation time in advance. Most practices will grant time off to team members as long as their shifts have been covered. The practice must establish a policy, include it in the manual, and enforce it. Team members who do not follow policy should be given a written warning. See the section on termination procedures in this chapter for guidance on documenting and enforcing procedures.

Team members should be made aware of the issues that arise when the practice is short staffed. Members must be held accountable for their shifts, and any absence (unless for an emergency or illness) is unacceptable. Team shortages contribute to increased stress levels, decreased team efficiency, and a worsening of patient and client care. They can also produce individual resentment, again leading to decreased team efficiency.

Jury Duty

When team members are summoned for jury duty, they are obligated by law to attend. School, work, or any other excuse is not allowed. Team members should be encouraged to have their shift covered before jury duty, and management should help with this coverage. Jury duty is a public service and should be served with pride.

PRACTICE POINT   Team members summoned for jury duty are required to do so by law and can be arrested for failure to appear.

Training Procedures

Training procedures should be clearly defined in the employee manual. Team members should be advised of the training schedule (if one is available) and when they are expected to master those skills (more information on developing a training program is provided later in this chapter). The manual should indicate whether there is a probationary period (generally 30 days) and the step that follows the probation. If the new employee does not succeed during the probationary period, the manual should indicate that the employee will be terminated. If the employee does succeed, the manual should indicate whether the team member will receive an evaluation and/or a raise. Some practices have a 30-day probationary period, give an evaluation at 30 days, then evaluate again at 90 days with a raise at that time. Manuals should also indicate how often evaluations will occur thereafter. It is recommended to provide yearly written evaluations for each team member, keeping copies in each team member's personnel file.

Noncompete Agreements

Veterinarians, groomers, or other team members who are paid on a production basis or who are significant income producers for the practice may be asked to sign a noncompete or restrictive covenant agreement (NCA). An NCA is a contract that protects the business and employer by preventing the employee from opening a business or taking employment at a location within certain number of miles of the practice. The purpose is to safeguard the veterinary practice when protectable interests are at risk. Owners have the right to protect tangible and intangible property. An example of intangible property is practice goodwill. Practice goodwill is the reputation within the community, with colleagues and staff, and in doctor and client/patient relationships. Intangible property, also known as *incorporeal property,* describes something that a person or corporation can have ownership of and can transfer ownership to another person or corporation, but has no physical substance. Tangible property is anything that can be touched and includes both real and personal property. Examples of tangible property are confidential information, client lists, and medical records. State laws vary regarding covenants, and they must be reasonable. The scope of activity is generally restricted and includes a time limitation and a geographic restraint. Historically, courts would not enforce covenants, and some are still reluctant to do so; they restrict a professional's ability to earn a living as well as restrict the public from the benefit of the competition. Courts are slowly changing and will critically analyze the above factors, including the restricted geographic location.

PRACTICE POINT   Noncompete agreements can be difficult to enforce in a court of law; therefore they should be drawn up with guidance from a lawyer.

Laws of Importance

Several legal topics need to be addressed and covered in the employee manual. These and other laws were discussed in detail earlier in this chapter.

Equal Opportunity Employment

A practice must follow Equal Opportunity Employment (EOE) guidelines. The practice cannot discriminate on the basis of race, color, sex, religion, or national origin and must state this to employees and potential employees.

Pregnancy

A practice cannot discriminate against pregnant team members. It is advised to state in the manual that team members are requested to inform management as soon as they are aware of the pregnancy so that all precautions can be addressed. A pregnant team member must decide what she can and cannot do. Safety issues can be addressed, such as radiation exposure and heavy lifting; however, the team member must decide her own safety level. She cannot be changed from technician status to reception status unless she requests to do so.

Sexual Harassment

Every team member must be protected from sexual harassment from both management and other team members. Sexual harassment occurs whenever unwelcomed sexual conduct is made a term or a condition of employment. It can occur when unwelcomed sexual conduct has the purpose or effect of interfering with an individual's work performance or creating an offensive work environment. It can also occur when a supervisor conditions the granting of an employment benefit upon the receipt of sexual favors. Unwelcomed sexual conduct can be in the form of jokes, suggestive comments, insults, threats, suggestive noises, whistles, cat calls, touching, pinching, brushing against someone, assault, or coerced sexual intercourse. Policies must be developed, stated, and followed to protect the practice from a potential lawsuit. Promotion, demotion, or pay based on sexual innuendo cannot be allowed and must be clearly stated. The manual should also indicate with whom the employee should discuss possible sexual harassment violations, and that the discussion will occur without the possibility of retaliation. Practices must have a zero tolerance policy when it comes to sexual harassment.

> **PRACTICE POINT** Sexual harassment cannot be tolerated in the practice and must be addressed immediately if a claim arises.

Safety and Security Procedures

Employees should receive safety training during the first few days of employment. Team safety should be of utmost importance. A safety program should be implemented and enforced. Chapter 21 covers the development and implementation of a safety program if one is not already in use.

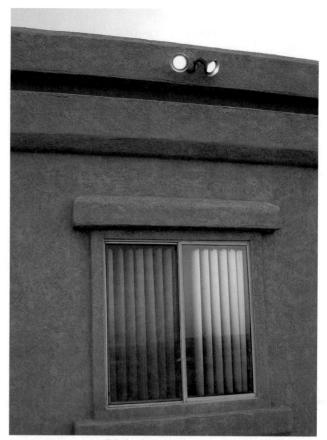

FIGURE 5-9 A well-lit building helps ensure the safety of employees and clients.

Security in and around the practice 24 hours a day is very important. The outside premises should be well lit and secure for team members who are walking pets (Figure 5-9). Security cameras may be needed depending on the location of the practice.

Employee entrance doors should be locked at all times, preventing the entry of clients or criminals. The door should only be locked from the outside, allowing access out the door in the event of an emergency.

The nature of the practice requires that staff members have access to the facility after hours. Consequently, security becomes an individual matter. Each team member has the responsibility to see that the practice is secured if he or she is the last person to leave. Keys should be issued to employees at the discretion of the practice manager. Keys must be returned at the end of employment or at the request of the practice manager.

Occupational Safety and Health Administration

OSHA recognizes and enforces employee safety. Rules and regulations have been implemented that employers must enforce (see Chapter 21).

> **PRACTICE POINT** Accidents must be reported immediately to upper management.

Reporting Accidents

Each accident should be reported to the owner and/or practice manager. Injuries can be serious and should not be hidden from management. When injuries occur, management should investigate and implement protocols to prevent the injury from reoccurring to another person. Proper forms must be completed when an injury has occurred, and the practice manager is responsible for ensuring that the forms are forwarded to the proper authorities when warranted.

Probationary Period

Many practices use a probationary period when hiring new employees. This trial period allows new team members to try the position and see if they are a match for the practice. The practice reserves the right to terminate the new employees at the end of the trial period if they do not appear to be fulfilling the job requirements. The probationary period should be clearly stated in the employee manual, including the length of the period, and that the practice reserves the right to end employment without cause. It can be detrimental to maintain employees who do not fit into the practice. Poor work ethic, poor performance, and negative attitudes are contagious, and if employees with these habits are kept for long-term employment, they can begin to affect the employees who are considered a "10."

Termination Procedures

Termination procedures are discussed in detail later in this chapter. However, the procedure should be discussed and clearly defined in the employee manual. Team members must be advised what to expect if the situation arises. Defined termination procedures also offer some protection to the practice if an unemployment claim or lawsuit ever arises.

EMPLOYEE PROCEDURE MANUAL

Developing an Employee Procedure Manual

An employee procedure manual not only helps train new employees, it also provides a guide to look up procedures as needed. Procedure manuals take time to develop and must be updated frequently to provide consistency with all team members (Box 5-11).

> **PRACTICE POINT** Employee procedural manuals help increase the knowledge and efficiency of the team.

Every procedure that is used in the practice should be listed. To start, team members may be asked to write up different procedures that are used on a daily basis. An outline can be useful to help organize procedures by department or technique, which then can be developed into a table of contents. The procedure manual can be organized in alphabetical order for easy and quick retrieval. Information included in each section should define the procedure, list the steps to accomplish the procedure, and include an explanation as to why the procedure is completed in that fashion. This allows team members to completely understand and be able to explain procedures to clients when needed. Figure 5-10 lists several topics that can be included in a manual.

Implementing an Employee Procedure Manual

When team members participate in creating an employee procedure manual, they are more likely to help implement it and make use of it. Once it has been completed, each team member should receive a copy, and a hard copy should be kept within the practice. It should be placed in a central location and be easy to find. Paperless practices can upload the employee procedure manual onto the computer system, allowing team members to access it from any computer in the clinic.

When new employees are hired, they must also receive their own copy. Each section can then be covered and explained over the course of several weeks. Covering all information within a short period of time will overwhelm new team members and they will be unlikely to remember what is covered in the manual. The procedure manual can be used to develop a training guide and schedule, covered later in this chapter. When team members question a protocol, they can reference the employee procedure manual. In many cases, certain techniques are used so infrequently that their protocols are forgotten.

Updating the Employee Procedure Manual

Each time a vaccine protocol, laboratory procedure, or surgical prep technique changes, the employee manual must be updated. The manual kept in the central location will change frequently; however, team members should receive a single sheet indicating the change. Employees should sign a form indicating they have received the update. Changes can be hard for some employees to implement. They may become resistant to the change, even though it has been formally established and they have signed the form indicating they are aware of the change. Some employees resist change because of their discomfort level with the change or new procedure. Training these employees with a different approach may improve compliance as well as ask why they oppose the change so much. They may have an insight that management has forgotten, and taking the new approach may help other employees implement the change better as well.

> **PRACTICE POINT** Employee procedural manuals must be updated when any protocol or procedure changes.

| **Box 5-11** | **Sample Table of Contents for Employee Procedure Manual** |

Animal bites
Artificial insemination
Bandages/splints/casts
   Pressure bandages
   Wound management
      Dry bandages
      Wet-to-dry bandages
   Splints/casts
Blood transfusions
   Oxyglobin
   Fresh frozen plasma
   Whole blood
      Equipment needed
Catheters
   Butterfly
   Foley catheters
   IV catheters
   Jugular catheters
   Polypropylene catheters
   Red rubber catheters
   Tom cat catheters
Common diseases
   Dog
   Cat
Common emergencies
   CPR
   Anaphylactic reaction
   Blocked cat
   Dyspneic animal
   Dystocia
   Gastric torsion
   Seizures
   Toxicities
Declaws
   Equipment
   Procedure
   Paper strips
Dentals
   Machine
   Gum disease
   Anatomy of the mouth
Determining age of cats and dogs
Diets
   Dogs
   Cats
   Ferrets
   Rabbits
   Reptiles
   Snakes
   Birds
   Special diets (Hills, Waltham, Purina)
Fluids
   Types
   Additives
   Catheter types and sizes
   Catheter use and maintenance
   Heparin bags and prep
   Administration of fluids
   Drip rate calculation

Heartworm disease
   Life cycle of the heartworm
   Treatment
   Prevention
Instruments
   Care and handling
   Autoclaving
   General pack
   Cold sterilization
   General cold pack
Kennel care
   Tech duties
   Cleaning procedures
   Blankets
Laboratory equipment and procedures
   Centrifuges
   Microscopes
   IDEXX Lasercyte Machine, T4
   Hemocytometer
   Refractometer
   Tonometer
   Diagnostic tests and lab work
      Bloodwork abbreviations
      Heartworm test
      Difil
      Parvo
      FELV
      FELV/FIV
      WBC
      HCT or PCV
      TP
      UA
      Fecal
      DTM
      Ear smear
      Ear mite check
      Skin scrape
      Staining slides
   Protocols for common bloodwork
      ACTH stim
      Bile acids
      Phenobarbital
      Thyroid
Logs
   Lab log
   Surgery log
   Controlled drug log
   Radiology log
Material Safety Date Sheets
   Location
   How to read
Medications
   Abbreviations
   Weight conversions
   Labels
   Administration
Neutering pets; see spaying/neutering pets
Pregnancy
   Care of female

Continued

Box 5-11	Sample Table of Contents for Employee Procedure Manual—cont'd

CPR, Cardiopulmonary resuscitation; *FELV,* feline leukemia; *FIV,* feline immunodeficiency virus; *WBC,* white blood cell count; *HCT,* hematocrit; *PCV,* packed cell volume; *TP,* total protein; *UA,* urinalysis; *DTM,* dermatophyte test medium; *ACTH stim;* adrenocorticotropic hormone stimulation; *NPO,* nothing by mouth.

PAYROLL

It is important for a manager to understand the entire payroll process. Becoming as organized as possible in its management will ensure a successful system. Payroll can be time consuming and tedious and must be maintained by a motivated, intelligent team member. That team member must be held accountable for correct payroll procedures and must ensure that all tax payments are submitted on time. The person who signs and prepares the payroll tax form is held accountable by the Internal Revenue Service (IRS); if any mistakes occur or payments are received late, that individual will be responsible for the late fees and corrections.

PRACTICE POINT The employee responsible for payroll and taxes is held accountable by the IRS for any mistakes that are made in or delay tax payments.

Pay periods are defined as the length of time covered by each payroll period and generally cover weekly, biweekly, or semimonthly periods. An example of 1 week would be Monday morning through Sunday night. A practice can determine what pay period works best as well as days of the week to start and stop the period.

Weekly pay periods pay employees once a week, generating 52 paychecks per year. The disadvantage to weekly pay periods is the administrative costs associated with processing payroll on a weekly basis. Biweekly payroll decreases administrative costs by processing payroll every other week, producing only 26 checks per year. Employees must learn how to balance their budgets to accommodate biweekly checks. Because there are not a balanced number of weeks in every month, there will be 2 months out of the year when payroll occurs three times within the month. This can make reports appear incorrect, as these months will appear less profitable, and should not be used in comparison with previous year-to-month analysis. If the months are analyzed, the increased payroll period should be noted. Semimonthly payroll eliminates this appearance in the analysis because payroll occurs evenly on the first and the fifteenth of each month and produces 24 pay periods per year.

Animal Bites:

Any bite is BAD! If you are bitten under any circumstances, you need to report it to Nancy and go to your doctor. Cats are the worst. They have the most bacteria and the worst bacteria. You must receive antibiotics from your doctor. If you do not, call Nancy. Be sure the doctor does not suture the wound closed.

Artificial Insemination:

In both dogs and cats, breeding can occur naturally between a male and a female, or by *artificial insemination (AI)*. To breed by AI, semen must be collected from the male and then either inserted directly into the female or deep-frozen for later use. The female must be in the proper stage of the estrous cycle. Once the semen is collected, it must be inserted into the female as soon as possible. If it is frozen it needs to warm to room temperature, be evaluated, and inserted into the female.

Equipment needed for AI:
- Rubber vulva
- Collection vial
- Slides to evaluate semen (place on microscope to warm slides)
- AI tube
- 12-mL syringe
- KY Jelly

Bandages/Splints/Casts:

Bandages: Bandages are used to protect an area (an incision), apply pressure to a specific area, or cover a wound. Bandages used to protect an area (e.g., after a dewclaw surgery) generally have a Telfa pad over the area, with some absorbent gauze and vet wrap. A bandage used to apply pressure (e.g., after a declaw surgery) requires absorbent gauze and vet wrap. If it is to apply pressure to the abdominal area, we may use an Ace bandage. For wound management, various types of bandages can be used. A **wet to dry bandage** is used when a wound cannot be sutured closed. A Kotex pad soaked with saline is applied to the wound, which is normally wrapped lightly with an Ace bandage. These bandages need to be changed at least twice daily. **A dry bandage** normally consists of a Telfa pad on the wound, which is wrapped with cotton bandage material, brown Kling gauze, then vet wrap. These bandages need to be changed frequently depending on the case and the doctor. A bandage must have "stirrups" (tape on the leg itself and wrapped around the bandage material). This helps stabilize the bandage to prevent it from slipping.

Splints/Casts: These are used to stabilize a broken bone. A splint may be used in place of a cast if there is an underlying wound dressing that needs to be changed frequently. Both splints and casts require a lot of padding to prevent pressure sores. First apply stirrups to both sides of the leg. Wrap the leg with cotton gauze high enough to protect the leg from the top of the cast or splint (always wrap from the toes toward the shoulder). Next, wrap the leg with brown Kling gauze, being sure not to wrap the leg too tight. If you are applying a splint, one stirrup should be taped onto the bandage and the other onto the splint. Secure the splint with additional tape as needed. Wrap the splint with brown Kling gauze and vet wrap. Be sure to check the toes daily for swelling. If

FIGURE 5-10 Sample pages from an employee procedures manual.

When determining payday, the day that team members receive their checks, it is important to allow sufficient time between the end of the pay period and payday for payroll preparation. Generally, 3 days is sufficient. If a bookkeeper or accountant is used, he or she may ask for less time.

Determining Staff Wages

Determining wages for different levels of staff can be a challenge, as a balance must be made between budgeting and maintaining an educated and dedicated staff. Team members must be compensated for their skill while there is any swelling, the splint needs to be redone. If you are applying a cast, soak the cast material in warm water for 1 minute. (Be sure to use gloves so that you do not get adhesive on your hands.) Apply the cast material and allow it to dry (approximately 3 to 5 minutes). Tape the stirrups onto the cast and wrap with vet wrap. ALWAYS leave space at the toes to check for swelling.

DO NOT ALLOW CASTS OR SPLINTS TO GET WET. If the animal must be outside, the foot can be wrapped in a plastic bag to protect the cast or splint. If the pet comes inside, remove the bag because sweaty paw pads will also get the splint or cast wet.

Blood Transfusions:

We have several different options when administering a transfusion. Once the method has been chosen, make sure all the products needed are available. If this is the first transfusion for the pet, the blood does not have to be cross-matched. If the pet has had prior transfusions, the blood must be matched to the donor. Reactions can occur in any animal. All patients must be monitored during and after the administration of the transfusion.

- *Plasma transfusion:* Fresh frozen plasma is used to treat animals with low protein or clotting factors. It must be ordered from the Animal Blood Bank. It is shipped overnight on ice and must be frozen until ready to use. Once you are ready to use it, thaw it to room temperature and use it within 24 hours. It is administered with a standard 15 d/mL IV infusion set.
- *Whole blood:* Whole blood is used to replace all blood components. It is generally donated from a staff member's pet. The doctor must determine that the donating pet is healthy, has not donated in the past 12 weeks, is parasite free, and is large enough to donate the amount of blood needed. The donor is placed on a table, and either the jugular vein or cephalic vein is clipped as for a catheter. A blood collection set is used. One end is inserted into the appropriate sized ACD bottle (a hemostat clip is placed on the line to prevent vacuum loss in the bottle). The 14-g needle is inserted into the vein (and secured as with an IV catheter and line). Once the blood flashes back, remove the hemostat and gently agitate the bottle while it is filling. Once the bottle is full, apply the hemostat onto the line again and remove the collection set from the donor pet. Apply a tight bandage to the site to prevent a hematoma if a cephalic vein is used. The donor pet should be fed a great meal after the donation. This donated blood is good for 3 weeks. It should be discarded after that. When administering the transfusion, a blood transfusion set is used. Prep the cephalic vein as you would for a general IV catheter. Insert the transfusion set into the collection bottle and allow the chamber to fill. Insert a catheter and flush with a heparin solution. Attach the transfusion set and administer at the recommended dose. Observe for any reaction.

  The following supplies are needed for whole blood transfusions:
  - Blood collection set
  - Blood administration set
  - ACD bottle
  - Catheter
  - Tape
  - Vet wrap
  - Treats for the blood donor

FIGURE 5-10, cont'd Sample pages from an employee procedures manual.

creating and maintaining an environment that is enjoyable for the staff. When considering wages, the benefits package that is available to the staff must be remembered (team members should be reminded of the benefits received during their annual review). The location of the practice within the United States also plays a factor in wage determination, as the cost of living in some areas is higher than in others. Practices in large cities, referral practices, and specialty centers will also have higher compensation rates than those in smaller cities and general practice.

PRACTICE POINT The cost of living continues to rise while the pay of long-term employees does not; a yearly evaluation system must be implemented to ensure raises are provided.

Catheters:

Butterfly: These catheters come with 25-g and 28-g needles. They are commonly used for subcutaneous fluids in exotic animals, ferrets, birds, and very small dogs and cats. We also use them to administer IV drugs to exotic pets. They are great for subcutaneous fluids when an animal is extremely wiggly; it allows movement without injuring the animal.

Foley catheters: These are generally used to do a cystogram (injecting dye into the bladder of a pet). Foley catheters have 2 ports: one to inject medication into and the other to inflate the balloon.

IV catheters: Selection of types of catheters and gauge depends on species and size, fragility of veins, length of time the catheter will be in place, and type of fluids administered. A 24-g catheter is commonly used for cats, a 22-g catheter for a small to medium dog, and a 20-g catheter for a large dog. A larger dog should also have a longer (2-inch catheter) versus the normal 1-inch catheter for medium and small dogs.

Jugular catheters: These are used to do transtracheal washes on pets. We commonly use 16-g and 18-g catheters.

Polypropylene catheters: We commonly use these catheters for blocked dogs. These catheters come in a variety of sizes in a large white tube. They are sterile in the tube, so be sure not to empty them or touch them when you remove one.

Red rubber catheters: These can be used for either tube feeding an animal or to insert into a blocked cat. They are individually packaged and come in sizes from 3 French to 14 French.

"Tom cat" catheters: These are used for blocked cats and come in one size. They are also packaged individually and are sterile in each package.

FIGURE 5-10, cont'd Sample pages from an employee procedures manual.

Box 5-12	**Common Team Positions in a Veterinary Clinic**

- Owner veterinarian
- Associate veterinarian
- Practice manager
- Registered/certified veterinary technician
- Office manager
- Veterinary assistants
- Receptionists
- Kennel assistant
- Groomer

To help a new practice determine a pay scale or an existing practice update its scale, a chart can be developed to show minimum, maximum, and average ranges for each position, as well as to determine any discrepancies a current practice may have in its pay scale system. It is critical to have consistent procedures for setting pay levels for each position. The first step is to list all the jobs in the practice and to rank them according to importance (Box 5-12). This allows the most important jobs to be ranked highest, providing the highest compensation. For new practices, this is ideal; for existing practices, it may reveal less important jobs receiving higher pay because the employee was recently hired. In general, wages have risen, but salaries of long-term employees have not. The second step is to chart what current employees are being paid. The third step is to insert the benchmark pay scales available from the American Animal Hospital Association (AAHA), Veterinary Hospital Managers Association (VHMA), or National Commission on Veterinary Economic Issues (NCVEI) to determine where the practice sits in the national average. As previously stated, the location of the practice in the United States is a factor in pay scales, but a practice should at least be at or above the 75th percentile. This will help recruit and retain excellent team members.

Veterinarians

Hiring a veterinarian for a practice is very important; not only should the person be able to fit into the practice, he or she has to be able to fit into the budget of the practice. To determine whether a practice can support another veterinarian, reports should be generated looking at the average number of clients seen on a yearly basis. To support a full-time–equivalent veterinarian, 800 to 1200 active clients are needed per year. Therefore the practice needs to see at least an additional 800 clients per year to justify a new veterinarian.

Once it has been determined that another veterinarian is needed and can be fairly compensated, then the practice must decide before hiring how it will be compensate the veterinarian and how much he or she will be compensated.

> ◎ **PRACTICE POINT** Veterinarians are paid by salary, production, or a combination of both.

Pro-sal, a combination of production and salary, is one form of compensation; salary only and production only are the other two types of salary commonly paid. If the practice commonly accepts after-hours emergencies, doctors may be paid additional money to compensate for their time. Under professional liability, veterinarians have a legal duty to accept emergencies or refer them to an emergency practice after hours.

Pro-Sal Formula

The most common form of compensation is a pro-sal formula, also referred to as the *production reconciliation hybrid*. This allows veterinarians to receive a base salary and a production bonus once a predetermined dollar amount has been reached. If this formula is chosen, the base salary must first be determined and is normally based on the veterinarian's experience. The production bonus then needs to be set; the practice must determine how much the veterinarian must produce before receiving the bonus. The practice should also decide what percentage of the production will be paid as a bonus and whether the bonus is paid on a monthly or quarterly basis.

An example of pro-sal is as follows:

A veterinarian is paid $60,000 base salary per year, with a 10% production bonus once production has reached $10,000 per month. Bonuses are paid monthly for the previous month's production. Payday is on the first and the fifteenth of each month.

To figure salary pay: **$60,000/24 (24 pay periods per year) = $2500 per check.** The veterinarian produced $33,000 for the previous month: **$33,000 × 10% = $3300.** The gross pay for the first is **$2500 + $3300 = $5800.** The gross pay for the fifteenth is $2500.

The definition of gross pay is the total amount earned before any taxes or other withholdings.

Salary

In brief, salary-compensated veterinarians receive a set amount, regardless of the amount of dollars produced. Some practices prefer to pay veterinarians a set salary as opposed to any other form of pay, as it seems to decrease the competition among veterinarians in the practice. It promotes a team environment, and all doctors and staff help each other accomplish all tasks, diagnoses, and treatments needed. A practice needs to determine a set salary for a veterinarian; again, this is generally based on his or her experience. As previously stated, veterinarians are exempt from overtime under FLSA. Hours should be monitored to prevent burnout.

> ◎ **PRACTICE POINT** Veterinarians are exempt from overtime wages, as defined by the FLSA.

An example of salary pay is similar to the example above; the veterinarian receives $60,000 in salary per year. Payday occurs on the first and the fifteenth of each month: $60,000/24 = $2500 per pay period.

Production

Production compensation pays a veterinarian a percentage of the amount of dollars produced. The practice must determine the percentage before hiring a veterinarian; average amounts are 18% to 25% in small-animal practice and 25% to 30% in large-animal practice. It is also necessary to determine what is paid as production. Medications, over-the-counter products, foods, diagnostics, and surgical procedures should all be considered. In general, veterinarians are paid just as the rest of the staff, either biweekly or on the first and the fifteenth of each month. A report is generated for each veterinarian indicating the dollar amount produced for that specific period. The dollar amount produced is then multiplied by the percentage determined and paid as gross salary.

A production-only salary can be easy to figure as well. A veterinarian is paid 20% of production of all services and products. Payday occurs on the first and the fifteenth of each month. The payroll manager should pull a report of that specific veterinarian's production from the first and the fourteenth of the month. If the veterinarian produced $15,000 during that period, $15,000 × 20% = $3000 gross pay. The second pay period report would run from the fifteenth to the thirtieth or thirty-first of the month. If the veterinarian produced $16,236 for that period, then $16236 × 20% = $3247.20 gross pay.

Production as the basis for salary can decrease the overall team spirit and promotes competition among veterinarians. Some veterinarians will perform diagnostic procedures that may not be necessary to increase their production numbers. This can lead to claims of gouging.

It also promotes competition between veterinarians in choosing wealthy clients and big cases over yearly exams, vaccines, and small procedures. It can also discourage veterinarians from participating in any procedures that do not produce an income or that only produce a small amount of income. If the practice offers healthy shelter-pet checks for a reduced cost, production-only veterinarians may choose not to see them.

The practice must determine which formula is going to work best for the practice. Some practices may find that competition is not a problem within the hospital and that either a pro-sal or production-only formula yields the best results. Others may find the salary formula to be the easiest and least time-consuming formula to use. The advantage to percentage-based compensation is that it can motivate veterinarians to work hard and produce more income. It emphasizes the medical and business aspect of veterinary medicine and compensates veterinarians for their successful efforts and the skills involved in practicing high-quality medicine. It can also eliminate opportunities for claims of discrimination because pay is based on production, not determined by management.

Practices must be well staffed and trained for a pro-sal or production formula to work efficiently. Veterinarians can effectively delegate duties, treatments, and diagnostics to technicians while they continue seeing patients. If they cannot delegate duties, they may become upset with management over the lack of staff training.

Emergency Pay

If emergencies are accepted after hours, veterinarians may be paid salary plus emergency pay. Some practices pay the set emergency fee per animal seen: an average of $35 to $50 per case before 11 PM and $50 to $75 after 11 PM. Other practices may pay 30% to 50% of the exam cost, plus a percentage of the diagnostics performed before the office opens. Yet another option may be to pay 10% of the exam fee and 18% to 22% of the total client transaction.

> **PRACTICE POINT** Veterinarians should be compensated in some fashion for emergency rotations.

Technicians

Credentialed technicians are usually compensated based on experience and should be paid on an hourly basis. Technicians are generally dedicated and will work hours in excess of 40 hours per week to ensure that the necessary duties, tasks, and treatments are completed for every patient. FLSA of 1938 states that all employees who work over 40 hours within a 1-week period must be paid overtime.

Practices may set an average start rate with a set number of years of experience to create consistency when hiring team members. Industry benchmarks are available from AAHA, VHMA, and NCVEI to help practices determine wage levels for technicians in each area of the United States.

Assistants, Receptionists, and Kennel Attendants

Many practices start team members without any experience at a minimum wage, allowing for raises as tasks and duties are mastered. Assistants without a certificate, receptionists, and kennel attendants generally do not have any veterinary experience, which is gained through the workplace environment. Some receptionists may be hired who have previous customer service experience, which should be considered when determining wages. Customer service skills are an invaluable resource to a practice and should not be overlooked.

Groomers

Some groomers are paid on a production percentage, just as veterinarians may be paid, whereas others may be paid hourly. Independent groomers may simply be paid a fee for each animal that is groomed; others may only rent the space within the veterinary practice.

> **PRACTICE POINT** Some groomers are considered independent contractors and are paid by the day rather than the hour.

Independent groomers must have their own tax identification numbers; therefore taxes are not taken out of the groomers' paychecks. They are responsible for paying their own federal and state taxes. At the end of the year, independent groomers receiving pay over $600 within the fiscal year must be issued a MISC-1099 form (when others are issued W-2s) for taxation purposes. The MISC-1099 cites all monies paid to the contractor on an untaxed basis. The groomer submits this MISC-1099 form with his or her taxes (Figure 5-11). (See the Evolve site that accompanies this text for the complete form.)

Determining Raises

Employees may receive raises on a scheduled basis. The practice should establish a policy as to when raises will be considered for all team members. Some practices may give raises after 3 months of employment, then on a yearly basis. Some practices give raises based on merit, whereas others give raises with the completion and mastering of skills. Cost-of-living raises must also be considered for those not receiving a raise based on merit or skill.

Raises should not be given at the same time employee evaluations are given; they tend to decrease the value of the evaluation. Evaluations should be completed first, and then raises can follow within a few months.

A budget should be developed that includes raises for employees. When a set dollar amount has been budgeted for raises, the amount can be distributed among team members. Lists can be developed rating team members, allowing a specific percentage or dollar amount increase. Those team members that go above and beyond the call of duty must be placed at the top of the list for the largest raises. Those with less skill and lower quality of work ethic can be placed at the end of the list. Veterinarians may be compensated based on production or receive a percentage increase, whichever the budget allows.

If the clinic's budget does not allow a set raise for employees, yet team members need to be rewarded for

9595 ☐ VOID ☐ CORRECTED

PAYER'S name, street address, city, state, ZIP code, and telephone no. Z Builders 123 Maple Avenue Oaktown, VA 22000 703-123-4567		1 Rents $ 2 Royalties $	OMB No. 1545-0115 2010 Form 1099-MISC	Miscellaneous Income
		3 Other income $	4 Federal income tax withheld $	Copy A For Internal Revenue Service Center File with Form 1096.
PAYER'S federal identification number 10-9999999	RECIPIENT'S identification number 123-00-6789	5 Fishing boat proceeds $	6 Medical and health care payments $	
RECIPIENT'S name Ronald Green dba/Y Drywall		7 Nonemployee compensation $ 5500.00	8 Substitute payments in lieu of dividends or interest $	For Privacy Act and Paperwork Reduction Act Notice, see the 2010 General Instructions for Certain Information Returns.
Street address (including apt. no.) 456 Flower Lane		9 Payer made direct sales of $5,000 or more of consumer products to a buyer (recipient) for resale ▶ ☐	10 Crop insurance proceeds $	
City, state, and ZIP code Oaktown, VA 22000		11	12	
Account number (see instructions)	2nd TIN not. ☐	13 Excess golden parachute payments $	14 Gross proceeds paid to an attorney $	
15a Section 409A deferrals $	15b Section 409A income $	16 State tax withheld $ $	17 State/Payer's state no.	18 State income $ $

Form 1099-MISC Cat. No. 14425J Department of the Treasury - Internal Revenue Service

FIGURE 5-11 IRS Form Misc-1099.

excellent work, then a one-time bonus can be given. A bonus allows team members to know they are appreciated, but affects the bottom line less than employee raises do. A bonus is a one-time payout, as opposed to a raise, which permanently increases expenditures. With that said, raises should not be overlooked because employees may seek employment at other practices offering higher pay.

> **PRACTICE POINT** Employee raises should be placed into the yearly budget; raises can then be allotted to team members without exceeding the yearly budget.

Managing Payroll

Payroll has many different aspects, and organization is the key to managing it successfully. Some practices have a bookkeeper or accountant manage payroll; others use internal office managers to complete the tasks.

Intuit QuickBooks is an excellent source for payroll software. Frequent tax updates are sent as well as tips for organizing payroll records. QuickBooks calculates the taxes that are withheld from the employee and those contributed by the employer. If direct deposit is used, a link is available to complete the deposit. When extra money is withheld from employees for insurance or retirement plans, QuickBooks establishes a sheet indicating what and how much should be withheld. Payroll sheets are developed for each employee, and taxes to be paid are calculated. Team members must take the time to enter the information initially, and QuickBooks does all the rest.

Calculating Payroll

Examples are used to help explain payroll calculations if a manual method is used instead of software.

Regular rate calculations:

Example A: Wanda is paid $10 per hour and works 34 hours per week. Payroll is paid every other Monday; therefore the work week is Monday, 12:00 AM through Sunday, 12:59 PM.

$$34 \text{ hours per week} \times 2 = 68 \text{ hours per 2-week period}$$

$$68 \text{ hours} \times \$10 = \$680 \text{ before taxes}$$

Overtime rate calculations:

Example B: This period, Ann has worked 44 hours during week 1 and 32 hours during week 2. She is paid $10 per hour; overtime is paid at $15 per hour (1½ times the regular rate).

Week 1: 40 hours × $10 = $400; 4 hours × $15 = $60

Week 2: 32 hours × $10 = $320

$400 + $60 + $320 = $780 before taxes

Example C: This period, Alex accrues 44 hours in week 1 and 52 hours during week 2.

Week 1: 40 hours × $10 = $400; 4 hours × $15 = $60

Week 2: 40 hours × $10 = $400; 12 hours × $15 = $180

$400 + $60 + $400 + $180 = $1040 before taxes

More examples of calculations are available in Chapter 24.

Records

Many states require employee payroll records be kept for an average of 7 years. They should be kept in a locked cabinet for confidentiality purposes (each practice must check its own state's law for the number of years records are required to be kept). Employees should receive a payroll check stub with each paycheck (those with direct deposit should receive a stub on the day of payroll). Payroll stubs should indicate the employee's name, wage, and gross income (income before taxes and other withholdings), along with Social Security and Medicare withholdings. Contributions to an sIRA or 401(k) program should also be stated, along with any withholdings for insurance. Payroll stubs for full-time employees may also state the vacation and sick hours available. A summary sheet for all employees should be kept on file for each payroll period.

Direct Deposit

With the technology available today, many practices and employees prefer to use direct deposit for payroll checks. The check is deposited directly into the employee's checking account on the date of payroll; the employee does not need to go to the bank to deposit the check.

> **PRACTICE POINT** Direct deposit of payroll checks saves time, paper, and money for the employer.

Practices may contact their bank for direct deposit procedures. Normally, an authorization form is submitted from each employee to the practice's bank. The form includes the employee's name, address, current bank, and checking account number. It should also be signed by the employee authorizing the direct deposit. The bank may also request a voided check to ensure the correct routing number is entered when the initial deposit is set up. Paycheck amounts are usually due to the bank 2 to 3 business days before payday. This ensures that the funds will be transferred on payday.

The advantages of direct deposit are numerous. Less paper is used, and it takes less time for the staff to write checks and place them in secured envelopes. Team members who do not have checking accounts may continue to request regular payroll checks; this should not be a problem because those checks can be written as they previously were.

Payroll Taxes

Several taxes are withheld from employees, and the employer is responsible for paying those as well as additional taxes. The practice bookkeeper, accountant, or team member responsible for payroll will determine this amount and must ensure that the taxes are paid on time. State revenue departments dislike late payments and often penalize heavily for those that are late.

Social Security and Medicare

Taxes withheld from an employee payroll checks include income tax, Social Security, and Medicare. Social Security and Medicare fall under the Federal Insurance Contribution Act (FICA), wherein 6.2% of the gross pay is withheld for Social Security and 0.145% is withheld for Medicare. The employer is responsible for contributing the same amount to FICA. The total employee income taxes, as well as the employee and employer portions of FICA, are paid to the IRS through a federal tax deposit (FTD) system.

> **PRACTICE POINT** Employers and employees are responsible for Medicare and Social Security contributions.

If an employee's gross pay is $1200, FICA would be $74.40 and the Social Security contribution would be $1.74.

$$($1200 \times 0.062) = $74.40 \text{ and } ($1200 \times 0.00145) = $1.74$$

FTDs are required and must be paid on either a monthly basis or a semiweekly basis. The amount of tax due within a select period determines whether practices must pay monthly or semiweekly. Form 8109 must be filled out with the deposit and can be submitted electronically or at the practice's banking institution (Figure 5-12).

Federal Unemployment Tax Act

In addition to reporting FICA contributions on Form 941, employers are also responsible for taxes under FUTA, which are reported on Form 940. These taxes are paid solely by the employer, not withheld or deducted from the employee. FUTA only taxes the first $7000 paid to an employee in 1 year; the rate is 0.008%. A few states do not have an unemployment program; therefore tax in these states may be slightly higher.

> **PRACTICE POINT** Employers are responsible for FUTA contributions.

AMOUNT OF DEPOSIT (Do NOT type, please print.)

DOLLARS   CENTS

MONTH TAX
YEAR ENDS →

EMPLOYER IDENTIFICATION NUMBER →

BANK NAME/
DATE STAMP

Name _____

Address _____

_____

City _____

State _____ ZIP _____

Telephone number ( )

IRS USE
ONLY

FOR BANK USE IN MICR ENCODING

Darken only one
TYPE OF TAX

941	945
1120	1042
943	990-T
720	990-PF
CT-1	944
940	

Darken only one
TAX PERIOD

1st Quarter
2nd Quarter
3rd Quarter
4th Quarter

86

Federal Tax Deposit Coupon
Form 8109-B (Rev. 12-2006)

- -

↑ ___ SEPARATE ALONG THIS LINE AND SUBMIT TO DEPOSITARY WITH PAYMENT ___ ↑   OMB NO. 1545-0257

What's new. The oval for Form 990-C has been deleted. Form 990-C has been replaced by Form 1120-C, U.S. Income Tax Return for Cooperative Associations. Filers of Form 1120-C must use the 1120 oval when completing Form 8109-B.

The type of tax ovals for the 1120, 1042, and 944 have been moved on the coupon. Read the type of tax to the right of the oval before you darken the oval.

Note. Except for the name, address, and telephone number, entries must be made in pencil. Use soft lead (for example, a #2 pencil) so that the entries can be read more accurately by optical scanning equipment. The name, address, and telephone number may be completed other than by hand. You cannot use photocopies of the coupons to make your deposits. Do not staple, tape, or fold the coupons.

The IRS encourages you to make federal tax deposits using the Electronic Federal Tax Payment System (EFTPS). For more information on EFTPS, go to www.eftps.gov or call 1-800-555-4477.

Purpose of form. Use Form 8109-B to make a tax deposit only in the following two situations.

1. You have not yet received your resupply of preprinted deposit coupons (Form 8109).

2. You are a new entity and have already been assigned an employer identification number (EIN), but you have not received your initial supply of preprinted deposit coupons (Form 8109). If you have not received your EIN, see *Exceptions* below.

Note. If you do not receive your resupply of deposit coupons and a deposit is due or you do not receive your initial supply within 5–6 weeks of receipt of your EIN, call 1-800-829-4933.

How to complete the form. Enter your name as shown on your return or other IRS correspondence, address, and EIN in the spaces provided. Do not make a name or address change on this form (see Form 8822, Change of Address). If you are required to file a Form 1120, 1120-C, 990-PF (with net investment income), 990-T, or 2438, enter the month in which your tax year ends in the MONTH TAX YEAR ENDS box. For example, if your tax year ends in January, enter 01; if it ends in December, enter 12. Make your entries for EIN and MONTH TAX YEAR ENDS (if applicable) as shown in Amount of deposit below.

Exceptions. If you have applied for an EIN, have not received it, and a deposit must be made, use Form 8109-B. Instead, send your payment to the IRS address where you file your return. Make your check or money order payable to the United States Treasury and show on it your name (as shown on Form SS-4, Application for Employer Identification Number), address, kind of tax, period covered, and date you applied for an EIN. Do not use Form 8109-B to deposit delinquent taxes assessed by the IRS. Pay those taxes directly to the IRS. See Pub. 15 (Circular E), Employer's Tax Guide, for information.

Amount of deposit. Enter the amount of the deposit in the space provided. Enter the amount legibly, forming the characters as shown below:

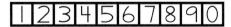

Hand print money amounts without using dollar signs, commas, a decimal point, or leading zeros. If the deposit is for whole dollars only, enter "00" in the CENTS boxes. For example, a deposit of $7,635.22 would be entered like this:

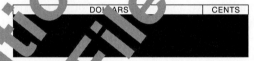

DOLLARS	CENTS

Caution. Darken only one space for TYPE OF TAX and only one space for TAX PERIOD. Darken the space to the left of the applicable form and tax period. Darkening the wrong space or multiple spaces may delay proper crediting of your account. See below for an explanation of Types of Tax and Marking the Proper Tax Period.

Types of Tax

Form 941   Employer's QUARTERLY Federal Tax Return (includes Forms 941-M, 941-PR, and 941-SS)

Form 943   Employer's Annual Tax Return for Agricultural Employees

Form 944   Employer's ANNUAL Federal Tax Return (includes Forms 944-PR, 944(SP), and 944-SS)

Form 945   Annual Return of Withheld Federal Income Tax

Form 720   Quarterly Federal Excise Tax Return

Form CT-1   Employer's Annual Railroad Retirement Tax Return

Form 940   Employer's Annual Federal Unemployment (FUTA) Return (includes Form 940-PR)

Form 1120   U.S. Corporation Income Tax Return (includes Form 1120 series of returns, such as new Form 1120-C, and Form 2438)

Form 990-T Exempt Organization Business Income Tax Return

Form 990-PF Return of Private Foundation or Section 4947(a)(1) Nonexempt Charitable Trust Treated as a Private Foundation

Form 1042   Annual Withholding Tax Return for U.S. Source Income of Foreign Persons

Marking the Proper Tax Period

Payroll taxes and withholding. For Forms 941, 940, 943, 944, 945, CT-1, and 1042, if your liability was incurred during:

- January 1 through March 31, darken the 1st quarter space;
- April 1 through June 30, darken the 2nd quarter space;
- July 1 through September 30, darken the 3rd quarter space; and
- October 1 through December 31, darken the 4th quarter space.

Note. If the liability was incurred during one quarter and deposited in another quarter, darken the space for the quarter in which the tax liability was incurred. For example, if the liability was incurred in March and deposited in April, darken the 1st quarter space.

Excise taxes. For Form 720, follow the instructions above for Forms 941, 940, etc. For Form 990-PF, with net investment income, follow the instructions on page 2 for Form 1120, 990-T, and 2438.

Department of the Treasury
Internal Revenue Service

Form **8109-B** (Rev. 12-2006)
Cat. No. 61042S

FIGURE 5-12 IRS Form 8109.

Income Taxes (Form 1120, 990-T, and 2438). To make an estimated tax deposit for any quarter of the current tax year, darken only the 1st quarter space.

Example 1. If your tax year ends on December 31, 2007, and a deposit for 2007 is being made between January 1 and December 31, 2007, darken the 1st quarter space.

Example 2. If your tax year ends on June 30, 2007, and a deposit for that fiscal year is being made between July 1, 2006, and June 30, 2007, darken the 1st quarter space.

To make a deposit for the prior tax year, darken only the 4th quarter space. This includes:

● Deposits of balance due shown on the return (Forms 1120, 990-T, and 990-PF).

● Deposits of balance due shown on Form 7004, Application for Automatic 6-Month Extension of Time To File Certain Business Income Tax, Information, and Other Returns (be sure to darken the 1120 or 1042 space as appropriate).

● Deposits of balance due (Forms 990-T and 990-PF filers) shown on Form 8868, Application for Extension of Time To File an Exempt Organization Return (be sure to darken the 990-T or 990-PF space as appropriate).

● Deposits of tax due shown on Form 2438, Undistributed Capital Gains Tax Return (darken the 1120 space).

Example 1. If your tax year ends on December 31, 2006, and a deposit for 2006 is being made after that date, darken the 4th quarter space.

Example 2. If your tax year ends on June 30, 2007, and a deposit for that fiscal year is being made after that date, darken the 4th quarter space.

How to ensure your deposit is credited to the correct account.

1. Make sure your name and EIN are correct.

2. Prepare only one coupon for each type of tax deposit.

3. Darken only one space for the type of tax you are depositing;

4. Darken only one space for the tax period for which you are making a deposit; and

5. Use separate FTD coupons for each return period.

Telephone number. We need your daytime telephone number to call if we have difficulty processing your deposit.

Miscellaneous. We use the "IRS USE ONLY" box to ensure proper crediting to your account. Do not darken this space when making a deposit.

How to make deposits. Mail or deliver the completed coupon with the amount of the deposit to an authorized depositary (financial institution) for federal taxes. Make your check or money order payable to that depositary. To help ensure proper crediting to your account, write your EIN, the type of tax (for example, Form 940), and the tax period to which the payment applies on your check or money order.

Authorized depositaries must accept cash, postal money orders drawn to the order of the depositary, or checks or drafts drawn on and to the order of the depositary. You can deposit taxes with a check drawn on another financial institution only if the depositary is willing to accept that form of payment.

If you prefer, you may mail your coupon and payment to Financial Agent, Federal Tax Deposit Processing, P.O. Box 970030, St. Louis, MO 63197. Make your check or money order payable to the Financial Agent.

Timeliness of deposits. The IRS determines whether deposits are on time by the date they are received by an authorized depositary. However, a deposit received by the authorized depositary after the due date will be considered timely if the taxpayer establishes that it was mailed in the United States in a properly addressed, postage prepaid envelope at least 2 days before the due date.

Note. If you are required to deposit any taxes more than once a month, any deposit of $20,000 or more must be received by its due date to be timely.

When to deposit. See the instructions for the applicable return. See Pub. 15 (Circular E) for deposit rules on employment taxes. Generally, you can get copies of forms and instructions by calling 1-800-TAX-FORM (1-800-829-3676) or by visiting IRS's website at *www.irs.gov*.

Penalties. You may be charged a penalty for not making deposits when due or in sufficient amounts, unless you have reasonable cause. This penalty may also apply if you mail or deliver federal tax deposits to unauthorized institutions or IRS offices, rather than to authorized depositaries. Additionally, a trust fund recovery penalty may be imposed on all persons who are determined by the IRS to be responsible for collecting, accounting for, and paying over employment and excise taxes, and who acted willfully in not doing so. For more information on penalties, see Pub. 15 (Circular E). See the Instructions for Form 720 for when these penalties apply to excise taxes.

Privacy Act and Paperwork Reduction Act Notice. Internal Revenue Code section 6302 requires certain persons to make periodic deposits of taxes. If you do not deposit electronically, you must provide the information requested on this form. IRC section 6109 requires you to provide your EIN. The information on this form is used to ensure that you are complying with the Internal Revenue laws and to ensure proper crediting of your deposit. Routine uses of this information include providing it to the Department of Justice for civil and criminal litigation, and to cities, states, and the District of Columbia for use in administering their tax laws. We may also disclose this information to federal and state agencies to enforce federal nontax criminal laws and to combat terrorism. We may give this information to other countries pursuant to tax treaties. Providing incomplete, incorrect, or fraudulent information may subject you to interest and penalties.

You are not required to provide the information requested on a form that is subject to the Paperwork Reduction Act unless the form displays a valid OMB control number. Books or records relating to a form or its instructions must be retained as long as their contents may become material in the administration of any Internal Revenue law. Generally, tax returns and return information are confidential, as required by IRC section 6103.

The time needed to complete and file this form will vary depending on individual circumstances. The estimated average time is 3 minutes. If you have comments concerning the accuracy of this time estimate or suggestions for making this form simpler, we would be happy to hear from you. You can write to the Internal Revenue Service, Tax Products Coordinating Committee, SE:W:CAR:MP:T:T:SP, IR-6406, 1111 Constitution Ave. NW, Washington, DC 20224. Do not send this form to this address. Instead, see the instructions under *How to make deposits* on this page.

 Printed on recycled paper

FIGURE 5-12, cont'd

Unemployment tax is generally paid quarterly; the amount of tax due depends on the schedule of payments. Just as with Form 941, payments are made electronically or at the practice's banking institution (Figures 5-13 and 5-14). (See the Evolve site that accompanies this text for complete forms.)

W-2 and W-4 Forms

Employees are required to fill out a W-4 form once they are hired for employment. The form asks questions to determine how many deductions should be withheld from the payroll check, along with requiring the employee's Social Security number, address, and signature. This form should be kept in the employee personnel file in case it is ever needed again, or if the employee wishes to change the number of deductions on the form (Figures 5-15 and 5-16). (See the Evolve site that accompanies this text for the complete form.)

At the end of the year, as taxes are prepared, the accountant or bookkeeper will produce W-2 forms that summarize the employees' earnings for the year. These forms include gross earnings and Social Security and Medicare, insurance, and retirement withholdings. These forms are due to employees no later than January 31 of each year.

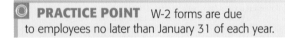

PRACTICE POINT W-2 forms are due to employees no later than January 31 of each year.

PERSONNEL FILES

There should be a file of confidential information on each employee. These files can be kept in a locking file cabinet that only the owner and practice manager can access. All information regarding an employee should be kept together and be well organized for easy retrieval.

The team member's resume may be located at the front of the file, followed by the W-4, the employee benefits form, and an emergency contact form. Raises, evaluations, reprimands, and any disciplinary history can be included next, followed by copies of any credentials the team member may have. Other documents may include job descriptions, interview reports, background verification reports, offer of employment letters, and training records. I-9 forms, garnishment orders, credit reports, and medical records should be stored in a separate file, again in a locked cabinet. It is recommended that these records be kept for a minimum of 7 years after an employee has left the practice in case employment verification should be needed by another employer, or in case of tax or payroll audits or job-related illnesses or injuries. State and local laws may vary regarding the length of years records must be kept; whichever period is longer should supersede the other.

CONTRACT EMPLOYEE VERSUS EMPLOYEE

Some veterinarians prefer to be contract employees instead of staff members. This is especially true for relief veterinarians. Contract employees, as stated above for groomers, are responsible for their own taxes. Therefore contract employees are paid a straight fee; taxes are not withheld from their paychecks.

PRACTICE POINT Contract employees must follow strict guidelines set by the IRS to remain contract employees rather than permanent employees.

The IRS is strict regarding the classification of contract employment versus employee. IRS code states that independent contractors are not required to follow instructions as to how to perform a task, duty, or job. The work must be performed at irregular intervals and cannot be full time. Contractors control their own hours and have the right to pursue other jobs. They must work without supervision and are paid by the job, not the hour. They are responsible for their own dues and licenses, which should be made available when contracted.

An example of an independent contractor would be a specialist who comes into a practice, performs surgery, and leaves. These doctors do not develop a client/patient relationship, are paid for the job performed, and generally bring their own technicians to assist. A relief veterinarian who covers for a short time, filling in for an absent veterinarian, is also an independent contractor. Veterinarians who work shifts for an emergency clinic must use caution if they choose to use the term *independent contractor.* They cannot continually work the same shift and cannot be considered to work full time.

Veterinarians who work as contract employees should have copies of all credentials, including state and controlled substance licenses and U.S. Department of Agriculture accreditation, on file. Verification of contract licenses should also be checked with the state board of veterinary medicine. It is the practice's responsibility to ensure that proper documentation is verified when hiring relief and contract veterinarians.

At the end of the year, any contract veterinarian receiving pay over $600 within the fiscal year must be issued an MISC-1099 form for taxation purposes (others are issued W-2s). A MISC-1099 cites all monies paid to the contractor on an untaxed basis. The veterinarian submits this MISC-1099 form with his or her taxes. (See Figure 5-11 for an example of a MISC-1099 form.)

If an independent contractor fails to file and pay his or her own taxes, and a practice used the contractor's services for over $600 and did not issue a MISC-1099 at the end of the year, the practice can be held responsible for all back taxes, interest, and penalty charges. It is imperative to contact a certified public accountant regarding

Form **940 for 2009:**   **Employer's Annual Federal Unemployment (FUTA) Tax Return**   850109

Department of the Treasury — Internal Revenue Service

OMB No. 1545-0028

(EIN)
Employer identification number ☐☐ – ☐☐☐☐☐☐☐

Name *(not your trade name)*

Trade name *(if any)*

Address
Number   Street   Suite or room number
City   State   ZIP code

Type of Return
(Check all that apply.)

☐ **a.** Amended
☐ **b.** Successor employer
☐ **c.** No payments to employees in 2009
☐ **d.** Final: Business closed or stopped paying wages

Read the separate instructions before you fill out this form. Please type or print within the boxes.

Part 1: Tell us about your return. If any line does NOT apply, leave it blank.

1   If you were required to pay your state unemployment tax in ...

1a One state only, write the state abbreviation . . . . **1a** ☐☐
   - OR -
1b More than one state (You are a multi-state employer) . . . . **1b** ☐ Check here. Fill out Schedule A.

2   If you paid wages in a state that is subject to **CREDIT REDUCTION** . . . . **2** ☐ Check here. Fill out Schedule A. (Form 940), Part 2.

Part 2: Determine your FUTA tax before adjustments for 2009. If any line does NOT apply, leave it blank.

3   Total payments to all employees . . . . **3** ▢

4   Payments exempt from FUTA tax . . . . **4** ▢

   Check all that apply: **4a** ☐ Fringe benefits   **4c** ☐ Retirement/Pension   **4e** ☐ Other
   4b ☐ Group-term life insurance   **4d** ☐ Dependent care

5   Total of payments made to each employee in excess of $7,000 . . . . **5** ▢

6   **Subtotal** (line 4 + line 5 = line 6) . . . . **6** ▢

7   Total taxable FUTA wages (line 3 – line 6 = line 7) . . . . . . **7** ▢

8   FUTA tax before adjustments (line 7 × .008 = line 8) . . . . **8** ▢

Part 3: Determine your adjustments. If any line does NOT apply, leave it blank.

9   If ALL of the taxable FUTA wages you paid were excluded from state unemployment tax, multiply line 7 by .054 (line 7 × .054 = line 9). Then go to line 12 . . . . **9** ▢

10   If SOME of the taxable FUTA wages you paid were excluded from state unemployment tax, OR you paid ANY state unemployment tax late (after the due date for filing Form 940), fill out the worksheet in the instructions. Enter the amount from line 7 of the worksheet . . . . . . **10** ▢

11   If credit reduction applies, enter the amount from line 3 of Schedule A (Form 940) . . . . . . **11** ▢

Part 4: Determine your FUTA tax and balance due or overpayment for 2009. If any line does NOT apply, leave it blank.

12   Total FUTA tax after adjustments (lines 8 + 9 + 10 + 11 = line 12) . . . . **12** ▢

13   FUTA tax deposited for the year, including any overpayment applied from a prior year . . **13** ▢

14   **Balance due** (If line 12 is more than line 13, enter the difference on line 14.)
   • If line 14 is more than $500, you must deposit your tax.
   • If line 14 is $500 or less, you may pay with this return. For more information on how to pay, see the separate instructions . . . . **14** ▢

15   **Overpayment** (If line 13 is more than line 12, enter the difference on line 15 and check a box below.) . . . . **15** ▢

Check one: ☐ Apply to next return.
            ☐ Send a refund.

▶ You **MUST** fill out both pages of this form and **SIGN** it.

Next ➡

For Privacy Act and Paperwork Reduction Act Notice, see the back of Form 940-V, Payment Voucher.   Cat. No. 11234O   Form **940** (2009)

FIGURE 5-13 IRS Form 940.

Form **941 for 2009:** Employer's QUARTERLY Federal Tax Return

950109

(Rev. April 2009) Department of the Treasury — Internal Revenue Service

OMB No. 1545-0029

(EIN)
Employer identification number ☐☐ — ☐☐☐☐☐☐☐

Name *(not your trade name)*

Trade name *(if any)*

Address

Number   Street   Suite or room number

City   State   ZIP code

Report for this Quarter of 2009
(Check one.)

☐ **1:** January, February, March

☐ **2:** April, May, June

☐ **3:** July, August, September

☐ **4:** October, November, December

Read the separate instructions before you complete Form 941. Type or print within the boxes.

Part 1: Answer these questions for this quarter.

1 Number of employees who received wages, tips, or other compensation for the pay period including: *Mar. 12* (Quarter 1), *June 12* (Quarter 2), *Sept. 12* (Quarter 3), *Dec. 12* (Quarter 4)   **1**

2 Wages, tips, and other compensation **2**

3 Income tax withheld from wages, tips, and other compensation **3**

4 If no wages, tips, and other compensation are subject to social security or Medicare tax   ☐ Check and go to line 6.

5 Taxable social security and Medicare wages and tips:

	Column 1		Column 2	
5a Taxable social security wages		× .124 =		
5b Taxable social security tips		× .124 =		
5c Taxable Medicare wages & tips		× .029 =		

5d Total social security and Medicare taxes (*Column 2*, lines 5a + 5b + 5c = line 5d) . .   **5d**

6 Total taxes before adjustments (lines 3 + 5d = line 6) **6**

7 **CURRENT QUARTER'S ADJUSTMENTS,** for example, a fractions of cents adjustment. See the instructions.

7a Current quarter's fractions of cents . . . .

7b Current quarter's sick pay . . . .

7c Current quarter's adjustments for tips and group-term life insurance

7d **TOTAL ADJUSTMENTS.** Combine all amounts on lines 7a through 7c **7d**

8 Total taxes after adjustments. Combine lines 6 and 7d **8**

9 Advance earned income credit (EIC) payments made to employees **9**

10 Total taxes after adjustment for advance EIC (line 8 – line 9 = line 10) **10**

11 Total deposits for this quarter, including overpayment applied from a prior quarter and overpayment applied from Form 941-X or Form 944-X . . . .

12a COBRA premium assistance payments (see instructions) . . . . .

12b Number of individuals provided COBRA premium assistance reported on line 12a . . . .

13 Add lines 11 and 12a **13**

14 Balance due. If line 10 is more than line 13, write the difference here **14**
For information on how to pay, see the instructions.

15 Overpayment. If line 13 is more than line 10, write the difference here

☐ Apply to next return.
Check one ☐ Send a refund.

▶ You **MUST** complete both pages of Form 941 and **SIGN** it.

Next ➡

For Privacy Act and Paperwork Reduction Act Notice, see the back of the Payment Voucher.   Cat. No. 17001Z   Form **941** (Rev. 4-2009)

FIGURE 5-14 IRS Form 941.

a Employee's social security number	OMB No. 1545-0008	Safe, accurate, FAST! Use IRS e-file. Visit the IRS website at www.irs.gov/efile
b Employer identification number (EIN)	1 Wages, tips, other compensation	2 Federal income tax withheld
c Employer's name, address, and ZIP code	3 Social security wages	4 Social security tax withheld
	5 Medicare wages and tips	6 Medicare tax withheld
	7 Social security tips	8 Allocated tips
d Control number	9 Advance EIC payment	10 Dependent care benefits
e Employee's first name and initial Last name Suff.	11 Nonqualified plans	12a See instructions for box 12 Code
	13 Statutory employee / Retirement plan / Third-party sick pay	12b Code
	14 Other	12c Code
		12d Code
f Employee's address and ZIP code		

15 State Employer's state ID number	16 State wages, tips, etc.	17 State income tax	18 Local wages, tips, etc.	19 Local income tax	20 Locality name

Form **W-2** **Wage and Tax Statement** **2010** Department of the Treasury—Internal Revenue Service

Copy B—To Be Filed With Employee's FEDERAL Tax Return.
This information is being furnished to the Internal Revenue Service.

FIGURE 5-15 IRS W-2 form.

the state and federal regulations that may apply to a practice when using a relief or contracted veterinarian.

PRACTICE POINT Any contract employee receiving over $600 in compensation from January 1 through December 31 must receive an MISC-1099 by January 31 of the following year.

It is also becoming popular for credentialed veterinary technicians to contract out their services. Technicians may provide relief services at hospitals that need coverage or provide consulting services. These are also considered contract employees who must also follow the aforementioned procedures.

TEAM TRAINING

There cannot be enough emphasis placed on the importance of team training. The success of a practice depends on the quality and quantity of training. New employees without any training should start with the basics, so as not to overwhelm them with information. New team members with experience should still follow a training protocol, taking care not to skip procedures and protocols. New employees with experience can breeze through training but are likely to miss critical practice protocols. Care should be taken to ensure this does not occur because this is where major mistakes can occur. Training should be fun and creative. Telling is not training, and it can also reduce the amount of information retained.

PRACTICE POINT Every team member should receive consistent team training to maintain skills and knowledge.

An excellent attitude is the No. 1 skill that is often forgotten. Practices overlook training and development of positive attitudes. A great attitude starts at the top and trickles down to the rest of the team. Owners, associates, and management must have a positive attitude every day; this encourages the rest of the team to follow. Positive attitudes are contagious and can lift the spirits of those around them; bad attitudes can foster failure.

Developing a Training Protocol

The creation of learning modules and skills lists that must be completed will help ensure that team members are trained properly. Each practice is different; development of these modules can be done on an individual basis.

Form W-4 (2010)

Purpose. Complete Form W-4 so that your employer can withhold the correct federal income tax from your pay. Consider completing a new Form W-4 each year and when your personal or financial situation changes.

Exemption from withholding. If you are exempt, complete **only** lines 1, 2, 3, 4, and 7 and sign the form to validate it. Your exemption for 2010 expires February 16, 2011. See Pub. 505, Tax Withholding and Estimated Tax.

Note. You cannot claim exemption from withholding if (a) your income exceeds $950 and includes more than $300 of unearned income (for example, interest and dividends) and (b) another person can claim you as a dependent on his or her tax return.

Basic instructions. If you are not exempt, complete the **Personal Allowances Worksheet** below. The worksheets on page 2 further adjust your withholding allowances based on itemized deductions, certain credits, adjustments to income, or two-earners/multiple jobs situations.

Complete all worksheets that apply. However, you may claim fewer (or zero) allowances. For regular wages, withholding must be based on allowances you claimed and may not be a flat amount or percentage of wages.

Head of household. Generally, you may claim head of household filing status on your tax return only if you are unmarried and pay more than 50% of the costs of keeping up a home for yourself and your dependent(s) or other qualifying individuals. See Pub. 501, Exemptions, Standard Deduction, and Filing Information, for information.

Tax credits. You can take projected tax credits into account in figuring your allowable number of withholding allowances. Credits for child or dependent care expenses and the child tax credit may be claimed using the **Personal Allowances Worksheet** below. See Pub. 919, How Do I Adjust My Tax Withholding, for information on converting your other credits into withholding allowances.

Nonwage income. If you have a large amount of nonwage income, such as interest or dividends, consider making estimated tax

payments using Form 1040-ES, Estimated Tax for Individuals. Otherwise, you may owe additional tax. If you have pension or annuity income, see Pub. 919 to find out if you should adjust your withholding on Form W-4 or W-4P.

Two earners or multiple jobs. If you have a working spouse or more than one job, figure the total number of allowances you are entitled to claim on all jobs using worksheets from only one Form W-4. Your withholding usually will be most accurate when all allowances are claimed on the Form W-4 for the highest paying job and zero allowances are claimed on the others. See Pub. 919 for details.

Nonresident alien. If you are a nonresident alien, see Notice 1392, Supplemental Form W-4 Instructions for Nonresident Aliens, before completing this form.

Check your withholding. After your Form W-4 takes effect, use Pub. 919 to see how the amount you are having withheld compares to your projected total tax for 2010. See Pub. 919, especially if your earnings exceed $130,000 (Single) or $180,000 (Married).

Personal Allowances Worksheet (Keep for your records.)

A Enter "1" for **yourself** if no one else can claim you as a dependent . . . . **A** _____

B Enter "1" if:
- You are single and have only one job; or
- You are married, have only one job, and your spouse does not work; or
- Your wages from a second job or your spouse's wages (or the total of both) are $1,500 or less.

B _____

C Enter "1" for your **spouse**. But, you may choose to enter "-0-" if you are married and have either a working spouse or more than one job. (Entering "-0-" may help you avoid having too little tax withheld.) . . . . **C** _____

D Enter number of **dependents** (other than your spouse or yourself) you will claim on your tax return . . . . . . **D** _____

E Enter "1" if you will file as **head of household** on your tax return (see conditions under **Head of household** above) . **E** _____

F Enter "1" if you have at least $1,800 of **child or dependent care expenses** for which you plan to claim a credit . . **F** _____
(**Note.** Do **not** include child support payments. See Pub. 503, Child and Dependent Care Expenses, for details.)

G **Child Tax Credit** (including additional child tax credit). See Pub. 972, Child Tax Credit, for more information.
- If your total income will be less than $61,000 ($90,000 if married), enter "2" for each eligible child; then **less** "1" if you have three or more eligible children.
- If your total income will be between $61,000 and $84,000 ($90,000 and $119,000 if married), enter "1" for each eligible child plus "1" **additional** if you have six or more eligible children. **G** _____

H Add lines A through G and enter total here. (**Note.** This may be different from the number of exemptions you claim on your tax return.) ▶ **H** _____

For accuracy, complete all worksheets that apply.
- If you plan to **itemize or claim adjustments to income** and want to reduce your withholding, see the **Deductions and Adjustments Worksheet** on page 2.
- If you have **more than one job** or are **married and you and your spouse both work** and the combined earnings from all jobs exceed $18,000 ($32,000 if married), see the **Two-Earners/Multiple Jobs Worksheet** on page 2 to avoid having too little tax withheld.
- If **neither** of the above situations applies, **stop here** and enter the number from line H on line 5 of Form W-4 below.

-------------------- Cut here and give Form W-4 to your employer. Keep the top part for your records. --------------------

Form W-4

Department of the Treasury
Internal Revenue Service

Employee's Withholding Allowance Certificate

▶ Whether you are entitled to claim a certain number of allowances or exemption from withholding is subject to review by the IRS. Your employer may be required to send a copy of this form to the IRS.

OMB No. 1545-0074

2010

1 Type or print your first name and middle initial.	Last name	2 Your social security number

Home address (number and street or rural route)	3 ☐ Single ☐ Married ☐ Married, but withhold at higher Single rate. **Note.** If married, but legally separated, or spouse is a nonresident alien, check the "Single" box.
City or town, state, and ZIP code	4 If your last name differs from that shown on your social security card, check here. You must call 1-800-772-1213 for a replacement card. ▶ ☐

5 Total number of allowances you are claiming (from line **H** above **or** from the applicable worksheet on page 2) **5** _____

6 Additional amount, if any, you want withheld from each paycheck . . . . **6** $ _____

7 I claim exemption from withholding for 2010, and I certify that I meet **both** of the following conditions for exemption.
- Last year I had a right to a refund of **all** federal income tax withheld because I had **no** tax liability **and**
- This year I expect a refund of **all** federal income tax withheld because I expect to have **no** tax liability.

If you meet both conditions, write "Exempt" here . . . . ▶ **7** _____

Under penalties of perjury, I declare that I have examined this certificate and to the best of my knowledge and belief, it is true, correct, and complete.

Employee's signature
(Form is not valid unless you sign it.) ▶ _____ Date ▶ _____

8 Employer's name and address (Employer: Complete lines 8 and 10 only if sending to the IRS.)	9 Office code (optional)	10 Employer identification number (EIN)

For Privacy Act and Paperwork Reduction Act Notice, see page 2. Cat. No. 10220Q Form **W-4** (2010)

FIGURE 5-16 IRS W-4 form.

Deductions and Adjustments Worksheet

Note. Use this worksheet *only* if you plan to itemize deductions or claim certain credits or adjustments to income.

1 Enter an estimate of your 2010 itemized deductions. These include qualifying home mortgage interest, charitable contributions, state and local taxes, medical expenses in excess of 7.5% of your income, and miscellaneous deductions . . . . **1** $ _____

2 Enter: { $11,400 if married filing jointly or qualifying widow(er) }
          { $8,400 if head of household } . . . . **2** $ _____
          { $5,700 if single or married filing separately }

3 **Subtract** line 2 from line 1. If zero or less, enter "-0-" . . . . **3** $ _____

4 Enter an estimate of your 2010 adjustments to income and any additional standard deduction. (Pub. 919) . . . . . . **4** $ _____

5 **Add** lines 3 and 4 and enter the total. (Include any amount for credits from *Worksheet 6* in Pub. 919.) . **5** $ _____

6 Enter an estimate of your 2010 nonwage income (such as dividends or interest) . . . . **6** $ _____

7 **Subtract** line 6 from line 5. If zero or less, enter "-0-" . . . . **7** $ _____

8 **Divide** the amount on line 7 by $3,650 and enter the result here. Drop any fraction . . . . . . **8** _____

9 Enter the number from the **Personal Allowances Worksheet,** line H, page 1 . . . . **9** _____

10 **Add** lines 8 and 9 and enter the total here. If you plan to use the **Two-Earners/Multiple Jobs Worksheet,** also enter this total on line 1 below. Otherwise, **stop here** and enter this total on Form W-4, line 5, page 1 **10** _____

Two-Earners/Multiple Jobs Worksheet (See *Two earners or multiple jobs* on page 1.)

Note. Use this worksheet *only* if the instructions under line H on page 1 direct you here.

1 Enter the number from line H, page 1 (or from line 10 above if you used the **Deductions and Adjustments Worksheet**) **1** _____

2 Find the number in **Table 1** below that applies to the **LOWEST** paying job and enter it here. **However,** if you are married filing jointly and wages from the highest paying job are $65,000 or less, do not enter more than "3." . . . . **2** _____

3 If line 1 is **more than or equal to** line 2, subtract line 2 from line 1. Enter the result here (if zero, enter "-0-") and on Form W-4, line 5, page 1. **Do not** use the rest of this worksheet . . . . **3** _____

Note. If line 1 is *less than* line 2, enter "-0-" on Form W-4, line 5, page 1. Complete lines 4–9 below to figure the additional withholding amount necessary to avoid a year-end tax bill.

4 Enter the number from line 2 of this worksheet . . . . **4** _____

5 Enter the number from line 1 of this worksheet . . . . **5** _____

6 **Subtract** line 5 from line 4 . . . . **6** _____

7 Find the amount in **Table 2** below that applies to the **HIGHEST** paying job and enter it here . . . . **7** $ _____

8 **Multiply** line 7 by line 6 and enter the result here. This is the additional annual withholding needed . . **8** $ _____

9 Divide line 8 by the number of pay periods remaining in 2010. For example, divide by 26 if you are paid every two weeks and you complete this form in December 2009. Enter the result here and on Form W-4, line 6, page 1. This is the additional amount to be withheld from each paycheck . . . . **9** $ _____

Table 1

Married Filing Jointly		All Others	
If wages from **LOWEST** paying job are—	Enter on line 2 above	If wages from **LOWEST** paying job are—	Enter on line 2 above
$0 - $7,000 -	0	$0 - $6,000 -	0
7,001 - 10,000 -	1	6,001 - 12,000 -	1
10,001 - 16,000 -	2	12,001 - 19,000 -	2
16,001 - 22,000 -	3	19,001 - 26,000 -	3
22,001 - 27,000 -	4	26,001 - 35,000 -	4
27,001 - 35,000 -	5	35,001 - 50,000 -	5
35,001 - 44,000 -	6	50,001 - 65,000 -	6
44,001 - 50,000 -	7	65,001 - 80,000 -	7
50,001 - 55,000 -	8	80,001 - 90,000 -	8
55,001 - 65,000 -	9	90,001 -120,000 -	9
65,001 - 72,000 -	10	120,001 and over	10
72,001 - 85,000 -	11		
85,001 -105,000 -	12		
105,001 -115,000 -	13		
115,001 -130,000 -	14		
130,001 - and over	15		

Table 2

Married Filing Jointly		All Others	
If wages from **HIGHEST** paying job are—	Enter on line 7 above	If wages from **HIGHEST** paying job are—	Enter on line 7 above
$0 - $65,000	$550	$0 - $35,000	$550
65,001 - 120,000	910	35,001 - 90,000	910
120,001 - 185,000	1,020	90,001 - 165,000	1,020
185,001 - 330,000	1,200	165,001 - 370,000	1,200
330,001 and over	1,280	370,001 and over	1,280

FIGURE 5-16, cont'd

Some protocols may work well in one practice but not in another. Changes can be made to protocols to continue to ensure the best quality of training. Training takes time and must be done in phases. Too much information will overload the new employee, who may not return to work the following day.

> **PRACTICE POINT** Phase training prevents new team members from becoming overwhelmed during the first few weeks of employment.

An excellent protocol has different levels of training and allows team members a reasonable amount of time to master the skills within each module. It is important that inexperienced team members understand why protocols are completed in such a manner, and that the protocols give examples of possible consequences of misinterpreted instructions. Skills should be detailed to ensure complete understanding of each skill. For example, customer service has a variety of skills under its umbrella: answering the phone courteously, greeting clients as they enter the practice, and answering questions a client may have (Box 5-13).

Training should occur during open hours. Hands-on training is much more effective than talking or reading, and when team members have to practice the skill over and over, and under the supervision of another team member, they are more likely to retain the information.

Basic modules for kennel assistants should include kennel duties and tasks. Included in a basic module would be cleaning techniques, chemicals, and the knowledge of diseases and their transmission. Animal handling, restraint, exercise, and basic nutrition may be addressed in modules to follow.

Veterinary assistants should be expected to know all the material for kennel assistants, a perfect example for module 1. The following modules can then cover surgery, laboratory, radiology, and pharmacology. Veterinary technicians are expected to know all the modules, allowing tasks to be added as the practice members become comfortable with the new team members' abilities. Credentialed technicians and those with a great deal of experience will be familiar with all the procedures; they should then use the time to become familiar with the practice protocols because those can vary from practice to practice.

> **PRACTICE POINT** Some team members may not need procedural training because they may have previous experience. However, protocols may be different and should be reviewed.

Phase training should be tailored to each new team member depending on experience. Modules contain a tremendous amount of information, and team members are expected to learn most of it and in a short time frame. Time should be taken to fully explain procedures and protocols to ensure the new employee fully understands them. It may be wise to explain the procedures and protocols multiple times, using a variety of methods for explanation.

New team members should be encouraged to read the employee procedures manual and the training modules. Once these are read, they can observe team members completing the skills, complete the skills themselves, and then be tested on the concept. Once a new team member has completed the first module with satisfaction, the second module can be started, with an estimated date of completion in mind.

It takes a *team* to train a *team*—and using *all* team members to train new employees improves efficiency greatly. Ten people training an individual produces much more knowledge than just one person doing training. However, one supervisor should be in charge of overseeing the testing procedure to ensure the employee can complete the procedures and techniques as expected. If any area needs improvement, it can be addressed at that time.

> **PRACTICE POINT** New members trained by a team have greater success than those trained by an individual.

Providing All Levels of Continuing Education

New employees are not the only team members who need training. Long-term and advanced assistants and technicians may not need the basic training that new employees do, but disease knowledge, treatments, and protocols may change frequently. If team members are not encouraged to attend outside continuing education seminars, then continuing education should be brought to the practice. Practices can incorporate manufacturers' representatives into the practice meeting schedule. Sales consultants have a variety of topics available and often allow the practice to pick topics they want to educate the staff about. Continuing education inspires and encourages team members to improve the quality and quantity of care they provide to both clients and patients. When team members receive quality education, they can educate the clients at a much higher level.

Role-Playing

A technique that yields a high success rate is role-playing. If a receptionist's or technician's job is to educate a client about heartworm disease, then team members should be able to recite the information to any other employee. Once they have mastered the words and the ability to convey the information to team members, then

Box 5-13	Phase Training

KENNEL ASSISTANT, MODULE 1

Policies and paperwork
- Employee personnel manual
- Employee procedures manual
- Employee expectations
- Professional ethics
- W-4, I-9, and benefits forms
- Time clock
- Mailbox
- Dress code

Cleaning
- Prevent transmission of disease
  - Which diseases are transmitted and how
- Isolation
  - Keep all isolation cleaning items in isolation
- Chemicals to clean with
  - Chlorhexidine
  - Vindicator
  - A-33
  - Clorox
- Chemicals not to clean with
  - Lysol
  - Ammonia
- Equipment
  - Scrub brushes
  - Mops and buckets
  - Brooms
- Technique
  - Scrubbing
  - Contact time
  - Rinsing and drying

Laundry
- Hot water
- Detergent and bleach

Towels and blankets
- Safety of blankets for patients
  - No holes or shredded blankets

Proper disposal of sharps
- Biohazard containers

Proper disposal of bodies
- Private burial
- Mass or private cremation

KENNEL ASSISTANT, MODULE 2

Nutrition
- Knowledge of different types of food
  - Puppy, maintenance, and senior formulas; prescription formulas
- Amount to feed each animal
  - Measure
- NPO
- PO

Hospital sheets
- Following treatments required

Walking patients safely
- Removing patients from cages/kennels safely
- Slip leash
- At least three times daily, more if indicated

- With IV fluids
- With bandaging material, casts, or other

Cats
- Clay litter
- Nonabsorbable litter
- Paper litter

KENNEL ASSISTANT MODULE 3

Hospital maintenance
- Trash
- Sweeping/mopping
- Cleanliness
  - Vents, fans, display shelving
  - Light fixtures
    - Working light bulbs and ballasts
  - Outside: weeds, animal waste and front porch appearance

KENNEL ASSISTANT MODULE 4

Restraint techniques
- Dogs and cats
- Psychological restraint
- Lifting appropriately
- Handling the fractious patient
- Lateral recumbency
- Sternal recumbency

Restraint for venipuncture (blood draw)
- Jugular
- Cephalic
- Saphenous
- Femoral

Use precautions when necessary
- Muzzles
- Slip leash
- Know when to hold tighter or use less restraint

Client concerns when restraining animals

E-collars

Normal vital signs
- Temperature
- Pulse
- Respiratory rate

Grooming
- Combing and brushing
- Ear cleaning
- Nail trimming
- Anal sac expression
- Bathing

VETERINARY ASSISTANT MODULE 1

Kennel assistant modules 1 through 4

VETERINARY ASSISTANT MODULE 2

Interaction with clients and patients
- Treat animals as if they were your own
- Make clients feel comfortable at all times
- Offer coffee or water to those who must wait extended periods of time
- Listen to what they say

Continued

Box 5-13   Phase Training—cont'd

- Show you care
- Offer to carry items and patients for clients
- Always provide an answer. If you don't have the answer, find the correct answer as soon as possible

Cleaning between patients
- Prevent transmission of disease
- Wash hands after each patient
- Clean table and exam room between each patient
- Clean any instruments used between patients

Animal care protocol
- Hospital sheets
- Proper food and proper feeding times for each patient
- Provide fresh water at all times, unless otherwise indicated
- Provide a clean blanket or towel at all times unless otherwise indicated
- Prevention of nosocomial infections
- Patient monitoring
  - Observe patient for any BM, urination, vomit, or abnormal condition. Indicate on hospital sheet and alert a veterinarian.
  - Patients should be monitored at all times while in the hospital

Performing medicated baths
- Be familiar with product and procedure for bathing
- Dermazole shampoo
- Pyopen shampoo
- Flea/tick dip
- Lime/sulfur dip

Medical records
- Reading and understanding medical records
- SOAP format
- Writing a complete medical record
- Abbreviations
  - Vomit, diarrhea, client, decline, patient, other common abbreviations used in practice
- Initials
- Filing of records
- Updating records

Exam room
- History taking
- Recording observations
- TPR
- Preparing room for veterinarian
- Cleanliness
- Stocking
- Sexing of animals
- Aging dogs and cats
- Mixing vaccines
- Filling syringes

Customer service
- Greeting clients with a smile
- Listening to what the client wants
- Satisfying customer needs
- Ensuring customers perceives the value in the services they received

Computer software
- Client information
- Patient history

- Invoicing
- Circle sheet or tracking sheet

Protocol and procedures
- Flow of patient appointments
- Exam room
- Surgical
- Vaccinations
- Dental care
- Laboratory testing
- Patient treatments

Common questions and concerns
- Heartworm disease and products carried
- Fleas and ticks; products carried
- Dietary/nutritional needs and products carried
- Shampoos and conditioners; products carried

VETERINARY ASSISTANT MODULE 3

Surgeries performed in practice
- Routine OVH/castrations
- Declaw
- Dewclaw
- Dental prophylaxis
- Orthopedic procedures
- Exploratory laparotomies

Surgical protocol
- Scheduling
- Surgery logs
- NPO
- Pre-anesthetic
- Anesthesia
  - Anesthetic planes
- Intubation
  - Selection of appropriate tube
  - Inflation of cuff
- Eye lubrication
  - Why
  - How
  - What lubrication to use
- IV fluids
  - Prepping site with aseptic technique
    - Clip
    - Clean
      - Betadine, alcohol, chlorhexidine
  - IV catheters
    - 18 g, 20 g, 22 g
    - Length
  - IV fluids
    - Normosol
    - NaCl
    - Dextrose
  - Securing
- Procedures
  - Sterile field
  - Opening packs
  - Suture material
    - Types of suture
    - Opening suture pack

Box 5-13 | Phase Training—cont'd

- Needles
  - Types of needles
  - Sterilizing
  - Opening
- Gowning the surgeon
- Monitoring the recovering patient
  - TPR
  - Removal of ET
  - Release instructions
- Equipment
  - Surgical table
    - Tilting, raising, and lowering
  - Monitors
    - Surgical monitor
    - Blood pressure machine
    - ECG
    - SPo$_2$
  - Anesthetic machine
  - Proper use
    - Proper administration of gases
    - Selecting appropriate anesthetic hoses
    - Refilling gas compartment
  - Surgical instruments and packs
    - Names and uses of individual instruments

Maintenance of equipment
- Change soda lime
- Change/maintain scavenger system
- Clean daily and check for leaks
  - Machine, including valves and bags
  - Anesthetic hoses
  - Masks
- Surgical laundry
- Cleaning of surgical suite
  - Table and lights
  - Counters

Autoclave protocol
- Use
- Pack preparation
  - Cleaning, lubricating, and maintaining instruments
- Preparation of individual instruments
- Proper labeling and taping
- Length of time autoclave is good for
- Maintenance
- Distilled water

VETERINARY ASSISTANT MODULE 4
X-ray
- Introduction
- Safety
- Equipment
  - Thyroid collar
  - Lead gloves
  - X-ray gown
  - Eye protection
  - Radiation badge
    - Proper use and placement
- Log
- Film

- Maintenance and use of cassettes
- Storage
- Filing of radiographs
- Identification
- Technique
  - Use of calipers
  - Understanding and determining kVp and mAs
  - Collimation
  - Anatomy of positions
    - D/V, V/D, A/P, lateral
    - Abdominal, thoracic
- Developer
  - Manual versus automatic versus digital
  - Maintenance of
  - Chemicals
    - Developing solution
    - Fix solution
  - Cleaning
  - Disposing of chemicals
- Ultrasound
- Endoscopy

Laboratory
- Common external parasites
  - Prepping for
    - Ear smear
    - Skin scrape
    - Cytology
- Common internal parasites
  - Collecting fecal samples
  - Prepping fecal
  - Reading fecal
- Equipment
  - HCT/PCV machine
    - Determining HCT
  - Chemistry machine
    - BUN, CREA, SGPT, ALT, BILI, GLU, CHOL, AMYL, PHOS, Ca, etc.
  - CBC machine
    - WBC, RBC, PLT, HCT
  - Electrolyte machine
    - Na, Cl, K
  - Microscope
    - How to use and clean
    - Different levels of power
    - Oil immersion
      - Cytologies
  - Refractometer
    - How to use and clean
    - Determining urine specific gravity and TP
  - Centrifuge
    - HCT, small and large
  - Tonometer
    - How to use, calibrate, and clean
  - Blood pressure machine
    - How to use
    - Measuring for correct cuff size
    - Doppler versus surgical monitor

Continued

Box 5-13   Phase Training—cont'd

- ECG machine
  - Location of clips
  - Alcohol on clips for better conduction
- Blood tubes
  - SST
    - Tests that cannot be drawn with SSTs
  - RTT
    - Serum used
  - LTT
    - EDTA anticoagulant
    - Plasma used
  - BTT
    - Citrate anticoagulant
    - Plasma used
  - GTT
    - Lithium heparin anticoagulant
    - Plasma used
- Using aseptic technique to obtain blood samples
- Testing available in house
  - CBC/chemistry/electrolytes/blood gases
  - Urinalysis
  - Heartworm 4DX (Heartworm, *E. canis*, Lyme, and anaplasmosis)
  - FeLV/FIV/HWT
  - Parvo
  - Spec CPL
- Testing available outside
  - Laboratory forms
  - Bile acids
  - Phenobarbital levels
  - ACTH stimulation
  - T4
    - Total T4
    - Equilibrium dialysis
    - Thyroid panels
- Maintenance of equipment
  - Daily
  - Weekly
  - Monthly

Stains
- Wright stain
- Diff-Quik
- New methylene blue
- Urinalysis stain

Urinalysis
- Collection of sample
  - Free catch
  - Cystocentesis
  - Catheterization
- Evaluation of
  - Microscopic
  - Stick
  - Specific gravity
- Urine culture and sensitivity
  - Collection of
  - Sample submission

Necropsy

- Material needed
- Sample submission

VETERINARY ASSISTANT MODULE 5
Patient discharge
- Discharge instructions
- Medications
- Pet's personal items: collars, blankets, and toys

Pharmacology
- Handling controlled substances
- Most common drugs used
  - Antibiotics
  - Antiinflammatory
  - Antihistamines
  - Cardiac
  - Ophthalmic
  - Otic
  - Gastrointestinal
  - Shampoos/conditioners
  - Skin care
  - Injectable medications
  - Tranquilizers
  - Thyroid
  - Miscellaneous
- Drug location
- Drug storage
  - Amber bottle versus clear bottle
- Drug use
- Potential drug interactions
- Normal dosing
- Normal instructions
- Labeling
- Counting
- Reading a prescription label
- Direction abbreviations
  - SID
  - BID
  - TID
  - QID
  - PRN
  - EOD
  - PO
  - IV
  - IM
  - SC

Reading the instructions to the owner
Administering medications to the patient
- Oral solution
- Pills or capsules
- Aural medication
- Ocular medication
- Topical medication

VETERINARY ASSISTANT MODULE 6
Patient treatments
- Injections
  - SC

Box 5-13 | Phase Training—cont'd

- IV
- IM
- Administering other medications
  - PO
  - AU/AD/AS
  - OU/OD/OS
  - Topically

Monitoring IV fluids and catheters
Developing patient hospitalization sheets
Developing patient release sheets

VETERINARY TECHNICIAN MODULE 1
- Kennel Assistant Modules 1 through 4

VETERINARY TECHNICIAN MODULE 2
- Veterinary Assistant Modules 1 and 2

VETERINARY TECHNICIAN MODULE 3
- Veterinary Assistant Module 3
- Place IV catheter
- Determine drip rate
- Induce and maintain anesthesia
- Monitor recovering surgical patients
- Perform dental prophylaxis

VETERINARY TECHNICIAN MODULE 4
- Veterinary Assistant Modules 4 and 5
- Obtain lab samples with aseptic technique
- Perform cystotomy
- Problem-solve x-ray techniques when needed

VETERINARY TECHNICIAN MODULE 5
- Veterinary Assistant Module 6

VETERINARY TECHNICIAN MODULE 6
- Develop leadership skills
- Provide CE for kennel and veterinary assistants
- Provide assistance with inventory control
- Provide accountability for products and supplies used
- Help develop protocols and procedures for practice
- Provide an excellent attitude that is contagious to the rest of the team

RECEPTIONIST TRAINING MODULE 1
- Policies and paperwork
  - Employee personnel manual
  - Employee procedures manual
  - W-4, I-9, and benefits forms
  - Time clock
  - Mailbox
  - Dress code
- Cleanliness of reception area

- Greeting clients
  - Responding to client questions and concerns
- Client service
- Telephone calls
  - Customer service
  - Friendly, positive tone
  - Length of time on hold

RECEPTIONIST TRAINING MODULE 2
- Procedures and protocols
  - Examinations
  - Vaccinations
  - Surgery
- Invoicing
  - Entering invoice
  - Reviewing invoice with client
  - Accepting payment
  - Change
  - Documenting transaction
- Appointments
  - Making
  - Accepting
  - Canceling/changing

RECEPTIONIST TRAINING MODULE 3
- Medical records
  - Creating new medical records
  - Updating patient records
  - Making entries in medical records
  - Filing
  - Retrieving
  - Reviewing for complete records
- Morning procedure
  - Checking clients in
  - Checking clients out
- Afternoon procedure
  - End-of-day procedures
- Computer software
  - Searching for history and past transactions
- Common questions and concerns
  - Heartworm disease and products carried
  - Fleas and ticks and products carried
  - Dietary nutritional needs and products carried
  - Shampoos and conditioners and products carried

RECEPTIONIST TRAINING MODULE 4
- Prescriptions
  - Medications
  - Abbreviations
  - Labeling
  - Reviewing instructions with clients

NPO, Nothing by mouth; *PO,* orally; *BM,* bowel movement; *SOAP,* subjective, objective, assessment, plan; *TPR,* temperature, pulse, and respiration; *OVH,* ovarian hysterectomy; *IV,* intravenous; *NaCl,* sodium chloride; *ET,* endotracheal tube; *ECG,* electrocardiogram; *SPo₂,* oxygen saturation; *kVp,* kilovolt peak; *mAs,* milliampere-second; *D/V,* dorsoventral; *V/D,* ventrodorsal; *A/P,* anteroposterior; *HCT,* hematocrit; *PCV,* packed cell volume; *BUN,* blood urea nitrogen; *CREA,* creatinine; *SGPT,* aspartate aminotransferase; *ALT,* alanine aminotransferase; *BILI,* bilirubin; *GLU,* glucose; *CHOL,* cholesterol; *AMYL,* amylase; *PHOS,* phosphatase; *Ca,* calcium; *WBC,* white blood cells; *RBC,* red blood cells; *PLT,* platelets; *Na,* sodium; *Cl,* chloride; *K,* potassium; *TP,* total protein; *SST,* serum separator tubes; *RTT,* red-topped tube; *LTT,* lavender-topped tube; *EDTA,* ethylene diamine tetraacetic acid; *BTT,* blue-topped tube; *GTT,* green-topped tube; *CBC,* complete blood count; *FELV,* feline leukemia virus; *FIV,* feline immunodeficiency virus; *HWT,* heartworm; *CPL,* cholesterol/phospholipid; *ACTH,* adrenocorticotropic hormone; *T4,* thyroid; *SID,* once daily; *BID,* twice daily; *TID,* three times daily; *QID,* four times daily; *PRN,* as needed; *EOD,* every other day; *IM,* intramuscular; *SC,* subcutaneous; *AU/AD/AS,* both ears/right ear/left ear; *OU/OD/OS,* both eyes/right eye/left eye; *CE,* continuing education.

they can educate any client. Team members are more nervous when having to role-play in front of their peers; this is an excellent test of their knowledge and confidence. They will come across as much more professional and educated in front of clients when they have confidence in the information they are conveying.

> **PRACTICE POINT** Role-playing can enhance every team member's ability to interact with clients.

Role-playing should be included in any training protocol. Receptionists will find it beneficial while making appointments or confronting upset clients. Assistants and technicians will find it beneficial when educating clients about diseases, and kennel assistants will become aware of potential problems in the kennel and how to fix them before they arise.

Methods to Retain Employees

Employee turnover rates not only affect the clinic financially but also decrease the team morale and efficiency as well. It takes a large amount of time and dedication to train employees. Training an employee reduces the amount of time spent with patients and clients, decreases the quality of care patients receive, and increases staff wages during the training period. A program to promote team spirit and satisfaction can take advantage of all these benefits. Job satisfaction includes respect for one another, recognition, achievement, and challenges.

Providing an environment that is open, friendly, and promotes communication is important. People spend the majority of their time at work. They should not have to be upset about coming to work, hate their jobs, or avoid team members because of an unfriendly work environment. Team members should be encouraged to talk with management about personnel issues without the fear of retaliation. Supervisors and practice owners should listen to team members and discuss issues with teams before they become a problem. Ask team members to complete an employee survey. Find out how they feel and what their concerns are, and address them. They will feel that their opinions count, and more than likely, if one employee has a problem with a topic, another does as well. Management may never know of the problem unless the team members are asked.

Each manager has his or her own techniques for conflict resolution. The ultimate goal should be to prevent and solve problems, not react and discipline. Creation of an enjoyable environment comes from the practice owners, associates, and managers. If harmony is nonexistent among these key individuals, the rest of the team cannot be expected to get along and enjoy their jobs. When team members are happy, the quality and quantity of patient and client care increase as well as the efficiency among the team members.

> **PRACTICE POINT** Team member retention is crucial to practice efficiency.

Salary is important to team members and should be kept within a reasonable range for the area. Team members cannot be expected to complete highly skilled tasks and procedures for minimum wage. However, if job satisfaction is high, salary may be less important. Benefits also contribute to salary; offering veterinary services at cost or at least a greatly reduced price may offset a lower salary.

Continuing education for team members is very important to increasing staff retention. Employees should be constantly fed new information to keep them motivated. Motivated employees seek new information on a daily basis, yearning for a challenge. Satisfying this craving for knowledge is a benefit for both the practice and the employer.

Team member involvement helps retain employees as well. If team members can be involved in decision making and help create and implement protocols and procedures, they are likely to feel needed. Team members take pride in tasks they had a role in developing and will ensure the success of those tasks. The practice benefits from team involvement as well; the ideas of the entire staff are better than the ideas of one or two. Sometimes, a new or improved idea can be created from ideas taken from several points of view, making for excellent problem prevention and solving.

Maintaining the same team also helps put clients at ease when they arrive at the practice. Clients know they will receive the same quality of care when they see the same team members each time. Receptionists know the client when they walk in the door, technicians know their pets' history, and they can leave their pets, if needed, knowing they will receive exceptional care. Client satisfaction of this magnitude will help increase the average client transaction, client retention, and client compliance.

Many ideas can be implemented to increase staff retention. As stated earlier, it must start with the management. Team appreciation is important and can be done several ways. Birthday cakes and cards are special; the entire team benefits from the joy and smiles singing "Happy Birthday" brings. Christmas-time holiday parties are expected and come at a stressful time of the year. Find other days to show employee appreciation. Inexpensive hiking trips can be planned; consider a night at the movies or special ice cream breaks in the middle of the day. Cruise deals can be found online for relatively inexpensive amounts. Trips taken together promote friendship and harmony outside the work environment. Trips can be more productive than a bonus given yearly and can include continuing education for the staff. The memories made from a trip far outweigh the money given in bonus form. Celebrate small victories frequently. Celebrating large victories places less emphasis on the "small stuff." Small stuff is important, too, and often is what keeps the practice rolling smoothly.

One of the most satisfying ideas for teams is to compliment an individual for a job well done as soon as it is accomplished. Many people only receive criticism, never a compliment. When team members receive compliments throughout the day, the spirit of the entire team is lifted a notch. Other team members will see the compliments and strive to achieve a compliment as well. Rarely do individuals become competitive at this stage because they know they are appreciated as well. It takes a team to be complete! Teams want feedback on their performance. If a correction is needed, it should be done privately and immediately followed with a compliment. Employees do not need to feel that they are only criticized.

> **PRACTICE POINT** Team compliments are essential to employee retention.

WORKERS' COMPENSATION INSURANCE

As stated earlier, workers' compensation insurance protects the employer from injuries individuals might receive while on the job. Injuries can include falls, animal bites, accidents, or exposure to harmful substances. Workers' compensation insurance is regulated by individual states, not the federal government; therefore not all states require coverage. Depending on the state, a business may be able to contribute to a state fund, a private insurance fund, or a combination of both. Some states also allow practices to be self-insured. It is advised to check with the state to ensure the practice is in compliance.

If an employee is bitten, falls, or injures himself or herself in any way on the jobsite, workers' compensation insurance pays for physician visits, medications, and hospitalization that may be required. Insurance will also pay the team member's wages if more than 5 days of work are lost due to the injury. Many practices do not require team members to visit a doctor when an accident has occurred because they are afraid that the cost of insurance will increase with each claim filed. However, if an injury worsens, and the team member does not seek medical attention, then the employer can be liable to pay for all medical costs. Workers' compensation may deny a claim if it is not filed within a specific number of days after the injury. All serious injuries, including dog and cat bites, should, at minimum, be examined by a physician to protect the employer against future liabilities.

> **PRACTICE POINT** Not all states require workers' compensation insurance; however, management should ensure employees are covered for accidents in some fashion.

If an employee becomes injured, a "first report of injury" form should be filled out. If medical attention is needed, the employee should be sent with the form provided by the company providing the insurance. The form should have the practice name, the policy number, and a place to input employee information. This paper can be presented to the medical office, which can then file the claim.

Once the medical visit has been completed, the practice can submit the first report of injury and the insurance form to the state division of labor as well as the insurance carrier. Workers' compensation should follow up with the rest of the documentation. If claims are not filed, the employee is responsible for the bill received from the medical office.

If the practice chooses not to carry workers' compensation insurance, the practice owner is exposed to liability. If a team member sustains an extensive injury on the job, the practice will be responsible for paying for the medical bills of the team member. Surgery can become costly, along with follow-up visits and physical therapy. Careful consideration should be taken if the practice chooses not to carry workers' compensation insurance.

THEFT AND EMBEZZLEMENT

Employee theft and embezzlement are the leading causes of unexplained inventory reduction and cash flow. Having excess inventory supplies available on the floor unfortunately invites employee theft. Team members see the extra supplies and think taking one box of Heartgard is not going to hurt the practice. However, if each employee took one box of heartworm preventative for each pet, the cost would be considerable. Theft normally does not stop with one box. Soon it becomes dog food or medication and, if the team member is not caught, can move to bigger, more expensive items. When employees purchase items, one team member should be responsible for entering charges for all employees. This can ensure correct charges for products and that all products are being charged for.

Team members can be crafty at embezzling cash. More than one person should be responsible for handling cash and balancing the cash drawer at the end of the night. Additionally, another person should be responsible for the deposits, and the office manager must balance the printed deposit slip to the daily total.

> **PRACTICE POINT** Employee theft and embezzlement occur, and steps must be taken on a regular basis to prevent such actions.

If employee theft or embezzlement is suspected, the practice attorney should be contacted for further advice. Some practices may install cameras to try to catch employees in the act. Proof of theft should be required. Once the practice has proof of the theft, the employee can be terminated. Practices must use caution when suspecting employee theft; a lawsuit can be initiated by the terminated employee if there is a lack of evidence.

TERMINATION

Termination procedures must be clearly stated and followed to protect the practice against an unemployment claim. In general, an employee is given a verbal warning and a method to correct the mistake, accident, or violation. The warning is documented in the personnel file, along with the date and the signature of the manager correcting the action (Figure 5-17). Three written warnings

---

ABC Veterinary Hospital

Employee Warning Notice

Employee Information

Employee Name: Date:
Employee ID: Job Title:
Manager: Department:

Type of Warning

☐ First Warning   ☐ Second Warning   ☐ Final Warning

Type of Offense

☐ Tardiness/Leaving Early   ☐ Absenteeism   ☐ Violation of Company Policies
☐ Substandard Work   ☐ Violation of Safety Rules ☐ Rudeness to Customers/Coworkers
☐ Other: _____

Details

Description of Infraction:

Plan for Improvement:

Consequences of Further Infractions:

Acknowledgement of Receipt of Warning

By signing this form, you confirm that you understand the information in this warning. You also confirm that you and your manager have discussed the warning and a plan for improvement. Signing this form does not necessarily indicate that you agree with this warning.

Employee signature   Date

Manager signature   Date

Witness signature (if employee understands warning but refuses to sign)   Date

FIGURE 5-17 Sample discipline form.

are then allowed, again each documented in the personnel file. Each written warning should be dated, along with the employee's and manager's signatures. The third written warning should also state that the next step is termination.

Termination must take place when a team member has been verbally warned and written up for unsatisfactory performance of duties, excessive tardiness and absenteeism, dishonest and unethical behavior, and/or criminal activity within the hospital (stealing or embezzlement) or outside the hospital (drug use).

The following guidelines should be used when the decision to terminate is final:

- Ensure that the employee was verbally corrected, all three written warnings are documented, and that the employee understood the correction and signed each entry.
- Do not fire employees while upset, angry, or in the midst of an argument. When emotions are high, incorrect words, phrases, and actions will be said or will take place. Wait until the emotions subside, and ensure correct termination procedures are followed. This will help protect the practice against wrongful dismissal complaints.
- If the employee has insurance through the practice, the Consolidated Omnibus Budget Reconciliation Act (COBRA) requires the practice to continue coverage for a specified time. COBRA also requires employers to continue coverage for former employees who have a medical condition that would prevent them from obtaining immediate coverage from a new employer.

Once a termination has been found to be warranted, time and procedure are of essence. The termination should occur at the end of the day, so that if any negative interaction occurs, it is less disruptive to clients and staff. Second, the employee's final paycheck should be prepared and given to the employee so that he or she does not have to return to the practice. Return of the door key should be requested at that time. The employee should sign termination papers, indicating the reason for termination. The entire procedure should be documented by the manager immediately, before any facts are forgotten. All documentation and paperwork should be placed in the employee's file and locked in a file cabinet. It is imperative to remember that all information regarding the termination should be kept confidential and not shared with other team members.

If an employee resigns, the practice should ask the employee to write a letter of resignation. If possible, the reason for leaving should be indicated as well as the final date of employment. An exit interview can be completed the last day of employment. Exit interviews can give the practice needed information: why the employee is resigning, his or her thoughts of items or ideas in the practice that need improvement, and ways the person might recommend or institute changes. These are just some ideas of how a practice can benefit from losing an employee.

 PRACTICE POINT   Correct termination procedures must be used when terminating an employee to protect the practice from potential unemployment claims.

Hospitals can develop their own termination procedures with more or fewer verbal and written warnings. Whatever method is chosen must be reasonable for both the employer and employee, defined in the employee personnel manual, and documented in the personnel file.

TROUBLESHOOTING AND PROBLEM-SOLVING SKILLS

A team uses a leader in many ways, one of those being as a troubleshooter. Troubleshooting problems before they occur can prevent a minor problem from becoming a major problem. Excellent managers and practice owners can envision the problem before it becomes one and institute measures of prevention. On the same topic, once a problem has developed, a team needs a leader to help solve the problem. All the team members should be included in evaluation of the problem. Once a solution has been developed, the entire team can enforce the change. The change is likely to be successful with the entire team promoting it.

VETERINARY PRACTICE and the LAW

According to federal Equal Opportunity Employment laws, it is illegal for a practice to discriminate in hiring on the basis of religion, race, sex, national origin, or age. Some states have also made it illegal to discriminate on the basis of sexual orientation. Under the Americans with Disabilities Act (ADA), employers must make reasonable accommodations to any individual with a physical or mental disability who is otherwise qualified to perform the tasks necessary for the job.

Employers must pay overtime to team members working more than 40 hours per week; those in violation may pay severe fines. Only those in administrative or professional positions may be paid salary; all other must be paid by the hour.

Self-Evaluation Questions

1. Give two examples of questions that cannot be asked during an interview.
2. What is the FLSA?
3. What is USERRA?
4. What is OSHA?
5. What posters are required to be posted in a practice?
6. Where should the required posters be posted?
7. What is the benefit of developing an employee manual?
8. What payroll taxes are employers responsible for?
9. What is a contract employee?
10. Why provide training in phases?

Recommended Reading

Garner C, Catanzaro T, Shirey J et al: *AAHA guide to creating an employee handbook*, ed 2, Denver, 1999, AAHA Press.

Heinke M: Beyond compensation: what to discuss when hiring a new associate, *DVM Magazine* May (3):51, 1997.

London SI: *How to comply with federal employment laws: a complete guide for employers written in plain English*, Rochester, NY, 2000, Vizia Enterprises.

Opperman M: Is it time to hire an associate? *Vet Econ* 35(3):66-68, 1994.

AAHA: *Financial and productivity pulsepoints*, ed 5, Lakewood, CO, 2009, AAHA Press.

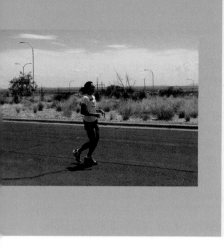

CHAPTER 6

Stress and Burnout

Chapter Outline

Stress Identification
    Positive and Negative Stress
    Choice, Control, and Consequences
    Stages of Stress
    Role of Neurotransmitters
    Personalities and Stress
    Identifying Stressors

Coping With Stress
Substance Abuse and Dependence
    Factors Affecting Substance Abuse
    Recognizing Substance Abuse
    Intervention
    Steps of Drug Intervention
Preventing Career Burnout

Learning Objectives

Mastery of the content in this chapter will enable the reader to:
• Identify stress.
• Explain the stages associated with stress.
• Identify common stressors.
• List methods used to control stress.

• Describe substance abuse.
• List methods of intervention.
• Identify characteristics associated with burnout.

Key Terms

Dependence
Intervention

Neurotransmitters
Stress

Stressors
Substance Abuse

Stress is responsible for a variety of effects in human beings, including physical illness, mental illness, and death. Stress has become accepted in today's society, and at times appears to be unavoidable. Many factors, such as irritable clients, complex cases, and a high volume of patients, can produce a high level of stress in veterinary medicine.

People choose to handle stress in different ways, either positively or negatively, such as with exercise (positive) or with drugs and alcohol (negative). Unfortunately, many choose to cope with stress through drugs and alcohol. Drugs and alcohol may relieve the emotional and physical effects of stress; however, the use of these substances generally creates more problems than they are worth. It is important to identify the source(s) associated with stress and attempt to control the situation. This will allow lower levels of stress, positively affecting physical and mental health.

STRESS IDENTIFICATION

Stress can be defined as the state produced when the body responds to any demand for adaption or adjustment. Stress produces stressors that can be identified as internal, external, or environmentally related. Internal stressors include a person's emotions and sensitivities. A person may be more sensitive to words or phrases said to them and may respond with more emotion than typical. External stressors may include limited time schedules and large workloads. Many people take on too many projects, filling their schedule and workloads to capacity, causing unusual stress and reactions. Environmental stressors many be as simple as hot or cold weather and complex noises. Too many alarms on a surgery monitor can cause a person to respond differently than others would.

Positive and Negative Stress

Stress comes in two forms: positive (good) stress and negative (bad) stress. Positive stress is the body's natural ability to learn how to cope with stress; it may energize a person to cope with the challenges presented. Good stress produces satisfaction and relief once the action or actions causing the stress are over. However, if positive stress continues for an unreasonable amount of time, it can turn into a negative stressor and affect the person

Box 6-1	Physical Problems That May Be Triggered by Stress

- Allergies
- Anxiety
- Asthma
- Backaches
- Chest pains
- Chronic fatigue
- Colitis
- Depression
- Dermatitis
- Dizziness
- Dry mouth
- Erratic breathing
- Facial tics
- Headaches
- Heart attack
- Heartburn
- Hypertension
- Hyperventilation
- Insomnia
- Muscle aches
- Nausea
- Nosebleeds
- Perspiration
- Sexual dysfunction
- Temporomandibular joint disorder
- Ulcers

negatively (Box 6-1). Good stress can result in an over-energized person who eventually becomes overworked, leading to exhaustion. A person who is exhausted ultimately becomes an overwhelmed individual. Bad stress can inadvertently affect a person physically, emotionally, and mentally. Bad stress affects blood pressure and heart rate and can make individuals respond in an unusual manner to normal situations. The normal situation of running out of milk may trigger a person's temper. Bad stress must be taken control of to prevent conflict between family and co-workers.

Choice, Control, and Consequences

Three factors affect good and bad stress: choice, control, and consequences. *Choice* is determined by the individual. An individual chooses to be involved in a project and chooses to have good stress associated with the project. For example, a technician chooses to remodel an exam room by applying new colors of paint, adding a border around the perimeter of the room, and staining the baseboards. The good stress provides satisfaction once the project is completed.

Control is how a person wishes to respond to and master stress. Clients and emergencies determine the schedule of a practice. The practice may set up the daily schedule, but walk-ins and emergencies ultimately change the schedule on a daily basis. The increased business and

complex cases add stress to each team member's daily routine; however, if team members can have a quick meeting to control the stress, then each member's stress level will decrease because a plan has been discussed and implemented. The team has taken control, ultimately reducing stress.

> **PRACTICE POINT** Individuals can control how to respond to stressful situations.

Consequence is the result of an action. For example, once cancer has been diagnosed, death is a likely outcome at some point in the patient's future. Therefore death is the consequence of the diagnosis. If the anticipated result is expected, the stress produced is a good stress (resulting in little effect on the heart rate and blood pressure). However, if an unexpected death results from anesthesia, bad stress results. Death is not a normal consequence of anesthesia and produces a large amount of stress on the staff.

Stages of Stress

The body automatically responds to stress mentally and physically. "Fight or flight" is the body's automatic response and is necessary for survival. Several stages exist in the fight or flight response: alarm, adaptation, exhaustion, and death. Stage 1, alarm, is the initial response to fight or flight. The body releases increased endorphins and hormones and the blood flow within the body is increased. This affects and increases the breathing rate, blood sugar levels, adrenal gland secretion, cortisone production, and perspiration. Adrenal gland secretion of epinephrine increases the individual's heart and respiratory rate. A prolonged increase in heart rate increases blood pressure, which ultimately has negative effects on the cardiac system. The adrenal glands' activity, over a prolonged period, may cause muscle tension and digestive tract disorders. Diarrhea, nausea, ulcers, and constipation can result from the adrenal glands' oversecretion. If stage 1 continues, the body learns to adapt to the conditions and tries to compensate for the abnormalities, resulting in stage 2, adaptation. After a prolonged period, the body adapts and becomes exhausted (stage 3), resulting in burnout, fatigue, and eventually death (stage 4).

Role of Neurotransmitters

During stressful situations, neurotransmitters in the brain are called on and can be oversecreted in a manner similar to hormone release and adrenal gland response during stage 1. Overproduction of neurotransmitters can cause anxiety, anger, and depression. After prolonged release, a person is no longer able to cope with normal stressors. This is when many turn to drugs or alcohol to try to eliminate the stress. Drugs and alcohol distort or eliminate the exchange of information in the brain, releasing the stress felt by these individuals.

Personalities and Stress

Personalities predispose people to experience stress differently. It is not known how personality affects stress, whether it is learned or genetic; however, personalities are grouped into types. The stress-prone personality is generally a "type A" personality. These individuals are perfectionists, often multitask, expect a high level of performance from themselves as well as their co-workers, and tend to be successful. Stress-prone individuals are at a higher risk for heart disease and hypertension (Figure 6-1). Stress-hardy personalities are less prone to stress, are in control of their lives, and do not have to be "the best." They often control and compartmentalize the stress and deal with it later. "Type B" personalities manage stress well, rarely letting others know they are suffering from any type of stress.

Identifying Stressors

Identifying stressors can help one cope with stress in a successful manner. Individuals in the veterinary field generally experience life-event, environmental, personal, client, and career stressors. Life-event stressors can include death, divorce, retirement, pregnancy, financial difficulties, and holidays. The list of life-event stressors that can affect an individual is endless, and each person will respond to each situation differently. For example, the holiday season can be extremely stressful for a person with financial difficulty or a large, overbearing family. Holidays may be peaceful and enjoyable for an individual with financial success and a small, close-knit family. How the person deals with the stress is individualized, as is whether they choose to control the situation or not.

Environmental stressors include climate, weather, pollution, crime, and traffic. In veterinary medicine, environmental stressors include noise levels, alarms, equipment, and inventory. Several noises and alarms may occur at once, including the ringing phones, barking dogs, and surgical monitor warnings. Equipment maintenance and breaks can be a huge stressor, especially for the technician who is in charge of maintaining and repairing equipment. Inventory shortages can be a stress to doctors, who may feel that supplies are always limited, preventing them from practicing the medicine they want.

Personal stressors may include lack of self-confidence and self-esteem. Team members who lack both self-confidence and self-esteem may have a harder time

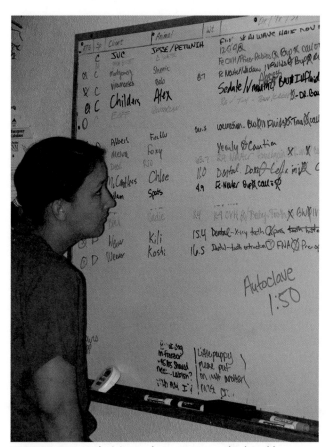

FIGURE 6-1 Technicians who are overworked and burnt out exhibit poor posture, unhappy facial expressions, and a lack of excitement in their position.

educating and taking care of clients as well as being successful in their personal lives.

Client stressors include clients who are angry, grieving, or "know-it-all" and the elderly. Angry clients make every team member's day miserable and are able to invoke every stressor. Grieving clients experience several emotions, including denial, anger, and eventually acceptance. Many times the team must cater to every stage and emotion of grief. This can add stress to each team member's daily routine, again invoking several other stressors. Know-it-all clients generally think they know more than the veterinarians themselves, although they have not attended veterinary school. These clients may choose to treat the patient themselves, regardless of the recommendations that have been made by the team. Teams should understand that they cannot control this type of client or their actions and should simply document the recommendations in the record. Some elderly clients want to talk about every animal they have owned, share every encounter the current pet has ever experienced, and want the best treatment available. Unfortunately, many cannot afford the best care available. The team may feel guilty and will sometimes makes concessions to help this type of client. Stress can be eliminated with this type of client, knowing that this client will take time and patience; preplanning would be of benefit to the staff. Satisfaction can be obtained from this type of stress when it is managed in the correct fashion.

> **PRACTICE POINT** Identifying stressors can help control the level of stress a person experiences.

Career stressors may include long hours, low pay, and unappreciated work ethic. Many technicians and veterinarians enter the profession with the understanding of low pay and long hours, but years of unappreciated work eventually have a compounding effect. Team members can take actions to minimize career stressors by controlling the situation. Team members must work together to eliminate long hours; each member should be responsible for capping his or her own hours. An individual can only put forth so many productive hours within a week's period. Pay scales can be evaluated and potentially increased by enhancing the skill set, knowledge, and value of each employee. Team members should consistently strive for higher levels of education, higher levels of care, and excellent levels of client education. An invaluable employee may receive higher compensation and be rewarded for the excellent work ethic put forth. Job satisfaction and dedication can decrease stress; again, long hours must be capped to prevent burnout.

COPING WITH STRESS

Once stressors have been identified, they must be analyzed as to which ones can be dealt with, coped with, and/or eliminated. Changes in lifestyle, mental and physical activities, and relaxation methods can be instituted to help eliminate, or at least reduce, stress (Figure 6-2). Nutrition, sleep, and exercise play a vital role in reducing stress and should be taken into consideration when making lifestyle changes.

Regular healthy eating habits are one of the best protectors against stress. Protein is especially helpful in counteracting the effects of stress on the body. Micronutrients from fruits and vegetables help improve the immune system, which is impaired as a side effect of stress. Since the blood glucose level is altered, individuals tend to overeat sugars, fats, and carbohydrates during stressful periods. These nutrients, although essential in small and limited amounts, are counterproductive in alleviating stress.

Sleep is imperative to reducing stress. Sleep needs vary from person to person and may change throughout the lifecycle. Most adults need 7 to 8 hours of sleep per night; each must learn the amount required to function properly, produce work at an acceptable level, and rise in the morning feeling refreshed. The REM (rapid eye movement) phase of sleep is also essential. Dreams occur during REM sleep, and it has been determined that this type of sleep is necessary to rest the body. Those who consume alcohol and use drugs do not experience a normal REM phase and therefore experience sleep deprivation.

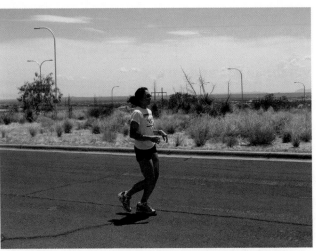

FIGURE 6-2 Exercise can alleviate stress and prevent a person from becoming burnt out in his or her profession.

Exercise reduces stress by reducing and releasing tension, restoring normal chemical balances, relieving mild depression, and decreasing the risk of cardiac disease. Exercise should be part of a normal daily routine and should include activities that are enjoyable. Each person enjoys activities on different levels; therefore finding one that satisfies both the mind and body is imperative. Many people enjoy running and the endorphins it produces, allowing the mind to solve problems and relieve stress as the body exerts energy. Others enjoy hiking, kayaking, weightlifting, or riding bikes. Any exercise program must be enjoyable to be beneficial. Each person must experiment and find the right activity.

Mental changes and activities can be initiated to reduce the effects of stress. Laughter, the best medicine, should be part of every person's day. Hobbies may be adopted, taking the mind away from stressors and allowing increased concentration on other topics. Music, reading, and art can also be forms of stress relief depending on the individual.

Expressing feelings is an excellent outlet for stress. Friends, family, and co-workers can be exceptional listeners for someone who needs to "vent." Once feelings are released, the stress level decreases. Talking with co-workers may not only elevate stress, but produce solutions to reduce the stress as well. Many times if one co-worker is experiencing stress associated with the practice, others are as well.

> **PRACTICE POINT** Individuals must have healthy eating and sleeping habits to effectively manage stress.

PRACTICE POINT Discussing stressful situations with friends or team members can reduce stress.

It is known that chronic and/or uninterrupted stress is very harmful. It is important therefore to take breaks and "decompress" (Figure 6-3). Walks can be taken instead of coffee breaks. Team members should use weekends to relax and avoid scheduling so many events that Monday mornings seem like a relief. Creating predictability at work and home provides structure and routine in one's life. Thinking and planning ahead allow various scenarios to be considered, good and bad, which may become realities at work or home. One cannot prevent the unexpected from happening; however, visualizing what is possible can provide a comfortable framework from which to respond. With this kind of preparation, stress can be turned into a positive force. Individuals can learn signals associated with stress and take measures to reduce them before they become a problem.

Stress-management counseling in the form of individual or group therapy is offered by various mental health care providers. Stress counseling and group discussion therapy have been shown to reduce stress symptoms and improve overall health and attitude.

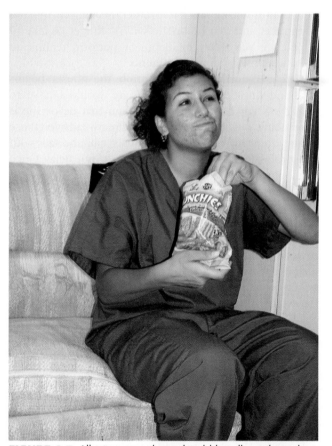

FIGURE 6-3 All team members should be allowed to take breaks on their shifts. Small breaks throughout the day can increase overall performance.

SUBSTANCE ABUSE AND DEPENDENCE

Not every person who uses drugs or alcohol to deal with stress is an abuser or becomes dependent on the product. However, the likelihood of dependence on the product is high. Substance abusers may use the drug or alcohol intermittently or on a regular basis. Either type of user may develop substance dependence. Stress has long been recognized as one of the most powerful triggers for drug or alcohol cravings and abuse.

PRACTICE POINT It has been proven that stress can induce drug and alcohol dependence.

Substance dependence is indicated by symptoms of tolerance to the effects of a drug and symptoms of withdrawal without the drug. The user eventually requires more substance to obtain the desired effects. When the individual is not using the substance, he or she may have symptoms such as cravings, anxiety, and/or depression. Once a user becomes dependent on a substance, he or she continues to use it regardless of the consequences. This is when individuals lose their families and jobs. The use of the substance has now become an addiction.

Factors Affecting Substance Abuse

Some risk factors for addiction have been determined; these include genes, chronic pain, sociocultural factors, and environment. Individuals who have families with a history of addictions must exercise caution at all times because the risk of addiction to alcohol or drugs is high. Individuals who suffer chronic pain have a higher chance of developing an addiction because it begins to take more substance to decrease the pain associated with chronic conditions. Sociocultural factors include age, occupation, ethnicity, and social class (including friends and acquaintances). Environmental factors include stresses associated with an occupation or family as well as the ability to access drugs. Individuals in the health care industry have a higher percent chance of becoming dependent on substances because of the availability and ease of access.

Recognizing Substance Abuse

It can be hard to recognize drug abuse or determine the correct time to intervene. Users hide the secret, keep it confidential, and eventually become isolated. These actions eventually lead to a feeling of helplessness; however, users justify the use of drugs due to the high levels of stress they may be enduring or the increased workload and fatigue that they experience.

Many substance abusers experience a change in behavior, practice poor personal hygiene, and dress in a sloppy, wrinkled, and unprofessional manner. They begin to withdraw from family, friends, and co-workers. They neglect their duties and cases, are disorganized, and exhibit poor judgment. Many start to write prescriptions for themselves, steal controlled substances from the practice, experience financial problems, and begin to have unexplained absences from work. This results in conflict and career instability.

It is important to intervene to protect clients and other team members. The practice may be at risk for malpractice suits because the impaired team member will make poor judgments. Those convicted of drug abuse can have their licenses revoked, which can prevent the license from ever being renewed.

> **PRACTICE POINT**   If a veterinarian or credentialed technician is charged with drug possession, his or her professional license can be revoked and never renewed.

Intervention

A drug intervention is a process that helps a drug addict recognize the extent of his or her problem. Individuals who are addicted to drugs or alcohol usually do not know their addiction is out of control. They tend to look at those around them as a measure of how right or wrong their actions are. Those who surround themselves with individuals who are caught up in the grasp of drug addiction are not able to see the drastic effects of their own dependence.

These individuals need objective feedback on their behavior. It is through a nonjudgmental, noncritical, systematic drug intervention process that the individuals are able to see their own lifestyle choices. When they truly understand the impact that their alcohol dependence or drug addiction has on others, they may begin to see they are hurting those around them.

The individual who is suspected of having a substance abuse problem may try to minimize his or her use, change the topic, joke about use, or say phrases such as "my substance use is no worse than anyone else's." Even if the individual begins to share some life problems that he or she has been experiencing, know that those problems will not get better unless the individual stops the use of alcohol or substances.

> **PRACTICE POINT**   Substance abusers may deny their drug or alcohol dependence; team members must intervene to change the abuser's lifestyle.

The goal of an intervention is for the addict to accept the reality of his or her addiction and to seek help. The process of conducting an intervention is a difficult and delicate matter. It is important that it is done correctly; otherwise the individual may feel cornered and become defensive. Advice from a trained professional is useful in determining the proper strategy and timing of a specific intervention.

If team members suspect that an individual has a problem with drugs or alcohol, they should get involved. It is the active involvement by concerned others that begins the process of lifestyle change. Intervention is the first step. Professional treatment is the second. Both are necessary steps for addicts to become free of their dependencies.

Steps of Drug Intervention

1. Time the drug abuse intervention. If possible, plan to talk with the addict when he or she is unimpaired. Choose a time when both the addict and the intervener are in a calm frame of mind and when a discussion can be done privately.
2. Be specific. Tell the co-worker that you are concerned about his or her drug or alcohol abuse and want to be supportive in getting help. Back up concerns with examples of the ways in which the drug abuse has caused problems for patients, clients, and co-workers, including any recent incidents.
3. State the consequences. The basic intent is to make the abuser's life more uncomfortable if he or she continues using drugs or alcohol. Let the abuser know that all measures will be taken to protect the staff, clients, and patients, and that he or she will no longer be able to practice veterinary medicine or perform technician duties while under the influence.
4. Listen. If, during an intervention, the abuser begins asking questions such as, "Where would I have to go?" or "For how long?" it is a sign that he or she is reaching out for help. Do not directly answer these questions. Instead, have the abuser call and talk with a professional. Offer support and do not delay. Once an agreement to seek professional help has been accomplished, seek admittance immediately.

Intervention is imperative; if a veterinarian or credentialed veterinary technician chooses not to accept help, then assistance must be obtained from the state board of veterinary medicine to remove the license. If a team member who is not licensed is the addict, he or she must be terminated to protect the integrity of the practice and the safety of fellow team members and patients.

PREVENTING CAREER BURNOUT

One of the most common causes of career change in veterinary medicine is burnout. Burnout can be defined as physical or emotional exhaustion, especially as a result of long-term stress. It is also an expression used to describe what might be better defined as depression or extreme exhaustion. Veterinarians and veterinary technicians are generally a very dedicated group and will work until the bitter end to ensure patients and clients are taken care of.

Teams sacrifice time from themselves to satisfy client and employer needs.

Negative attitudes are more contagious than positive attitudes, and clients will perceive the negativity. The end result may be lost clients, lost revenue and, ultimately, loss of valuable team members. Physical symptoms of burnout include ulcers, fatigue, overeating, gastroenteritis, cardiac abnormalities, backaches, and nausea. Behavioral issues associated with burnout include withdrawal, increased alcohol intake, agitation, depression, distraction, and increased spending.

> **PRACTICE POINT** Burnout affects every member of the practice: clients, staff, and owners.

Burnout victims hate to go to work; they have lost the enthusiasm and passion that drove them into the veterinary profession. Often the one suffering from burnout is the last person to identify and admit that burnout has occurred. Team workers, family, and friends can identify burnout much earlier; however, the victim cannot change until acceptance of the condition has occurred.

Breaks and vacations are a necessity to reinvigorate the team, individuals, and practice owners. They should be looked at as an investment, not a loss, because the invigoration brings new ideas, motivation, and enthusiasm back to the business. Continuing education can be stimulating, rejuvenating, and exciting for the entire team and is considered an investment as well as prevention for burnout.

Boundaries must be set for work and personal items. A team worker's personal life cannot be sacrificed for the sake of the practice. Time must be taken to enjoy activities outside the practice; family, health, and fun must be listed as priorities.

> **PRACTICE POINT** Vacations are necessary to prevent burnout.

Exercise programs may be instituted for the entire team. It can take a lot of motivation to invigorate team members who have not exercised regularly, but the benefits that each team member will receive will be extremely rewarding. The exercise team leader may save a life by instituting an exercise program and save a valuable employee from leaving the profession.

Assistants may look into schools to receive credentials. This may allow an increase in salary, responsibilities, and knowledge. Education never devalues a person; it increases the value to the team and to the individual and allows the continuous challenge of climbing the ladder within a career. Credentialed technicians may look toward specialty boards, community-involved events, and continuing education for challenges and rewards. Since many practices lack an experienced practice manager, a technician may take the management challenge and develop methods to improve the practice financially. The possibilities are endless; it is up to the individual to seek challenges, prevent burnout, and continue to motivate others to succeed in a potentially rewarding career.

What Would You Do/Not Do?

Alex, a longtime employee, is scheduled to work 34 hours per week but has been accumulating more than 44 hours a week by covering other employees' shifts. While it is great that he is helpful in preventing the practice from being shorthanded, it is beginning to take a toll on Alex's personality. Generally, Alex is very friendly and provides excellent customer service. The clients usually rave about his service, until recently. The office manager has received client complaints about Alex's rude behavior; one comment from a client stated he did not have time to explain a procedure. Another client stated that he made her feel stupid because she did not understand the vaccination schedule when she asked for clarification.

What Should the Office Manager Do?

The office manager must address the negative attitude that has overcome Alex and ask what has happened recently that has affected him so much. Alex may be having personal issues that have shortened his temper, but he may be unaware how he has affected others around him. After asking what has happened, the office manager may ask him how a change can improve the situation. Alex may penalize himself enough and change his behavior without any penalty from the practice. If Alex becomes defensive about his attitude, he may be encouraged to take some vacation time to relax and unwind. If he does not wish to take time off for himself, he may be advised to decrease his hours until things work out for him, leaving him under less stress. Good managers protect their employees from burning out by asking questions and learning about problems and methods to prevent them. Many times ineffective managers are quick to blame and criticize; this creates resentment and unhappiness in a workplace environment.

VETERINARY PRACTICE and the LAW

Team members who work excess hours and burn out on the profession do not take the time to discuss procedures, diseases, and conditions with clients. Exhausted team members have short tempers with clients and do not provide clients with information sufficient for making informed consent. Short tempers and poor nonverbal communication prevent clients from asking questions and may prevent clients from returning to the practice in the future. Veterinarians and team members who do not clearly communicate with clients are at a higher risk of having a complaint filed with the state veterinary board. Complaints must be fully investigated and may result in license revocation.

Stress and burnout must be prevented before they begin. Full-time employees should take vacation as it is allotted; vacations provide relaxation and rejuvenation on return to the practice. Continuing education also rejuvenates employees and stimulates interest in new topics. All team members should protect one another and watch for symptoms of fatigue, exhaustion, and burnout.

Self-Evaluation Questions

1. What symptoms physically occur in someone under undue stress?
2. How does good stress differ from bad stress?
3. What factors affect stress?
4. What three methods can reduce stress?
5. What stressors may affect someone in the veterinary profession?
6. What is substance abuse?
7. What factors have been determined to increase the likelihood of a substance abuse?
8. By what evidence does an individual reveal that he or she is a substance abuser?
9. Why should one intervene if substance abuse is suspected?
10. What can happen to a professional convicted of drug use?

Recommended Reading

Almeida DM, Kesser RC: Everyday stressors and gender differences in daily stress, *J Pers Soc Psych* 75:670-680, 1998.

Heinke MM: *Practice made perfect: a guide to veterinary practice management*, Lakewood, CO, 2001, AAHA Press.

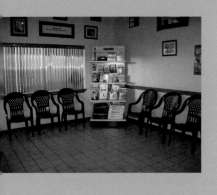

Practice Design

Chapter Outline

Principles of Time and Motion
Body Positioning
Ergonomics
Health and Safety of Reception Team Members
Design and Function of Effective Practices
Creating Comfortable Reception Areas

Creating Comfortable Exam Rooms
Consultation Rooms
Retail Area
Middle Area
Treatment Area

Learning Objectives

Mastery of the content in this chapter will enable the reader to:
- Discuss motion economy.
- Clarify how to complete tasks more efficiently.
- Distinguish proper body position.
- Define ergonomics.

- Describe the design and function of effective practices.
- Develop comfortable reception areas.
- Develop comfortable consultation rooms.
- Develop an effective retail area.

Key Terms

Ergonomics
Maintenance Diets

Motion Economy
Therapeutic Diets

Time and Motion

Many veterinary practices are located in older buildings and are beginning to look at remodeling, upgrading, or moving into a new building. Many things must be taken into consideration when moving to a new building. Selecting a location that is easy to find for both new and existing clients will increase the growth of the practice. The building should look clean and professional from the outside (Figure 7-1). The hospital or practice sign should be easy to see and read from the street (Figure 7-2). Team members will be responsible for the input of ideas to increase efficiency at the new or updated location; this demands an understanding of the principles of motion economy and the placement of equipment to create an environment that helps the team work in a smarter way and more comfortably. The goal of motion economy is to be more efficient, not to work harder and more strenuously.

PRINCIPLES OF TIME AND MOTION

When determining the placement of office equipment and supplies, the principles of time and motion should be considered. Time and motion refer to the amount of time and degree of motion required to perform a given task. This is important in the receptionist's office and exam rooms of a general practice. Many studies have been completed to understand how to minimize the amount of time and motion it takes to perform basic tasks. To improve motion economy, it is necessary to eliminate unnecessary steps or tasks, rearrange equipment, organize procedures, and simplify tasks. The principles of motion economy can aid in accomplishing these goals, thereby reducing stress and increasing productivity within the practice (Box 7-1).

BODY POSITIONING

Receptionists should consider sitting whenever possible to eliminate undue stress on the back, neck, and legs. Improper posture while standing can lead to fatigue, which can decrease productivity. While seated in a chair, a person should have the thighs parallel to the floor, the lower legs vertical, and the feet firmly on the floor (Figure 7-3). While using the keyboard, the arms should be positioned so that the forearms and wrists are as horizontal as possible. The back and neck should be erect, with the upper arms perpendicular to the floor. It should be remembered that the receptionist should always face clients; a team member's back can appear rude and unapproachable.

Technicians working on the floor all day must have a correct body posture to reduce future back problems. Body posture should be straight, with no slumping. Team competitions can be held to correct others' body posture on a daily basis. Team members must also remember to lift with their legs, not their backs, to prevent back injuries. Most back problems are due to continual, long-term, incorrect lifting procedures; therefore injuries may not be felt for years. Management must initiate and enforce correct lifting procedures to protect the team from future painful conditions.

ERGONOMICS

Ergonomics is the science that studies the relationship between people and their work environments. Interrelated physical and psychological factors are involved in

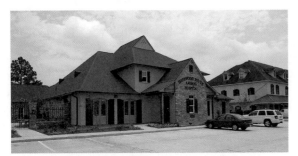

FIGURE 7-1 The client parking lot should be clearly designated and clean. (From Bassert JM, McCurnin DM: *McCurnin's clinical textbook for veterinary technicians*, ed 7, St Louis, 2010, Saunders Elsevier.)

the creation of a stress-free work environment. By understanding the abilities that people have and their work patterns, it is possible to design an environment that conforms to the work needs of team members. The appropriate use of design can make a job much more productive and efficient while reducing work-related injuries and discomforts.

Physiologic factors include color, lighting, acoustics, heating and cooling, space, furniture, and equipment. Poor lighting can play a large factor in team member inefficiencies; improper lighting causes eye strain, misinterpreted hospital sheets and records, or missed parasites on a pet.

Acoustics can play a vital role in kennel assistants' duties because they spend most of their time within the kennel ward. Barking dogs with a piercing tone can wear down even the best attitude, decreasing the efficiency of the team member (let alone a recovering patient!). When working in noisy areas for extended periods of time, personal hearing protectors can be worn (Figure 7-4).

Heating and cooling have an effect on clients and team members as well as patients. Clients may become irritated easier when the facilities are hot; team members may not work as efficiently when it is either too hot or too cold. Patients may not recover as well in cold environments and may need additional blankets to maintain body temperature, thus decreasing the efficiency of the team.

Smaller spaces always decrease the efficiency of a team, as does too large a space with wasted room. When designing a practice, whether remodeling an old or new building, space efficiency matters.

Color plays a large role in how a client perceives the practice and the team. An attractive, cheerful, and efficient reception area confirms the confidence the practice has conveyed to the client. A dark, dirty, and cluttered

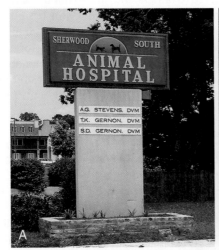
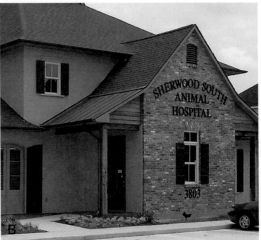

FIGURE 7-2 **A,** Hospital signs should be professional and clearly visible from the street. **B,** Signs directly on the building may also be used. (From Bassert JM, McCurnin DM: *McCurnin's clinical textbook for veterinary technicians,* ed 7, St Louis, 2010, Saunders Elsevier.)

Box 7-1	Applying the Principle of Motion Economy in the Business Office

- Position objects as close to the point of use as possible.
- Use motions that require the least amount of movement.
- Minimize the number of materials used for a given procedure.
- Use smooth, continuous movements, not zigzag motions.
- Organize materials in a logical sequence.
- Use ergonomically designed chairs to provide good body posture.
- Provide lighting that eliminates shadows.
- Provide work areas that are at elbow level.
- Computer screens should be positioned within 10 to 40 degrees of horizontal.

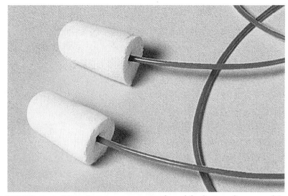

FIGURE 7-4 Hearing protectors should always be used in noisy kennels. (From Bassert JM, McCurnin DM: *McCurnin's clinical textbook for veterinary technicians,* ed 7, St Louis, 2010, Saunders Elsevier.)

HEALTH AND SAFETY OF RECEPTION TEAM MEMBERS

A variety of factors can affect the health and safety of receptionists. For example, spending hours a day looking at a computer screen can result in eye strain and fatigue. Repetitive keyboarding can lead to wrist discomfort and possible bursitis or tendonitis. Inappropriate body posture can lead to back discomfort. To help relieve eye strain, computer monitors should have appropriate lighting and be placed at an angle to decrease glare on the screen. The use of an ergonomically designed mouse and keyboard can decrease fatigue in the wrist, and an ergonomically designed chair can help facilitate correct body posture while seated at a desk (Figure 7-5).

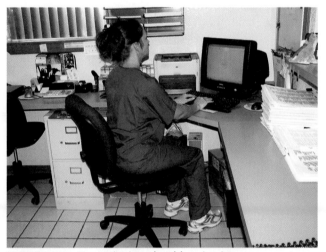

FIGURE 7-3 Receptionists should maintain proper posture by keeping their feet flat on the floor, legs perpendicular, and back straight.

DESIGN AND FUNCTION OF EFFECTIVE PRACTICES

The size, type of practice, and services offered are three main factors that affect the design and efficiency of a hospital. The primary goal is to develop a solution that optimizes the efficiency of the team while providing clients and patients with a high standard of care.

Most practices are divided into three parts: the front, middle, and back. The front generally consists of the reception area and exam room. The middle refers to the laboratory, pharmacy, and treatment area, and the back refers to kennel wards and storage area.

CREATING COMFORTABLE RECEPTION AREAS

The reception area is the gateway to the practice and provides the clients with the first impression of the hospital (Figure 7-6). Overcrowding and congestion always occur in the reception area, especially as clients arrive for appointments and to pick up patients or medications. Congestion doubles as clients check out with their pets. This congestion can lead to undesirable pet interaction and client dissatisfaction.

reception area can bring doubts or mistrust to the client. Light colors with warm hues can create a cheerful setting, while cool colors, such as light green and blue, can produce a tranquil setting. Tranquil settings can benefit both the team and the client during difficult and stressful situations.

Physical factors include the use of proper equipment to help prevent injury. Office chairs should have a broad base with four to five casters for proper balance. They should also have a well-padded seat with back support. Computer monitors should be placed at the appropriate height and distance from the receptionist to prevent eye and neck strain. Computer keyboards should have an ergonomic design and should also be placed at the proper height to prevent bursitis or tendonitis. Technicians should always use proper restraint equipment when indicated and get help when lifting or transporting large and heavy animals or equipment.

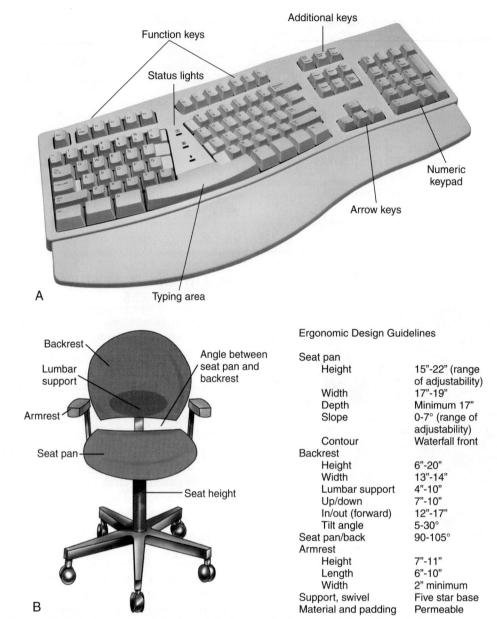

FIGURE 7-5 **A**, An ergonomic keyboard. **B**, Ergonomic design guidelines for a chair (measurements relative to chair seat). (*A* From Finkbeiner B, Finkbeiner C: *Practice management for the dental team,* ed 6, St Louis, 2006, Mosby Elsevier; *B* from Jacobs K: *Ergonomics for therapists,* ed 3, St Louis, 2008, Mosby Elsevier.)

It can be advisable to develop separate waiting areas for dog and cat patients, reducing the stress on both the owners and pets. A practice may also have separate check-in and check-out areas, reducing the congestion associated with both procedures. If a practice boards or grooms patients, a separate entrance may benefit both clients and team members.

A warm atmosphere can be created with comfortable chairs, nice artwork on the walls, and plants. Chairs should be made of a material that is easy to clean, does not stain, and is durable. Seats should have some space between them. Clients do not like to sit right next to each other, especially those with large dogs. Plants should be hung from the ceiling or on the wall to prevent dogs from urinating on them. A restroom should be provided off the reception area for the convenience of clients.

Photos albums can be created of team members and their pets. Photos may include professional portraits as well as spontaneous photos, showing activities team members participate in with their pets outside the office. Photo albums can also be created of clients and their pets. Clients should be asked for permission to place photos in the album. A practice photo album can also be created, showing different rooms of the practice, activities that occur in those rooms, and team members performing activities. Many clients wonder what it looks like behind the scenes and what occurs once their pet leaves the exam room; this is a wonderful creation to appease their mind. Picture collages also warm up rooms, giving clients something to look at while they wait.

CREATING COMFORTABLE EXAM ROOMS

Exam rooms are frequently white, dirty, and smell of the previous patient. Cleanliness is imperative to owners and should be to the entire team. Rooms should be swept and mopped after each patient to decrease the chance of transmitting disease. Cleanliness also prevents the transmission of odors. Warm, neutral tones calm clients. Practices may add nicely framed pictures or client education posters. Thumb tacks should not be used to hang posters; holes in the wall and torn posters devalue the practice. Wall borders also add a nice touch to rooms, along with comfortable chairs that allow clients to sit

near patients on the examination table. Rooms should not be cluttered with models, treats, or diagnostic equipment (Figure 7-7). Countertops and sinks should be clean at all times.

CONSULTATION ROOMS

Consultation rooms are very nice to have for clients who arrive at the practice and need to discuss patient care with doctors and technicians. They can also be used for euthanasia. Rooms should be quiet, away from high traffic areas, and provide a sense of comfort. Nicely framed pictures may line the room, as well as a comfortable couch or chair. A radiograph viewer may be added for consultation purposes, as well as models for client education. Exam room tables may be left out, as this room is strictly for consultations, not exams. If a euthanasia is performed, the patient may have a nice, comfortable blanket on the floor or be held in the arms of the client.

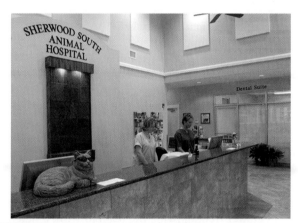

FIGURE 7-6 A reception area should give a warm, comfortable feeling to clients and staff. (From Bassert JM, McCurnin DM: *McCurnin's clinical textbook for veterinary technicians,* ed 7, St Louis, 2010, Saunders Elsevier.)

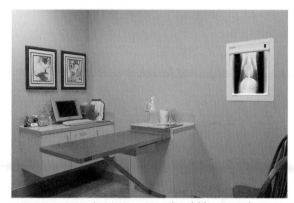

FIGURE 7-7 Examination rooms should be warmly decorated, clean, and in excellent condition. (From Bassert JM, McCurnin DM: *McCurnin's clinical textbook for veterinary technicians,* ed 7, St Louis, 2010, Saunders Elsevier.)

What Would You Do/Not Do?

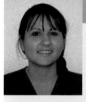

Lori, a veterinary technician, recently attended continuing education and learned about the benefits of adding colors to exam and treatment rooms. The rooms in her practice are white and always appear dirty. She envisions a colorful exam room with a border of puppies and kittens. To her, the color should be a soft, calming color. She learned that calming colors will help ease client tensions when they are in the rooms. Lori is afraid to approach the practice manager with her idea for fear of rejection.

What Should Lori Do?
Lori should put a proposal together that lists all of the elements she learned in continuing education. She could research the best possible colors and find a border that

would match the color combination that she has in mind. Second, she could put an estimate together of the total cost to paint the room, including her labor, paint, and materials. Once all of this information is together, she can propose her plan to the practice manager and owner, who may be excited and have ideas to add as well. Team members should always feel that their ideas and contributions are important and not be afraid to present them. Practice managers appreciate team members who are independently motivated and willing to go the extra step to add a personal touch to the practice.

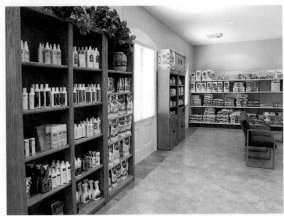

FIGURE 7-8 Professional display in reception area. (From Bassert JM, McCurnin DM: *McCurnin's clinical textbook for veterinary technicians,* ed 7, St Louis, 2010, Saunders Elsevier.)

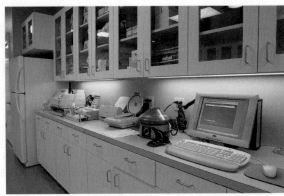

FIGURE 7-9 The laboratory is located just beyond the examination rooms. (From Bassert JM, McCurnin DM: *McCurnin's clinical textbook for veterinary technicians,* ed 7, St Louis, 2010, Saunders Elsevier.)

RETAIL AREA

Retail areas are great for drawing attention to products the practice promotes; however, extra attention needs to be given to this area to prevent theft (Figure 7-8). Retail areas that can be placed behind the reception area may hold more valuable items such as collars or leashes; cheaper toys and smaller items can be placed in the reception area. Therapeutic diets should be placed behind the counter, allowing maintenance diets to remain in the reception area. Many practices have limited space to carry excess products, so care must be taken when choosing what products will be carried. It should be determined what and how the practice will benefit if it chooses to carry a product. However, clients look to veterinary practices for recommendations of products to purchase, food to feed, and toys that should be allowed for their pet. An appropriate balance must be determined within each practice.

MIDDLE AREA

The middle area of a veterinary practice generally includes the pharmacy and laboratory areas, which must also function in an efficient manner (Figures 7-9 and 7-10). If the pharmacy and laboratory share the same space, there must be enough room for computers, laboratory equipment, prescription filling, and a location to write on records. Equipment should be placed in ergonomically efficient locations, reducing the workload of team members as they complete tasks associated with the laboratory area. Laboratory equipment must be placed far enough apart to allow fans to efficiently cool the equipment. Electrical outlets should not be overloaded, which can cause a fire hazard.

TREATMENT AREA

The treatment is generally referred to as "the back" of the practice and encompasses radiology (Figure 7-11), surgery (Figure 7-12), the treatment area (Figure 7-13), and the kennel and isolation wards. Floors should have an anti-slip surface, reducing accidental slipping on wet floors. The treatment area should be set up to allow traffic to flow freely and uncongested. Treatment tables should be positioned to allow team members to work from any angle; therefore placement of tables in the center of a room works well. Electrical outlets can be placed in the ceiling if needed, reducing the number of cords that a team member might trip on. The treatment area must remain clutter free, allowing the team to work efficiently, especially when space is limited.

⚖ VETERINARY PRACTICE and THE LAW

When developing, designing, or remodeling a practice, the Americans with Disabilities Act must be considered. This act is a federal law that protects those with disabilities, including team members and clients. Clients must be able to have full access to the facility; this includes parking lot ramps, bathroom access (wide doors and handrails), and wide doors for wheelchair access to all rooms.

Team members with disabilities cannot be discriminated against if they can complete the job requirements as listed in the job description section of the employee manual. By law, employers must make reasonable accommodations to enable the employee to perform the listed job duties. Reasonable accommodations may include making existing facilities used by employees readily accessible and usable by individuals with disabilities.

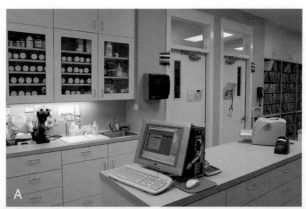

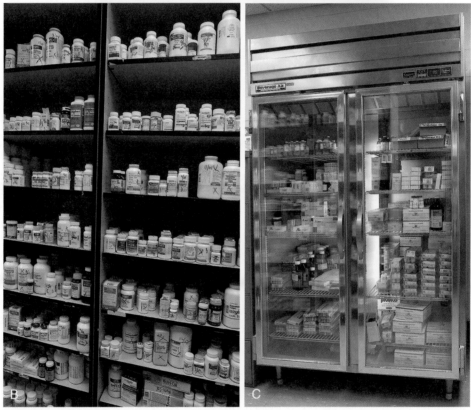

FIGURE 7-10 **A**, Pharmacy is located near examination rooms and inpatient treatment area. **B**, Drug shelf storage in pharmacy. **C**, Glass door refrigerator for storage of vaccines and biologics. (From Bassert JM, McCurnin DM: *McCurnin's clinical textbook for veterinary technicians*, ed 7, St Louis, 2010, Saunders Elsevier.)

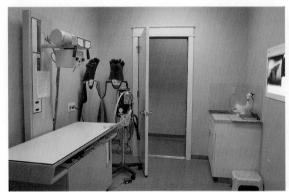

FIGURE 7-11 Radiology room with x-ray machine and protective equipment hanging on the wall. The automatic film processor is not visible through the open door. (From Bassert JM, McCurnin DM: *McCurnin's clinical textbook for veterinary technicians,* ed 7, St Louis, 2010, Saunders Elsevier.)

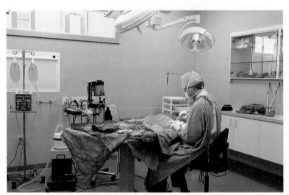

FIGURE 7-12 Surgical room with one door for both entrance and exit, ceiling-mounted lights, and minimal countertops. (From Bassert JM, McCurnin DM: *McCurnin's clinical textbook for veterinary technicians,* ed 7, St Louis, 2010, Saunders Elsevier.)

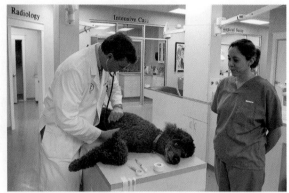

FIGURE 7-13 Centralized treatment area accommodates both outpatient and inpatient treatment. (From Bassert JM, McCurnin DM: *McCurnin's clinical textbook for veterinary technicians,* ed 7, St Louis, 2010, Saunders Elsevier.)

Self-Evaluation Questions

1. What is the goal of motion economy?
2. What are the principles of time and motion?
3. What is ergonomics?
4. What factors contribute to ergonomics?
5. Why is creating a comfortable reception area so important?

Recommended Reading

Bridger RS: *Introduction to ergonomics,* ed 3, Boca Raton, FL, 2008, CRC Press.

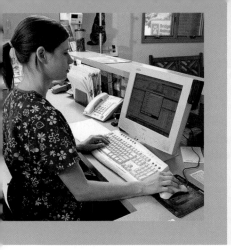

CHAPTER 8

Technology in the Office

Chapter Outline

Information Systems
Hardware
Software
Selecting Hardware
    Location, Location,
       Location
    Types of Computers
    Processor Selection
    Printer Selection
    Servers

Selecting Software
Cost Analysis
Software Implementation
Internet Security
Backing Up the System
Other Technology
    Digital Cameras
    Scanners and Copiers

Learning Objectives

Mastery of the content in this chapter will enable the reader to:

- Differentiate between hardware and software.
- Determine the appropriate computer hardware to meet the requirements of the practice.
- Identify veterinary software that will best serve the practice.
- Create an appropriate hardware and software implementation schedule for the staff.

- Define methods used to protect the computer system with appropriate security features.
- Explain the importance of daily backup procedures.
- Discuss methods that allow office technology to be used to the fullest potential.

Key Terms

Adware
Backup Devices
Broadband
Card Reader
CD
CD/DVD
Cookies
Cost Analysis
CPU
Data
Data Conversion
Desktop
Digital Camera
Docking Station
DSL
DVD
External Hard Drive
Firewall
Floppy Disk Drive
Gigabyte
Graphics Card

Hacker
Handwriting Recognition
Hard Drive
Hardware
Host
Internet
Inventory Management Software
IP Address
Keyboard
Label Printer
Laptop
MAC
Desktop
Megabyte
Microphone
Modem
Monitor
Mouse
Network Card
PC
Pop-ups

Printer
Processor Speed
RAM
Scanners
Server
Software
Sound Card
Spam
Spam Filter
Speakers
Spyware
Tablet
Trojan Horse
USB
Video Graphics Card
Virus
Voice Recognition
Wireless LAN Access Point
Worm
Zip Drive

Over the last decade, the veterinary profession has benefited from the advances made in computer technology, including faster processors, increases in the amount of information that can be stored, and greater networking capacities. The prudent selection of technology equipment is a major component of veterinary practice productivity and efficiency. The ultimate goal is to develop an effective automated information and processing system that can evolve with practice growth and that will be able to utilize new technology as it is developed.

Computers are used to maintain the functions of the practice on several levels. The electronic office is a workplace where computers and other electronic equipment carry out many of the office's routine tasks. This equipment also provides more options for gathering, processing, displaying, and storing information. Box 8-1 gives some examples of applications of technology that are used on a daily basis in veterinary practices.

The technology revolution that led to the information age has had a profound effect on the business office. The use of electronic office technology in the veterinary practice allows the team to be more efficient and organized. It can help automate routine tasks, improve cash flow, and increase accuracy. Today, a patient's radiograph can be sent virtually (i.e., by computer) to a specialist as soon as it is taken and before the client leaves the practice. This results in improved patient and client care, increased productivity, and reduced stress on team members.

INFORMATION SYSTEMS

An information system is a collection of elements that provide accurate, timely, and useful information. To understand the procedure of an information system, one must understand the basic terminology related to the concept. A glossary of terms, definitions, and pictures helps define electronic office equipment and is useful when selecting products (Box 8-2).

Several components make up a computer system. Hardware, software, and data are important and can

Box 8-1	Applications of Technology in the Veterinary Practice

- Online continuing education
- Computerized appointment system
- Consultation with specialists and experts
- Credit card processing
- Digital photographs
- Digital radiographs
- Electronic/paperless medical records
- Email reminders
- Online office procedural manuals
- Supply purchases
- Web page design and maintenance

factor into the decision-making process when choosing to purchase either of the first two. A computerized hospital information system is a significant investment, and the overall plan must integrate hardware, software, training, and ongoing management control. To receive an excellent return on investment, the integration of these elements is crucial.

> **PRACTICE POINT** Computer hardware and software represent an expense that will yield the highest return on investment for the practice.

HARDWARE

Hardware refers to the actual physical equipment of a computer. The central piece of hardware in the information system is the computer. A computer is a device that electronically accepts data, processes the data arithmetically and logically, produces output from the processing, and stores the results for future use. The word *computer* is often used as a general term for the entire system. In reality, the computer is the actual workhorse of the system.

Computers are generally classified in three categories: mainframe, minicomputers, and microcomputers. The mainframe computer is a large system that handles numerous users, stores large amounts of data, and processes data at very high speeds. This type of computer may be found in a veterinary sales distribution office in which many sales are processed at the same time.

A minicomputer is compact and has a lower processing speed and more limited storage capacity than those of a mainframe. It is, however, more powerful than a microcomputer. This system is generally found in veterinary practices in which computer resources are shared. This system may be implemented in a centralized area, with several computers in outlying areas of the practice linked into it.

A microcomputer, or personal computer, is the smallest of the computer systems and is self-contained with regard to the circuitry and components. These systems are also popular in smaller veterinary practices and can be connected together to form a local area network (LAN).

Most computers are made up of a central processing unit (CPU), monitor, keyboard, mouse, graphics and video cards, CD and DVD drives, backup devices, and printers. It is also imperative to consider a power supply that has a surge protector included as well as a backup battery system if the electricity fails for more than a few minutes. The CPU is the central unit of the computer, and the monitor allows visualization of software applications. A mouse allows navigation through software applications, and a keyboard allows the user to type commands for the software. Graphics and video cards are used to produce outstanding quality and detail in the monitor. CD or DVD drives allow programs to be installed or information to be saved. Other backup devices may

Box 8-2   Technology Terms

Backup Device: Device that copies information from the CPU and stores it for retrieval in the event of computer malfunction. Backup devices can be either internal or external.

Broadband: High-speed Internet connection that can transmit information 40 times as fast as telephone and modem connection.

Card Reader/Writer: A card reader/writer is useful for transferring data directly to and from a removable flash memory card. Examples of flash cards are those used in a camera or music player.

Central Processing Unit (CPU): The brain of the computer; located in the main unit.

CD: Device for storing data; stores approximately 650 to 700 MB (megabytes) of information.

CD/DVD Drives: Newer computers are built with a DVD drive than can read CDs or DVDs. CDs or DVDs cannot be recorded or written over; they can only be read by the driver. If one plans to write music, audio files, or documents onto a CD or DVD, then CD/RW or DVD/RW should be considered. RW stands for *rewritable.* This allows the CD or DVD to be rewritten once the information has been recorded once. A DVD has a capacity of at least 4.7 GB (gigabytes) versus the 650 MB capacity of a CD. Drives can be either internal or external.

Desktop: Computer that sits on the top of a desk; not considered a portable unit.

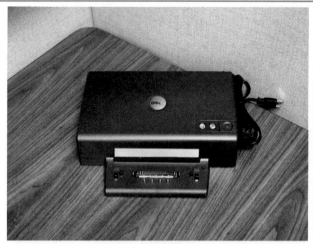

Docking station

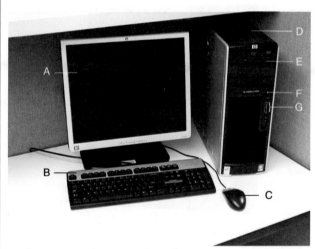

Desktop. **A**, Monitor. **B**, Keyboard. **C**, Mouse. **D**, Computer. **E**, CD/DVD drive. **F**, Power. **G**, USB ports.

Digital Camera: A camera that can capture images without the use of film. Images are then transferred to the computer with a connection wire. Photos can then be printed from the computer or stored for future use. Digital cameras come in a variety of megapixels. The higher the megapixel count, the better the resolution of the photo. A digital camera can be an effective marketing tool in a veterinary practice.

Digital Subscriber Line (DSL): High-speed Internet connection that uses the same wires as a telephone.

Digital Versatile Disc (DVD): Device for storing data that can hold more information than a CD.

Docking Station: Stationary device that allows a tablet to function as a desktop computer.

External Hard Drive: An external hard drive is a storage drive that allows data to be stored outside the computer. External hard drives are protected in heavy black cases and can create an extra storage space or contain a complete backup of the computer system.

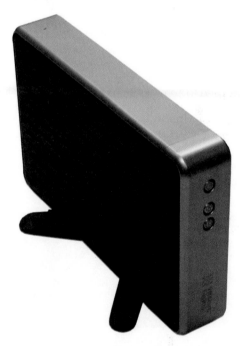

External hard drive

Floppy Disk Drive: Floppy disks are used to back up and transfer data or load applications onto a computer. Floppy disk drives are becoming obsolete because most programs are now written to CDs and DVDs. A standard-sized floppy disk drive is 3.5 inches, and a disk holds only 1.44 MB of information.

Gigabyte (GB): Measure of computer data storage; approximately 1 billion bytes.

Box 8-2 | **Technology Terms—cont'd**

Graphics Card: Card inserted into the CPU that determines the level of detail at which video images will appear on the monitor.

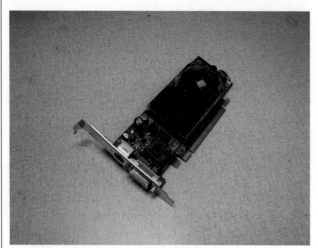

Graphics card

Handwriting Recognition: Technology that allows the computer to convert touch screen writing into printed words.
Hard Drive: A hard drive stores all data and can hold more than 100 GB of information.
Joystick/Wheel/Game Controller: Used to play games, these devices provide realistic game play with feedback, programmable buttons, and specialized levers.
Keyboard: The keyboard is one of the most important devices used to communicate with the computer. It should have at least 101 keys on it and have a USB connection to plug into the computer. Some users prefer wireless keyboards, especially when a smaller desk space is being utilized. For team members who use the keyboard for a majority of the day, an ergonomic keyboard may be considered.

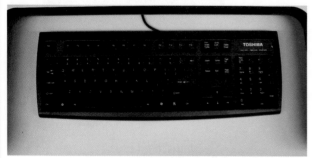

Keyboard

Label Printer: Printers designed to produce labels for bottles, containers, or envelopes.

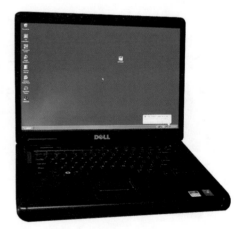

Label printer

Laptop: A portable computer.

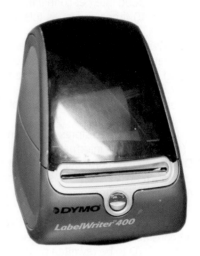

Laptop computer

Continued

Box 8-2   Technology Terms—cont'd

Megabyte: Measure of computer data storage; approximately 1 million bytes.

Microphone: Used to record sound.

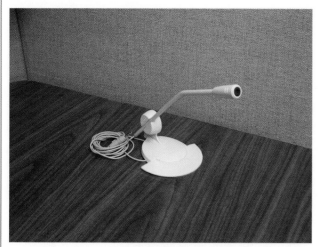

Microphone

Modem: A device used to connect to the Internet as well as send and receive faxes via a phone line. The modem converts digital data to analog data to send to the end user; the modem also converts analog information back to digital when it is received.

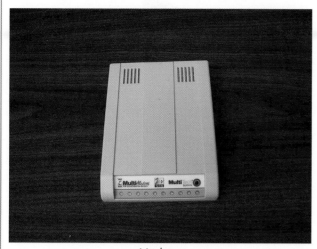

Modem

Monitor: The monitor is used to view documents, read email, and view pictures. A minimum of a 17-inch screen is advised; however, if digital photos will be reviewed, a 19- or 21-inch monitor is recommended. Flat panel screens are excellent space savers and provide a high-quality picture.

Mouse: A mouse allows navigation through applications on the computer. The mouse allows the user to point and click. A mouse can be cordless, which may benefit some users. Others prefer a mouse with an ergonomic design and an optical sensor. An optical sensor allows the mouse to be used without a mouse pad, which may be useful if working in a small desk space.

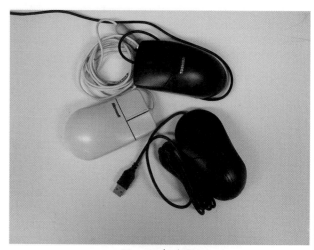

Mouse devices

Network Card: A network card allows connection to a network or DSL for Internet connection. If a server is in use for the practice software system, each computer will need to have a network card to allow the computers to communicate with each other.

Printer: Laser and inkjet printers are available. Laser printers print faster and with higher quality than an inkjet printer, and the ink generally costs less for a laser printer. Photograph printers are more expensive and print with a higher resolution. Printers should have a USB connection.

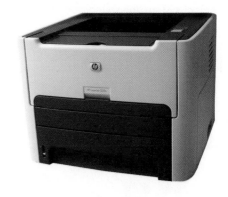

Laser printer

Continued

Box 8-2	Technology Terms—cont'd

Processor Speed: The processor speed is the speed at which the brain of the computer can sort information and produce results.

Random Access Memory (RAM): The short-term memory of a computer. RAM plays a vital role in the speed of the computer. 512 MB or more is recommended for optimal use.

Scanner: A scanner can be used to scan documents or photos into the computer. Scanners are generally flat-bed scanners; they should have a color depth of at least 48 bits and a resolution of at least 1200 × 2400 dpi. The higher the color depth, the more accurate the color. A higher resolution picks up more subtle gradations of color.

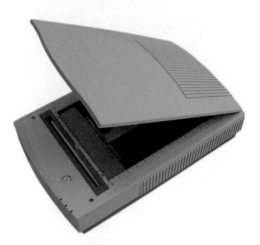

Scanner

Server: A server serves information to the computers to which it is connected. When users connect to a server, they can access programs, files, and other information.

Sound Card: Sound cards are responsible for playing sounds and recording audio. Most sound cards available today are capable of recording and playing digital audio. If the computer will be used extensively for game playing or as an entertainment system, the sound card can be upgraded.

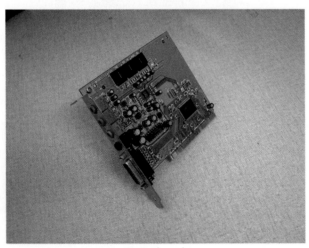

Sound card

Speakers: Speakers emanate sound and, as mentioned, if the computer will be used for game playing or used for presentations, the speakers can be upgraded for a higher quality sound.

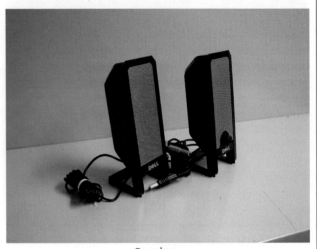

Speakers

Tablet: Portable computer that allows touch screen and handwriting recognition.

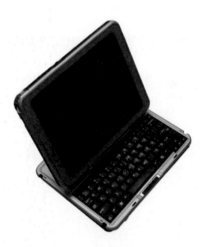

Tablet computer

Continued

Box 8-2	Technology Terms—cont'd

Video Graphics Card (VGC): A video graphics cards enables the computer to display high-quality and clear graphics. If the computer will be used for extensive graphic work, the VGC may be upgraded for enhanced performance.

PC Video Camera: A PC video camera is a small camera that allows the capture of images and display of live video. Cameras sit on a monitor or desk.

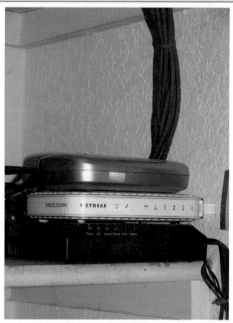

Wireless router

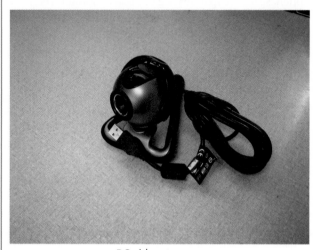

PC video camera

Zip Drive: A zip drive allows the backup of data and important files. An alternative to backing up files on a zip drive is to back up files on a CD-RW or DVD-RW.

USB (Universal Serial Bus): The most common type of computer port used to connect keyboards, printers, scanners, Internet, or external drives.

USB Flash (Jump) Drive: A USB drive allows information to be stored on it and used on different computers. The drive fits into the USB port and can hold up to 4 GB of information.

Voice Recognition: Technology that allows a computer to input information from spoken commands.

Wireless LAN Access Point: A wireless LAN access point allows several computers to access a network or Internet connection though a single cable modem or DSL connection. Each device requires a wireless card.

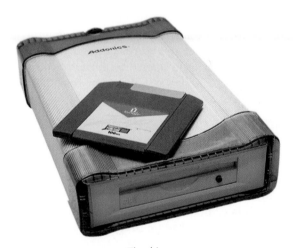

Zip drive

already be located on the machine or can be connected externally; they can save large amounts of information as needed. It is often recommended to regularly back up the entire system onto an external device in case the computer system crashes. A power supply should always have a surge protector; if the electricity surges, it may short out the computer system, losing all the information stored on the computer.

SOFTWARE

Software is the system or program the computer follows. Each software company has different recommendations for hardware guidelines.

PRACTICE POINT The most common software applications available are Microsoft Windows and Mac OS X.

Microsoft Windows supports most veterinary practice applications. Computers that use this operating system are generally referred to as *PCs*, as opposed to Macs, which are made by Apple, Inc., and typically use a different operating system. Some veterinary practice software applications can also be run on a Mac; the relevant software company should be consulted to ensure compatibility.

Operating outdated software on outdated hardware decreases the efficiency of a practice. Older hardware is slower and less compatible with the technology that is available today. Modern software selection and high-tech hardware will have a positive impact on every aspect of the practice. Compatible hardware and software packages can streamline the business and increase the efficiency of every team member, including the veterinarian. Reports can be developed that have a positive effect on the marketing aspect of the practice, education materials can be developed for each individual client, and reminders can be generated at a faster pace than with previous methods. Software and hardware investments will show a greater return on investment than any other capital expense in the veterinary practice.

SELECTING HARDWARE

When first starting out, it is better to start small and simple, knowing that computer technology changes on a continual basis. Computers can become outdated in 6 months; therefore it is advisable to buy only for the immediate need. Once the user is comfortable with the computer and wishes to upgrade, a higher quality computer and more complex system can be researched and purchased.

Location, Location, Location

If a practice wishes to buy several computers for the practice and place them throughout the practice, terminal locations must be determined. Common locations include the receptionist station, pharmacy area, doctor's office, practice manager's office, and treatment area. Practices that are preparing to go paperless should also place a computer in each exam room, surgery laboratory, and radiology room. Practices should ask team members which locations would best increase efficiency and decrease wasted time. Teams should also determine the number of computers needed to increase efficiency while also maintaining budget requirements.

> **PRACTICE POINT** The location of a computer can increase the efficiency of team members.

Types of Computers

Three types of computers may be considered for use in the practice: desktop, laptop, or tablet. Desktop computers are the most durable and least expensive. They are large and bulky and may take up more room than a space has to offer. Laptops are more expensive and fragile, but they are portable, smaller, and great for a practice that needs to be mobile. Tablets, a newer technology, are handheld and offer handwriting recognition as well as touch screen capability. Again, teams should determine the type of computer that will provide the most efficient use of space and time while remaining within budget guidelines.

Processor Selection

Once the type of computer has been chosen, the user must determine which type of processor will be the best option for the practice. Slower and cheaper processors include Celeron and Athelon; faster and more expensive processors include Pentium III and Pentium IV. Software companies will verify the type of processor recommended to run their veterinary software. The difference in cost may be minimal, making it worth purchasing a higher quality and faster processor.

> **PRACTICE POINT** Pentium III and IV processors are faster and more efficient than others on the market.

Printer Selection

A decision must also be made as to which type of printer will suit the practice best. Laser and inkjet printers are the most efficient in terms of speed and ink usage. The printers responsible for invoices should be durable, quick, and use the smallest possible amount of ink. Color printers are generally more expensive to purchase, and ink refill cartridges can be costly. Color printers should be reserved for use in the business office. Label printers should be placed in the pharmacy area for better efficiency. Veterinary software packages will make recommendations of label printers to use with their particular software.

Servers

If a practice chooses to have several computers in the hospital, it is best to have them linked together. Each computer should have its own CPU; however, to allow the computers to work well together, they should be linked to a shared CPU for more efficiency. If only two computers are linked together, then the computer with more memory and a faster processor should be the main server. However, either computer in this example could be used as the server. In practices where five or more computers are linked, it may be recommended to use a separate server. This will allow information to be processed at a quicker, more efficient rate.

> **PRACTICE POINT** Servers allow computers to share information quickly and efficiently.

Computers can be linked together via a wireless internet or through cabling that may be run through the walls of the building. A computer consultant should be contacted to determine the best method for each practice. Many older buildings have thick walls that can prevent efficient transmission of wireless waves; therefore wired terminals may be necessary. If a practice has an attic crawl space, wires can be dropped in almost any location, allowing the installation of computers anywhere the practice deems helpful.

SELECTING SOFTWARE

Many factors should be considered when researching software applications for veterinary practices. Hardware requirements, software support, education, and customization of software are a few elements that should be taken into account. Support is defined as the technical assistance offered by the company that helps facilitate the proper use of the software. This includes troubleshooting and problem resolution. Two of the most important factors include the hours of availability for tech support and how long it takes for the company to respond to practices in need of help (Box 8-3).

Education and training must be provided by the company for team members to properly use the software and maximize its efficiency. Training can vary from, "Here's the manual," to an on-site trainer.

> **PRACTICE POINT** Proper on-site training of software increases the use and efficiency of systems and team members.

Customization is defined as the ability of the software to adapt to the specific needs of the practice. For optimal efficiency, team members should be able to modify features with little or no assistance from the company. If the company needs to modify features, additional costs may be incurred and the team efficiency may be decreased.

Many practices may need to utilize multiple types of software packages to meet their needs, as many applications do not cover all aspects needed. Veterinary software is excellent at providing medical records, transactions, and reports relating to production. Accounting and management software may be needed to handle budget planning and payroll administration, whereas picture archival and compression software may be needed for digital radiography and ultrasonography (Box 8-4).

To help determine the type of software that would best suit a practice, a list should be developed of the practice's needs and wants. Team members can brainstorm for ideas to increase the efficiency of the team, and then research can be undertaken on software that meets those needs. What are some areas in which problems always occur? Lost records? Incomplete records? Lost charges? Clients having to wait for invoicing? Inventory management? Forgotten reminders? These are all questions that can be asked of team members.

It is wise to use software companies that have been in business for a number of years because technical support and upgrades in the future are imperative. Many practices have purchased cheap software from fly-by-night companies that are no longer in business. Recommendations

Box 8-3	Suggestions for Successful Software Selection

- Accessible client account data
- Accessible management data
- Clarity of user manuals
- Client education-based documents
- Complete audit trail
- Cost
- Data conversion abilities
- Interaction with other software applications
- Inventory management
- Long-term company
- Medical records
- Payroll
- Recalls/reminders
- Reduction of paperwork
- Reports generated
- Security features
- Technical support
- Training
- User friendly
- Veterinary software

Box 8-4	Veterinary Software Web Addresses
Avimark	www.avimark.net
Animal Intelligence	www.animalintelligence.com
CornerStone-Idexx	www.idexx.com/animalhealth/computersystems/vpm
DVM Manager	www.dvmmgr.com
DVM Max	www.dvmax.com
Impromed	www.impromed.com
Intravet	www.intravet.com
VetTech Software	www.vet-software.com

Not an exclusive list.

can be solicited from other practices, and software applications can be reviewed online and at veterinary conventions. Sales representatives should be willing to give demonstrations of their product in the practice, allowing all team members to ask questions and determine the effectiveness of the software.

> **PRACTICE POINT**   Software can be costly; however, cheaper software is not better, and quality of software should not be compromised.

Demonstrations can also be loaded onto the computer with a CD or DVD or via the Internet. Those given by a representative in person will be more thorough; however, demonstrations given by a DVD may allow more interaction with the software. If a user can figure out the software without a personal demonstration, then the software is probably very user friendly. This is another benefit that should be seriously considered. Many team members, especially those who are older, do not have the computer skills that most members of the younger generation possess. A program must be user friendly and easy to navigate to be efficient for all team members.

> **PRACTICE POINT**   Software representatives should provide team members with demonstrations and allow questions to be asked when searching for the perfect software.

Sales representatives should be asked for a list of practices that currently use their software. These practices should be called to verify their experience with the company's technical support, the years of service that the company has been in business, and the extent of satisfaction that the practice has with the software.

Based on the information received from several demonstrations, the needs and wants list may need to be changed and updated. Security features should be a top concern as well. Access should be limited to certain areas of the software. Only managers and owners should have access to passwords, pricing, confidential information, or deletion of certain items. It is important that these areas are protected so that malicious activity or accidental changes cannot occur.

Medical records entry, storage, and retrieval may vary from one software product to the next, but none will be as flexible as a handwritten medical record. Chapter 14 offers more detail on computerized medical records. Practices wishing to go paperless tend to be more efficient and knowledgeable with computer systems. Paperless records prevent the loss of records and allow all radiographs and lab work results to be downloaded into the patients' files. Radiographs and lab work can be pulled up in any exam room for clients to view. The only paper required is to print invoices for clients. A major

disadvantage is the possibility of a computer malfunction or power outage, either of which could cripple the practice. It is therefore imperative to back up computers on a daily basis, both on site and off site (Figure 8-1).

Inventory management can be accomplished with most veterinary software versions. Chapter 15 offers great detail on inventory management and methods to implement a successful system. Veterinary inventory software will allow the input of invoices when supplies are received and will deplete quantities when clients are charged out. This is an excellent system for products that are sold outright but can create problems for supplies that are used to produce a service. An example might be an injection: a solution is drawn up into a 3-mL syringe, but the doctor prefers a new needle to be placed on the syringe for the administration of the injection. How does one keep track of the extra needle used for the injection? This is why it is imperative that a physical inventory and order quantity check be done to verify supply quantities (Figure 8-2).

Reports can be generated from software management but will usually need to be exported into another type of accounting software for financial management. Veterinary software reports are great for reporting the average doctor and client transactions, determining areas of profit in the practice, or comparing data from year to year. However, to produce profit and loss statements or any other financial reports, information may need to be exported into accounting software, such as QuickBooks or Peachtree (Figures 8-3 through 8-5).

> **PRACTICE POINT**   Production reports are essential to the management of the practice.

COST ANALYSIS

When considering hardware and software requirements, it is important that a budget be determined. Efficient software systems can be costly, and it should be remembered that cheaper software systems may not produce the best results.

Costs should also be included when preparing the practice for a new computer system or upgrade. The cost of running new cables or electrical lines must be considered as well as the actual computer installation costs. Both hardware and software configuration may need to be completed by a local computer master to ensure they are compatible.

Most software companies offer data conversion as an option to transfer records into the new software. Team members may still need to make small adjustments to client and patient records during the transition.

> **PRACTICE POINT**   All costs must be included when creating a budget for computer hardware and software upgrades, including those for setup and maintenance.

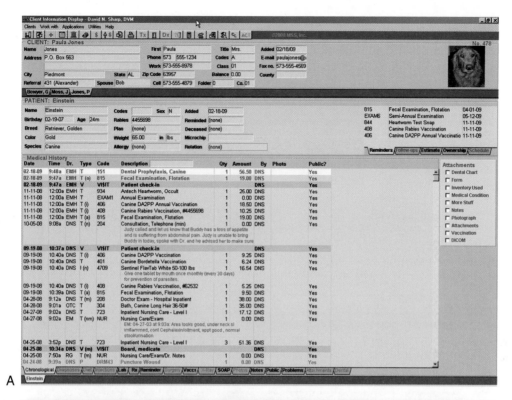

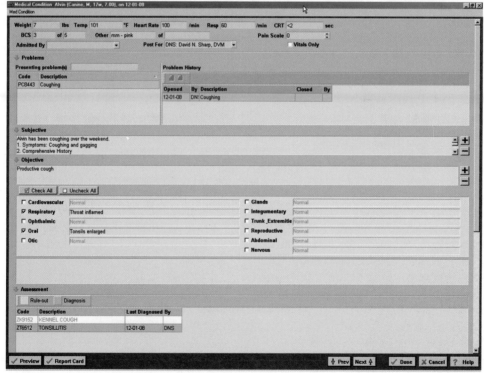

FIGURE 8-1 A and **B,** Sample screens from a paperless medical record. (Courtesy McAllister Software Systems, Inc., Piedmont, Mo.)

Other initial costs may include any remodeling that needs to be completed to accommodate the new computers and/or printers and any additional supplies needed to start up the new system.

Recurring costs may include maintenance and support fees for the software system, and the replacement of any hardware components that fail in the future. The average life of a computer system is generally 4 to 7 years, after which time new technology will likely be available to once again increase the efficiency if the practice.

Many companies offer software that "will be able to complete" tasks in the future; however, those features

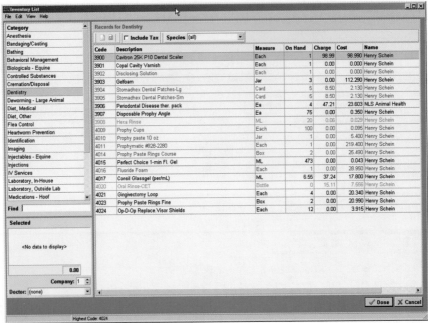

FIGURE 8-2 Example of an inventory list. (Courtesy McAllister Software Systems, Inc., Piedmont, Mo.)

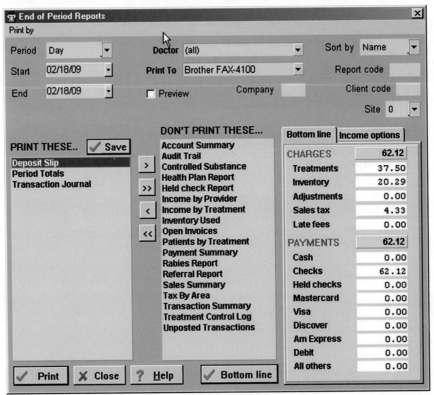

FIGURE 8-3 Example of an end-of-period report. (Courtesy McAllister Software Systems, Inc., Piedmont, Mo.)

are currently unavailable. Practices should use caution when looking at applications such as this. The company may not be around in the future; furthermore, a practice needs those applications now as well as in the future

Computer hardware should be supported locally; software can be supported over the phone and via an Internet connection. It is impossible to run software on hardware that is broken, and it is essential to have a computer technician available to repair or replace computer hardware when needed. Occasionally, it may be cheaper to replace a computer than to try and repair it. Unfortunately, the downside is having to reload software

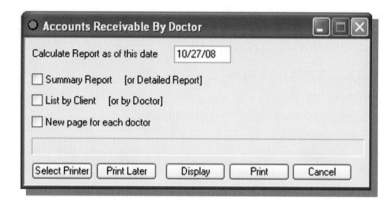

Accounts Receivable by Doctor   INTRAVET VETERINARY CARE

As of 10/27/2008

Doctor	Current	30 Days	60 Days	90 Days	Total
IntraVet Animal Hospital		52.21	52.21		104.42
Marisa Covey, DVM	968.07		679.74	850.68	2498.49
Marley Winston, DVM	106.50	511.56	220.00	112.80	950.86
Wayne Dalton, DVM		519.59	0.91	424.91	945.41
Boarding Drop Off / Pick up				49.78	49.78
David Kyle, DVM		576.10	3.55		579.65
Total Distributed Receivables	1074.57	1659.46	956.41	1438.17	5128.61
Total Undistributed Receivables	45.27	66.83	21.94		134.04
Total Balance Due					5262.65

Doctor	AccNo	Client	Current	30 Days	60 Days	90 Days	Total
IntraVet Animal Hospital	5284	Ross Perot			52.21		52.21
	5035	Andy Wolf		52.21			52.21
Marisa Covey, DVM	28	Tom Brokaw			130.53		130.53
	5341	Charlie Brown				253.22	253.22
	71	Keenen Carson	84.12				84.12
	104	Veronica Casper			24.71		24.71
	5069	Kirk Herbstreit	86.35				86.35
	59	Marley Johnson	496.67				496.67
	4764	Caitlyn Mosview				369.00	369.00
	5321	Kari Ann Moustin	300.93				300.93
	85	Andrew Ross				228.46	228.46
	92	Doug Zinn			524.50		524.50
Marley Winston, DVM	5115	Julia Childs			220.00		220.00
	5069	Kirk Herbstreit	106.35				106.35
	100	Irwin Hilton		360.00			360.00
	5051	Austin Powers				110.05	110.05
	69	Chloe Sartin	0.15				0.15
	5132	Felix Unger		151.56			151.56
	92	Doug Zinn				2.75	2.75
Wayne Dalton, DVM	5341	Charlie Brown		318.59			318.59
	4744	Tom Ellsesser				298.68	298.68
	5137	Glen Mason				126.23	126.23
	243	Kirk Matthews		201.00			201.00
	5318	Carl Noriega			0.91		0.91
David Kyle, DVM	5228	Charlie Islay			3.55		3.55
	5334	Chloe McCale	20.00				20.00
	5351	Carl McCarren	556.10				556.10

FIGURE 8-4 Example of an accounts receivable report. (Courtesy IntraVet, Effingham, Ill.)

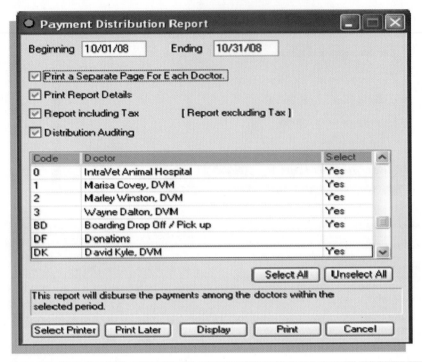

FIGURE 8-5 Example of a payment distribution report. (Courtesy IntraVet, Effingham, Ill.)

applications. Software issues can be handled by technical support via the Web. Most computers are or can be connected to the Internet by broadband or DSL. This allows technical support to diagnose and fix software hazards immediately, usually within a few minutes of connection.

Information should be backed up onto a CD, DVD or external hard drive at the end of each day. Power surges or computer failure may occur at any time and can be due to multiple problems. It cannot be assumed that since a computer system is new, failures will not occur. It is also recommended to back up information off site on a daily basis in case something should happen to the building, such as theft or fire. This would allow immediate information retrieval and reloading in the event of a catastrophe.

SOFTWARE IMPLEMENTATION

A change in software can cause great anxiety for a veterinary team. Team members who have been a part of the practice for an extended period will have the most difficulty with the change. Those who do not have extensive experience with computers may also have a hard time with the new process and may need extra assistance regarding training.

> **PRACTICE POINT** Software change can be stressful to team members and clients and should be completed in phases.

The software company should provide in-house training for a predetermined amount of time for all team members. Half-day or full-day training seminars are needed so that the team can learn about the software program. Teams should be able to practice entering client data so that there is little stress on them when the software is up and running. Appointments should be kept to a minimum during this period to allow the staff to adjust. The pace can then be slowly increased back to normal levels.

If many applications are available on the software, practices may wish to add them in phases. Team members can easily become overwhelmed when using new software and make mistakes that would not normally occur. If a practice is changing to a new software program with the ultimate goal of becoming a paperless practice, then the change should take place in either two or three phases. The first phase could be to implement the new hardware in all areas of the practice. Phase two would include the change to the new software program, allowing 6 months to 1 year for the staff to adjust to the new system. The third phase would be to reach the final goal of becoming paperless.

Practices that have not used computers previously will take more time to implement changes. Team members should first be trained on the use of computers in general and become familiar with the basic Microsoft operations. Courses are available through community colleges to enhance the learning experience. Second, training personnel from the software company should be notified of the slower transition, allowing them to invest more time and proper training techniques to assist in the change. Third, team members should realize the benefit the new computer system will have on the practice and have patience during the transition. Once team members reap the benefits from the increased efficiency, the system will be used with less frustration and anxiety.

Managers should plan to attend continuing education seminars given by the software company to continue learning about the software. Many programs have tools and settings that the practice has never used or even knew existed. Continuing education will allow the continued progressive use of software, integrating new technology every year to help enhance the value to the practice.

> **PRACTICE POINT** Continuing education on software use is imperative because new technology is released yearly.

INTERNET SECURITY

Most computer systems will have access to the World Wide Web, especially if the practice maintains a Web site. Doctors may use the Internet to send referrals, including radiographs, videos, and bloodwork results. They may also look up information for complex cases or consult with a specialist.

The Internet can be harmful to computer systems; therefore precautions should be taken to prevent a catastrophe from occurring. There is no such thing as a completely safe Web site or safe computer system because hackers have gained access to many of them. Firewalls, antivirus programs, and different levels of passwords are the major precautions that can be taken to protect a computer system. Emails and attachments from unknown senders should not be opened, and Web sites with uncertainty should not be accessed. Even when all protection available is utilized, it is still possible to be victimized by unwanted worms, viruses, and hackers (Boxes 8-5 and 8-6).

Firewalls are an excellent source of protection. They check every piece of information that comes in and goes out of a computer system. Firewalls are often already installed on operating systems; they simply need to be enabled to start their job. It takes a small amount of time for firewalls to become efficient and recognize malicious programs.

Excellent antivirus programs include Norton and McAfee antivirus software. Both programs screen for

---

Box 8-5 Internet Security Terms

Adware: A program or software that installs itself onto the computer without the user's knowledge. Adware plays a role in advertising; it collects information about the user, as well as Web sites visited, and uses this information to display pop-up advertisements that may interest the user.

Cookies: Cookies are messages given to the browser with information that has been collected about the user when visiting Web sites. When the user returns to the Web site, the browser remembers the user and can present the user with a customized Web site.

Firewall: Device that regulates what comes in and out of the computer. The device will reject invalid programs.

Hacker: An individual or group of people that intentionally attempts to break into computer systems and install worms, viruses, or other dangerous software. They may also alter information, cause damage, and erase programs.

Host: A computer that is connected to a network or the Internet. Each host has a unique IP address.

Internet: A network that connects millions of users to various Web sites.

IP Address: A specific number that identifies the user's computer.

Pop-ups: Windows that pop onto the user's screen soliciting unwanted information.

Spam: Emails that are not considered useful and that can be damaging to the user.

Spam Filter: A device that filters spam, preventing it from infiltrating the user's computer.

Spyware: Software that secretly gathers information from the user's computer and transmits it to the source.

Trojan Horse: A destructive program, usually attached to an email, that inhibits the computer.

Virus: A program loaded onto a computer and runs against the user's wishes. Viruses are usually able to replicate and send themselves on to other sites. Viruses tend to use up all the memory available on a computer, decreasing the processing speed or stopping the system.

Web Browser: Application used to locate and browse Web sites.

Worm: A program that replicates itself over a computer network and performs malicious actions that can shut the computer system down.

Box 8-6 Internet Safety Practices

- Do not open a site if there is any question about its authenticity.
- Do not open email or download attachments from unknown senders.
- Avoid deals that are too good to be true.
- Spybot is software that will search a computer for malicious software and deletes it.
- Never use passwords that include personal items such as birthdays, house numbers, or Social Security numbers.
- Change passwords frequently.
- Create passwords that include letters, numbers, and symbols. The greater the combination, the harder it is to hack.

---

have downloaded onto the computer system. Chapter 8 covers more detailed information of security features available for computer systems.

> **PRACTICE POINT** Internet security is imperative to protect the system from malicious individuals.

BACKING UP THE SYSTEM

Backing up the system cannot be emphasized enough. A computer can crash for any reason, including malfunction, electrical surge, theft, natural disaster, or malicious damage. Systems should be backed up each night, after the practice closes, onto a CD, DVD, or external hard drive (software systems will provide a recommendation as to which source to use). This disk should be removed and stored in the safe in case fire, flood, or theft should occur. This disk will allow information to be loaded onto a new system if needed. It is also ideal to back up the system off site. This can be done via the Internet or with a second disk that is taken to a safe storage place off premises.

If a computer crash occurs in the middle of the day, technical support should be called to see if any lost information since the last backup can be retrieved. If information cannot be retrieved, information will need to be re-entered. This is why a daily backup is imperative.

OTHER TECHNOLOGY

In addition to the computer systems described, other technologies are prevalent in the practice today and include telephone systems, voice mail equipment, fax machines, copy machines, calculators, scanners, digital cameras, and time clocks.

Digital Cameras

Digital cameras and printers are a nice addition to the practice. They can be used to enhance client education, market the practice, or add information to the medical

---

viruses and have firewalls and anti-spam programs. Most software programs include a trial period, which must be renewed once it expires. It is important to renew these subscriptions because updates are automatically sent to the computer so that it may recognize newly developed viruses.

Antivirus software should be set up so that it automatically scans all files on a regular basis. This allows continuous scans of files, seeking any viruses that may

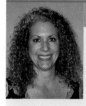

What Would You Do/Not Do?

The practice manger receives a call early one morning from the city police department that the alarm had been triggered at the veterinary practice. The manager informs them that nobody should be on premises at this time of night, and she would meet the officers at the practice. Upon arrival, they see that the practice has been vandalized and the computers have been stolen. The phones were smashed, along with the emergency lights. Apparently when the criminals broke into the practice, they thought the emergency lights were the security system and when they could not get the alarm to stop, they broke the lights. Since the alarm continued, they only grabbed the computers and fled the scene. The practice manager panics, thinking they will not be able to operate the business the following day without computers.

What Should the Practice Manager Do?

If backup procedures were followed correctly at the end of the evening shift, the computer system was backed up onto a DVD or an off-site location. A computer can be temporarily moved from an exam room or treatment area to the front office to provide a temporary practice server for the computer system until another computer can be purchased. The stored DVD can be uploaded into the temporary computer, allowing business to continue as usual; no information was lost in the theft. A "plan B" should always be available in case of emergency or natural disaster. Having a backup plan prevents stress overload in tense situations such as this.

---

record. Cameras can be used to take photos before and after dental prophylaxis to show the owners the difference in the teeth once the procedure has been completed. A pet that has a condition that will take time to improve may have a diagnostic photo taken; when it returns for a recheck, the photo can be compared looking for any signs of improvement. Many software packages allow the importation of pet photos for the medical record; the photo can be taken each year and imported into the record. One photo can also be given to the owners.

 PRACTICE POINT   Digital cameras are an excellent marketing tool as well as a record enhancer.

Digital cameras are available in a range of megapixel capabilities; the higher the megapixels, the better the resolution of the photo. Price also increases with the number of megapixels the camera has; therefore choosing the megapixel capability that will suit the practice is important. Some digital cameras are sold with individual printers; others must be purchased separately. Photo printers can be costly, and so can the ink and paper to refill them. Teams should determine to what extent a camera and printer would be used and research the products that are available in the selected price range.

Scanners and Copiers

Scanners and copiers are essential to a veterinary practice on a daily basis. Scanners may be used to scan in previous medical records, authorization forms, or photos. They may also be used to scan laboratory results into a file to email to a specialist. A copier may be used to copy records, client education information, or accounts payable invoices.

The extent that these pieces of equipment will be used will determine the type of product to purchase. If a scanner will be used multiple times a day and needs to capture clearer resolution, then a larger, more expensive scanner should be purchased. If many copies will be produced on a daily basis, then a larger, more efficient copy machine will be required. If smaller machines are purchased to save money, the level of satisfaction will be low. Smaller machines are not equipped to handle large workloads and will stop working sooner. Smaller machines also provide lower quality and take longer to process. This decreases the overall efficiency of the team as well as profits because another machine will need to be purchased sooner.

VETERINARY PRACTICE and the LAW

As more client and patient information is stored on computers and shared on computer networks that can often be accessed from a veterinarian's home, security and privacy have become major issues. Social Security numbers and driver's license numbers should never be stored on a shared network.

Each individual who has access to a computer should have a unique password, which should be changed on a regular basis. The password is a set of alphanumeric characters that allow a user to log on the system or specific parts of the computer system. Individuals should not share passwords with others.

Individuals should have access only to the types of information or applications that fall within their job descriptions. System security should be designed in such a way that each security level permits access to only the applications and databases that are required for the team member to complete job duties.

Self-Evaluation Questions

1. What is a CPU?
2. What is a server?
3. What is the benefit of having computers connected to each other?
4. What comprises a computer?
5. What considerations should be given when selecting software?
6. What is Spybot?
7. Why back up the system daily?
8. Which is more efficient, a CD or DVD? Why?
9. Why are floppy disks becoming obsolete?
10. What benefits would the practice receive from the implementation of a digital camera?

Recommended Reading

Heinke MM: *Practice made perfect: a guide to veterinary practice management,* Lakewood, CO, 2001, AAHA Press.

McCurnin D, Bassert JA, Byard V: *Clinical textbook for veterinary technicians,* ed 7, St Louis, 2010, Elsevier.

Sheridan JP, McCafferty O: *The business of veterinary practice,* Tarrytown, NY, 1993, Pergamon Press.

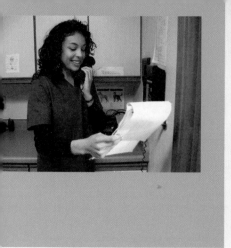

Outside Diagnostic Laboratory Services

Chapter Outline

Choosing a Diagnostic Laboratory
Sample Submission
Laboratory Forms
Sample Shipment

Sample Pickup
Results
Fees
Client Service

Learning Objectives

Mastery of the content in this chapter will enable the reader to:
- Identify the correct sample needed for specific testing.
- List methods used to preserve samples correctly.
- List methods used to label samples correctly.
- Identify laboratory forms.

- Define methods used to submit samples safely to the lab.
- Describe an appropriate fee structure for outside laboratory services.

Key Terms

Aerobic
Anaerobic
Anticoagulants
Cytology

EDTA
Food and Drug Administration (FDA)
Formalin
Histopathology

National Committee for Clinical
  Laboratory Standards (NCCLS)
Plasma
Serum

Outside laboratories are any laboratories to which patient samples are submitted. Some practices may use several outside labs for a variety of tests. It is important that measures are implemented to ensure that the correct forms are sent to each lab and that samples are prepared according to lab standards and sent correctly, either on ice or dry. Samples must also be packaged correctly so that they do not break during shipment.

Many practices continue to use in-house laboratory services for general chemistries and complete blood counts (CBC). In-house laboratory equipment is essential for receiving immediate results, especially in critical cases. For optimal results, in-house equipment must be consistently checked for quality control while performing maintenance. Many in-house laboratories can increase the bottom line of the practice, and equipment must be chosen with that in mind. For all tests that cannot be completed in-house, an outside service must be chosen.

CHOOSING A DIAGNOSTIC LABORATORY

Choosing a diagnostic laboratory can be a challenge because many factors are involved in the decision. First and foremost, the diagnostic laboratory must offer services and tests that the veterinarian is looking for. Some laboratories specialize in specific tests and have the newest technology available. For example, the Gastrointestinal Laboratory at Texas A&M University specializes in gastroenterology-related tests, and many other diagnostic laboratories will submit samples to this specific lab because of their testing protocol and results.

PRACTICE POINT The choice of an outside laboratory should be based on customer service, quick result turnaround time, and consistency of results.

Standard laboratory services should include analysis for biochemical profiles, CBCs, cultures, cytology, and histopathology. Many laboratories offer services that extend beyond those listed, enabling veterinarians to provide better service to their clients.

Laboratories should abide by guidelines set forth by the National Committee for Clinical Laboratory Standards (NCCLS) and adhere to the strict guidelines outlined by the Food and Drug Administration (FDA). All labs being considered should continually monitor and perform quality controls for accuracy and reproducibility by internal and external quality assurance programs.

SAMPLE SUBMISSION

Correct sample submission is absolutely critical for the tests required. Many tests require serum, not plasma, for accurate testing. Tests that require plasma may require the sample to be spun with a specific anticoagulant. Serum is produced when a red-topped tube is centrifuged, separating the red blood cells and coagulation proteins from the liquid portion of the blood. Red-topped tubes should be allowed to clot for 15 to 20 minutes before centrifugation. The sample can then be spun for 10 to 15 minutes at 2500 rpm. The serum can then be removed from the clot and placed in a plain glass red-topped tube for transport. If a serum separator tube (SST) has been used, there is no need to remove the serum. Do not use serum separator tubes for therapeutic monitoring, such as digoxin, phenobarbital, or theophylline levels.

EDTA (ethylenediamine tetraacetic acid) is an anticoagulant that is added to a lavender-topped tube, preventing clotting of the blood. Plasma can then be obtained by centrifuging the sample and removing the liquid portion of the sample without any red blood cells. Other common anticoagulants include lithium heparin, sodium heparin, and potassium citrate (Figure 9-1 and Table 9-1).

> ◎ **PRACTICE POINT**   Anticoagulant products include EDTA, lithium heparin, and potassium citrate.

Tissue samples submitted to the lab for histopathology require fixation. Formalin is a preservative that maintains the tissue characteristics for transport. Larger tissues may be partially cut, allowing the formalin to penetrate thicker tissues. The specimen container should contain 10% formalin at 10 times the volume of the tissue. Never reuse a sample submission jar because it may contain residuals of the previous specimen and is often labeled with the old patient information.

Formalin should be used with caution because it is a known carcinogen. It should not be inhaled, and gloves and eye protection should be worn when handling the chemical. Most laboratories provide practices with prefilled formalin jars, which decrease the risk to the team members handling the chemical. If formalin is supplied

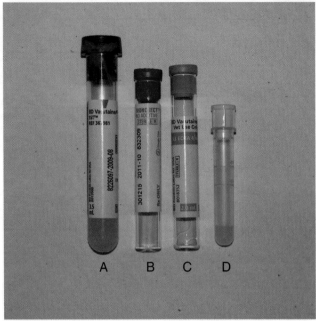

FIGURE 9-1   Various blood tubes. **A**, Serum separator tube. **B**, Red-topped tube. **C**, Lavender-topped tube. **D**, Green-topped tube with serum separator.

in a gallon container, jars should be filled under a hood or in a well-ventilated area. See Chapter 21 for more information regarding the handling of formalin.

> ◎ **PRACTICE POINT**   Do not submit cytology samples with histopathology samples preserved in formalin.

Cytology samples submitted to laboratories may need to be stained or unstained, depending on the test and the facility. Laboratory procedure books should be consulted before sample preparation to ensure the correct cytology is submitted. Cytology slides should never be shipped in the same bag as a formalin container because the fumes are known to degrade cytology samples.

Samples submitted for cultures must also indicate the source of the sample as well as specify whether an anaerobic or aerobic culture should be performed. Anaerobic is a technical word that literally means *without air*, whereas aerobic refers to *with air*. The veterinarian should indicate which culture is preferred, depending on the location of the sample. Aerobic samples should be kept refrigerated until pickup, then shipped with a cold pack. Anaerobic cultures should be kept at room temperature and processed within 48 hours of sample collection.

Each sample (blood tubes, biopsy jars, and slide containers) must be clearly marked with the patient's name, date, and type of specimen (urine, serum, plasma, etc.). All lids and/or caps must be secured to prevent the sample

Table 9-1	Common Laboratory Tests				
Type of Testing	Specimen	Container	Additives		Storage
Chemistries	Serum	RTT	None		Refrigerate
	Serum	SST	None		Refrigerate
Immunology	Serum	RTT, SST	None		Refrigerate
Endocrinology	Serum	RTT	None		Refrigerate
Phenobarbital	Serum	RTT	None		Refrigerate
Digoxin	Serum	RTT	None		Refrigerate
Theophylline	Serum	RTT	None		Refrigerate
Hematology	Whole blood	LTT	Anticoagulant EDTA		Refrigerate
Coagulation	Citrated plasma	BTT	Anticoagulant		Frozen
PT and PTT			Sodium citrate		

RTT, Red-topped tube; *SST,* serum separator tube; *LTT,* lavender-topped tube; *BTT,* blue-topped tube; *PT,* prothrombin time; *PTT,* partial thromboplastin time.

What Would You Do/Not Do?

Harry, a 13-year-old Chihuahua, is presented for lethargy and weight loss. Dr. Dreamer examines the dog and advises the technician to pull blood for a CBC/chemistry panel to be sent to the lab. Sophia draws the blood as told and prepares the sample for submission to the lab. All laboratory work is sent by a courier service to a lab outside the state; therefore it must be packaged well to prevent damage during shipment.

The following morning, the results are received on the fax machine; however, they indicate that one of the blood tubes broke during shipment, preventing the chemistry

samples from being run. Dr. Dreamer is furious at Sophia and insists that she call the owner herself.

What Should Sophia Do?

Sophia knew the importance of protecting samples during shipment; she must call and inform the owner of the broken sample. She must assure the owners that Harry has enough blood for a second sample and that she will wait for them on her lunch hour to accommodate them at a convenient time. She should then package the sample correctly, ensuring it will be well protected during shipping.

---

from leaking or formalin from spilling. A protective, absorbent material should be wrapped around individual samples to prevent the sample from being broken during shipment. Slides should be packaged in a slide container to prevent the glass from breaking.

LABORATORY FORMS

Forms must be filled out correctly for the lab to return correct and sufficient data. Vital information includes species, age, gender, breed, patient name, client name, date, and the submitting doctor's name. The specified test must be marked correctly. If pathology samples are being submitted, the history of the pathology is very important. Pathologists look at the history, as well as the patient, to help determine a diagnosis. Without this critical information, a misdiagnosis may be made. Various submission forms are shown in Figures 9-2, 9-3, and 9-4.

Copies of submission forms should be kept for records. IDEXX and Antech provide carbonless submission forms, whereas others may not. Copies should be made so that the team will know which tests where submitted and on which date. Samples may become lost in the mail or the wrong test may be performed. This allows team members

to track samples and hold team members accountable if the wrong test code was submitted.

SAMPLE SHIPMENT

Proper sample shipment is absolutely critical when submitting samples. Instructions must be followed for various tests to be completed. Some samples only need to be submitted with an ice pack to keep the sample cool during shipment. Other samples must be sent frozen, and some do not need to be chilled at all. All samples should remain in the refrigerator for storage until the courier has arrived to pick them up. Keeping the samples chilled preserves cell function. During the winter months, samples must be protected from freezing during shipment. Samples may be submitted with a bag of hot saline solution and can be insulated by wrapping them in layers of newspaper or bubble wrap (Figure 9-5).

Depending on the laboratory and the veterinarian's need for rapid results, some shipments may need to be sent overnight to the lab, whereas others may simply be sent by Priority Mail. All procedures should be verified with the laboratory by team members to ensure the best sample submission and result turnaround time.

FOR LAB USE ONLY

COLLECTION DATE

IDEXX LABORATORIES

Customer Service
888-433-9987

Mark an "X" here for ASAP

Please send duplicate results to:

Account # _____
Practice Name _____
Patient ID# (optional)

C601923

OWNER LAST NAME

PATIENT NAME

SEX
☐ Male
☐ Female
☐ Spay/Neut.

SPECIES
☐ Canine
☐ Feline
☐ Avian
☐ Equine
☐ Other

AGE: _____ Years _____ Months

BREED _____

VETERINARIAN(S)

[ ] SOULES
[ ] _____

☐ Check here for BASIC CBC

CANINE / FELINE GENERAL PROFILES
All profiles require serum and lavender top

☐ 53	Comprehensive Canine *Chem 25, Amyl/Lip, CBC, T4, HW*	(R/S, L)
☐ 66	Feline Viral Plus *Chem 25, CBC, T4, FeL V, FIV, FIP*	(R/S, L)
☐ 54	Feline Combo *Chem 25, CBC, FeL V, FIV*	(R/S, L)
☐ 74	Feline Combo Plus *Chem 25, CBC, T4, FeL V, FIV*	(R/S, L)
☐ 885	Comprehensive Feline *Chem 25, Amy/Lip, CBC, T4, FeL V, FIV, FIP*	(R/S, L)
☐ 75	Total Health Plus *Chem 25, Amy/Lip, CBC, T4*	(R/S, L)
☐ 46	HealthChek Plus *Chem 25, CBC, T4*	(R/S, L)
☐ 1	HealthChek *Chem 25, CBC*	(R/S, L)
☐ 1013	Total Health *Chem 25, Amyl/Lip, CBC*	(R/S, L)
☐ 1294	Chem 11, CBC	(R/S, L)
☐ 1272	Chem 21, CBC	(R/S, L)
☐ 1850	Adult Screen *-Chems 25, CBC, UA*	(R/S, L, U)
☐ 865	Senior Screen *-Chems 25, T4, CBC, UA*	(R/S, L, U)

SPECIAL TEST REQUESTS
Code #   Test Name

FECALS/WELLNESS
☐ 5010 Fecal Ova and Parasites
☐ 72440 Lab 4Dx
☐ 26049999 Canine Easy Annual 1 *(Chem 10, sCBC, Lab 4Dx, Fecal O & P)*
☐ 26139999 Feline Easy Annual *(Chem 10, sCBC, Feline HW Ab)*
☐ 2463 O & P, Giardia Antigen by Elisa

CANINE TESTS
☐ 7246 Lyme Quant C6
☐ 1849 Spec cPL
☐ 2337 HealthChek with Spec cPL
☐ 2625 Canine Diarrhea Panel

FELINE TESTS
☐ 2626 Feline Diarrhea Panel
☐ 2512 Feline Upper Respiratory Panel
☐ 1717 Feline Hemotropic Mycoplasma

HEMATOLOGY
☐ 300 CBC - Comprehensive (L)
☐ 319 Buffy Coat Smear (L)
☐ 309 Platelet Count (L)
☐ 6 Coag Profile (BTT, L)
  (CBC, PT, PTT, PLT, FIB Quant)
☐ 56 Coag Panel #1 *(PT, PTT, PLT)* (BTT, L)
☐ 311 PT (BTT)
☐ 312 PTT (BTT)

ENDOCRINOLOGY
☐ 13 Thyroid Panel #1 *(T3, T4)* (R/S)
☐ 851 Thyroid Panel #2 *(T4, FT4 ED)* (R/S)
☐ 804 T4 (R/S)
☐ 849 FT4 ED (R/S)
☐ 119 ACTH Stimulation (pre & post) (R/S)
☐ 274 Dex Suppression (pre & post 8 hr.) (R/S)
☐ 275 Dex Suppression (pre & post 4 & 8 hr.) (R/S)
☐ 245 Fructosamine (R/S/L/GN)
☐ 806 Progesterone (R)

GENERAL CHEMISTRIES
☐ 257 Bile Acids Panel (Pre & 2 hr Post) (R/S)
☐ 111 Chem25 (R/S)
☐ 1113 Chem27 (R/S)
☐ 1271 Chem21 (R/S)
☐ 1293 Chem11 (R/S)

LARGE ANIMAL PROFILES
☐ 11 Large Animal Profile (R/S, L)
  Chems, CBC, FIB
☐ 316 Inflammatory Profile (R/S, L)
  CBC, Plasma Protein, FIB

ADD TO ANY PROFILE *(R/S unless otherwise indicated)*

☐ 8531	TSH	☐ 22	T4
☐ 7231	Canine Heartworm Antigen	☐ 7101	FeCoV (FIP)
☐ 850	Free T4 ED	☐ 72461	Lyme Quant C6
☐ 1045	FeLV Ag + FIV Ab	☐ 18491	Spec cPL
☐ 2570	Bile Acids (single)		
☐ 997	Urine Pro/Creat Ratio (U)		
☐ 9101	Urinalysis ☐ Cysto ☐ Other (U)		

WHITE COPY - LABORATORY • YELLOW COPY - HOSPITAL

IMPORTANT! Please provide history:

HISTOPATHOLOGY
☐ 601 Biopsy with Microscopic Description
☐ 608 Biopsy (No Microscopic Description)

# of sites/lesions/organs _____

# of specimens/tissues submitted _____

DORSAL   VENTRAL

Prev. Date & Accession # _____

CYTOLOGY
Source required: _____
☐ 605 Cytology with Microscopic Description
☐ 600 Cytology (No Microscopic Description)
☐ 607 Bone Marrow with Microscopic Description
☐ 900 CSF Analysis (Includes Cytology)
☐ 905 Fluid Analysis, Body (Includes Cytology)
☐ 906 Fluid Analysis, Joint (Includes Cytology)

THERAPEUTIC DRUG MONITORING
☐ 1000 Phenobarbitol (red top only)
☐ 1001 Digoxin (red top only)

URINE / STONE ANALYSIS
☐ 909 Stone Analysis (Chemical) (STN)
☐ 90900 Stone Analysis (Crystallographic) (STN)
☐ 910 Urinalysis ☐ Cysto ☐ Other (U)
☐ 910 U/A ☐ 943 Culture if indicated *(check both boxes)*
  ☐ Cysto ☐ Other
☐ 4035 Culture ONLY
  ☐ Cysto ☐ Other
☐ 994 Urine Protein / Creatinine Ratio (U)
☐ 946 Urine Cortisol / Creatinine Ratio (U)

MICROBIOLOGY
Source required: _____
☐ 400 Aerobic Culture & Suscept (C)
☐ 427 Aerobic Culture ID only (C)
☐ 401 Anaerobic & Aerobic C & S (ANC, C)
☐ 4022 Salmonella & Campylobacter Fecal Culture (F)
☐ 4035 Urine Culture & MIC ☐ Cysto ☐ Other (U)
☐ 405 Fungal Culture (C/SC)
☐ 1394 Comprehensive UA & Culture ☐ Cysto ☐ Other (U)

IMMUNOLOGY / SEROLOGY
☐ 24 FeLV Ag (ELISA) & FIV Ab (ELISA) (R/S)
☐ 723 Heartworm Ag - Canine (R/S, L)
☐ 707 Coggins, EIA (AGID) (R/S)
☐ 7077 Coggins, EIA (ELISA) (R/S)
☐ 303 Coombs (L)
☐ 709 FeLV Ag (ELISA) (R/S)
☐ 717 FeLV Ag (IFA) (L)
☐ 710 FeCoV (FIP) (R/S)
☐ 702 Brucella Screen (K9) (R/S)
☐ 7246 Lyme Quant C6 (K9) (R/S)
☐ 1849 Spec cPL (K9) (R/S)

AVIAN / EXOTIC
☐ Panel # _____
☐ 435 Avian / Reptile Aerobic C&S (C)
☐ 415 Exotic Respiratory Screen (C&S, Fungal) (C)
☐ 4023 Avian Fecal Culture (C&S, Gram Stain) (C/F)

REV 06-08

FIGURE 9-2 IDEXX submission form. (Courtesy IDEXX Laboratories, Inc., Westbrook, Maine.)

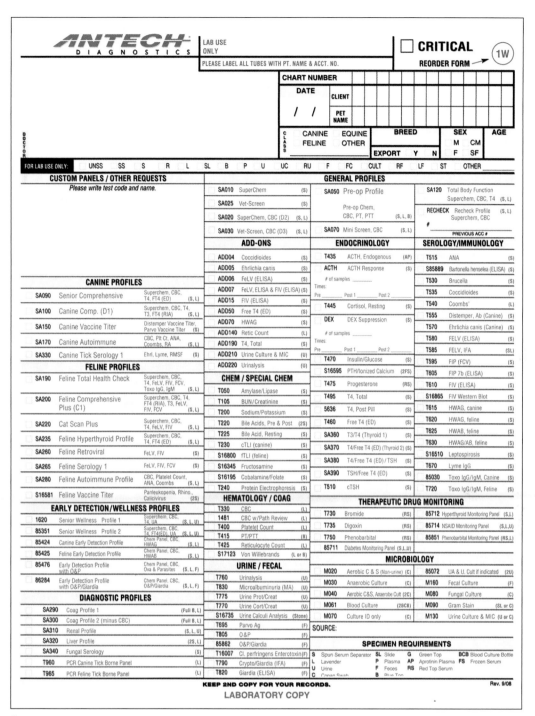

A

FIGURE 9-3 A through **C,** Antech submission forms. (Courtesy ANTECH Diagnostics, Los Angeles, Calif.)

ANTECH DIAGNOSTICS

☐ **CRITICAL** REORDER FORM ②

LAB USE

DATE / /

CLIENT

PET NAME

CHART NUMBER

SEX	AGE	SPECIES
☐ M ☐ F		

CLASS

AVIAN
- ☐ (PAS) PASSERINE
- ☐ (PS) PSITTACINE
- ☐ (RA) RATITE
- ☐ OTHER _____

REPTILE
- ☐ (IG) IGUANA
- ☐ (SN) SNAKE
- ☐ (TUR) TURTLE

SMALL MAMMAL
- ☐ (FT) FERRET
- ☐ (L) RABBIT
- ☐ (RO) RODENT

OTHER
- ☐ _____
- ☐ _____
- ☐ _____

FOR LAB USE ONLY: ☐ GRGU ☐ GRGS ☐ GRV ☐ HCT ☐ USSV ☐ SSV ☐ RV ☐ LV ☐ FSL ☐ RU

DOCTOR / CUSTOM PANELS

AVIAN PROFILES

☐ AE020 **Comprehensive Avian Profile**
(GRT-S, BS, 2 HCT)
CBC
Albumin CPK K
AST (SGOT) Globulin Na
Calcium Glucose T. Protein
Chloride Phos Uric Acid
Cholesterol

☐ AE030 **Comp. Avian Post Purchase**
(2 GRT-S, 1 GRT-NS, BS, 2 HCT, Cult, F, 2 FS)
- Comp. Avian Profile
- Chlamydophila Ab (EBA)
- Giardia ELISA Ag
- Gram Stain (Fecal)
- PBFD PCR (Blood)
- Polyoma PCR (Swab)
- Protein Electrophoresis

☐ AE050 **Standard Avian Profile**
(GRT-S, BS, 2 HCT)
CBC
AST (SGOT) Phos
Calcium T. Protein
CPK Uric Acid
Glucose

☐ AE060 **Mini Avian Post Purchase**
(2 GRT-S, BS, 2 HCT, 2 FS)
- Comp. Avian Profile
- Gram Stain (Fecal)
- Protein Electrophoresis

☐ AE080 **Feather Picker Profile**
(1 GRT-S, 1 GRT-NS, BS, 2 HCT, CS (Skin), F, 2 FS)
- Comp. Avian Profile
- Culture (Skin)
- Gram Stain (Fecal)
- Giardia ELISA Ag
- PBFD PCR
- Protein Electrophoresis

☐ AE090 **Hepatic Profile**
(3 GRT-S, BS, 2 HCT)
- Comp. Avian Profile
- Bile Acid
- Chlamydophila Ab (EBA)
- Protein Electrophoresis

☐ AE110 **PU/PD Profile**
(2 GRT-S, BS, 2 HCT, U)
- Comp. Avian Profile
- Protein Electrophoresis
- Urinalysis

☐ AE140 **Respiratory Profile**
(3 GRT-S, BS, 2 HCT)
- Comp. Avian Profile
- Aspergillus Ab
- Chlamydophila Ab (EBA)
- Protein Electrophoresis

☐ 85206 **Chlamydophila Profile**
(1 GRT-S, 1 GRT-NS, Cult)
- Chlamydophila Ab EBA (IgM)
- Chlamydophila Ab IFA (IgG)
- Chlamydophila PCR (Blood)
- Chlamydophila PCR (Swab)

☐ 85188 **Polyoma Profile**
(1 GRT-S, 1 GRT-NS, Cult)
- Polyoma Ab
- Polyoma PCR (Blood)
- Polyoma PCR (Cloacal Swab)

☐ 85359 **Aspergillus Profile**
(1 GRT-S)
- Aspergillus Ab
- Aspergillus Ag
- Protein Electrophoresis

☐ RECHECKAE **RECHECK**
Recheck Profile
Comp. Avian Profile
_____
PREVIOUS ACC #

REPTILIAN PROFILES

☐ AE160 **Comp. Reptilian Profile**
(GRT-S, BS, 2 HCT)
CBC
Albumin CPK Na
AST (SGOT) Globulin T. Protein
BUN Glucose Uric Acid
Calcium Phos
Chloride K

☐ AE180 **Standard Reptilian Profile**
(GRT-S, BS, 2 HCT)
CBC
AST (SGOT) Glucose Uric Acid
Calcium Phos
CPK T. Protein

MAMMALIAN PROFILES

☐ AE200 **Comp. Mammalian Profile**
(GRT-S, LT)
CBC
Albumin Cholesterol K
Alk Phos Creatinine Na
ALT (SGPT) CPK T. Bili
AST (SGOT) Globulin
BUN Glucose
Calcium Phos
Chloride T. Protein

☐ AE220 **Standard Mammalian Profile**
(GRT-S, LT)
CBC
Alk Phos Creatinine T. Protein
ALT (SGPT) Glucose
BUN Phos
Calcium T. Bili

☐ AE230 **Geriatric / Weak Ferret**
(2 GRT-S, LT, U)
- Comp. Mammalian Profile
- Insulin Level
- Urinalysis

☐ AE240 **Rabbit Neurologic Profile**
(2 GRT-S, LT)
- Comp. Mammalian Profile
- Encephalitozoon Ab
- Pasteurella Ab

☐ AE250 **Rabbit Respiratory Profile**
(2 GRT-S, LT, CS (Nasal))
- Comp. Mammalian Profile
- Culture (Deep Nasal)
- Pasteurella Ab

☐ S17116 **Adrenal Androgen Profile**
(SST)
- Estradiol
- 17-OH-Progesterone
- Androstenedione

INDIVIDUAL TESTS

☐ S16011 Aspergillus Ab (GRT-S)
☐ 85358 Aspergillus Ag (GRT-S)
☐ AE260 Bile Acid (GRT-S)
☐ AE270 Avian CBC/Diff. *(See Directory)*
☐ AE275 Mammalian CBC/Differential
CHLAMYDOPHILA (Psittacosis)
☐ AE280 Antigen ELISA (Cult-Feces)
☐ S16670 Antibody EBA (GRT-S)
☐ S16788 PCR (GRT-NS)
☐ S16672 PCR (Cult)

OTHER REQUESTS:

INDIVIDUAL TESTS

☐ S16322 Distemper Ab, Ferret (GRT-S)
☐ S16877 Encephalitozoon Ab (GRT-S)
☐ T805 Fecal Flotation and O & P (F)
☐ T820 Giardia ELISA Ag (F)
☐ T470 Insulin Level (GRT-S)
☐ AE290 Lead Level (GRT)
☐ S16789 Mycoplasma PCR (Cult)
☐ S16600 Pasteurella Ab (GRT-S)
☐ S16601 Pasteurella PCR (Cult)
☐ S16085 PBFD PCR (GRT-NS)
☐ T400 Platelet Count, Manual
☐ S16625 Polyoma PCR (GRT-NS)
☐ S16626 Polyoma PCR (Cult)
☐ S16628 Polyoma Ab (GRT-S)
☐ AE300 Protein Electrophoresis (GRT-S)
☐ T425 Reticulocyte Count (LT)
☐ S16095 Sexing –Avian (GRT-NS)
☐ T760 Urinalysis (U)
☐ 85448 West Nile Virus Ab (GRT-S)
☐ 85449 West Nile Virus PCR (LT, Tissue)
☐ S16012 Zinc Level - (GRT-S)

MICROBIOLOGY
Source:

☐ M010 Acid Fast Stain (Air Dried smear)
☐ M020 Aerobic Culture (CS)
☐ M030 Anaerobic Culture (CS)
☐ M040 Aerobic & Anaerobic Culture (CS)
☐ M050 Aerobic & Fungal Culture (2 CS)
☐ M070 Culture ID Only (CS)
☐ M080 Fungal Culture (CS)
☐ M090 Gram Stain - (FS, CS)
☐ M110 Mycoplasma Culture - (See Directory)

Please List Testing Priority
1.
2.
3.
4.
5.
6.
7.

KEY
GRT-NS Not Spun. Green top microtainer tube (heparinized, with or without separator gel)
GRT-S Spun. Green top microtainer tube (heparinized, with separator gel)
BS Blood smear (slide)
F Fecal sample (pea size)
FS Fecal smear (slide)
Cult Culturette
CS Copan swab
U Urine
LT Lavender top microtainer tube (EDTA)
HCT Heparinized hematocrit tube
SST Serum separator microtainer tube

REV. 10/02

B

FIGURE 9-3, cont'd

ANTECH
DIAGNOSTICS

LAB USE ONLY

REORDER FORM → 3W

DATE	CLIENT														
/ /	PET NAME														
DOCTOR															
CHART #															

SPECIES:
☐ CANINE ☐ EQUINE
☐ FELINE ☐ AVIAN
Other _____

BREED | AGE | SEX
☐ M ☐ CM
☐ F ☐ SF

CHOOSE A PATHOLOGIST: If you would like to direct this case to a specific pathologist, please write name in this box. Please note that this is subject to the availability of the pathologist at the time of sample receipt. If the pathologist is unavailable, it will be forwarded to another Antech pathologist.

REQUESTED PATHOLOGIST
1.
2.
3.

HISTOPATHOLOGY / CYTOLOGY

☐ CYTO   Cytology (Source: _____)

☐ FLUA   Fluid Analysis with Cytology (_____)

☐ CSF   CSF with Cytology

☐ BONE   Bone Marrow Cytology

☐ BUFFY   Buffy Coat Smear

☐ FBX   Biopsy, Written
          (Includes Microscopic Description,
          Microscopic Findings, Prognosis & Comment)

☐ MBX   Biopsy, Mini
          (Includes Microscopic Findings, Prognosis
          & Comment)

☐ BMCB   Bone Marrow Core Biopsy
          (Includes Microscopic Description,
          Microscopic Findings, Prognosis & Comment)

☐ STAT   BIOPSY STAT FEE (see Service Directory for details)

☐ DERM   Dermatopathology
          (Biopsy & Dermatologist Recommendations)

Type of Biopsy: ☐ Excisional   ☐ Incisional
                      ☐ Needle   ☐ Endoscopic

All tissue(s) submitted? ☐ Yes ☐ No

Number of Containers Submitted: _____

☐ 30 mL ☐ 60 mL ☐ 100 mL ☐ 32 oz.

Number of Specimens Submitted: _____

Source/Site: _____

Previous Biopsy/Cytology Submitted? ☐ Yes ☐ No

Reference Number: _____

LOCATION

DORSAL VIEW

R   L

VENTRAL VIEW

PATIENT HISTORY

PLEASE NOTE:
This section is critical for Biopsy/Cytology interpretation.

_____

FOR LABORATORY USE
(Please do not write in this space)

1. No. of containers received: _____

2. Tissues received: _____

*LABEL EACH CONTAINER SUBMITTED WITH CLINIC NAME, CLIENT AND PATIENT NAME, AND TISSUE SOURCE.   (Rev. 7/03)

C

LABORATORY COPY

FIGURE 9-3, cont'd

GASTROINTESTINAL LABORATORY

CLINIC DETAILS

Veterinarian: _____

Clinic/Hospital: _____

Address: _____

City:_____ State:_____ ZIP:_____

Clinic E-mail Address:_____
(E-MAILED RESULTS WILL OFTEN BE AVAILABLE SEVERAL HOURS BEFORE FAXES ARE SENT)

Telephone:_____ Fax: _____

Preferred reporting method: ☐ **E-mail**   ☐ **Fax**   ☐ **Fax & E-mail**

DATE:

LABORATORY USE ONLY

Date Received: _____

Accession #: _____

Check #: _____

Charges: _____

Amt. Received: _____

PATIENT DETAILS

Owner's Name: _____

Animal's Name: _____

Species (circle):   Dog   Cat   Other (   )   Breed: _____

Age:_____ Years   Sex: M   F   MC   FS

Your Internal Identifier: _____

IMPORTANT NOTES

Most assays are species-specific; you **MUST** indicate a species in patient details.

SEPARATE SERUM FROM CLOT BEFORE SHIPPING

Both hemolysis and lipemia may interfere with test performance.

TEST(S) ORDERED - PLEASE CHECK BOXES

Serum TLI, PLI, Cobalamin, Folate (2.0 mL serum, fasting) $ 00 .... ☐
Serum TLI, Cobalamin, Folate (1.0 mL serum, fasting) $ 00 .... ☐
Serum PLI, Cobalamin, Folate (1.0 mL serum, fasting) $ 00 .... ☐
Serum TLI, PLI (1.0 mL serum, fasting) $ 00 .... ☐
Serum Cobalamin, Folate (1.0 mL serum, fasting) $ 00 .... ☐
Serum TLI (1.0 mL serum, fasting) $ 00 .... ☐
Serum PLI† (0.5 mL serum, fasting) $ 00 .... ☐

Canine C-Reactive Protein (0.5 mL serum, fasting) $ 00 .... ☐
Serum Bile Acids: Pre-feeding (1.0 mL serum, fasting) $ 00 .... ☐
                       Post-feeding (1.0 mL serum, 2 hours postfeeding) $ 00 .... ☐
Serum Gastrin (0.5 ml serum, fasting) $ 00 .... ☐
Triglycerides (0.5 ml serum, fasting) $ 00 .... ☐

PCR testing: *Tritrichomonas foetus* $ 00 .... ☐
                 Campylobacter spp. (*C. jejuni, C. coli, C. upsaliensis, C. helveticus*) $ 00 .... ☐
                 Heterobilharzia americana $ 00 .... ☐
                 Clostridium perfringens enterotoxin gene $ 00 .... ☐

Fecal α_1-Proteinase Inhibitor (**Canine or Feline**)* $ 00 .... ☐

For ordering supplies please fill out the line below and fax to the laboratory:
5 sets of three preweighed fecal tubes: (   ) boxes at $25.00 each for α_1-PI

Use ONLY FedEx or UPS for all shipping. **Do not use the U.S. Postal Service; this may cause delay in deliveries.**

*Fecal specimens for α_1-Proteinase Inhibitor are **only** accepted in our containers. Samples must be **frozen** in these tubes and **shipped frozen** to the laboratory by overnight carrier. **This test is species specific; indicate species in patient details.**

†Serum PLI (Spec cPL or Spec fPL) will be run only within panels or alone as a follow-up test.

TOTAL CHARGES FOR THIS ANIMAL   **$**
PAYMENT METHOD: ☐ Check Enclosed (make payable to GI Lab - TAMU)   ☐ Please Bill Me

We can not accept packages that are marked "Bill Receiver". Please use our pre-printed shipping labels to save on shipping! Call (979) 862-2861 for more information.   Prices valid as of 01/01/2009

FIGURE 9-4 Texas A&M submission form. (Courtesy Jörg M. Steiner, Texas A&M University, College Station, Texas.)

SAMPLE PICKUP

Sample pickup is also an important factor in submitting samples to labs. If most samples are sent to one lab in particular, the lab should provide a courier service for sample pickup. Depending on the location of the laboratory facility, the lab may send its own courier, or samples may be shipped by another agent, such as FedEx, UPS, or DHL. Timing of sample pickup can also help a practice decide which lab to choose. It is ideal to have samples picked up late in the day, allowing any samples collected during the day to be sent. Results can be received the following morning. When samples are picked up midday, anything collected after pickup must wait until the following day to be sent to the lab. This causes delayed results, decreasing the quality of patient care. Studies indicate that red blood cell morphology and platelet parameters change with delayed analysis. Laboratories strive to provide the best service available, and courier pickup is one of those services. Ask the laboratory representative for the latest possible pickup; if that time is not ideal, search for other labs and ask what they can offer as far as sample pickup.

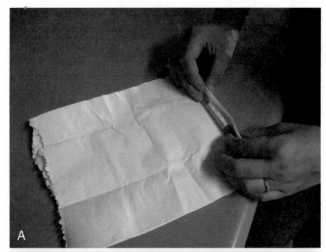

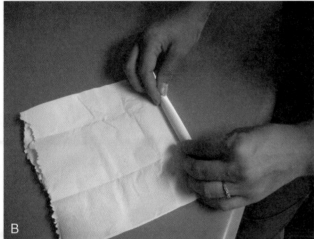

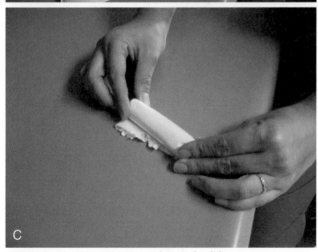

FIGURE 9-5 Protecting samples to the laboratory.

> ◎ **PRACTICE POINT** Sample pickup scheduled late in the business day is best for the practice and clients.

RESULTS

Results should be received in a timely fashion. Specialized tests may take longer to run; however, laboratory description books should indicate the time frame required.

If results are delayed, a lab representative should call the practice and communicate the delay.

Results should offer a variety of information. Alongside the patient results, a reference range will be listed. This reference range indicates the normal ranges for that particular piece of equipment. Flags can also indicate patient results outside the normal range, drawing attention to specific abnormalities. If a patient's CBC appears abnormal, a pathology review should automatically be indicated. Having a pathologist review the smear can increase the time until results are received. Some labs require the veterinary practice to request a review when abnormalities are present. This can increase the time for patient diagnosis and treatment; therefore it is a benefit when a laboratory automatically initiates a pathology review. Cytology and histopathology reviews should be received by the practice in a timely manner. All tissue samples should automatically have the margins reviewed, indicating whether tumor cells have spread beyond the margin of the tissues.

> ◎ **PRACTICE POINT** Results should include the normal values for that particular species.

Laboratory reports should be detailed and provide current, progressive information for the veterinarian, especially in pathology cases. It saves the veterinary team time when lab reports include specific disease and treatment indicators with regard to sample results (Figures 9-6, 9-7, and 9-8).

Results may be reported by fax, phone, or Internet. Practices with computer medical records may choose to have results automatically populated into the correct medical record. Alerts are set for the team when results are available. It is imperative that correct patient information be submitted when this option is chosen or results will become lost if they are autopopulated into another patient's record.

> ◎ **PRACTICE POINT** Laboratory results can be automatically downloaded into patient records, saving team members time and helping avoid lost results.

FEES

Fees vary from lab to lab. Some labs may compete for the practice's business, thereby allowing special pricing on the most common profiles. Specialized testing can become fairly expensive, especially when one lab forwards the sample to another. Research may be done to find the "best" lab available for running specific tests. A team member can call that lab and receive specific pricing information as well as details on shipping the sample and the turnaround time for results. This can save the practice and client a large amount of money.

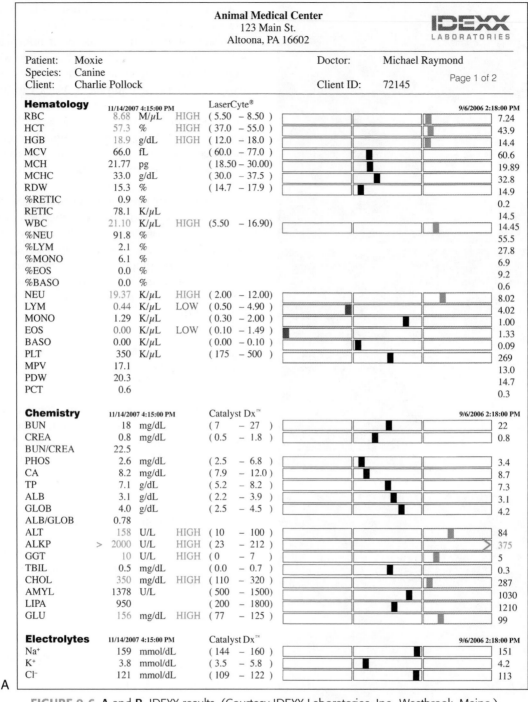

Animal Medical Center
123 Main St.
Altoona, PA 16602

IDEXX LABORATORIES

Patient:	Moxie	Doctor:	Michael Raymond	
Species:	Canine			Page 1 of 2
Client:	Charlie Pollock	Client ID:	72145	

Hematology   11/14/2007 4:15:00 PM   LaserCyte®   9/6/2006 2:18:00 PM

RBC	8.68	M/µL	HIGH	(5.50 – 8.50)		7.24
HCT	57.3	%	HIGH	(37.0 – 55.0)		43.9
HGB	18.9	g/dL	HIGH	(12.0 – 18.0)		14.4
MCV	66.0	fL		(60.0 – 77.0)		60.6
MCH	21.77	pg		(18.50 – 30.00)		19.89
MCHC	33.0	g/dL		(30.0 – 37.5)		32.8
RDW	15.3	%		(14.7 – 17.9)		14.9
%RETIC	0.9	%				0.2
RETIC	78.1	K/µL				14.5
WBC	21.10	K/µL	HIGH	(5.50 – 16.90)		14.45
%NEU	91.8	%				55.5
%LYM	2.1	%				27.8
%MONO	6.1	%				6.9
%EOS	0.0	%				9.2
%BASO	0.0	%				0.6
NEU	19.37	K/µL	HIGH	(2.00 – 12.00)		8.02
LYM	0.44	K/µL	LOW	(0.50 – 4.90)		4.02
MONO	1.29	K/µL		(0.30 – 2.00)		1.00
EOS	0.00	K/µL	LOW	(0.10 – 1.49)		1.33
BASO	0.00	K/µL		(0.00 – 0.10)		0.09
PLT	350	K/µL		(175 – 500)		269
MPV	17.1					13.0
PDW	20.3					14.7
PCT	0.6					0.3

Chemistry   11/14/2007 4:15:00 PM   Catalyst Dx™   9/6/2006 2:18:00 PM

BUN	18	mg/dL		(7 – 27)		22
CREA	0.8	mg/dL		(0.5 – 1.8)		0.8
BUN/CREA	22.5					
PHOS	2.6	mg/dL		(2.5 – 6.8)		3.4
CA	8.2	mg/dL		(7.9 – 12.0)		8.7
TP	7.1	g/dL		(5.2 – 8.2)		7.3
ALB	3.1	g/dL		(2.2 – 3.9)		3.1
GLOB	4.0	g/dL		(2.5 – 4.5)		4.2
ALB/GLOB	0.78					
ALT	158	U/L	HIGH	(10 – 100)		84
ALKP	> 2000	U/L	HIGH	(23 – 212)		375
GGT	10	U/L	HIGH	(0 – 7)		5
TBIL	0.5	mg/dL		(0.0 – 0.7)		0.3
CHOL	350	mg/dL	HIGH	(110 – 320)		287
AMYL	1378	U/L		(500 – 1500)		1030
LIPA	950			(200 – 1800)		1210
GLU	156	mg/dL	HIGH	(77 – 125)		99

Electrolytes   11/14/2007 4:15:00 PM   Catalyst Dx™   9/6/2006 2:18:00 PM

Na⁺	159	mmol/dL		(144 – 160)		151
K⁺	3.8	mmol/dL		(3.5 – 5.8)		4.2
Cl⁻	121	mmol/dL		(109 – 122)		113

A

FIGURE 9-6 A and **B,** IDEXX results. (Courtesy IDEXX Laboratories, Inc., Westbrook, Maine.)

○ **PRACTICE POINT**   Client costs for laboratory analysis should include the supplies used to obtain the sample.

For the practice to recover hidden costs associated with laboratory analysis, the practice must double the cost of the testing to the client. Costs that must be considered include:
• The time it takes the team members to draw and prepare the samples.

• The cost of supplies used to obtain the sample if they are not provided by the lab. Supplies may include a syringe and needle, formalin if purchased by the gallon, and slides used for cytologies.
• Some laboratories may add a fuel surcharge to the monthly statement.
• Shipping fees if samples are submitted to labs other than those used for general analysis. This may include overnight fees to FedEx or UPS.

Animal Medical Center
123 Main St.
Altoona, PA 16602

IDEXX LABORATORIES

Patient:	Moxie	
Species:	Canine	
Client:	Charlie Pollock	

Doctor:	Michael Raymond	
Client ID:	72145	Page 2 of 2

Immunoassay   11/14/2007 4:15:00 PM   SNAPshot Dx™   9/6/2006 2:18:00 PM

T_4 1.3 μg/dL   1.8

< 0.8	μg/dL	Low
0.8 - 1.5	μg/dL	Equivocal
1.6 - 5.0	μg/dL	Normal
>5.0	μg/dL	High
3.0 - 6.0	μg/dL	Therapeutic Range

CORTISOL (Low-Dose Dexamethasone Suppression)

Baseline	6.5	μg/dL
4 hour	1.4	μg/dL
8 hour	4.0	μg/dL

4-Hour	8-Hour	Interpretation
<1 μg/dL	<1 μg/dL	Normal
1 – 1.5 μg/dL	1 – 1.5 μg/dL	Inconclusive, consider repeating in 6–8 weeks
>1.5 μg/dL and >50% of baseline	>1.5 μg/dL and >50% of baseline	In the presence of supporting clinical signs, results are consistent with Cushing's Disease; consider HDDST to rule out adrenal tumor
<1.5 μg/dL or <50% of baseline	>1.5 μg/dL and >50% of baseline	Consistent with PDH
>1.5 μg/dL and >50% of baseline	>1.5 μg/dL and <50% of baseline	Consistent with PDH

Urinalysis   11/14/2007 4:15:00 PM   IDEXX VetLab® UA™   9/6/2006 2:18:00 PM

Urine SG	1.020	
pH	6.0	6.5
LEU	neg	neg
PRO	1+	neg
GLU	neg	neg
KET	neg	neg
UBG	1+	norm
BIL	neg	neg
BLD	neg	neg

*Confirm all leukocyte results with microscopy

09-68073-00

B

FIGURE 9-6, cont'd

CLIENT SERVICE

Client service is a very important factor when choosing outside laboratories. Team members often place calls looking for specific results, lab codes, or supplies. It is important that the call is answered in a timely manner, that lab personnel are friendly, and that they provide the answers needed. Veterinarians often need to consult with a pathologist or specialist regarding cases and results of previously submitted lab work. Most labs will provide a consult free of charge if a sample has been submitted on that case. Once a veterinarian has placed a call to the consult line, the lab should return the call to the veterinarian within one business day. Again, laboratories strive to provide the best service available, and consult calls should be returned immediately.

Most laboratories will provide veterinary practices with supplies for submitting samples, free of charge. Supplies include blood tubes, histopathology jars, sample submission bags, and forms. If any additional materials are needed, a call to customer service will take care of the request (Box 9-1).

ANTECH DIAGNOSTICS 13633 N. Cave Creek Phoenix AZ 85022 Phone: 800-745-4725

Client #
Chart #

Accession No. PXBC04335299	Doctor	Owner	Pet Name	Received
Species Canine	Breed Great Pyrenees	Sex CM	Pet Age 2Y	Reported

Test Requested	Results		Reference Range	Units
SUPERCHEM				
AST (SGOT)	31		15-66	IU/L
ALT (SGPT)	86		12-118	IU/L
Total Bilirubin	0.1		0.1-0.3	mg/dL
Alkaline Phosphatase	19		5-131	IU/L
GGT	1		1-12	IU/L
Total Protein	6.4		5.0-7.4	g/dL
Albumin	3.9		2.7-4.4	g/dL
Globulin	2.5		1.6-3.6	g/dL
A/G Ratio	1.6		0.8-2.0	
Cholesterol	239		92-324	mg/dL
BUN	20		6-25	mg/dL
Creatinine	1.3		0.5-1.6	mg/dL
BUN/Creatinine Ratio	15		4-27	
Phosphorus	4.9		2.5-6.0	mg/dL
Calcium	10.3		8.9-11.4	mg/dL
Glucose	98		70-138	mg/dL
Amylase	540		290-1125	IU/L
Lipase	457		77-695	IU/L
Sodium	153		139-154	mEq/L
Potassium	4.7		3.6-5.5	mEq/L
Na/K Ratio	33		27-38	
Chloride	115		102-120	mEq/L
CPK	84		59-895	IU/L
Triglyceride	66		29-291	mg/dL
Osmolality, Calculated	319 (HIGH)		277-311	mOSm/kg
Magnesium	1.6		1.5-2.5	mEq/L.
COMPLETE BLOOD COUNT				
WBC	5.7		4.0-15.5	$10^3/\mu L$
RBC	6.6		4.8-9.3	$10^6/\mu L$
HGB	16.4		12.1-20.3	g/dL
HCT	47		36-60	%
MCV	70		58-79	fL
MCH	24.7		19-28	pg
MCHC	35		30-38	%
Comment				
RBC MORPHOLOGY	NORMAL			

Differential	Absolute	%		
Neutrophils	3420	60	2060-10600	/μL
Lymphocytes	1653	29	690-4500	/μL
Monocytes	342	6	0-840	/μL
Eosinophils	285	5	0-1200	/μL
Basophils	0	0	0-150	/μL
Platelet Estimate	Adequate			
Platelet Count	290		170-400	$10^3/\mu L$

FIGURE 9-7 ANTECH results. (Courtesy ANTECH Diagnostics, Los Angeles, Calif.)

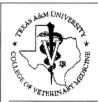
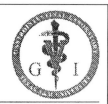

Gastrointestinal Laboratory
Dr. J.M. Steiner
Department of Small Animal Medicine and Surgery
Texas A&M University
4474 TAMU
College Station, TX 77843-4474

Website User IDs:
GI Lab Assigned Clinic ID: 3421

Phone:
Fax:
Animal Name:
Owner Name:
Species:
Date Rec'd:

Veterinary Clinic Tracking Number: GI Lab Accession: 269911

Test	Result	Control Range	Assay Date
Cobalamin Fasting	285 ng/L	251-908	09/18/08

    Interpretation: Low end of normal range. Suggestive of distal small intestinal disease. Recheck and/or consider cobalamin supplementation. Http://www.cvm.tamu.edu/gilab/research/cobalamin.shtml

Folate Fasting	11.5 ug/L	7.7-24.4	09/18/08

    Interpretation: Result is within the normal range.

Pancreatic Lipase Immunoreactivity Fasting	122 ug/L	0-200	09/18/08

    Interpretation: Result within the reference range.

TLI Fasting	18.9 ug/L	5.7-45.2	09/18/08

    Interpretation: Result is within the normal range.

Comments: Please note- the PLI test was repeated to verify the results.

Important
Notices:
    Have you received our latest newsletter yet?

    If you are willing to help with our fund-raising campaign by placing flyers in your waiting room, please contact us at 979-862-2860 or [gidevelop@cvm.tamu.edu].

    We do not accept shipments of samples with shipping billed payable to receiver. Samples submitted in this fashion will be billed additional charges for clerical time and handling.

GI Lab Contact Information

Phone: 979 862 2861   Email: gilab@cvm.tamu.edu
Fax: 979 862 2864   www.cvm.tamu.edu/gilab

FIGURE 9-8 Texas A&M results. (Courtesy Jörg M. Steiner, Texas A&M University, College Station Texas.)

Box 9-1	Outside Laboratories and Their Specialties

Michigan State University (endocrinology)
Diagnostic Center for Population and Animal Health
4125 Beaumont Road
Lansing, MI 48910
www.animalhealth.mes.edu

Kansas State Veterinary Diagnostic Lab (rabies antibody titer)
1200 Denison Avenue
Manhattan, KS 66506
www.vet.k-state.edu/rabies

Colorado State University Diagnostic Lab (serology/PCR)
300 West Drake
Fort Collins, CO 80523
www.cvmbs.colostate.edu/dlab

Cornell University (drug levels, serology, parasitology)
Animal Health Diagnostic Center
Upper Tower Road
Ithaca, NY 14853

Midwest Animal Blood Services (blood typing)
4983 Bird Avenue
Stockbridge, MI 49285

University of California-Davis (serology/polymerase chain reaction)
Endo Lab: Department of Population Health and Reproduction
Tupper Hall, Room 114
School of Veterinary Medicine
Davis, CA 95016

Texas A&M GI Lab (gastrointestinal)
4474 TAMU
College Station, TX 77843
www.TVMDLweb.tamu.edu

Vita-Tech Laboratories (parasitology)
2316 Delaware Avenue
Buffalo, NY 14216

VETERINARY PRACTICE and the LAW

Certain hazardous and perishable items may be mailed through the U.S. Postal Service but are subject to specific packaging and labeling requirements. Diagnostic clinical samples that are liquid or contained in a liquid must be mailed in a sturdy, securely sealed, water-tight container cushioned in a secondary container. There must be enough cushioning to absorb all the material if the primary container breaks. If hazardous chemicals are used (formalin) the container must be marked with a biohazard symbol.

Self-Evaluation Questions

1. How should lab samples be packaged for shipment?
2. What is serum?
3. What tests use serum?
4. What is plasma?
5. What is an anaerobic bacterium?
6. Why shouldn't cytology samples be submitted along with samples preserved in formalin?
7. Why should samples be submitted on ice?
8. What information needs to be recorded on the laboratory sheet?
9. What factors should be considered when choosing an outside laboratory?

Recommended Reading

Cowell R: *Veterinary clinical pathology secrets*, St Louis, 2004, Mosby Elsevier.

Duncan JR, Prasse KW, Mahaffey EA: *Veterinary laboratory medicine*, ed 4, Hoboken, NJ, 2003, Wiley.

Hendrix C, Sirosis M: *Laboratory procedures for veterinary technicians*, ed 5, St Louis, 2007, Mosby Elsevier.

Sirosis M: *Principles and practices of veterinary technology*, ed 2, St Louis, 2004, Mosby Elsevier.

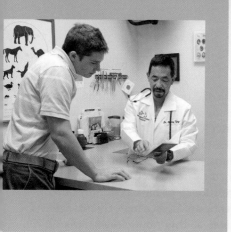

Marketing

Learning Objectives

Mastery of the content in this chapter will enable the reader to:
- Define different methods of marketing.
- Identify effective marketing techniques.
- Explain and implement ethical marketing.
- Compare marketing plans.
- List effective methods for Web site development.
- Describe a pet portal system.
- Discuss the benefits of gift certificates.

Key Terms

Assertive Marketing
Branding
Community Service
Company-Supported Web Site
Cost-Benefit Analysis
Direct Marketing
Domain Name

External Marketing
FTP
Host-the-Site Web Site
Indirect Marketing
Internal Marketing
Lead Time
On-Site Hosting Web Site

On-Hold Messaging
Open House
Pet Portals
Target Marketing
URL
Web Site

Marketing is an integral part of the success of a practice. Various forms of marketing occur on a daily basis without conscious thought. Client education, clean facilities, and a superb team all contribute to indirect forms of marketing. Direct marketing may include Yellow Pages advertisements, newspaper advertisements, and newsletters. Internal marketing is directed toward current clients and includes reminders, postcards, and recalls. External marketing is geared toward potential clients and educates them about the services the practice offers.

In the monthly budget, 2% to 3% should be allocated to marketing, whether for internal, external, direct, or indirect services. Team members may not be aware of the marketing skills they already possess; these skills can be enhanced on a daily basis.

Practices should determine what qualities make them unique. Great medical and professional services no longer set one veterinary hospital apart from others. Every practice provides professional service and good medicine. Is the staff unique? Is the practice located in a prime location? Do the practice hours differ from those of other veterinary hospitals in the area? Determining what makes the hospital unique will help make any marketing program a success.

Each practice may want to consider a SWOT analysis. SWOT is defined as *s*trengths, *w*eaknesses, *o*pportunities, and *t*hreats. Strengths and weaknesses are internal and focus on the practice, whereas opportunities and threats evaluate the external market. A SWOT analysis can help a practice determine what makes it unique.

Practices can create a signature customer service. Client service is a must; positive word-of-mouth is the most successful form of free marketing. Team members must drive home the value of the service to the client. Client confidence in the medical skills and professional services provided by a practice is the primary driver of value, along with friendly staff. Secondary drivers include compassion, education, and cleanliness. These all lead to superior customer service and client satisfaction.

> **PRACTICE POINT** The "4 P's" of marketing are *p*roduct, *p*lace, *p*rice, and *p*romotion.

Product marketing includes both professional services and products that the practice sells. The team must understand and believe in the services and products provided; otherwise, the marketing effort could fail. An example would be acupuncture. Many veterinarians and team members are unaware of the benefits acupuncture may provide to patients. If one veterinarian in the practice promotes and provides acupuncture services but the remaining team members are unaware of the benefits, then the service may fail in the practice. Products are just as important. Team members should receive training on the products that the practice wishes to carry. These include diets, ear cleaning supplies, and shampoos. Manufacturer and distributor representatives love to provide education to practices. Ask the representative to provide a luncheon seminar to help educate the team regarding new products the practice carries.

Place: The practice should be located in a convenient location with easy access. "Location, location, location" is the phrase that is always heard, and that is just as important for veterinary practices as for anything else. Parking lots should be easy to pull into, without any barriers or obstructions to avoid. If the parking lot is always overflowing, additional lot space may be acquired, allowing additional parking spaces to be added. Existing practices that do not have an ideal location may consider adding services and products that other practices in the immediate area do not provide. External marketing plans can focus on those areas to draw clients to a less-than-ideal location. Existing practices may also add

signage and increased perimeter lighting to draw attention to the practice.

Price: Price can be a factor for some clients, and the practice can decide on which services it wishes to provide competitive prices. Price shoppers generally shop for the best prices on routine surgeries, dental prophylaxis, examinations, and vaccinations. Diagnostic testing, hospital procedures, and medications are not shopped services, and relationships have generally been developed by the time they are prescribed. Clients will accept or decline services at this point, regardless of cost. Practices do not want to be the cheapest service in town, nor should they offer less service in order to compete. If a practice believes in high-quality medicine, then clients should be charged for it. Once clients perceive the value of the excellent service and medicine, they will be clients for life.

Practices may wish to consider gathering competitive intelligence information from other practices in the area to differentiate themselves from others. By differentiating, the practice can set itself apart from other hospitals in the community. This can ultimately increase sales and profits by attracting new clients as well as helping retain old clients.

Promotion: Promotion includes the mechanism used to promote products and services within and outside the veterinary practice. This can include direct and indirect marketing or internal and external marketing. All are discussed in the following sections. Many veterinary manufacturers or distributors will support clinic marketing techniques with additional incentives. Some companies may provide free product samples, whereas others will provide incentives to the staff to increase sales.

It should be remembered that the goal of the practice is to offer high-quality medicine (professional, medical, and client oriented) regardless of the specials that may be offered by companies. Marketing techniques and specials should be analyzed to ensure they are in line with the practice's mission, goals, and practice philosophies.

> **PRACTICE POINT** Marketing strategies must be analyzed on a yearly basis, making changes where needed.

Practices should analyze their marketing strategy on a yearly basis. Are current methods working? Have service and sales increased with current marketing techniques? If not, where has the marketing failed? Internally? Lack of new clients? Practice managers should be able to track before-and-after results and make changes as needed. Only 2% to 3% of a budget is not a tremendous amount of money to spend; therefore the allocation of funds to a particular segment is vital, as is ensuring the segment's success.

BRANDING THE PRACTICE

Branding is defining the practice with a logo, phrase, and/or hospital name. Each practice should develop a symbol that clients can associate with the practice. Whenever they see the symbol, they think of ABC Veterinary Hospital. An example is Target stores. Target is branded with a red and white target. When a commercial plays on the television and the red target logo appears, people know that the commercial is a Target commercial before the word Target appears. This is known as *branding,* and it is a clever marketing tool for a veterinary hospital to use. Practices may also use a short and easy phrase. For example, "ABC Veterinary Hospital, where quality and compassion count," offers three important points within one sentence. It lists the name of the practice and two important aspects of the practice.

Once logos, symbols, or phrases have been developed, they should be placed on every item that has the practice name. This includes letterhead, business cards, client education materials, Web sites, client information sheets, brochures, and any advertising that is done on a public and professional level. Clients must be able to associate the logos and symbols with the practice. The association can take years to develop but will be rewarding once it has been achieved.

INDIRECT MARKETING

Indirect marketing centers on the clients the practice currently serves. Client education has been discussed in other chapters and is highlighted later in this chapter. Client education serves as the greatest indirect marketing tool that can be used. Educating clients regarding the professional services their pet needs is imperative. Client education materials must be sent home with every client at every visit. This includes puppy and kitten exams, boosters, yearly exams, and senior exams. All clients must be informed about heartworm disease, internal and external parasites (as well as their zoonotic potential), nutrition, and obesity management. If a patient has been diagnosed with a condition or disease, the client must receive printed materials to take home and review. Materials should include information about the disease as well as treatment options that are available. Clients become overloaded with information when they are visiting a practice and will retain only 20% of the information provided. Sending home information reiterates the information and allows a more successful communication with other household members (spouse, significant other, children).

All team members should receive training on services, procedures, and protocols on a continuing basis. When team members can explain procedures with confidence and without hesitation, clients will accept the services that have been recommended. Facilities must be kept clean and odor free. Clients perceive value and service, along with cleanliness, as top priorities when seeking service for their pets. If a practice has heavy animal or cleaning agent odors, they may never return. Trash containers should be emptied several times a day because they are a significant contributor to odors circulating in the practice. Smaller trash cans should be used, mandating frequent emptying. Pet eliminations must be cleaned immediately, regardless of whether they occur in the reception, treatment, or kennel area. Odors circulate quickly and, unfortunately, efficiently! Walls, baseboards, and door frames must be washed weekly and pictures and fans should be dusted daily. Anatomic models must be free of dust and lint and counters clear of clutter.

> **PRACTICE POINT** A spotlessly clean facility is a form of indirect marketing.

Professional, clean, and friendly team members encourage clients to feel comfortable and ask questions. When clients are comfortable, they will not only return to the practice in the future, they will also recommend the practice to their friends, family, and co-workers. Clients must be greeted upon entry and assisted when leaving. Team members wearing name badges inform the client of who they are as well as their positions within the practice. This is comforting to clients who wish to know who they are working with. Team members wearing clean, wrinkle-free uniforms appear professional and approachable, which encourages client interaction.

> **PRACTICE POINT** Name badges should be worn at all times, allowing the client to know who is caring for their pets.

Team members can also establish courteous and reliable relationships with clients to help promote indirect marketing. Many businesses do not address clients by name. Addressing clients and pets by name is a very effective customer service/marketing tool. When they are addressed directly by name, they feel special. "Good morning, Ms. Thurman. How are you and Fluffy doing today?" is an excellent greeting for both the client and pet. When the pet's name and history are addressed, the client's confidence in the practice increases, leading to better overall satisfaction with the practice.

All the above directly contribute to an increase in client communication. Client communication is the key to increasing client compliance and client retention. As stated above, communication with clients by client education is imperative. Clients must understand procedures and feel comfortable with the recommendations being made. Team members who maintain eye contact and have an open body posture when talking with owners relay a message of confidence. If eye contact is not made and team members have folded arms, the client may neither perceive the value of the service being recommended nor have confidence in the team. If there is lack of confidence, client retention and compliance will decrease.

> **PRACTICE POINT**   Clients must have confidence in the team to accept recommendations.

Creating a staff board that lists all team members and placing it in the reception area allows clients to know who is on the team. A staff board may list the employees' first names, along with any credentials they may have. Pictures may also be included. Doctors can be listed with DVM (or VMD, depending on the graduating school) and technicians with RVT, CVT, or LVT, along with any other degrees that have been received. Often, team members will have completed a bachelor's or associate's program in college. The practice managers may be a CVPM, and assistants may also be certified. All team members, including kennel personnel, should be listed, so as to inform clients who is caring for their pets. Last names should not be listed due to security precautions.

Client compliance is discussed in Chapter 11; however, the key point to remember is that client compliance is the driving force behind client retention, client recommendations, and client satisfaction. Educating the client is imperative, as previously stated. Team members must make recommendations to every client, regardless of their perception of the client's financial situation. Establishing a written protocol of policies and procedures, along with following up on cases, will help increase client compliance. Recommendations and compliance should be tracked, allowing revisions to be made to help increase client compliance. Indirect marketing to current clients takes many shapes and values; every

facet must be explored to maximize each practice's potential (Figure 10-1).

DIRECT MARKETING

For many years, the human medical professions have efficiently leveraged direct marketing tools, whereas the veterinary medical community has been slow to adopt these methods. However, as competition for a successful practice has risen, so has the use of direct marketing techniques. In previous years, many communities have only had one or two veterinary practices serving them, and direct marketing was not needed. In today's world, the number of practices has risen, and working to ensure survival of the business is reality. Direct marketing is now needed more than ever to keep a practice viable.

> **PRACTICE POINT**   Direct marketing techniques must be kept fair and ethical.

Direct marketing is the most popular form of marketing and has been around for years. The Yellow Pages are a classic example of direct marketing. The practice must make the general public aware of the services that are available as well as the doctors who are on staff. Newspaper advertising also notifies the public of any specials or notices the veterinary hospital wishes to publish. It is important to keep in mind the benefit that the practice may receive from the advertising must be weighed against the cost of the ad. Advantages and disadvantages of phone book advertising and newspaper ads are discussed in the external marketing section of this chapter. It is important to remember that direct marketing is targeted to potential and existing clients whom the practice wishes to serve.

Recommendation Compliance Report				ABC Veterinary Clinic
Period: 01/01/08-01/01/09				
Code	Description	#of Recommendations	# of Compliances	(%)
R0001	Rabies	910	607	(66.7)
R0002	DHPP	791	298	(37.67)
R0003	Bordetella	126	61	(48.41)
R0004	Heartworm Prev	1088	544	(50.00)
R0005	Dental Prophylaxis	754	398	(52.79)
R0005	Pre Anesth BW	950	367	(38.63)
R0006	General Health BW	1589	1061	(67.77)
R0007	Senior Screening	790	421	(53.29)
R0008	Therapeutic Food	984	398	(40.45)

FIGURE 10-1 Sample report tracking client compliance.

What Would You Do/Not Do?

The local association of veterinarians has been approached by the newspaper to provide a weekly veterinary topic that will be printed every Monday in the business section of the newspaper. One specific veterinarian has announced that he would be responsible for writing the topics each week. Other veterinarians are concerned that he may use this as an opportunity to promote his veterinary practice instead of the community of veterinarians as a whole.

What Should the Practice Do?

If more than one veterinarian or practice has concerns with one individual being responsible for the articles, then the concerns must be addressed openly. Most likely, if one practice has concerns, others do as well but are hesitant to voice their opinions for fear of a confrontation. Concerned practices may offer a solution: one individual may be responsible for writing the article, whereas others can rotate the responsibility of proofreading the article and adding any other information that may be needed. This allows several individuals to include their thoughts while educating the community about topics in veterinary medicine.

Box 10-1	Examples of Internal Marketing

- Recalls
- Clean, updated, and pleasant-smelling office
- Open discussions with team members and clients
- Staff identification
- Staff enthusiasm
- Newsletter
- Timely replies to client requests
- Client education
- Telephone etiquette
- Client acknowledgment
- Professional appearance

INTERNAL MARKETING

Internal marketing has been discussed in previous chapters and includes reminders, recalls, appointments, and newsletters sent to current clients. The goal of internal marketing is to retain current clients. This can be accomplished in several ways; reminders can be sent for different reasons, including yearly exams, vaccinations, heartworm preventive refills, or yearly bloodwork. The key to successful internal marketing is listening to the client. By listening, team members can determine their wants and needs. Practices can use tools to help implement internal marketing techniques, but team members must listen to and satisfy the needs of each client (Box 10-1).

Reminders

Reminders should appear professional and be free of errors. If reminders are handwritten, the writing should be clear and easy to read. Reminder cards must have the basic information included on each card: pet's name, the date the reminder is due, and what the pet is due for. The clinic information must include the name, address, phone number, Web site, and logo of the veterinary clinic. It is also imperative to state that clients should call to make an appointment. Some clients assume that

because they received the reminder, they can come any time. They are then upset at the wait time when they arrive as walk-ins. Reminders are discussed in further detail in Chapter 11 (Figure 10-2).

Reminders should be sent no more than 4 weeks in advance of the due date because clients may forget the appointment they have made or simply disregard the reminder because it was sent far in advance. Reminder systems are programmed to delete the reminder if the client has arrived for an appointment before the due date. However, if reminders have been printed too early, the reminder will be sent regardless and the client is left feeling confused because he or she just visited in the clinic. They may call the reception team and question the accuracy of the staff, because "they were just there."

> **PRACTICE POINT**   Reminders should be sent on a biweekly basis and not more than 4 weeks in advance of the service due date.

Some reminder systems are also set up to generate second and third reminders for noncompliant clients who have not returned (Figure 10-3). Again, if reminders are printed too early, another reminder will be printed indicating the noncompliance. Clients who do not respond to reminders should be called; this will allow the staff to check on the pet, answer any concerns the owner may have, and schedule an appointment. Often, clients are extremely busy and have not taken the time to schedule an appointment and will appreciate that the practice has called. By making these calls, the practice has added a personalized touch to customer service. Customer service is centered on relationship building, connecting, and engaging with the client (Figure 10-4).

Recalls

Recalls should be completed for every patient that has visited the practice in the previous few days, regardless of whether it was for a yearly exam, vaccines, or an ear

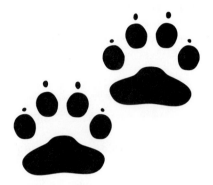

ABC Veterinary Clinic

Our records indicate that your pet is past due for vaccines. In order to provide the best care for your pet, please make an appointment as soon as possible.

Dr. Nancy Dreamer
Dr. Sue Garden
Dr. Katie Love

Reminder

Please call to make an
appointment today!
555-333-1900
2399 Saturn Circle
Anytown, USA
www.abcveterinaryclinic.com

Healthcare that lets your pets live longer healthier lives!

FIGURE 10-2 Sample reminder.

infection. The team member in charge of recalls can check on a patient after vaccinations to make sure there was no reaction to the vaccines. If the pet received medications, team members can follow up to ensure the pet is improving and is not having any problems with medications that were dispensed. If a pet had surgery, team members should always follow up and review the release instructions, ensuring the client fully understands them (e.g., no exercise for 7 days postoperatively). Telephone calls allow owners to ask questions that they may not have thought to ask while at the hospital or address new concerns that have arisen. Team members can also verify that the client was satisfied with the visit and schedule a follow-up exam if needed. See Chapter 11 for more information on recalls.

Newsletters

Newsletters can include information regarding vaccine protocol changes and discussions on behavior, disease, or nutrition. Clients love to receive information that they can read at home, and a newsletter will help satisfy this need.

PRACTICE POINT Newsletters are excellent ideas for both internal and external marketing techniques.

Newsletters do not have to be fancy; simple information within the space of four pages is plenty. Too much information can overwhelm owners. Information to include should be practical and easy to understand.

If diseases are a topic to be covered, they should be discussed in layman's terms. If clients do not understand it, they will not read it and the money spent on it has been wasted. Newsletters should be fun and colorful, while maintaining the goal of educating clients, to increase client compliance (Figure 10-5). Tips for the day, quote of the week, and fascinating facts are just a few pieces of information that can be included in a newsletter. Community-service events and animal-related organizations can also be acknowledged on the last page of newsletters because half the page will be used for mailing purposes.

Pictures can be included in newsletters; however, the quality of the print must be excellent. Copied pictures do not reproduce well and, as previously stated, poor-quality newsletters are correlated to poor professional veterinary service. Drawings reproduce well and can be included. Microsoft Publisher provides nice preset designs that can be used to develop newsletters, or a graphics designer can be contacted for professional setup and layout.

Veterinary manufacturers and software companies also offer to send out newsletters to clients with the practice name and address. These newsletters are professional, colorful, and eye catching and cost a minimal amount (if anything) to send out. Most are sent from a central location in the United States and arrive at the clients' homes quarterly. Mailing lists can either be uploaded from the practices' veterinary software and forwarded to the company, or team members can print labels and affix them to the newsletters themselves.

REMINDER COMPLIANCE REPORT

This report will show how many reminders were due for a specific date range, how many were satisfied and the overall percentage of satisfaction. It will include inactive pets (as they may have complied or not complied during that date range) and those set up not to receive reminders.

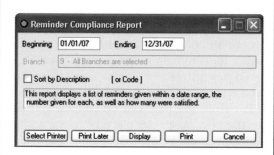

Reminder Compliance Report		INTRAVET VETERINARY CARE		
For period: 01/01/2007 - 12/31/2007				
Code	Description	Number of reminders due	Number of compliances	Percentage
LI147	AHH I drug monitor	7	2	28.57
VA115	Bordetella intranasal	103	40	38.83
VA117	Corona virus vaccine	2	0	0.00
VA125	DA2PP adult vaccination	143	62	43.36
VA120	DA2PP puppy vaccination	14	8	64.29
MI900	Dental recommended 6 mo	43	25	58.14
VA121	DPV vaccine	1	1	100.00
VA155	FeLV vaccination adult	81	37	45.68
VA160	FeLV vaccination kitten	5	4	80.00
VA150	FVRCP - feline vaccination	96	47	48.96
VA145	FVRCP - kitten vaccination	2	2	100.00
AP455	Heartgard refill	90	55	61.11
LI300	Heartworm/Ehr/Lyme snap	84	43	51.19
LABR	Labwork recommended	14	2	14.29
LI500	MAT.fecal flotation	192	79	41.15
VA300	Porphyromonas vaccine Ye	5	2	40.00
VA105	Rabies canine 3 year	100	43	43.00
VA110	Rabies feline 1 year	79	35	44.30
VA100	Rabies puppy 1 year	4	1	25.00
TOTALS:		**1065**	**489**	**45.92**

REMINDER COMPLIANCE BY RECALL REPORT

This report looks at reminders as a whole to measure our overall reminder efficiency. The breakdown lists compliance vs. non-compliance and presents information about why the reminders may or may not have been satisfied. There are specific factors that can affect the numbers reported on this report.

NOTE: Recently converted data may show inflated numbers for manually cleared reminders, due to how reminders are converted.

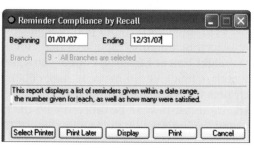

Reminder Compliance by Recall Report INTRAVET VETERINARY CARE

For period: 01/01/2007 - 12/31/2007

Total number of reminders due:	1065
Total number of satisfied reminders:	489

Compliance		**45.92% (489)**
15.49%	(165)	Satisfied before a reminder could be sent.
10.52%	(112)	Satisfied after 1 reminder.
10.52%	(112)	Satisfied after 2 reminders.
7.70%	(82)	Satisfied after 3 reminders.
1.69%	(18)	Satisfied after 4 reminders.

Non Compliance		**54.08% (576)**
9.58%	(102)	Did not receive a reminder and were not satisfied.
44.51%	(474)	Received a reminder and were not satisfied.

Notes: Out of 489 cleared reminders, 0.20% (1) were manually cleared.
Out of 576 non compliances, 4.51% (26) were from patients setup not to receive reminders

COMPLIANCE REPORTS

FIGURE 10-3 Sample reminder compliance report. (Courtesy IntraVet, Dublin, Ohio.)

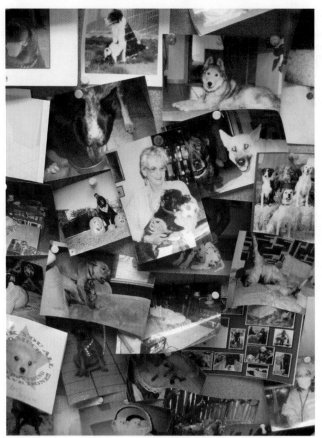

FIGURE 10-4 Collage of client and patient pictures.

Topics cover a variety of client education materials and generally have games to play, drawings for kids to color, and trivia for the clients. Team members can ask their sales representatives for any information their company may have regarding this excellent marketing tool.

Other Ideas for Internal Marketing

Many practices have been creative in using internal marketing techniques to continue to please their clients. Welcome cards can be sent to new clients, along with a DVD giving the new client a tour of the practice. The DVD can include team members in action, surgery, and client interaction. The DVD does not have to be long; the goal is simply to introduce the client to the practice. DVDs can easily be made with technology available today, and reproduction of the DVD is inexpensive. This idea for internal marketing is very effective at creating a long-lasting relationship and establishing the kind of doctor-practice-client bond for which all practices should strive.

> ⦿ **PRACTICE POINT** Internal marketing techniques are aimed at the current clientele a practice serves.

"Thank you for the referral" letters can be sent to current clients who have referred a new client to the practice. Practices may wish to simply send a card, or perhaps include a gift card to a local coffee house or grocery store as a token of appreciation. Any acknowledgement will be greatly appreciated by the client. Condolence cards are always appreciated by clients when they have lost a pet. The entire team can sign the card and add a little note expressing their thoughts. Special clients and clients in the top 20% of the accounts should receive flowers or a plant. These clients have obviously spent money helping their pets, and the practice should take the extra step to express their condolence. Sending flowers to all clients can become costly; therefore seeking other ideas to help remember the pet is a good idea. Painted paw prints or clay paw imprints are inexpensive and easy to accomplish and are appreciated by owners. Hair from the paw can be clipped and paint applied to the paw. A special piece of paper with the Rainbow Bridge poem printed on it can be applied to the paw, allowing the outline of the paw to be transmitted to the paper. Once dried, it can be mailed to the owner. Clay paw imprints are just as easy to accomplish, but may cost more than paw prints. See Chapter 12 for more ideas on how to remember patients.

A pet that has suffered and survived a traumatic experience or injury might receive a purple heart for its courage (Figure 10-6). Purple hearts make clients feel great and are an excellent conversation piece. Once again, the practice name is brought up in conversation as to why and how the pet received the Purple Heart. Pet bandannas are relatively cheap to produce, and clients usually put them on pets by with excitement (Figure 10-7). Purple hearts or bandannas can have the practice information on it, along with a catchy phrase like, "I survived!" A phrase like this initiates conversations, as friends will ask, "What did Fifi survive?"

A Weight Management Hall of Fame can be instituted with before-and-after photos. A short story can be posted on the successful endeavor with both the client and the pet posing for the after photo. Halls of fame should be placed in a highly-visible area that all clients can see. A weight Hall of Fame can engage conversation in the reception area and can motivate other clients to enter their pets in a weight-loss program.

Pediatric toothbrushes can be ordered with the practice name and logo printed on the handle (Figure 10-8). Toothbrushes can be placed in puppy and kitten kits, in dental kits, or simply given to owners when the team is talking about dental disease. Leashes can also be printed with the practice name and logo. Luggage tags can be designed with the practice information and placed on animal carriers when cats or small dogs have been dropped off. The client's name can be placed on the back of the tag and tied to the handle of the carrier. The carrier will always have identification on it when the

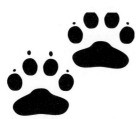

ABC VETERINARY CLINIC

THE PAW PRINT

Dr. Nancy Dreamer
Dr. Sue Beam
Dr. Frances Love

February is National Pet Dental Month!

JOIN THE FIGHT AGAINST ORAL DISEASE!

For most of us, caring for our teeth and gums has been part of our family routine for as long as we can remember. Just like you, your pet needs dental care too - regular, professional care from your veterinarian. Preventative care is important to keep plaque removed. Daily brushing and feeding special pet foods can also help.

WHAT CAUSES PERIODONTAL DISEASE?

Plaque is a colorless film that contains large amounts of bacteria. If left unchecked, plaque mineralizes into tartar, destroys gums, and results in the loss of tissue and bone that support the teeth. Preventative oral care can reduce the formation of plaque and help maintain proper oral health throughout your pet's life.

CONTRIBUTING FACTORS:

- Poor Oral Hygiene
- Breed
- Age
- Genetics

SIGNS OF PERIODONTAL DISEASE:

All pets are at risk for developing dental problems. Once your pet displays the signs listed on page 2, serious dental disease may be present. Don't wait for these signs. Start a preventative program today!

Continued page 2

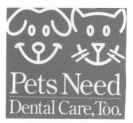

Pets Need Dental Care, Too.

Highway 70 Construction Update

With the new construction on Highway 70 approaching Saturn Circle, clients will encounter brief periods when access to the clinic is difficult. The project plan is to build an overpass at the intersection of Roadrunner and Highway 70. A one-way frontage road will run on either side of the highway. Once the overpass is completed, eastbound clients can drive under the overpass and access the clinic from the westbound frontage road.

In the meantime, Saturn Circle should remain accessible from Highway 70 or Del Rey Blvd.

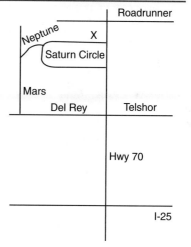

FIGURE 10-5 Sample newsletter.

owner returns, and the name of the practice is clearly visible for friends and family to see.

Marketing messages can be printed at the base of receipts to inform clients about important topics. Newsletters, Web site tools, or information regarding puppy classes can be summarized, helping promote the practice's internal marketing tools. The invoice in Figure 10-9 uses the opportunity to promote puppy classes that the practice provides.

Target marketing is directed toward current clients with a special breed, species, or age of animal and/or one with a particular disease or condition (obesity, diabetes, arthritis). Practices can determine the needs, wants, and concerns of a specific group of clients and develop a target strategy based on those results. Another way to benefit from target marketing is to stay attuned to the news media. Team members can listen to breaking news stories regarding veterinary-related issues. For example, tick-borne diseases may be on the increase, with the news media reporting the story. A postcard can be generated listing the risk factors and symptoms of tick-borne diseases and promoting tick-prevention products.

If the practice has decided to increase dental awareness for 1 month out of the year, clients with pets older

National Pet Dental Month...

Signs of Periodontal Disease:

- Bad breath
- Yellow-brown crust around the gum line
- Red and irritated gums
- Pain while eating
- Pawing at the mouth
- Change of chewing or eating habits
- Bleeding gums
- Tooth loss
- Subdued behavior
- Excessive drooling

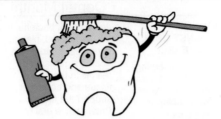

Brushing your pet's teeth daily helps reduce the amount of tartar and plaque buildup!

Good oral health may also require a pet food formulated to clean teeth and reduce the symptoms of periodontal disease. Foods available include:

- Science Diet Oral Care
- Science Diet T/D
- Friskies Dental Diet

Tips on brushing your pet's teeth

- Introduce a brushing program gradually; this may take several weeks.
- Make the initial sessions brief but positive.
- At first, dip your finger into beef bouillon for a dog or tuna water for a cat and rub your finger over your pet's teeth.
- Gradually introduce a finger brush rather than a toothbrush.
- When it is time to graduate to a toothpaste for pets, put a small amount on your finger brush and let you pet taste it.
- **BE SURE TO USE A TOOTHPASTE FOR PETS. HUMAN TOOTHPASTE CAN BE TOXIC TO YOUR PET.**

Springtime Is Here, And So Is Parvovirus!

Canine parvovirus is an acute systemic illness characterized by vomiting, bloody diarrhea, and lethargy. Parvo attacks rapidly dividing cells in the gastrointestinal tract, making the pet vomit and have diarrhea. It also affects the bone marrow. Parvovirus affects unvaccinated dogs, starting as early as 6 weeks of age. A puppy may be exposed to parvovirus and harbor the virus for 5-7 days before showing symptoms. The onset of symptoms may be sudden, and if left untreated, can be fatal.

Parvovirus can stay in the ground for 2 years and infect unvaccinated puppies and dogs. If an area has been contaminated with parvo, clean the area with a dilute Clorox solution and rinse well. Hospitalization is the best method available for treating patients with parvo. IV fluids, antibiotic injections, and supportive therapy help prevent this virus from becoming fatal.

The best way to prevent parvovirus is to vaccinate puppies starting at 6 weeks of age. It is recommended to vaccinate puppies every 3-4 weeks until the pet is 12 weeks of age. If a puppy is over 12 weeks of age, we recommend an initial vaccine and a booster 3-4 weeks after the first vaccine is given.

We recommend that all vaccines be boostered annually.

Page 2   THE PAW PRINT

FIGURE 10-5, cont'd Sample newsletter.

than 5 years may be targeted to receive dental health information. Other ideas of target marketing may include allergy patients and a postcard bringing their attention to the newest dermatologic antihistamine or steroidal drugs or heartworm disease and a special on a heartworm preventive (Figure 10-10).

Team members should be able to select a particular species or breed in the veterinary software and create a list with client names, addresses, and pet names. The list can then be exported into a spreadsheet, allowing mailing labels to be generated. These labels can be affixed to postcards. The dental postcard can be sent to canine patients older than 7 years or another target audience,

educating clients about dental disease and requesting them to make an appointment for an immediate dental prophylaxis (Figure 10-11).

> **PRACTICE POINT** Target marketing can be an extremely successful technique used to increase particular services that the practice offers.

If postcards, newsletters, or other advertising brochures have been developed, all team members should be made aware of the advertisement. Examples of postcards, newsletters, and brochures should be given to, and reviewed with, team members before the mailing.

Spaying and Neutering Your Pet: Population Control

Do you know how many puppies or kittens are produced from a single mother over a period of 72 months? **13,120!** For every person born, **15 dogs and 45 cats are born!** Pet overpopulation is a big problem. In order to keep up with the current flood of puppies and kittens, every person would have to own 2 dogs and 6 cats during their entire lifetime! That means a household of 5 would harbor **10 dogs and 30 cats!**

The number of dogs and cats in the United States exceeds the capacity of what our society can care for. As a result, many healthy pets are euthanized or become the victims of accidents, starvation, or disease.

Spay Day USA is March 1 to March 31. All spays and neuters are discounted for the entire month of March. All you have to do is call and make an appointment. You will be helping your pet and helping control the pet population!

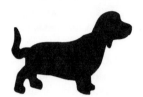

Statistics courtesy of Dona Ana Humane Society.

The Health Benefits of Spaying or Neutering Your Pet

Many studies indicate that pets live longer healthier lives when they have been spayed or neutered! Female pets that are spayed before they exhibit their first heat have less than a 1% chance of developing mammary cancer in their senior years. If they are spayed after their first heat, the chance of mammary cancer increases to 13%! Pets that have not been spayed are also at a higher risk of having pyometra, an infection of the uterus. Treatment for pyometra requires an emergency surgery; however, this potentially fatal infection is completely preventable by having your pet spayed.
Male pets also have an increased risk of having prostate or testicular cancer in their senior years if they are not neutered.

- Spaying and neutering makes pets more affectionate companions and makes male cats less likely to spray and mark their territory.
- A spay or neuter surgery is a one-time cost that is relatively small when compared to the benefits. It is a small price to pay for the health of your pet and the prevention of unwanted animals!

Information courtesy of the Humane Society of the United States.

MYTHS AND FACTS ABOUT SPAYING OR NEUTERING YOUR PET:

- "My pet will get fat and lazy": Most pets become overweight from being overfed and not getting enough exercise.
- "But my pet is purebred": 1 out of every 4 animals brought to the shelter is also purebred.
- "I want my dog to be protective": Spaying or neutering does not affect a dogs natural instinct to protect the home and family.
- "I don't wan't my male pet to feel like less of a male": Pet's don't have any concept of sexual identity or ego.

Page 3

FIGURE 10-5, cont'd Sample newsletter.

If the information is sent out before a review, a client will inevitably receive it and bring it to the attention of the staff. It is embarrassing and degrading to team members to find out from clients about a special the practice is promoting.

The cost of mailing letters, postcards, or newsletters must be evaluated with a cost versus benefit ratio. Producing these items can be costly, along with the cost of mailing them. It should be determined whether the mailing will produce a greater profit than the cost itself. Email is a cheap form of advertising; collecting email addresses from clients is a creative way to increase internal marketing techniques at a greatly reduced cost. Email messages can be bright, colorful, and grab the attention of clients, just as any printed piece of material would. Some clients may prefer to receive email instead of "snail mail." Anti-spam laws and legal requirements should be reviewed before sending emails to ensure the practice is within legal boundaries.

Box 10-2 shows a cost versus benefit ratio to analyze the benefit of creating a target market for dentals. If a practice wishes to increase the number of dentals by 100 during a 1-month period and chooses to target dogs older than 7 years, then all costs associated with creating the target must be determined. Box 10-2 shows that it will cost the practice $120 to produce and mail 100 cards. Costs in this figure include the paper, ink, and labels and the labor used to produce these cards. Labor

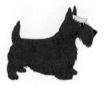

FIGURE 10-5, cont'd Sample newsletter.

in this formula includes the manager's time at $15 per hour, plus an additional 20% that the practice pays in taxes on this employee for payroll taxes (20% is an approximate number). This figure states that the practice charges $157 for a basic dental (this cost does not include any additional charges that may be accumulated for the procedure, including radiographs, extractions, the application of Doxirobe gel, antibiotics, or pain medication). The costs associated with producing a basic dental are approximately $89.60. This includes the technician's time of 1 hour (as well as the 20% payroll tax), drugs, an estimated equipment usage fee, and 10% allocated to practice overhead. An estimated equipment usage fee is the amount that it costs the practice to use that piece of equipment until it is paid off.

An overhead fee includes electricity, mortgage, insurance, and so forth. The practice profit from a basic dental is $67.40. Therefore two dentals must be completed to break even.

> **PRACTICE POINT** A cost/benefit ratio should be performed before target marketing, ensuring that the cost of the promotion can be easily recovered.

If a practice has a 50% response to the target cards and increases the number of dentals to 50 for the 1-month period, the potential gross revenue is $7850 (50 × $157 = $7850). Subtract the original target cost of $120 and the gross generated from the target program is $7730. Imagine if the response was 100%!

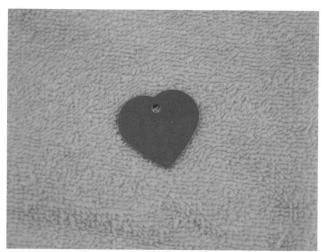

FIGURE 10-6 Purple heart.

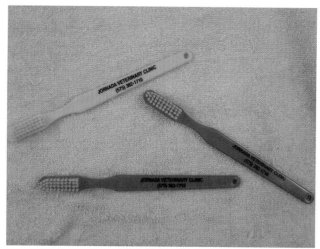

FIGURE 10-8 Pediatric toothbrushes.

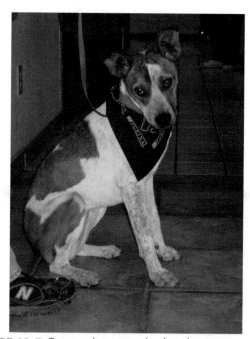

FIGURE 10-7 Pet wearing a practice bandanna.

Many veterinary manufacturers may sponsor such target programs by providing a postcard and stamp. Team members simply generate a label, which dramatically reduces the costs associated with such programs and significantly increases the bottom line. Practices must analyze the information contained in these postcards, ensuring the information contained is in line with the practice's high quality of medicine and marketing techniques. A postcard or newsletter may contain information or phrases that are not supported by the practice, which can be detrimental.

"Exam room report cards" can be sent home with clients. Preprinted report cards can easily be marked for normal and abnormal results. Abnormal findings can be summarized. Any procedures or follow-up exams that

---

Box 10-2   **Example of Cost/Benefit Ratio**

TARGET MARKETING COST/BENEFIT ANALYSIS
Target: Increase the number of dentals by 100 for a 1-month period
Cost of a basic dental procedure: $157
Cost associated with production of target:
Labor: Estimated at 3 hours, $15/hour with 20% overhead for taxes
$3 \times \$15 \times 20\% = \$54$
Postage: $0.42 \times 100 = \$42$
Paper: 0.40/paper (4 cards per paper)
   $0.40/4 = 0.10/card = 0.10 \times 100 = \$10$
Ink: $19.99/cartridge; one cartridge produces 200 postcards
$19.99/200 = 0.10/card = 0.10 \times 100 = \$10$
Labels: $19.99/500 labels = 0.04/card $0.04 \times 100 = \$4$
Total cost to target clients: $120
Cost associated with producing a basic dental:
Labor: 1 hour; $12/hour with 20% overhead for taxes
   $\$12 \times 20\% = \$14.40$ $14.40
Drugs: $5.50
Equipment use $54
Overhead (10%) $15.70
Total cost associated with a dental $89.60
Profit associated with 1 dental $= \$157 - \$89.60 = \$67.40$

---

may be necessary can be prioritized for the client, indicating the most important procedure first. Report cards give clients something to take home. They can review the findings with other family members to better ensure that correct information is communicated. Clients tend to become overwhelmed with information in exam rooms; this will help them remember correct information and increase client compliance (Figure 10-12).

PRACTICE POINT   Exam room report cards give clients something to take home from the day's visit.

ABC Veterinary Clinic
2399 Saturn Circle
Anytown, USA 89000
555-555-5555

Maria Rogers
6454 Downtown Circle
Anytown, USA 89001   Account # 21312

"Scruffy" Rogers
Age: 9 years
Weight: 45#
Reminders: DHPP due 5/10/10
            Rabies due 5/10/11
            Heartworm Test due 5/10/09

Invoice Number: 10090
Date: 04/28/08
Dr. Nancy Dreamer

Date	Service	Unit	Extended Cost
04/28/09	Exam with Vaccinations	1	0.00
04/28/09	Distemper, Adenovirus,	1	$45.99
04/28/09	Parainfluenza, Parvo	1	
04/28/09	Strongid	1	$5.99
04/28/09	HG Puppy Kit	1	$0.00
04/28/09	Nail Trim	1	$0.00
04/28/09	Biohazard Fee	1	$3.00

	Subtotal	$54.98
	Tax 6.25%	$ 3.44
	Invoice Total	$58.42

Puppy Obedience Training Classes Begin May 15, 2009!
Call to reserve your space now!

FIGURE 10-9 Sample invoice with a marketing statement at the bottom.

Mailing owners copies of lab work results is also a form of internal marketing. A sheet can be included that summarizes abnormal results and the need to follow up. Electrocardiograms, urinalysis, ultrasounds, and bloodwork can all be sent to clients. This can also help increase client compliance because the owner may be able to better understand the abnormal results. A preprinted sheet should also be sent, informing the owner which organ each test evaluates. A brief summary may be included regarding what may be causing the abnormality (Figure 10-13).

PRACTICE POINT Sending a copy of lab work results to clients with a brief explanation of the tests performed is an internal marketing technique that will strengthen the client bond.

Special activities and open houses that celebrate certain events can market the practice to both current and prospective clients. Open houses can be used to promote

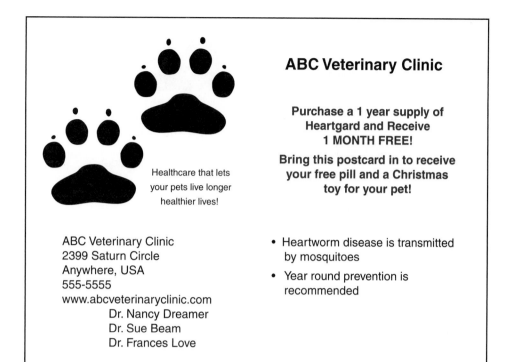

ABC Veterinary Clinic

**Purchase a 1 year supply of
Heartgard and Receive
1 MONTH FREE!**

**Bring this postcard in to receive
your free pill and a Christmas
toy for your pet!**

Healthcare that lets
your pets live longer
healthier lives!

ABC Veterinary Clinic
2399 Saturn Circle
Anywhere, USA
555-5555
www.abcveterinaryclinic.com
Dr. Nancy Dreamer
Dr. Sue Beam
Dr. Frances Love

- Heartworm disease is transmitted
  by mosquitoes
- Year round prevention is
  recommended

FIGURE 10-10 Sample heartworm preventive reminder.

National Pet Week, National Veterinary Technician Week, the practice anniversary, the welcoming of a new doctor, or the renovation of the practice.

Open houses can be simple or elaborate, depending on the budget set aside for the promotion. The American Veterinary Medical Association (AVMA), National Association of Veterinary Technicians in America (NAVTA), and veterinary manufacturers can be contacted for more information, sponsorship, and signage to help promote the celebration. Advertising helps make such events more successful (Figure 10-14).

Special events can be hosted during open houses, such as pet walks, pet shows, and talks regarding pet health. Competitions for prizes can be developed with categories such as cutest pet, longest nosed pet, or best tricks. Simple, short talks can also be given regarding nutrition, training techniques, and animal husbandry.

Internal marketing techniques can be used in many ways and should be explored to help bring the practice to the next level.

EXTERNAL MARKETING

As with direct marketing, the goal of external marketing is to advertise the practice's services to potential clients. Examples include the Yellow Pages, newspaper advertising, and Web sites and may also apply to newsletters if they are delivered to grooming shops, boarding facilities, doggy daycare centers, or pet stores. Having a large,

professional, eye-catching sign that is illuminated at night also helps promote the practice.

> **PRACTICE POINT** External marketing techniques are aimed at potential clients.

Participating in community service and activities is also a form of external marketing while helping to educate the public (Box 10-3).

The key to external marketing is to determine prospective clients and patients and use the best method to attract them. External marketing does not generally elicit immediate results. Consistent and repetitive messaging must be directed toward potential clients to obtain results; therefore, if the practice wishes to increase business, external and direct marketing approaches are recommended to achieve this goal.

Feedback mechanisms may be used to determine the effectiveness of marketing techniques. "How did you hear about us?" may be listed on a client/patient information sheet or included in a survey offered to clients after their first visit. This and other mechanisms can ultimately be used in a cost/benefit analysis to help determine which marketing techniques may or may not be used in the future.

Marketing must be kept ethical, fair, and professional. The AVMA code of ethics states that advertising by veterinarians is ethical when there are no false, deceptive, or misleading statements or claims. A false, deceptive, or misleading statement or claim is one that communicates

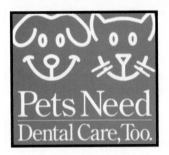

February is National Dental Month

You're invited to bring your pet in for a
FREE oral exam!

- Signs of periodontal disease include:
    - Bad bath
    - Yellow-brown crust on teeth
    - Bleeding gums
    - Tooth loss
    - Abnormal drooling
- Bacteria associated with periodontal disease may affect the liver, kidneys, and the heart!
- Schedule an appointment for your free oral exam today!

Offer good through February 20

10% of ALL dental procedures through February 26

Helping pets live longer healthier lives!

Dr. Nancy Dreamer
Dr. Sue Beam
Dr. Frances Love

ABC Veterinary Clinic
2399 Saturn Circle
Anywhere, USA
555-5555

FIGURE 10-11 Sample dental reminder.

false information or is intended, through a material omission, to leave a false impression. Testimonials or endorsements are advertising, and they should comply with the guidelines for advertising. In addition, testimonials and endorsements of professional products or services by veterinarians are considered unethical unless they comply with the following:

1. The endorser must be a bona fide user of the product or service.
2. There must be adequate substantiation that the results obtained by the endorser are representative of what veterinarians may expect in actual conditions of use.
3. Any financial, business, or other relationship between the endorser and the seller of a product or service must be fully disclosed.
4. When reprints of scientific articles are used with advertising, the reprints must remain unchanged and be presented in their entirety.

The principles that apply to advertising, testimonials, and endorsements also apply to veterinarians and their communication with clients.

Choosing how to advertise in the Yellow Pages takes extra thought and consideration. Many factors should be addressed before making a decision regarding what size of ad to purchase. The overall cost of advertising in the Yellow Pages can be expensive and is relative to the size of ad chosen. Yellow Pages advertising provides long-term advertising for practices and serves the extended community. Advertisements can range from a single line with the name and phone number of the practice to a large color, full-page display ad. Practices that are in a small area and have relatively little competition do not need large ads. Simply stating the facts is all that is needed: hours of operation, doctors on staff, species served, address, phone number, and Web site. If there are several veterinary clinics in the area, then a larger ad may be needed, adding the services that are provided and any special offers the practice may have. A large ad can be overwhelming and may cause clients to overlook it. Caution should be used when developing the ad, and all opinions should be considered before submitting the ad for publication. In some areas of the United States, several companies produce Yellow Pages books that target the same audience. Practices may have to advertise in each book; therefore a budget should be established for each publication to prevent overspending on advertising. For effective marketing, it should be determined which book is most commonly used in the area, and the most expensive ad placed with that particular company.

PRACTICE POINT Yellow Pages ads are an effective external marketing technique.

- Office tours
- Lectures
- Phone directories
- Newsletter
- Outdoor building sign
- Business cards
- Media advertising
- Open house
- Web site

Lead times can be long for each of these publications. Generally, ads must be ready for submission 6 months before publication, and any changes or additions must wait until the next publication. This can be detrimental to new businesses or those adding new doctors. Maintaining contact with the phone book sales representative may help facilitate the latest possible date to submit the ad.

Newspaper ads can come in the form of client education. Many newspapers have sections available in which a practice can purchase space and submit an article educating the general public about a particular disease. The ad may state to visit ABC Veterinary Hospital for more information. Other forms of advertising may include a boxed ad introducing a new veterinarian, service, or product. Newspaper ads can have several disadvantages, including the location of the ad in the newspaper. Ads are generally spread throughout the newspaper at the discretion of the graphic development team; this can lead to readers missing the ad due to obscure placement. Some ads can appear dated and reproduce poorly. Unfortunately, the poor quality can reflect on the value of the practice. If an ad is chosen to be run, all team members should be familiar with it.

PRACTICE POINT Newspaper articles can be informative while advertising the services the practice offers.

Community service events create a win-win situation for all those involved. The practice team members may have one or two organizations that they participate in, and in which they can involve the practice as well. The practice owners may have an organization that they wish to donate to within the community. Either way, it is free advertising for the practice and lets the community know that the veterinary team supports community events.

Some ideas of community service may include a "lump and bump" screening at the local farmers' market on Saturday mornings. A veterinarian and technician can educate potential clients about the seriousness of lumps on pets. Many people bring pets to farmers' markets; this is an excellent place to hand out literature and educate the public. Team members can also participate

in dental screenings for pets at local events; many people do not know the significance of dental disease in their pets. Attending career days at local schools is also a form of external marketing. Team members can create "kid packs" that include a surgical cap and mask as well as a business card and literature on heartworm disease or any other potential risks that are high in the area. They can be placed in a bag that has the practice information printed on it.

PRACTICE POINT Participation in community service events is an effective external marketing technique that can be personally gratifying.

Speaking at career days can have a lasting impact on children. Showing interesting radiographs and allowing children to auscultate a dog's heart can stimulate interest and help foster their education. Community service at this level is highly recommended and satisfying.

Practices may also wish to be more involved in community service events around the holidays, participating in food drives, or clothing campaigns for kids, or collecting Christmas presents for a particular family. Instead of buying gifts for each team member, the team can buy a present for a child in a homeless family that the practice adopts through a local homeless shelter. The team can take the presents to the family or shelter; seeing the surprise on a family's faces at this time of year is very rewarding! Shelters generally acknowledge contributors in a local newspaper ad after the holidays.

External marketing can be accomplished in several ways, and often at a nominal price. The goal is to increase business by attracting potential clients to the practice, but it can be rewarding at the same time.

WEB SITES

Technology has accelerated, and many clients use the Internet to search for information. Clients want information on the practice, including professional services that are offered, doctors, hours of operation, and a map to locate the office. Clients also want to be able to refill prescriptions, make appointments, and order products at any time of the day or night. They want reliable information on diseases, vaccination protocols, and procedures recommended by the practice. Web sites allow direct, indirect, and external marketing at all levels.

Web sites can be fun, educational, and a challenge, all in one. They should be visually engaging, attractive, easy to navigate, and interactive. Some practices may elect to hire a design company to develop and maintain a site; others may choose to develop and maintain a Web site themselves. Whichever the practice chooses, it must appear professional, be reliable, and be updated frequently. It should not look like any other veterinary Web site in the vicinity.

_____'s Report Card

Owner's Name _____ Date _____

Vaccination Program

❑ Up to Date
❑ Vac. due: PARVO_____; DHLP-C_____; Bordetella_____; LYME_____;FCVR/C_____; Feleuk_____; FIP_____; Rabies_____
❑ Vac. given: PARVO_____; DHLP-C_____; Bordetella_____; LYME_____;FCVR/C_____; Feleuk_____; FIP_____; Rabies_____

1. Coat & Skin
❑ Appear Normal ❑ Oily   ❑ Itchy
❑ Dull   ❑ Shedding   ❑ Parasites
❑ Scaly   ❑ Matted   ❑ Other ____
❑ Dry   ❑ Tumors   _____

2. Eyes
❑ Appear Normal   ❑ Infection
❑ Discharge   ❑ Cataract: L___ R _____
❑ Inflamed   ❑ Other _____
❑ Eyelid Deformities _____

3. Ears
❑ Appear Normal   ❑ Tumor: L___ R___
❑ Inflamed   ❑ Excessive Hair
❑ Itchy   ❑ Other _____
❑ Mites   _____

4. Nose & Throat
❑ Appear Normal   ❑ Inflamed Tonsils
❑ Nasal Discharge ❑ Enlarged Lymph Glands
❑ Inflamed Throat ❑ Other _____

5. Mouth, Teeth, Gums
❑ Appear Normal   ❑ Inflamed Lips
❑ Broken Teeth   ❑ Loose Teeth
❑ Tartar Buildup ❑ Pyorreah
❑ Tumors   ❑ Other
❑ Ulcers

6. Legs & Paws
❑ Appear Normal   ❑ Joint Problems
❑ Lameness   ❑ Nail Problems
❑ Damaged Ligaments ❑ Other _____

7. Heart
❑ Appears Normal ❑ Slow   ❑ Other ____
❑ Murmur   ❑ Fast   _____

8. Abdomen
❑ Appears Normal   ❑ Abnormal Mass
❑ Enlarged Organs ❑ Tense/Painful
❑ Fluid   ❑ Other _____

9. Lungs
❑ Appear Normal   ❑ Breathing Difficulty
❑ Abnormal Sound   ❑ Rapid Respiration
❑ Coughing   ❑ Other _____
❑ Congestion   _____

10. Gastrointestinal System
❑ Appears Normal   ❑ Abnormal Feces
❑ Excessive Gas   ❑ Parasites
❑ Vomiting Problem ❑ Other _____
❑ Anorexia   _____

11. Urogenital System
❑ Appears Normal   ❑ Enlarged Prostate
❑ Abnormal Urination ❑ Mammary Tumors
❑ Genital Discharge ❑ Anal Sacs _____
❑ Abnormal Testicles

12. Weight _____ lbs
❑ Normal Range   ❑ Thin
❑ Heavy   ❑ Other _____

13. Diet
❑ Excellent   ❑ Vitamins Needed
❑ Good   ❑ Improvement necessary

Dogs
Last Heartworm Test
Date _____
Htwm Prevention
_____
Intestinal Parasites Tested
Date _____
Flea Control
Pet _____
Yard _____
House _____

Cats
Feline Leukemia Test
Date _____ Pos Neg
Feline Aids Test
Date _____ Pos Neg
Intestine Parasites
Checked _____
Outdoors ____ Hrs/day
Flea Control
Cat _____
Home _____
_____
Drug Allergies??
_____
_____
_____

Professional Services
_____
_____
_____
_____
_____
_____
_____
_____
_____
_____
_____
_____

Special Instructions/Recommendations
_____
_____
_____
_____
_____
_____
_____
_____
_____

Examination Needed_____   Days/Months
Next Appointment _____ @____AM/PM

FIGURE 10-12 Sample exam room report card. (Courtesy American Animal Hospital Association, Lakewood, Colo.)

Bloodwork Summary

Today your pet had bloodwork completed. Below is a list of the tests that were completed, along with the organ or body part that is being evaluated with that test. You will also find a brief description of what may be causing the abnormality associated with that value. This is not a complete list and is just a summary; please ask our team members if you have any questions.

Pre-Anesthetic Bloodwork: An abbreviated profile that is recommended prior to anesthesia.

Test	Organ	Common possible causes of abnormal values
BUN	Kidney	Increased = kidney disease
CREA	Kidney	Increased = kidney disease
ALT	Liver	Increased = liver disease
SGPT	Liver	Increased = liver disease
GLU	Pancreas	Increased = diabetes, stress
Total protein	Various	Decreased = protein loss; increased = dehydration; various causes
WBC	White blood cells	Increased = infection
RBC	Red blood cells	Decreased: various
HCT	RBC volume	Decreased: limmune mediated/tick-borne disease
Platelets	Clotting function	Decreased: clotting abnormality
Urinalysis:		
Specific gravity	Kidney	Decreased: kidney disease, dehydration
WBC	Bladder	Infection
RBC	Bladder	Inflammation
Glucose	Pancreas	Diabetes
Ketones	Pancreas	Diabetes
Protein	Bladder/kidney	Protein loss
pH	Bladder	Increased or Decreased: urinary stones
Crystals	Bladder	Urinary stones
Casts	Bladder/kidney	
Bacteria	Bladder	Infection
ECG	Heart	Heart disease

FIGURE 10-13 Summary of lab work results and explanation of tests.

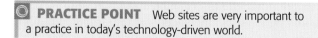 **PRACTICE POINT** Web sites are very important to a practice in today's technology-driven world.

Developing a Web Site

There are three major options for Web site creation: host the site, on-site hosting, and company-supported hosting. Hosting the site generally means that it is developed and maintained by the practice, which can be done with the practice server or by renting space on another server. Web site space is very competitive, with many companies offering space, so it is generally cheap to rent space. The pages are created using Web design software and uploaded to the server through file transfer protocol (FTP). Practices have full control over content and can update it at will. Many different Web page software applications are available. When looking for software, a top choice is one that is user friendly, has a tutorial, and has a variety of designs available to build pages. Developing a Web site is time consuming and takes practice; however, the return on investment is well worth it.

On-site hosting is an option for practices that do not wish to fully design their own Web site. Practices can manipulate predesigned Web content directly on a preexisting site or upload content to their own site. The advantage is already having predesigned content; the

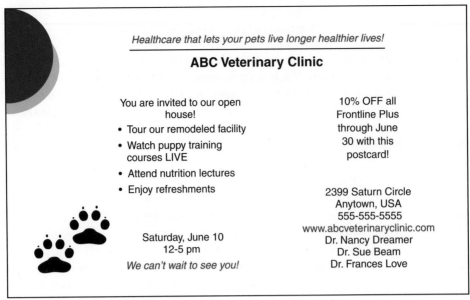

FIGURE 10-14 Open house postcard.

disadvantage is that other practices will likely have the same or similarly designed Web sites.

Company-supported Web sites are typically created by a design company and the practices may have little or no access to the content provided. Updates and changes must be done by the company. Smaller companies that employ webmasters may be able to design practice Web sites and make changes as requested by the practice relatively easily. It is up the practice to submit the information to the webmaster and to ensure that all information that has been included is correct.

PRACTICE POINT Web sites should be fun, easy to navigate, and filled with information the clients can use.

Pages should include the same design on each page. As stated above, the logo and phrase should be included on the heading of each page. Pages should be easy to navigate and have a "back" and "home" option on each.

Box 10-4 lists some important topics that can be included in Web page design. Even if a webmaster is employed to develop and maintain a site for the practice, it is still the team members who must gather information to be posted. It is also the responsibility of the team members to supply the webmaster with updated information regarding protocol changes, staff or doctor changes, and added professional services. Content is most important and cannot be delegated to a webmaster.

The introduction page is very important. A picture of the front of the building helps introduce the practice to potential clients and refamiliarizes existing clients. A welcome message is an excellent tool that allows a short summary of the products and services provided and the practice philosophy.

Box 10-4	Important Topics for Web Pages

- Hours of operation
- Doctors
- Staff members
- Achievements/awards
- Procedures
- Professional services offered
- Hot topics: diseases that are prevalent in the area
- Prescription refills
- Retail center
- Monthly special
- Community service
- Newsletter
- Pet of the month
- Client surveys
- Client testimonials
- Virtual tour
- Frequent forms
- Ask-a-tech column

A variety of pictures should be included in Web design. A site can have too much information listed and clients will skim over the information and not read it. Pictures should be strategically placed with information bordering them. They should include a variety of species, with a variety of colors and ages. Pictures must be clear and uncluttered. The software will recommend what format pictures should be saved in for best uploading.

The Web site address should be the name of the veterinary hospital if at all possible. For example, ABC Veterinary Hospital should have an Internet address of ABCVeterinaryHospital.com. This allows clients to find the address easily and also allows the hospital name to be included in the key words of the address. A URL, or uniform resource locator, is the address of the

Web site on the World Wide Web. The address is composed of numbers and periods and is unique to each site. However, the Web site must have a domain name for people to be able to locate it. Many companies sell domain names, all of which are regulated by one organization, the Internet Corporation for Assigned Names and Numbers (ICANN). This is a private nonprofit organization that manages the domain name system. A domain name may need to be purchased to secure the Web site address for the practice. If that particular name is already used by another facility, something creative should be added, such as adding the city to the address (ABCVeterinaryHospitalChicago.com).

Within the design software, the Web page allows key words to be entered that will attract potential clients to the site when they are surfing the Web. Key words that should be entered include the species the practice treats, professional services that are available, and last names of the doctors on staff. Some software versions only allow a specific number of words; therefore prioritizing the words is imperative.

All Web sites must have an email contact address; email should go to the webmaster or the practice manager in case problems or questions arise. The email address should be checked on a daily basis for any correspondence that may have arrived in the inbox.

> **PRACTICE POINT**   Hyperlinks are addresses within the Web site that direct clients to a new page, either within the Web site or on another Web site.

Web sites can also include hyperlinks, which are images or highlighted portions of a text on a Web page that are linked to other Web pages, either on the same site or another Web site. This allows clients to move to other locations within the Web site more easily, or to move to other Web sites that have been linked with the practice site. Practices may wish to provide hyperlinks to businesses that they recommend; groomers, pet shops, or boarding kennels are common hyperlinks.

Web sites should follow a three-click rule; information that clients are looking for should be found in just three clicks. Studies suggest that the longer it takes people to find information, the less likely they are to stay on the current Web site. Web sites should be informative, fun, and easy to navigate.

Pet Portals

Pet portals are third-party online marketing retailers that sell items that the practice authorizes at the price the practice sets. Although monthly rental fees are charged to the practice, these can be a large profit center for the business. The benefits of pet portals is that the practice does not have to carry the products in the office, therefore decreasing ordering, holding, and other inventory-related costs. Clients can shop online at any time and feel they can trust the products that are available on the practice's Web site.

Pharmacy refill requests can also be managed through pet portals. Clients can request prescription refills, team members can approve the refills, and the third-party company will manage the refills and send them directly to the clients. The pet portal service sends a check to the practice monthly or quarterly with the profits. Clients can also make appointments through pet portals and see their vaccination history or reminder status. Pet portals allow clients to have the interaction they want and deserve through the Internet.

Marketing the Web Site

Once the Web site has been developed, the address should be published on every business item, along with the logo and phrase. Business cards, brochures, client education materials, prescription labels, and newsletters should list the address.

> **PRACTICE POINT**   To help promote the Web site, Web addresses must be printed on everything the practice produces.

Newsletters can also direct clients to hot topics that are listed on the Web site. The Web site is a business developer and should be marketed that way. Clients need to know the site exists, and driving them to it is important. If a webmaster is being paid to maintain the Web site and pet portals are being used, the Web site must produce enough money to pay for its maintenance and upkeep.

BUSINESS CARDS

Business cards are designed to be an easy reference for clients. They should be professionally printed with minimal information. Cards with too much information appear cluttered and disorganized. The cards should include the basic information: name of the practice, address, phone number, doctors on staff, Web site address, and the practice logo and catchphrase. If the practice employs more than three doctors, more than one business card may be needed. A professional graphic designer should be consulted to create the best design for the hospital. The back of business cards can be used as appointment cards. The pet's name and appointment date can be listed on the back; this allows clients easy retrieval of both the business information and appointment time.

MAGNETS

Business cards can also be placed on magnets. Clients can place the magnets on their refrigerators. Friends and family will see these magnets and may strike up a conversation regarding the practice and the veterinary services offered. This is an excellent way to market the veterinary hospital at minimal cost. Professional printing houses can produce magnets in mass quantities, or packages of magnets can be purchased at local office supply stores, and team members can glue business cards onto the magnet. Team members may try producing their own, asking how clients and team members like them. If it is a good idea for the practice, then a mass production order can be placed.

PRACTICE BROCHURES

People only retain 20% of what they hear but 30% of what they read. Fun and colorful brochures will help clients retain the information the practice wishes to educate current and potential clients about (Box 10-5).

> **PRACTICE POINT**   Practice brochures are an effective method to educate clients about services offered.

The goal of a brochure is to state the mission of the practice, introduce the doctors (and also the staff if space allows), and list the professional services the practice offers (Figure 10-15). The purpose of the mission statement is to state the reason for the practice's existence. "ABC Animal Hospital strives to provide excellent quality and care for our patients and clients. Each animal deserves special attention at every visit," is an example of a mission statement a practice may choose to list at the beginning of a brochure.

Doctors may be listed next, with a small biography of each listed next to his or her picture. Clients like to be able to place a name with a face, and knowing something personal about the doctor helps build a trusting

relationship from the beginning. Biographies may include where the doctors went to school, how long they have been in practice, and perhaps favorite hobbies. The biography should be short and concise; too much writing can distract the reader, who will skip to the next section of the brochure.

Professional services should be listed with bullet points to emphasize the importance of each service. Current and potential clients often do not know what services veterinary practices provide. This is an excellent area to introduce them to the services that are available to help their pet live a longer life. Services should be limited to one or two words if possible.

The hours of operation are essential, along with the address, phone number, Web address, and logo. A map can also be placed on the back of the brochure in case it is passed on by a current client to a friend or co-worker.

Brochures should be trifolded to the standard brochure size. Pictures should be placed throughout the publication to break up the writing. Again, too much writing can deflect readers' attention and they will not read the brochure. This defeats the purpose of educating clients about the practice.

Brochures should be designed by a professional graphic designer to produce an eye-catching, educational brochure. The purpose of the brochure is to market the practice. Clients will relate a poorly produced brochure to poor professional veterinary service. Strive to have the best brochure possible and spend the extra money (a one-time fee) to have it done correctly.

> **PRACTICE POINT**   Practice brochures should be professionally designed and printed to portray the practice's professional image.

Professionally printed brochures are also essential. In-clinic laser printers do not print with as high a quality as printing houses do. Brochures should be printed on a thicker stock of paper than copy paper; this will also help draw attention to the brochure. Again, the extra money spent for the professional appearance pays off in the end. Clients relate high-quality brochures and marketing techniques to high-quality medicine.

CLIENT EDUCATION MATERIALS

As stated earlier, clients retain only 20% of what is told to them but 30% of material they read. It is therefore imperative to send clients home with education materials. Client education sheets may include preprinted brochures from manufacturers discussing topics such as heartworm disease or preventable diseases. They may also include information on the condition with which a particular pet has just been diagnosed.

Box 10-5   Highlights for Practice Brochures

- State-of-the-art laboratory facility
- Modern surgical facilities
- Radiology services
- Dental services
- Ophthalmology services
- PennHIP certification
- Preventive care
- Intensive care
- Oxygen therapy
- Senior pet health care
- Avian/exotic/reptiles
- Home Again microchip implantation
- Pain management
- Allergy testing
- Artificial insemination
- Early drop-off service
- Variety of specialty foods, including Science Diet, Waltham, and Purina

Method of Payment

Payment is expected at time of service. We accept cash, personal checks, and major credit cards. We also offer Care Credit, a credit card used exclusively for veterinary services. Simply fill out an application with our receptionist and you will be notified within the hour if you are accepted.

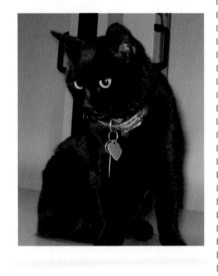

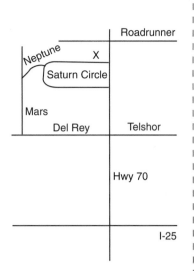

Roadrunner

Neptune   X

Saturn Circle

Mars

Del Rey   Telshor

Hwy 70

I-25

2399 Saturn Circle
Anywhere, USA
555-555-5555
www.abcveterinaryclinic.com

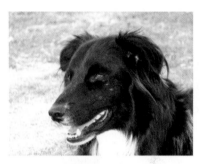

**ABC
Veterinary
Clinic**

Complete Healthcare for your pet

FIGURE 10-15 Sample practice marketing brochure.

Some veterinary practice software produces such handouts with the client and pet names, the practice name, the doctor that is seeing the patient, and the date of diagnosis. These are informative sheets that explain the disease, its symptoms, and the possible treatments. They are professional in appearance, easy to read, and quick to produce. If the practice does not have software to produce such handouts, then materials may need to be produced by team members (Figure 10-16).

When creating such pieces, it is important to keep in mind that they must appear professional, be error free, and contain language that clients can understand. They should be short, simple, and easy to read. If clients do not understand the words or if the brochure is too long, clients may toss the information to the side and not read the material once they have arrived home. All client education materials should have the practice name, address, phone number, and Web address included at the top of the sheet. Some client education sheets may need to be modified when new products or procedures have been developed; it is important to review the materials on a yearly basis looking for needed changes. Practices do not

want to make one recommendation when the information they hand out recommends another (Figure 10-17).

> **PRACTICE POINT** Client education materials must be reviewed annually, making changes as needed.

Clients will also share materials with other family members once they have arrived home. Medicine confuses many people, and they may be unable to explain the disease, diagnosis, or medications to others once they have left the practice. If it is in writing, the confusion decreases, communication is clearer, and fewer mistakes will made by the client. Clients will also be more likely to follow and accept recommendations because they understand the disease and the treatment options. Practices cannot provide enough education to clients; practices should strive to send every client home with at least one piece of client education material to help improve client knowledge and compliance. Any documents sent home with clients must be recorded for future referencing.

Welcome!

Welcome to ABC Veterinary Clinic! Our caring staff is here to provide your pet with the highest quality of surgery and medical care. We take pride in providing an environment that is safe, efficient, and friendly for you and your pet. That's why your thoughts are important to us. You know your pet best, so please advise us of any changes your pet may be experiencing, and please ask any questions!

Meet our doctors!

Nancy Dreamer, DVM

Sue Beam, DVM

Frances Love, DVM

Services Provided

- **State-of-the-Art Laboratory Facility**
- **Modern Surgical Facilities**
- **Radiology Services**
- **Dental Services**
- **Ophthalmology Services**
- **Preventative Care**
- **Intensive Care**
- **Oxygen Therapy**
- **Senior Pet Healthcare**
- **Avian/Exotic/Reptile Care**
- **Microchip Implantation**
- **Pain Management**
- **Allergy Testing**
- **Early Drop-Off Service Available**
- **Variety of Specialty Foods, Including Science Diet, Waltham, and Purina**

Avian/Exotic Reptile Medicine

Many diseases common in birds, exotics, and reptiles are not readily apparent until they have reached an advanced stage. Our emphasis is on preventative healthcare through proper nutrition and early detection of disease through diagnostic lab work.

Annual Exams

Yearly physical exams are important to your pet's health. These exams may detect diseases or health conditions that you may be unaware of. During physical exams we evaluate your pet's history and exposure rate, and we will recommend a vaccine protocol tailored to your pet's particular needs.

Heartworm Prevention

We recommend year-round heartworm prevention for all dogs and outdoor cats. Please ask for more information.

Mon-Thur: 8:00 am-7:00 pm
Fri: 8:00 am-4:00 pm
Emergencies are seen at
Veterinary Emergency
Services: 222-9098

FIGURE 10-15, cont'd

ON-HOLD MESSAGING

When clients are placed on hold, time seems to pass slowly. The client may only be on hold for 1 minute, but it seems like 5 minutes! It makes sense to be able to use this time to advertise the services the practice offers. This can be accomplished in several ways. Several companies produce CDs that can be played on a system while clients are on hold. Messages can be developed specifically for the practice and include the practice name as well as the names of the doctors. New messages are produced on a quarterly basis and can change with the seasons. Other CDs may have up to 80 different messages that can be chosen from, and the practice can pick the top 40 to play through the system. Topics may include heartworm disease, special diets, special procedures, dentals, antifreeze toxicity, chocolate toxicity, heat stroke, or plant poisonings. The choice is unlimited and special CDs can be made for each individual practice.

The practice can purchase a one-disk CD player/receiver unit that allows programming. This programming allows the practice to choose the messages to be played and repeats itself when finished playing. The CD plays constantly; therefore, each time a call is placed on hold, the caller will hear a different message. The CD player is plugged into the central phone system, and the volume can be adjusted from the receiver. It is imperative that the message be at the correct volume. If it is too loud, clients will pull the phone away from their ears and not listen to the message; if it is too quiet, they will not be able to hear the message. Team members can call the first phone line of the clinic and place it on hold; while on hold and listening to the message, the volume can be adjusted.

> **PRACTICE POINT** On-hold messaging is an effective internal and external marketing technique.

DONATIONS

Many schools, organizations, and individuals will seek donations for events they are sponsoring or attending. Although donations to local events and organizations go

Account number:	Patient:	Age:
Phone number:	Species:	Sex:
	Breed:	Tag:
	Color:	Weight:
	Doctor:	

ANAL SAC DISEASE

What are the anal sacs?

Popularly called anal glands, these are two small pouches located on either side of the anus at approximately the four o'clock and eight o'clock positions. The sacs are lined with numerous specialized sebaceous (sweat) glands that produce a foul-smelling secretion. Each sac is connected to the outside by a small duct that opens just inside the anus.

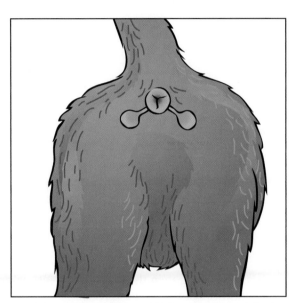

What is their function?

The secretion acts as a territorial marker—a dog's calling card. The sacs are present in both male and female dogs and are normally emptied when the dog defecates. This is why dogs are so interested in smelling one another's feces.

Why are the anal sacs causing a problem in my dog?

Anal sac disease is very common in dogs. The sacs frequently become impacted, usually due to blockage of the ducts. The secretion within the impacted sacs will thicken and the sacs will become swollen and distended. It is then painful for your dog to pass feces. The secreted material within the anal sacs forms an ideal medium for bacterial growth, allowing abscesses to form. Pain increases and sometimes a red, hot swelling will appear on one or both sides of the anus at the site of abscessation. If the abscess bursts, it will release a quantity of greenish yellow or bloody pus. If left untreated, the infection can quickly spread and cause severe damage to the anus and rectum.

How will I know if my dog has anal sac problems?

The first sign is often scooting or dragging the rear along the ground. There may be excessive licking or biting, often at the root of the tail rather than the anal area. Anal sac impaction and infection is very painful. Even normally gentle dogs may snap or growl if you touch the tail or anus when they have anal sac disease. If the anal sac ruptures, you may see blood or pus draining from the rectum.

What should I do?

Problems with the anal gland are common in all dogs, regardless of size or breed. If you are concerned that your pet may have an anal sac problem, call your veterinarian at once. Treatment for impaction involves flushing and removal of the solidified material. Since this condition is painful, many pets will require a sedative or an anesthetic for this treatment.

FIGURE 10-16 Sample client education flyer. (Courtesy Lifelearn, Guelph, Ont, Canada.)

to good causes, a predetermined amount should be set aside in the budget each year. It is very easy to go over budget when donating because many students are great at pleading their cases. Spreading the donation budget over a 12-month period will help prevent the practice from donating more than it can afford.

In exchange for donations, it is reasonable to expect some advertising. Some schools may place the contributor's name on a T-shirt or calendar, or recognize larger contributions at sporting events.

When a donation is given to a nonprofit organization, a receipt should be generated for the practice. This receipt should be kept for year-end tax purposes. Donations are an excellent source of external marketing, but a maximum amount should be set each year.

ABC Veterinary Clinic
2399 Saturn Circle
Anytown, USA
555-555-5555
www.abcveterinaryclinic.com

Dr. Nancy Dreamer, Dr. Sue Beam , Dr. Frances Love

Postoperative Drain Placement Care

A drain was placed in your pet today to help the wound heal from the inside out. Drainage from the site will occur around the drain. Please keep the area as clean as possible.

- Place a warm, soapy washcloth over the drain area. Leave on area for 5 minutes. This will help loosen drainage material on the skin.
- Wipe away all drainage, crusts, or scabs that may be on the skin and around the tube.
- Slightly pull the tube up and down.
- Clean the area twice daily.

From 3 to 5 Days after the drain tube has been placed, you will return to our clinic to have it removed. Once removed,

- Continue to use a warm, soapy washcloth to keep the area clean.
- Remove scabs that have formed on the area so that the wound can heal from the inside out.
- Continue cleaning the wound twice daily for 3 days after drain removal.

FIGURE 10-17 Sample in-house client education sheet.

GIFT CERTIFICATES

As with donations, gift certificates can be created to give to nonprofit charities for door prizes, raffles, or drawings. Charities are grateful that the practice would donate gift certificates; in reality, potential clients may or may not use the gift certificates they have won. The practice is the winner in this situation. The name of the practice is announced several times, and they will receive a receipt for the total value of the gift certificates that were given to the organization. The practice may gain a new client, and there is no loss if a gift certificate is not used (Figure 10-18).

> **PRACTICE POINT** Gift certificates can be more effective than donations to nonprofit organizations.

Gift certificates can be used to give away services or products. One example is to print a gift certificate for a yearly exam and vaccines. When a client uses this certificate, he or she is likely to purchase more services or products. He may choose to have a heartworm test and purchase heartworm preventive while at the practice, or may add a collar and a leash while checking out at the counter. Although the exam and vaccines were provided at no charge, the practice made a profit on the additional services and products the client chose. If the recipient is a new client, then the practice has just gained a new client through the gift certificate.

IMPLEMENTING A MARKETING AND TRAINING PROGRAM FOR TEAM MEMBERS

Marketing techniques will not overcome the effects of poor client relations within a practice. Unless effective client communication and client orientation are practiced on a client-by-client basis, marketing will be unsuccessful. The exam room is the center of marketing efforts. Practices must develop consistent protocols and deliver the same message. This same message must be repeated several times in the same visit for the client to retain the information.

> **PRACTICE POINT** Repetitive, consistent information must be provided to clients to increase client compliance.

Once communication and client education have been mastered, then helping team members to focus on and understand the human-animal bond is a great place to start developing marketing skills. Once team members understand the needs and wants of clients, they can become better communicators. Team members must believe in the services they are recommending; they should want

ABC Veterinary Clinic

Gift Certificate

2399 Saturn Circle
Anywhere, USA
555-555-5555

Dr. Nancy Dreamer
Dr. Sue Beam
Dr. Frances Love

The 2010 Pet Expo and Showdown

This certificate entitles you to vaccines and a yearly exam for one pet

Authorized by _____ Number _____ Expires _____

Certificate is not redeemable for cash   www.abcveterinaryclinic.com

FIGURE 10-18 Sample gift certificate.

to complete those services for their own pets. If they do not follow recommendations for themselves, they will not be successful at recommending them to clients, nor will clients accept the recommendations.

Listening to clients is another key component to effective marketing programs. If teams do not listen to clients, they will not understand what their needs are. This ultimately leads to client dissatisfaction and decreased compliance. Client needs and wants may include professional services as well as emotional and consumer needs.

Positive body language is just as effective as listening. Team members should have open arms, wear smiles on their faces, and make eye contact. Folded arms and frowns will prevent clients from asking questions and create a negative atmosphere. Lack of eye contact shows a lack of confidence in the recommendation and can result in client refusal of the service. If possible, maintain physical neutrality; if the client is standing, the team member should also be standing while speaking the client. If a client is sitting, the team member should sit next to the client to prevent speaking (physically) down to him or her.

Assertive marketing can be defined as providing clients with the information they need to accept the practice recommendations. Team members should provide the facts about and benefits of the recommended service. Assertive marketing techniques can include showing advantages for the pet and the client, along with explaining the reason for providing the procedure now rather than later, and detailing the consequences of not accepting the recommendation.

Team members should not be shy when making recommendations. Powerful words can be used in conversation. For example, "Your pet needs bloodwork," or "Your pet deserves a dental," will usually cause clients to accept the recommendation. Team members

should never be shy or embarrassed about the recommendation they are making; if they are, they need to be educated on the importance of the service they are providing.

SEIZE THE OPPORTUNITY!

Marketing techniques give the practice the ability to inform the community what the practice is about. Practices should take the opportunity to provide current and potential clients with information regarding veterinary services and recognize the team for their unique abilities. Practices must stand out in the crowd and separate themselves from the rest of the pack. Simply providing veterinary services is no longer good enough. Teams must be creative, informative, and compassionate to help the practice excel at the next level. All these goals can be achieved through some degree of marketing. A professional graphic designer and webmaster can help practices appear more professional, which increases the value to the client. Seize the opportunity while the opportunity exists!

VETERINARY PRACTICE and the LAW

When marketing products or procedures, it is unethical for veterinarians to promote, sell, prescribe, dispense, or use secret remedies or any other product for which they do not know the ingredient formula. It is also unethical for veterinarians to use or permit the use of their names, signatures, or professional status in connection with the resale of ethical products in a manner that violates those directions or conditions specified by the manufacturer to ensure the safe and efficacious use of the product. Veterinarians cannot prescribe or dispense prescription products in the absence of a valid client-patient relationship.

Self-Evaluation Questions

1. What is internal marketing? Give an example.
2. What is external marketing? Give an example.
3. What example can be applied to both internal and external marketing?
4. Why is a Web site essential in today's market?
5. What information should be included in client education materials?
6. Why should a practice be branded?
7. What is a pet portal?
8. What is the purpose of reminders and recalls?
9. Why is indirect marketing so important?
10. How would a practice brochure benefit the practice?

Recommended Reading

Heinke MM: *Practice made perfect: a guide to veterinary practice management*, Lakewood, CO, 2001, AAHA Press.

Massonnier SP: *Marketing your veterinary practice II*, St Louis, 1997, Mosby.

McCurnin D: *Veterinary practice management*, Philadelphia, 1988, JB Lippincott.

Opperman M: *The art of veterinary practice management*, Lenexa, KS, 1999, Veterinary Medicine Publishing Group.

Remillard J: Essentials of internal practice promotion. In Chubb D (ed): *Business management for the veterinary practice*, Denver, CO, 1995, Chubb Communications.

Sheridan JP, McCafferty O: *The business of veterinary practice*, Tarrytown, NY, 1993, Pergamon Press.

Communication Management

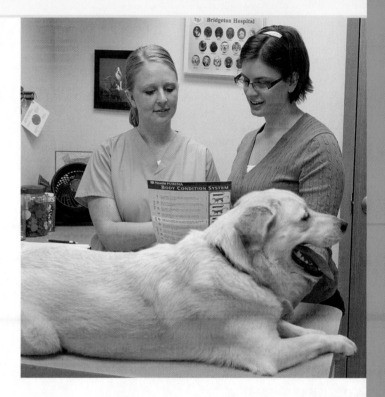

Clients drive the practice; the team takes the practice to the next level. Without clients, practices cannot make the next level. Client communication is essential to the successful practice and must be the primary commitment of all team members. Client communication involves speaking with, educating, listening, and understanding client wants and needs. If client satisfaction is not met, clients will not return. Not only will they not return, they will tell 10 people why they were not satisfied with the practice.

There are many barriers to client communication, and team members must develop methods to overcome these barriers. Some barriers may exist because of ethnicity, gender, or language differences. Other barriers may be factors that are out of the practice's control: the client may be having a financially difficult time, suffering from a medical condition, or experiencing a divorce or loss of a family member. Whatever the barrier is, methods exist to help clients understand what their pets need for medical treatment. Estimates should always be created for clients because this is the top complaint filed with state veterinary boards. Clients do not know what the charge or the final outcome of the case is going to be. If clients are fully advised of the services their pets need and they understand the value of the service, receive an estimate, and are consistently updated with changes, their satisfaction level will be met.

The "verbal image" of team members is critical to client communication. If a team member appears to lack confidence in recommendations, does not have the information to answer client questions, or has decreased levels of eye contact, the recommendations made will likely not be accepted. Team members must be confident in their recommendations, provide information to back up the recommendation, make eye contact, and have confident body posture. Techniques can be implemented to strengthen each team member's verbal image and body language.

Clients undergoing the grieving process experience a number of emotions that may be addressed by the veterinary health care team member. The human-animal bond develops over time and is strong, which explains why clients experience such pain with the loss of a pet. Team members can help clients through this incredibly tough time by providing emotional support.

Client Communications

Chapter Outline

Learning Objectives

Mastery of the content in this chapter will enable the reader to:
- Describe the importance of written client materials.
- Describe the importance of professional verbal skills.
- List methods used to communicate in a positive, professional manner.
- Identify methods used to educate clients with a variety of techniques.
- Describe the importance of providing estimates for clients.
- Define client needs.
- Clarify barriers that prevent effective client communication.
- List methods that can improve verbal image.

Key Terms

Body Language
Client Communication
Client Compliance
Client Grievances

Client Retention
Client Survey
Estimates
Informational Brochure

Recalls
Reminders
Verbal Image

Communication is one of the most important aspects of working with veterinary clients. It is extremely important that clients fully understand procedures that are being performed on their pets. They must also be educated on the proper care of their animals throughout the various life stages. All of this must be relayed in a professional manner.

Client communication comes in a variety of forms. It starts in the front office with the reception team. Greeting clients as they enter the practice communicates that the staff acknowledges their presence. Communication should occur in a positive, friendly manner, which enhances the practice image. Communication includes both verbal and written forms in the exam rooms. The veterinarians, technicians, and assistants must educate the client with words that can be understood, but must take care to not offend. Many clients want to learn the information but do not understand medical terminology. The amount of information given to clients can be based on the clients' knowledge and skill (Figure 11-1).

Written communication includes all client education materials. Clients should take home information with every visit. After puppy and kitten exams, clients should be sent home with material informing them about internal parasites and vaccination schedules. Clients bringing pets in for follow-up booster examinations may be sent home with information on nutrition as well as on the benefits of spaying and neutering. The last visit may include information on the prevention of obesity and dental disease. Yearly exam patients may need to be educated on weight-loss programs and nutritional and behavioral issues. Senior patients should be educated on the importance of monitoring bloodwork and frequent,

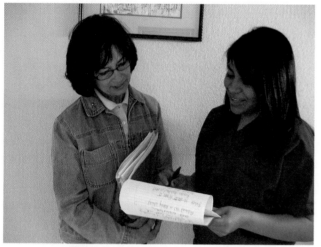

FIGURE 11-1 A technician educating a client.

regular exams. Each client should receive a report card explaining the normal and abnormal findings for his or her pet and what follow-up procedures or treatments are recommended (see Figure 10-11).

Surgical patients must receive postoperative discharge instructions. These instructions may vary by procedure, but all clients must be informed as to when to start food, medications, and activity.

Boarding clients will appreciate receiving report cards on their pets, which may include information on the pets' appetite, activity level, and attitude (Figure 11-2).

Any patient that is diagnosed with a disease or condition should be given information to take home and review regarding the disease and any treatments available. If the clients have any questions, they can call the practice and verify information before scheduling an appointment for the treatment.

VERBAL AND WRITTEN SKILLS

Team members should be able to communicate well with clients verbally. Specific words may be chosen when talking with clients to project the professional

---

Report Card

For _____   Arrival _____

Date _____   Departure _____

How I Ate:

_____ I devoured my food!

_____ I ate some of my food.

_____ I didn't feel like eating much.

My personality:

_____ I was very friendly.

_____ I was shy.

_____ I was quiet.

_____ I was talkative.

How I Played:

_____ I was so excited, I played like crazy.

_____ I was shy.

_____ It took me awhile to feel comfortable.

_____ I need to work on my "petiquette."

Potty Time:

_____ I went regularly.

_____ I went infrequently.

My Behavior Was:

_____ **A**bsolutely wonderful!

_____ **B**etter than most.

_____ **C**ould have been better.

_____ **D**id my best.

_____ **F**orget it. I will be good next time!

Comments: _____

_____

_____

_____

_____

_____

Thank you for boarding with us.

FIGURE 11-2 Sample boarding report card.

image of the practice. Lower and deeper voice tones make team members appear more confident and authoritative, whereas high-pitched tones sound insecure and immature. With practice, deeper tones can be established, enhancing each team member's value. Chapter 2 discusses telephone etiquette and effective voice tones as well as how the speed of talking can affect a conversation. Client perception starts when a call is placed to the practice and is definitely affected by the tone of the conversation.

> **PRACTICE POINT** Role-play client education topics to enhance the verbal image of team members.

Employees should role-play client education topics. Many employees do not realize the number of times filler sounds such as "um" are in a sentence until they are counted. A team member may also record a conversation and listen to the recording. Listening to one another is an excellent training tool. Reducing the number of "ums" in a sentence will increase client trust and compliance. Enhancing the staff's verbal skills will help take the veterinary practice to the next level.

Clients will always have questions about their pets' health care. It is important to remember that clients are asking these questions because they do not know the answers; team members must not judge clients for asking questions. Team members forget that topics that are very basic to the team are new to an owner. Teams must not get frustrated answering these questions for clients. A client service manual is suggested to help new team members learn the appropriate answers to client questions. This includes correct verbiage, correct pronunciation, and the skill to respond to such questions. Chapter 23 covers the most common diseases and procedures that team members should be familiar with. This will help improve client communication.

Once a team member has gained experience and knowledge about veterinary medicine, his or her confidence is noted by the client. Clients begin to feel they can trust the information that has been provided to them, and they develop a trusting relationship with that team member. Team member confidence is a great asset to the practice and should be a top training priority for all employees. Professional appearance also helps increase confidence; clean, unwrinkled uniforms will help project authority and credibility. Team members who are compassionate, concerned, and interested in patients come across as more confident and will stimulate clients to ask more questions.

When delivering bad news to clients, it should be done in a professional, tactful environment. Team members should be empathetic and expect clients to be upset, angry, or emotional. Being prepared for the situation will help the team member diffuse it. Many times, it is the veterinarian that will deliver the news; however, team members should be ready in case they need to take the place of the doctor. Team members should speak slowly and listen to the clients' response. Client may not fully understand the conversation; therefore it may be necessary to repeat the information. Written information should also be sent home with clients to ensure complete understanding.

> **PRACTICE POINT** Clients receiving bad news should be taken to a quiet, comforting room to speak with the doctor.

Letter Etiquette

It is extremely important that staff members have excellent writing skills. Chapter 14 reviews the importance of completing medical records in a professional, legible manner. Team members must be able to verbally communicate procedures with clients, along with writing professional, educational, and clear discharge instructions for owners. The goal of written communications is to prevent miscommunications before they occur, prevent the owner from asking the same questions several times, and represent the business, ultimately increasing sales and professional services.

> **PRACTICE POINT** Hospital communications depend on the excellent verbal and written communication skills of every team member.

Team members must be able to write effective letters for different aspects of the practice. Collections letters, vaccine reaction letters, and letters of acclimation are just few letters that a doctor may request. Pets that have had a severe vaccine reaction in the past may have been advised to withhold vaccinations in the future. A letter may be required by the city or county as to why the client is not in compliance with the law. Airlines may require a letter of acclimation, indicating that a pet is healthy enough to fly at temperatures below 40° F or higher than 80° F. It is important to only state the facts; do not embellish to make the letter longer.

Letters should include the date, the client's name, the pet's name, and the doctor's name. The pet's species, gender, and whether it has been altered may need to be added depending on the letter. The problem needs to be addressed, along with the resolution. The doctor can then sign the letter. Letters should be kept short and to the point.

Email Etiquette

Correspondence by email is becoming a popular choice of communication for clients. Email etiquette is just as important as letter writing and verbal skills. It must always be remembered that email can go anywhere, to anyone. Therefore emails should be kept short and sweet. If a consultation is needed, the client should be advised to make an appointment with a veterinarian to discuss the case. Clients may take suggestions in email as insults, starting a terrible line of communications. Emotions cannot be read in email; therefore a face-to-face visit is much more beneficial. On the business side of email, clients are not charged for the time the team or a veterinarian spends responding to emails.

CLIENT COMPLIANCE

There are many categories that contribute to client compliance. Client compliance is defined as the number or percentage of clients who accept recommendations made by the veterinary health care team. Verbal and written skills, reminders and recalls, marketing, education, and understanding client and patient needs are only a few areas that contribute to client compliance.

Before client compliance can develop, clients must receive excellent service. They need to have a reason to return to the veterinary practice. Trust, satisfaction, and quality of service must be established; the veterinarian-client relationship can span a lifetime and serve a variety of pets. Positive attitudes from team members who believe in the medicine the practice provides radiates to clients. Client trust can be encouraged, resulting in higher client compliance. Excellent medicine and a team-based veterinary practice provide client satisfaction and a high quality of service.

Client compliance can be increased by verbal and written communications. Informing clients about diseases and treatment protocols encourages owners to accept recommendations. This information comes in the form of discussions with the client as well as any client education material available. Following up on the case can also increase compliance, along with reminders that are sent out on a regular basis.

> **PRACTICE POINT** Client education is the driving force of client compliance.

Reminders and Recall Systems

Many software programs can automatically generate reminders and recalls for the veterinary team. Smaller practices may handwrite reminders on a monthly basis. Reminders are simply that; they remind owners that pets are due for a procedure. Practices may elect to send out reminders for a variety of services, including yearly exams and/or vaccines (based on the current vaccination protocol), heartworm testing, and/or a fecal analysis (depending on the location of the practice in the United States). Practices may also send out reminders for yearly laboratory work, including testing for hypothyroidism, phenobarbital levels, or bile acids for patients that are on long-term medications that may have potential side effects if not monitored closely. From a marketing perspective, hospitals may send out reminders for senior care exams or dental month (see Chapter 10). Communications can also be sent to remind clients to refill their pets' medication, including heartworm preventive and medications that treat hypothyroidism or hyperthyroidism, seizures, and/or allergies (Figures 11-3 and 11-4).

Reminders must be clear, concise, and to the point. If a client makes an appointment for an exam, the reminder must clearly indicate that necessity; otherwise a client may walk into the practice without an appointment for an examination. Grammar and spelling must be correct,

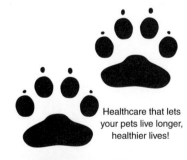

ABC Veterinary Clinic

Healthcare that lets your pets live longer, healthier lives!

ABC Veterinary Clinic
1234 Saturn Circle
Anytown, MN 12345
555-555-5555
www.abcveterinaryclinic.com

Dr. Nancy Dreamer
Dr. Sue Beam
Dr. Frances Love

- All Heartworm Preventive Is 10% OFF!
- Ask About the New Pro-Heart Injection!

10% OFF!

Our records indicate that your pet(s) are due for a refill of heartworm preventive. Come into our office by May 31 and receive 10% off your prescription refill.
Call your refill in before arriving and it will be ready for pickup.

FIGURE 11-3 Reminder cards are a good way to maintain client relationships.

and the message must be inviting. A simple reminder can help maintain the relationship that the practice has worked hard to establish with a client.

Reminder cards can be ordered from a variety of software companies or supply houses. Some systems may require a specific type of card to fit system or printer requirements; however, a variety of choices are available to choose from. Dogs, cats, puppies, and horses posing in different outfits and performing different tricks should grab a client's attention. Chapter 10 includes more helpful reminder ideas. Manufacturers also supply reminders for their particular product or service. Merial, Novartis, and Pfizer supply reminders for their vaccines, heartworm preventives, and products.

> **PRACTICE POINT** Statements on reminders should be short, sweet, and to the point. They should clearly indicate that the client needs to make an appointment for his or her pet.

Reminders can also come in the form of phone calls. Clients should be called the day before their appointments to remind them of surgical procedures or appointments that have been scheduled. Clients can be reminded of the surgical protocol to follow at that time as well. Those whose pets are due for yearly exams, lab work, and vaccinations should also be called as a friendly reminder. If a client needs to reschedule his or her appointment, it can be done at that time, allowing the team to fill the appointment spot with another patient.

Reminder systems (whether manual or automatic) must be programmed to remove patients once they have died. It is emotionally distressing for a client to receive a reminder for a pet that has died, especially if the loss occurred at the veterinary hospital. It is not uncommon for a pet to suddenly die at home and for the owner not to inform the hospital of the death until receiving an appointment reminder. Team members should be empathetic, apologize, and guarantee that the owner will not receive another reminder.

In today's high-tech world, veterinary practices can send reminders by email, text messages, and cell phones. This is a relatively inexpensive way to connect with clients and remind them of services that are due for their pets. Computer software systems can be programmed to send either printed cards or email reminders, allowing many reminders to be sent at once. Follow-up reminders can then be generated for those who did not respond to the initial notice.

Recalls are lists that are generated by veterinary software systems to remind staff to call certain clients to check on patients (Figure 11-5). Recalls can be created for surgical patients, pets that have received vaccines, or any patient that has been in the hospital for a period of time. Software systems allow team members to set a specific number of days for the recall to be generated. Certain charged services can also be linked to a recall generator, thereby creating a recall each time one of those services is entered. Each day, reception teams can print lists and call clients to see how patients are progressing. This is a great time to ensure that the client was satisfied with the services and answer any remaining questions. If the client has any concerns or the pet has not progressed as expected, an appointment can be made with a specific doctor to recheck the patient. Always document in the record the telephone conversation and how the pet is recovering. This allows team

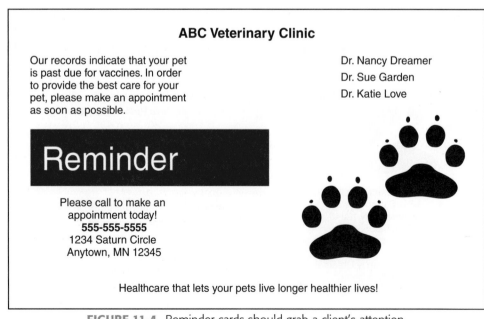

FIGURE 11-4, Reminder cards should grab a client's attention.

Recall List					ABC Animal Clinic
Printed for dates 3/3/09-3/3/09					
Account #	Client	Patient	Phone	Procedure	Doctor
428	Sharon Bean	Miss Kitty	123-458-0901	Fe OVH	ND
17266	Steve Doolittle	Lucky	345-234-1234	K9 OVH	ND
17266	Steve Doolittle	Cookie	345-234-1234	K9 OVH	ND
3427	Desiree Cloud	Scamp	456-123-1234	Dental	SM
6785	Nancy Shade	Wheeler	123-567-8901	K9 OVH	ND

FIGURE 11-5 Recall lists remind staff members to call and check on patients.

members to follow the case if the client needs to return for a recheck.

Manual recall lists can also be generated by practices that do not use specialized software. A list can be kept in a small notebook with the client information and a brief reminder of the procedure. This is a well-organized way in which to help follow up with clients. Again, appointments can be made at this time if needed, and these conversations must be documented in the record.

> **PRACTICE POINT** Recalls are generated to help team members follow up on patient care.

Educational Information

There are many ideas that can increase client compliance, but it must be reiterated that client compliance starts with client education. If a client does not understand a procedure or have a trusting relationship with a veterinary hospital, the recommendations will not be followed. Educational information can come in a variety of forms; speaking with the client, writing information down, and/or printing out information for the client to take home are the most efficient methods for providing information (Figures 11-6 and 11-7). Clients will also search the Internet to get more information. Today's Internet is full of information; however, it is sometimes incorrect. Veterinary practices must understand the client is being proactive on the pet's account in searching for current information; a practice must embrace the idea and filter the information as much as possible. Providing clients with written materials to take home and read will increase their knowledge and trust of the veterinary practice (Figure 11-8). The more information that is received from the practice, the less they will search on the Internet. Clients will not remember all the information they were advised of while they were in the clinic. The more printed information they receive, the more they will retain once they get home and review it. Team members should be available to answer basic client questions; once the client has gained enough

experience on the topic, a veterinarian may be needed to answer further questions.

Practices can print customized brochures, handouts, and personalized client instructions to provide the most current and correct information to clients. Veterinary software programs may have educational materials that print the client and doctor names; a specific topic is entered into the computer and the document is printed (Figures 11-9 and 11-10). The benefit to these computer-based documents is the customization that can be done to make them truly client-oriented pieces of material. Many client education manuals are also available for purchase from educational companies. These manuals are generally loosely bound in a binder; the information needed can be removed and copied, then returned to the binder (Figure 11-9, *B*). Practices can also produce brochures that are unique to the individual practice. Graphic designers can create professional-looking brochures for a nominal fee. Team members with design experience can use Microsoft Publisher to produce professional-looking brochures and print them on a small color printer in the office. Only a small number of brochures should be printed so that changes can be made to the brochure since procedures may change throughout the course of the year. Chapter 10 includes more information on producing a quality educational brochure.

Messages may need to be repeated several times for clients to retain the information. Clients tend to suffer from sensory overload with all the information they receive in a veterinary practice; therefore it is imperative that information be concise, correct, and simple to read. Studies indicate that 90% of new information learned will be lost within 30 minutes if not reinforced. Repeat, repeat, repeat. The more clients hear and read a message, the more they will retain the information.

Manufacturers also provide a variety of professional posters that relate to current medical topics; these come at no charge to practices that use their products (Figure 11-11). These posters can be changed on a regular basis, providing a new look to the clients each time they arrive at the practice.

Dental Report Card

Last name_____ Pet _____ Date _____

Just like human beings, dogs are susceptible to plaque and tartar buildup that can lead to gingivitis and periodontitis, a chronic form of the disease that can be painful.

Periodontal disease, which includes gingivitis and periodontitis, is an inflammation and/or infection of the gums and bone around a dog's teeth. It is caused by bacteria that accumulate in the mouth, forming soft plaque that later hardens into tartar. If untreated, periodontal disease can eventually lead to tooth loss.

Over time, plaque and tartar buildup can lead to inflammation of the gums around the dog's teeth: **gingivitis.**

Periodontitis is a potentially irreversible infection that, if left untreated, can result in the destruction of gum and bone and other tissues around the teeth. In most severe cases, periodontitis can ultimately lead to loss of teeth, fracture of the jawbones, and other serious consequences that can dramatically affect quality of life and overall health. Whenever possible, preventing disease is preferable to treating it!

Dental disease can also lead to cardiac and/or kidney disease. The bacteria that collect in your pet's mouth also circulate throughout the body, contributing to a variety of other diseases.

The good news is that periodontal disease can be prevented with a good dental care program, including:

- Daily home oral care: brushing your pet's teeth can be fun!
- Dental toys: rope toys, rawhides that are dissolvable, and Denta-Bones. Remember, hard toys can fracture teeth. Any chew toy should be slightly pliable.
- NEVER give you pet beef, chicken, or pork bones!
- Veterinary dental cleaning as advised.

Stage 1—Gingivitis

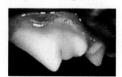

Plaque and tartar buildup can lead to an infection causing inflammation of the gums around the dog's teeth. Gum tissue around the teeth can become inflamed and swollen.

Stage 2—Mild Periodontitis

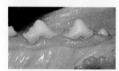

Inflammation progresses to an infection that starts to destroy gum and bone tissue around the teeth. This can lead to discomfort for the dog, and bad breath may be noticeable.

Stage 3—Moderate Periodontitis

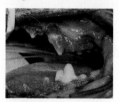

The continuing infection destroys more tissue around the teeth, often causing bleeding of gums and loosening of teeth. The discomfort and pain can affect eating habits.

Stage 4—Severe Periodontitis

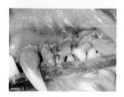

Extensive infection is tearing down even more of the attachment tissues (gum and bone). Teeth are at risk of being lost.

FIGURE 11-6 Client education is important to client compliance.

> **⊙ PRACTICE POINT**   Nonverbal communication can affect client compliance.

BODY LANGUAGE

Being able to read and understand a client helps to increase client compliance. Trust and compliance can also be built when clients are able to read team members. Body language is a nonverbal form of communication that plays a key role in client education. Body language accounts for almost 60% of communication! Following are a few key characteristics of body language.

Folded Arms

When a person has folded arms, it generally indicates that they are defensive and unwilling to accept recommendations or advice. If a team member is approached by a client and the team member has folded arms, the client may

feel uncomfortable about asking questions (role-playing will help teach team members to unfold arms while in the practice). A client with folded arms may be unwilling to accept recommendations and may have some underlying issues with the service provided (Figure 11-12). A team member can correct this situation easily by handing the client something to hold. A brochure, a model of a joint (e.g., hip, knee, elbow), or anything else will force the person to unfold the arms; this will gradually open the lines for communication. Once this has occurred, the team member can continue educating the client and ask if there is any other information that the client needs. Team members should also make sure at this point that all the client's concerns have been addressed.

Body Posture

A team member's body posture sends a message to the client. If a team member enters an exam room slumped over, with head down and shoulders folded in, the client is going

Jornada Veterinary Clinic
2399 Saturn Circle
Anywhere, NM 88012

Overweight Management Feeding Program

Recheck

Date: 08/04/2008
Client: Margarite Brice
Patient: FERGUS
Current weight: 76.9 lbs, 34.95 kg
Current body condition score: 8

Recommended daily intake: 397.91 Kcal/day*
Feeding recommendation: 1-1/4 cups of PVD OM Overweight Management® (Dry) plus 39 Kcals of treats (about 1 OM Biscuit).
1-1/2 cups.

* This recommendation is based on your dog's response to the weight management program, including change in weight and number of days since the last visit.

Projected Weight Loss
This diet may result in a 1.0% weight loss of 0.769 lbs, or 0.349 kg per week.

Week of:	Lbs	Kg
08/04/2008	76.9	34.95
08/11/2008	76.1	34.60
08/18/2008	75.4	34.25
08/25/2008	74.6	33.90
09/01/2008	73.8	33.55

Diet description: PVD OM Overweight Management® (Dry)
Purina Veterinary Diets®
OM Overweight Management® (Dry) brand CANINE FORMULA
- Reduced calorie diet to help dogs safely lose or maintain weight
- Formulated with low fat, high fiber, and exceptional palatability
- Formulated to achieve a high protein/calorie ratio
- Available in dry and canned forms

This recommendation is a guideline based on average energy needs. Individual pets may have different energy requirements because of environmental conditions, activity levels, age, genetics, and breed size.

It is VERY important to have FERGUS rechecked in 2-4 weeks to determine special individual energy requirements.

FERGUS's next appointment is on _____ at _____

FIGURE 11-7 Purina overweight management document. (Courtesy Nestle Purina, St. Louis, Mo.)

to feel that the team member lacks confidence and skill and does not enjoy his or her job (Figure 11-13). The client may not accept the recommendations that are advised simply because of the team member's poor body posture. Team members who are slumped over are likely to have quiet voices, lack energy, and appear unmotivated. Instead, team members should enter exam rooms with their heads up, a straight body posture, and shoulders back. This attitude will boast confidence, excitement, and skill. Clients will accept the recommendations that are made and develop a firm relationship with the team (Figure 11-14).

Eye Contact

While educating clients, maintain eye contact with them at all times. Lack of eye contact is perceived as diminished skill, knowledge, and confidence. When team members maintain eye contact, the client will feel more comfortable about accepting recommendations.

ESTIMATES

All clients should be provided with an estimate of procedures and services that will be performed on their pets (Figure 11-15). Estimates are a major part of client

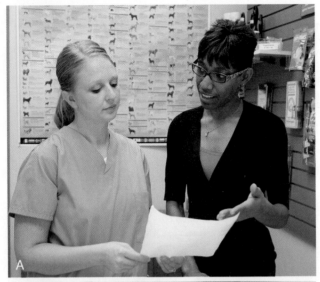

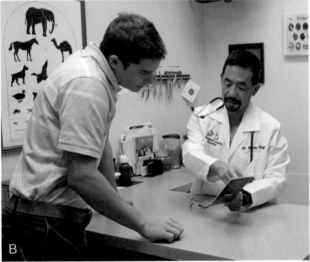

FIGURE 11-8 Written information provided by the veterinary technician (**A**) and the veterinarian (**B**) will increase client understanding and encourage client compliance.

communication and are the most common complaint for state board investigators when clients air grievances against veterinary practices. Clients must be educated regarding the procedures their pets are going to receive. Second, they must fully accept the estimate provided. If any charges or procedures change from the original estimate, the client should be called and informed. Estimates can be established for simple outpatient procedures such as yearly exams, anal sac expressions, or nail trims. Estimates should also be provided for inpatient procedures such as routine spays, neuters, and laceration repairs. Patients that are to be admitted to the hospital must have estimates provided, and the client must be updated daily regarding the total amount as well as changes that occur as the patient has further diagnostics completed. Clients should sign estimates, indicating that

they agree to the procedures and are financially responsible for the charges (Figure 11-16).

> **PRACTICE POINT**   Every client should be provided with an estimate, regardless of whether the client states no desire for one.

Estimates should persuade clients to ask questions and encourage discussion regarding the medicine their pets will be receiving. They can also foster the discussion of deposits and the hospitals payment policy. Some clients will need time to think about the estimate provided and discuss financing options with a spouse. Clients may need to call the practice back with approval or decline of diagnostics based on that discussion.

Team members should be trained to give accurate estimates and to remind clients that estimates can change based on diagnosis, treatment, and progression or regression of the patient. Estimates given over the phone should always include an exam; clients should then be informed that another estimate will be provided once a tentative diagnosis has been made. Incorrect estimates given over the phone can give clients false information and hope, in the end increasing client frustration and dissatisfaction.

ENSURING CLIENT UNDERSTANDING

Client education is central to client compliance. Clients who do not understand a policy, procedure, or service will not comply with recommendations. Clients cannot ask for services they are unaware of, nor can they ask for services that they do not comprehend. Client education can fail for many reasons, including lack of team member time, concern, or compassion, poorly educated staff, or the unwillingness of clients to comply.

Clients, as do team members, learn and understand information in a variety of ways. Some may learn better with visual aids: pictures, videos, and illustrations. Others may learn better with verbal communication. Team members must be able to determine what the most successful way will be to educate an individual client. Client education should be a positive, enthusiastic experience. Words should be simple and understandable. Many clients are embarrassed to admit that they do not understand medical terms. If they do not understand the terms, they will not comprehend the information provided. A combination of materials should be available to aid in client education. Customized brochures from manufacturers, posters, videos, and CDs that clients can take home will help reiterate information that was presented while the client was in the practice. Skeletal models and both normal and abnormal radiographs will help the clients visualize the procedure or abnormality affecting their pets.

What Would You Do/Not Do?

Megan, a veterinary technician, is checking in a 15-year-old cat. Conner has been vomiting for the last couple of days, but still seems to have interest in eating and has normal bowel movements. Megan continues gathering the history on the patient and begins to take Conner's temperature. Ms. Coffman, Conner's owner, abruptly states, "He does not have a fever! He does not need his temperature taken! Why do you guys insist on always taking his temperature! All you do is make him uncomfortable! He already hates coming to this place as it is!" Megan, surprised by the sudden outburst, slowly places the thermometer on the table, collects the medical record and leaves the room, without saying anything.

What Should Megan Have Done?

First, Megan could have let Ms. Coffman know that it is hospital policy that all patients presented to the hospital are required to have a temperature taken, and that this must be completed before the veterinarian enters the room. She could explain that temperature is a vital sign, and that vital signs often change with disease. She may also state that it is common for patients to have a fever with an infection. Giving this explanation might have allowed her to continue with the process of taking the temperature.

Alternatively, Megan could have asked her supervisor to help her, who then would have explained the protocol to Ms. Coffman. Megan was already upset by the comment and might have needed someone in a superior position to help explain the procedure in a clearer manner.

> **PRACTICE POINT**   Individuals have different learning abilities. Being able to educate clients with a variety of techniques will help increase client understanding.

Clients should be educated in a quiet and safe environment. Distractions from their pets, other clients, and team members can occur and can prevent the client from paying attention. These cause clients to focus on activities going on around them instead of the information that is being presented.

UNDERSTANDING CLIENT AND PATIENT NEEDS

Team members who understand both clients and patients to the fullest extent will be the best employees. Many team members can excel at one but not the other, and it takes time, practice, and patience to excel at both. There are different types of clients. Calm, honest, and happy clients may be considered one type. Mean, arrogant, and "know it all" clients can be another. Some can be angry at the world and untrustworthy, and sometimes lack funds. Another type may lack funds but are happy and willing to accept the best recommendations available for their financial situation. Different approaches are needed to best handle the various types of clients, and patient care must never be forgotten, whatever the client's personality type. Each patient must receive the best possible medicine regardless of its owner's type, and being able to mix the two can be a challenge. When communicating with clients, different techniques may be necessary to maximize communications. Some clients may need basic words; others may understand medical terminology. Some clients require choices; others cannot be given options and must be told what to do. Team members should be able to read clients within 30 seconds and determine the best communication technique for a given situation.

> **PRACTICE POINT**   Team members who comprehend client and patient needs are exceptional employees.

The first type—calm, honest, and happy—are the clients every team member dreams of serving. These individuals allow the team to practice the best medicine because they follow recommendations and are polite to work with. They appreciate education and want to learn about their pets' conditions; they will look up information on the Internet and ask questions.

The second type—mean, arrogant, and know it all—can be extremely frustrating for team members. These people are angry at the world; if team members can remember that, then the comments made by these clients will not be taken personally. Know-it-all clients can be easy to deal with; simply hand them correct, printed information to correct their mistaken information. Once they get home and read the information, they can correct themselves instead of the team trying to make that change.

The angry patient who lacks funds can be the most degrading for team members to deal with. These are the clients who may exclaim to team members, "You don't care about my animal! All you care about is the money!" They want to be able to charge the service and then never return to pay. They can belittle the staff quickly; managers should step in and stop this action immediately. Team members do not deserve this treatment, and clients of this mentality should be "fired." Veterinary team members are in their profession because they love animals and *want* to do what is best for patients, regardless of a client's finances.

The final type of client can be rewarding but sometimes frustrating for some team members. Clients who are lacking in funds cannot follow the best recommendations for their pet. However, these clients love their pets and will do what they can with the limited finances available. These clients are honest about their finances and usually will pay any services that they have charged. Making options available for these clients is rewarding. Finding a solution that works for the client, the pet, and the team can be challenging, but the client will be grateful for the service provided.

	Patient: TAYLOR	Age:	N/A
	Species: CANINE	Sex:	FE
	Breed: Red Heeler	Tag:	528
Account number: 4572	Color: Red	Weight:	
Phone number:	Doctor:		

LUXATING PATELLA

What is a luxating patella?
The patella, or kneecap, is normally located in the center of the knee joint. The term *luxating* means "out of place" or "dislocated." Therefore, a luxating patella is a kneecap that moves out of its normal location.

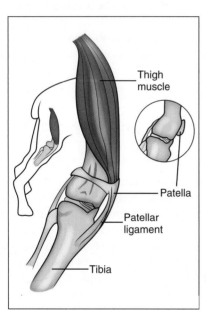

What causes a patellar luxation?
The muscles of the thigh attach to the top of the kneecap. There is a ligament, the *patellar ligament*, running from the bottom of the kneecap to a point on the tibia (the bone in the lower leg) just below the knee joint. When the thigh muscles contract, force is transmitted through the patella and patellar ligament to a point on the top of the tibia. This results in extension or straightening of the knee. The patella stays in the center of the leg because the point of attachment of the patellar ligament is on the midline and because the patella slides in a groove on the lower end of the femur (the bone between the knee and hip) called the *trochlear groove.*

The patella usually luxates because the point of attachment of the patellar ligament is not on the midline of the tibia. It is almost always located too far medial (toward the middle of the body). As the thigh muscles contract, the force is pulled medially, or to the inside of the knee.

After several months or years of this abnormal movement, the inner side of the trochlear groove in the femur wears down. Once the side of the groove wears down, the patella is then free to dislocate. When this occurs, the dog has difficulty bearing weight on the leg. It may learn how to kick the leg and snap the patella back into its normal location. However, because the side of the groove is gone, it easily dislocates again.

Does a luxating patella cause any long-term problems for my dog?
Some dogs can tolerate this problem for many years, even for all of their lives. However, this weakness in the knee predisposes the knee to other injuries, especially torn cruciate ligaments. With advancing age, arthritic changes may take place in the joint, causing pain.

Can a luxating patella be corrected?
Surgery should be performed if your dog has a persistent lameness or if other knee injuries occur secondary to the luxating patella.

A

FIGURE 11-9 A, Sample client information handout.

Acute Colitis

Acute colitis is a sudden inflammation of the colon. The most common signs are diarrhea and straining to defecate. The stools are often soft and contain blood or mucus. The condition can be caused by infection, eating garbage or foreign materials, intestinal parasites, changes in diet, and even emotional upsets.

Because the exact cause is often difficult to determine, the condition is usually treated symptomatically the first time. If there are recurrences, a more extensive search for the cause is advised.

Important Points in Treatment:

1. Lab tests are often necessary to diagnose the condition and monitor the effectiveness of treatment.

2. Give all medications as directed. Please call the doctor if you cannot give the medication.

3. Diet: _____ Feed a normal diet
   _____ Feed a prescription diet _____
   _____ A special diet: feed mixture of 4 parts boiled white rice to 1 part boiled ground beef, turkey, or chicken. Feed small amounts every 4-6 hours or as follows: _____
   _____
   _____

4. Activity: _____ Allow normal activity
   _____ Restrict activity as follows: _____
   _____
   _____

5. Water: _____ Allow free access to fresh water at all times.
   _____ Restrict water intake as follows: _____
   _____
   _____

Notify the doctor if any of the following occurs:
- Your pet refuses to eat the recommended food.
- Your pet's symptoms reoccur after an apparent recovery.
- Your pet is reluctant to eat and/or loses weight.
- There is a change in your pet's health.

B

FIGURE 11-9, cont'd **B,** Sample client information handout.

PRACTICE POINT Do not allow clients to ruin the day. Learn and grow from the experience!

PRACTICE POINT Clients want appreciation and to be listened to, along with help, honesty, care, and understanding.

What Do Clients Really Want?

Before team members can relate to clients, they must be able to identify what clients really want. Veterinary practices may elect to send out a survey to clients to ask what they want in a veterinary hospital. Typical responses can be classified into several categories: appreciation, listening, help, honesty, care, and understanding.

Clients want to be *appreciated* for coming to a specific veterinary practice and not another. Clients want to be appreciated when recommending new clients. Furthermore, clients want to be appreciated for the care they have given their animals.

Clients want team members to *listen*. Clients want to tell stories about their pets (for some, this is their "child") and to be appreciated for telling them. Team members can be poor listeners when they are only thinking of the next question to ask. It is important to listen, remain nonjudgmental, and avoid making assumptions.

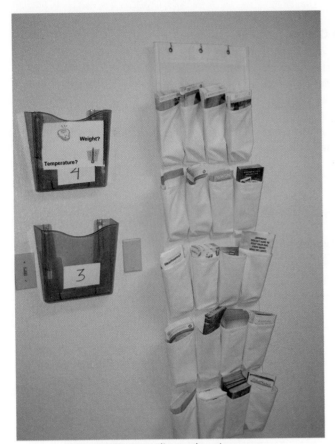

FIGURE 11-10 Client education center.

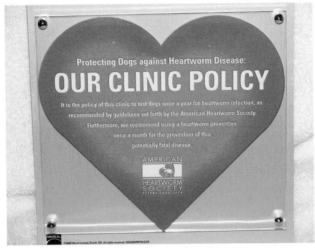

FIGURE 11-11 Client education poster.

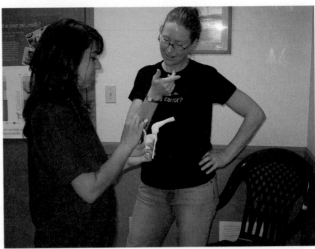

FIGURE 11-12 Technician educating a client by handing her a model.

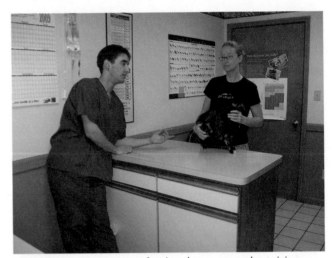

FIGURE 11-13 An unprofessional team member giving information to a client.

Open-ended questions should be asked; who, what, when, where, and why will help the team *listen* to the clients' answers.

Clients want *help* without asking for it. Excellent team members will take the extra step to help clients to the car with their pets or a bag of food. Helping clients establishes an excellent client-practice bond.

Clients want *honesty.* They do not want to be lied to or advised of only one treatment option regarding their pet. They want the clear-cut truth, to receive education about all options available, and be referred to a specialist when needed. If a team member does not know the answer to a question that has been asked, clients want them to honestly find an answer, not just respond "I don't know."

Clients want to know that the staff *cares* about their pets. They want the receptionist to care when they call, and they want the kennel attendant to care when they pick their pet up.

Last, but not least, clients want *understanding.* They want the team to understand their particular situation, whether it is financial or personal. The majority of clients are willing to pay for services, regardless of price, if the team satisfies their *wants.* The client has perceived

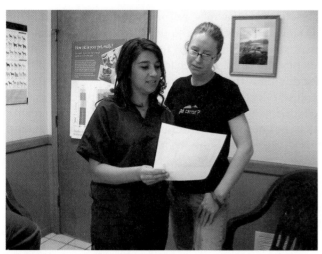

FIGURE 11-14 A professional team member standing up straight with shoulders held back.

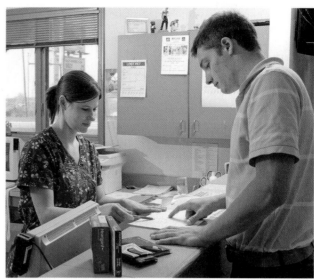

FIGURE 11-15 Estimates should be explained to clients in detail so they fully understand their costs and the hospital payment policies.

ABC Veterinary Clinic
123 Saturn Circle
Anytown, MN 12345
(555) 555-5555

CHARGE ESTIMATION

Account: 19902
Date: 07/31/09
Page: 1

Sharon White	Phone (123) 678-6789		Patient: Marshmallow
Code	Service/Item	Qty	Amount
0216	Office call	1	$35.54
0920	IV catheter	1	$37.90
0924	IV fluids per liter	2-3	$31.28-$46.92
0916	IV care daily	2	$38.48
909	Hospitalization, routine	1-2	$32.48-65.68
4150	Urinary catheter	1	$32.48
0302	Anesthesia	1	$104.36
3815	General health profile	1	$91.24

ESTIMATE TOTAL $403.76-$422.60

THIS IS ONLY AN ESTIMATE AND DOES NOT INLCUDE SALES TAX. The actual diagnostic treatment plan may require more medications and/or procedures. The range of estimate may vary. This estimate is valid for 30 days only.

I have read and understand this estimate. I understand that I must leave a deposit before the procedure, and the balance must be paid when my pet is released from the hospital.

Signature _____ Date _____

FIGURE 11-16 Sample estimate.

and understood the value of the practice when all of the "wants" have been met.

Client Surveys

Surveys can either be mailed to clients or given to them as they are checking out with the receptionist. Surveys can be kept short and simple; this allows the team to know whether they are satisfying client needs. Shorter surveys will be completed more often than those that are lengthy. Client surveys are an easy monitoring solution to help understand clients' satisfaction and level of comfort with the services the practice provides. Clients maintain the business; therefore it is imperative to make sure they are satisfied and receive value for the service provided. If clients are unsatisfied, practices want to be notified and given the opportunity to address the problem. Hospitals do not want to lose clients or have negative comments made about them throughout the community. It is very important to strive for a high level of satisfaction from every client (Figure 11-17).

Handling Client Complaints and Grievances

Clients may be frustrated for a variety of reasons that are not related to the veterinary practice. Others may be frustrated because they do not feel they were provided the best medicine. Whatever the client complaint is, it must be handled appropriately, professionally, and quickly.

Team members cannot become defensive when discussing complaint issues with clients. When team members get defensive, the intensity and emotion of the conversation rise, and clients become more upset. Instead, team members should immediately take the distraught or angry client to another room. Emotions can be more intense when other people are around; therefore taking clients to a quiet room can quickly diffuse the intensity. Team members should listen to what the client has to say. Eye contact should be maintained throughout the conversation. Let the client air the complaint before asking any questions. Once the client has finished, the team member should repeat what was said, ensuring no miscommunication arises. Once the client and team member agree on the event that has occurred, the team member may offer some solutions to satisfy the client. Once clients are able to voice their concerns, their anger tends to drop a level. Once it is repeated back to them and it appears the team member has understood their side of the story, the anger level drops another level. When solutions are offered, clients feel satisfied that their problems will be handled appropriately.

> **PRACTICE POINT**   Team members can diffuse a client's anger simply by listening.

Solutions that may be presented to clients may be as simple as adjusting the invoice. Other solutions that may satisfy clients are to let them know a new policy or procedure may be enacted because of this particular dilemma, that team member education will increase, and/or client education will change to prevent this from occurring again. Clients are satisfied when they realize that they can make a difference. Although it may be hard for a team member to say "thank you" after a client discussion of this caliber, it is necessary; *thank you* is a powerful phrase to a client.

At times, the client may not understand the procedure or service that was performed, and regardless of the steps the team member takes to calm the client, the client will remain irate. If a client becomes abusive toward a team member despite the team member having taken every step possible to calm the person, the client should be asked to leave the premises. A discussion can continue when the emotions have subsided. If a client will not leave the property when asked, the police should be called immediately. Staff and client safety should always be a concern. People in today's society cannot be trusted to not harm others. A client may be under the influence of an illegal substance or may have some psychological issues that are uncontrolled. Once the client's emotions have subsided, a telephone call can be made by team members to find a solution to the issue at hand.

> **PRACTICE POINT**   To help calm an angry client, listen, understand, and provide solutions to solve the issue.

It must be realized by all team members that arguing and confrontation will not resolve a conflict. If a team member has become emotionally involved in an unresolved discussion, another team member must step in and remove the initial member from the confrontation. Emotions will escalate quickly; other clients will hear the argument and staff stress levels will grow. It is important for the entire team to prevent discussions from becoming this emotional.

> **PRACTICE POINT**   Team members should use distraught clients as a learning experience and correct their actions to prevent the same miscommunication from occurring again.

When clients present problems to team members, it should be taken as a learning experience. Clients perceive actions, conversations, and procedures differently than team members do. If one client perceives an action one way, others may as well. It is important to be proactive and prevent problems from arising, rather

---

Client Survey

We appreciate your business at ABC Veterinary Clinic and value your suggestions for improvement. Please take a few moments to fill out our survey and return it to the hospital.

Please rate the following questions from 1 (superior) to 5 (unacceptable).

I received an appointment that was convenient for me.	1 2 3 4 5
The hospital was clean when I arrived.	1 2 3 4 5
The receptionist acknowledged me immediately.	1 2 3 4 5
The veterinary technician was friendly.	1 2 3 4 5
The veterinary technician was knowledgeable.	1 2 3 4 5
The veterinarian was friendly.	1 2 3 4 5
The veterinarian was knowledgeable.	1 2 3 4 5
I received materials to take home and review.	1 2 3 4 5
My pet received exceptional care.	1 2 3 4 5
The staff cares about my pet.	1 2 3 4 5
The services are reasonably priced.	1 2 3 4 5

What can we do to improve our services for you? _____
_____
_____
_____

If one of our team members provided exceptional care today, please let us know so that we may recognize that person: _____
_____
_____

FIGURE 11-17 Client surveys are a good way to determine whether client needs are being met.

than being reactive and solving problems only after clients have become upset.

BARRIERS TO CLIENT COMMUNICATIONS

There are different barriers that must be overcome with clients to increase client communications. Characteristics differ immensely in the previously mentioned list of client types; however, handling each type of client is relatively the same. Clients may appear nervous, defensive, or embarrassed. They may have language or cultural differences or may be hearing impaired. Team members may prejudge a client and make assumptions before an estimate is discussed with the client. This may prevent the best medicine from being offered to the client. Another barrier, as previously discussed, is listening. Team members must listen to the meaning of the client's words and be able to understand the client's perspective. Once these barriers have been identified and overcome, the communication can continue, and more effectively.

Clients may become defensive or embarrassed when they feel they have not given their pet the best care or cannot afford the best care. Clients may have crossed arms, avoid making eye contact with team members, or only interact with the team when questions are asked. A caring, empathetic team member can easily break this barrier by finding something to compliment the pet on. Suddenly, clients may feel a small sense of pride and may become more open to suggestions and advice.

In most parts of the country, some clients will be of a different culture or language from team members. It is important to try to understand clients' cultural differences and elements of their language to provide the best possible medicine to all clients. A specific team member might have a friend or an acquaintance that can educate the staff on a specific culture in the local area, as well as teach a few key terms in that particular language. It may also be of benefit to have a translator available to try to accommodate these clients. Nonverbal behavior varies from culture to culture. Differences are often expressed through gestures, eye contact, interpersonal distance, and touch. A client with folded arms may be insecure of the situation due to cultural differences rather than being upset. Again, this can be overcome by giving the client something to hold while team members are educating them on an important health care topic.

> **PRACTICE POINT** Give a client a brochure or a model to hold to encourage the person to be more open to discussion.

Another barrier to communication can come from team members. It can be extremely difficult to discuss an obese pet with an obese owner. It can also be difficult to discuss dental disease with a client who has bad teeth or no teeth at all. Situations of this sort can be overcome by role-playing different scenarios. Some clients may have more compassion for their pets than themselves and are willing to place Fluffy on a diet when the health benefits are discussed. By educating the client on the benefits of taking Fluffy outside for daily walks, the client will benefit. Many people show love for their pets by giving treats; however, a team member can show owners other ways to show love for their pets.

IMPROVING VERBAL IMAGE

The success of the veterinary practice depends on client compliance. Client compliance depends on client education and acceptance of recommendations. Clients will not accept recommendations from uneducated, unmotivated team members. The client-patient relationship will not be established without confidence, skill, and understanding from team members. By providing continuing education for all employees, team members will be able to discuss procedures, protocols, and diseases much more thoroughly. Team members will learn correct definitions and pronunciations and be able to educate clients with a higher level of confidence. For example, staff members can pick a word of the day and educate others as to the correct definition and pronunciation. Once it has been mastered, team members can use the word in sentences throughout the day. Role-playing and continuing education for team members will help the knowledge, enthusiasm, and proficiency of each individual on the team.

CLIENT RETENTION

Client development and retention are critical elements that lead to a successful practice. Excellent client communication plays a major role in satisfying clients. The veterinary team plays a significant role in building and maintaining the human-animal bond. Team members educate clients about health care issues from the first visit. Reminders, recalls, and client education can have a positive effect on this bond, which ultimately leads to client satisfaction and retention.

Some clients will leave a practice for reasons beyond the practice's control. Some clients may move, change jobs, or lose a pet. Some clients may have not established a relationship with the practice and are willing to try another practice because it is closer to their home. In general, a small-animal practice will lose 10% to 15% of clients each year. It should be a goal to retain 70% to 75% over a 3-year period.

> **PRACTICE POINT** Every team member plays a significant role in client retention.

To retain clients, team members must know the clients' goals and practices must meet or exceed these goals. Positive experiences should be created for each client. Once the goals have been met and a positive experience has been created, customers are satisfied. Customer satisfaction equals loyal customers who recommend the practice to family, friends, and co-workers.

VETERINARY PRACTICE and the LAW

After a surgical procedure, it is the responsibility of the team member releasing the patient to ensure the client fully understands the release document. Each topic must be addressed with the client: when to offer food and water, when to allow activity, how to care for the surgical area, when to start the medications, and when to return for a recheck. If medications are dispensed, the owner should be shown how to give the medication. If the patient is able to receive the medication while in the office, the first dose should be demonstrated and given.

Postoperative instructions should be printed on a carbonless copy form. Once the instructions have been reviewed with the owner, the owner should sign the top copy, indicating receipt of the release sheet. If a follow-up appointment has been scheduled, the time and date can be written on the release sheet and the bottom copy given to the owner. The original document can then be filed with the medical record.

This ensures that clients have complete understanding of the release instructions and provides proof that they have received a copy. Verbal release instructions are not sufficient; written documentation must exist.

Self-Evaluation Questions

1. Why are verbal and written skills imperative in veterinary medicine?
2. What is client compliance and how can it be achieved?
3. What are the benefits of a reminder system?
4. Create an example that can enhance client education.
5. What would be an appropriate body stance when addressing clients?
6. Why is body posture important?
7. How should an angry client be handled?
8. How can common barriers be overcome?
9. Why are estimates important?
10. How can individual verbal image be improved?

Recommended Reading

Heinke MM: *Practice made perfect: a guide to veterinary practice management*, Lakewood, CO, 2001, AAHA Press.

McCurnin D, Bassert JA, Lukins RL: *Clinical textbook for veterinary technicians*, ed 7, St Louis, 2010, Saunders Elsevier.

Opperman M: *The art of veterinary practice management*, Lenexa, KS, 1999, Veterinary Medicine Publishing Group.

Sirosis M: *Principles and practices of veterinary technology*, ed 2, St Louis, 2004, Mosby Elsevier.

Thill JV, Bover CL: *Excellence in business communication*, ed 8, Upper Saddle River, NJ, 2008, Prentice Hall.

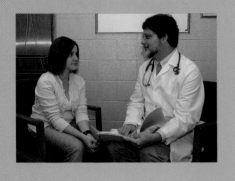

CHAPTER 12

Interacting with a Grieving Client

Chapter Outline

Understanding the Human-Animal Bond
Understanding Euthanasia
The Euthanasia Procedure
Pet Memorials

Cremations
    Owners Picking up Remains
Understanding and Dealing With Grief

Learning Objectives

Mastery of the content in this chapter will enable the reader to:
- Define the human-animal bond.
- Differentiate between quality and quantity of life.
- Identify the euthanasia process.
- List types of pet memorials that are available.

- Define the five stages of grief.
- Discuss client solutions to help cope with the loss.
- Explain euthanasia to children.
- Define pet depression.

Key Terms

Anger
Bargaining
Cremation
Denial

Depression
Euthanasia
Human-Animal Bond

UNDERSTANDING THE HUMAN-ANIMAL BOND

The human-animal bond is an emotional bond that forms as a benefit to both humans and animals (Figure 12-1). Each party treats the other with mutual respect, trust, devotion, and love. To some clients, pets are their children; to others, pets are their best friends. Whichever connection has been developed, it is generally a long-lasting relationship (Figure 12-2).

> ⊙ **PRACTICE POINT** The human-animal bond is defined as a description of the emotion a human feels toward an animal. This emotion enables a connection that can be expressed as affection and a sense of understanding between animal and human.

This bond is strengthened by the veterinary health care team. Each time the client visits, the bond is strengthened as the owner receives further education on how to help care for his or her pet. Team members who are empathetic and encourage the human-animal bond are cherished and tend to be requested by clients. These team members are usually employed over the long term by a veterinary practice and may have the experience of seeing a pet for its first visit and following its progress until its last visit. These team members will face grieving issues with long-term clients.

Sometimes, clients may come to the veterinary practice to euthanize an animal because they are unable to see their current veterinarian. Although these clients have not established a relationship with the staff, team members must remember the clients are grieving. Clients show grief in different ways, and team members may see the worst of the grieving process. Some clients may appear angry with the team when, in reality, this may be the way the client deals with the pain of losing a pet. If a pet is euthanized or dies in the hospital, clients may appear frustrated and accuse the hospital of not providing the best service possible. An excellent way to handle clients of this type is to listen. Active listeners keep eye contact and nod their heads in understanding. Let the clients talk about their frustrations. Once they can discuss the dilemma,

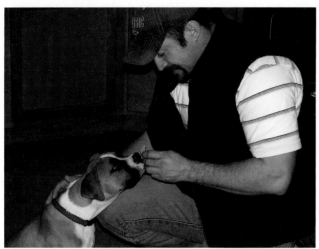

FIGURE 12-1 The human-animal bond is typically a strong and long-lasting one.

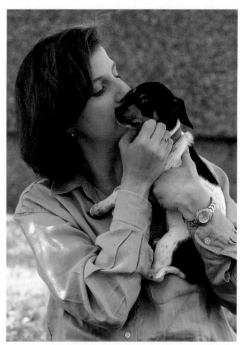

FIGURE 12-2 The decision to bond with a new animal should be left to the client experiencing the loss. Bonding with a new pet should be viewed as a tribute to the love and companionship shared with the previous animal. (From Bassert JM, McCurnin DM: *McCurnin's clinical textbook for veterinary technicians,* ed 7, St Louis, 2010, Saunders Elsevier.)

their anger begins to resolve, especially when they feel team members understand their frustration. This is not the time to become defensive for the team; it is the time to listen and respond with simple responses such as, "I understand your frustration, Mrs. Smith, I will certainly look into this," or, "I know you loved Fluffy, Mrs. Smith. She was very special. You provided the best care possible. I will take care of these issues." The veterinary team provided the best medicine possible, but the state of grief distorts the thought process.

UNDERSTANDING EUTHANASIA

Making the decision to euthanize a pet can be extremely difficult for clients. Some clients may not believe in euthanasia, whereas others do not believe in allowing a pet to suffer. The true definition of euthanasia comes from the Greek terms *eu,* meaning good or right, and *thanatos,* meaning death. Therefore euthanasia refers to an easy and painless death.

Clients should be educated regarding the euthanasia process so that they can make well-educated decisions. A team member should never tell a client "Now is the time to euthanize." Clients can misconstrue that statement and feel that the staff member made them euthanize their pet. Suggestions can be given, and simple statements can be made such as, "It would not be a wrong decision if you made the choice to euthanize Fluffy."

> **PRACTICE POINT** Quality of life should be considered over quantity of life when debating euthanasia of a pet.

Clients should be able to fully understand and differentiate quality versus quantity of life for their pets.

Quality being the enjoyable aspect; the pet can still move around, eat and drink, and have bowel movements and urinate appropriately. Quantity of life is the time frame of the animal's life; at times an owner will be keeping the animal alive for personal reasons or will be waiting for a specific moment to make the decision. Clients may make decisions based on increasing the length of time the pet can survive rather than the quality of life while the pet survives.

THE EUTHANASIA PROCEDURE

Clients may call and ask questions regarding the euthanasia procedure at the veterinary hospital. They may ask if a house call can be made, if an appointment to bring the pet in is required, or if they can just walk in. Many practices do not perform house calls, and the client may be referred to a veterinarian who does. If a client chooses to come in to the practice, the team member should advise the client of what to expect. Most clients have not experienced a euthanasia procedure and therefore do not know what to expect. If team members take the time to educate them before they get to the practice, they are a little more prepared for what is a life-changing experience. Making an appointment may be practice policy; however, some clients may be unable to abide by this policy when it comes to euthanizing their pet. It is an extremely overwhelming decision to make, and having to wait until a scheduled appointment time may be difficult. It is making an appointment for death. Walk-ins should be accommodated when possible.

When a client arrives at the clinic for euthanasia of a pet, every attempt should be made to get him or her into a quiet room as soon as possible. Many practices have separate rooms used only for this purpose. Team members need to remember that this is a very difficult time for a client, who may not understand everything that is explained. The euthanasia process should be explained again, including the options that exist for the body (many hospitals offer private cremations, mass cremations, or burial services at a local pet cemetery). The owner must sign the release form, and all charges should be taken care of at this point. Figure 2-10, *H* in Chapter 2 is an example of a euthanasia release form. Team members should ensure that the name the on the file matches the name on the euthanasia form.

> **PRACTICE POINT**   Euthanasia forms must be signed by the client before the process begins.

If a pet is hospitalized and its owner wishes to have the pet euthanized but is not present to sign a euthanasia release form, the owner should state the wish to have the pet euthanized to two different team members. Both team members must write in the record that the client requested euthanasia and that this was verified by them. This will protect the practice in the event that a client states that he or she did not authorize the euthanasia.

The euthanasia procedure varies from hospital to hospital; however, the same general ideas apply overall. The pet may have a catheter placed intravenously so that the vein is easier to access while in the euthanasia room with the client. Some practices may give a tranquilizer that relaxes the pet. This also allows the owner to stay with the pet and "say goodbye" (Figure 12-3). When the owner is ready, a euthanasia solution is injected into the vein; most solutions are an overdose of a barbiturate. This causes the heart to stop beating and the respirations to cease. When the heart is no longer audible, the patient has died. Clients should be advised that pets may lose their bowels and urinate when the muscles relax. They should also understand that pets generally do not close their eyes when they die and that this is normal.

If a patient has died in the hospital and a client would like to visit the pet, every attempt should be made to make the animal as presentable as possible. All catheters and bandaging materials should be removed, and any blood, feces, or urine should be wiped away. The eyes can be glued shut for a more peaceful appearance. The rectal area can be placed in a waterproof sack in case the bowels are released, and the pet should be wrapped

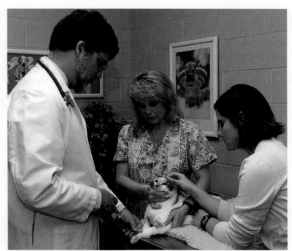

FIGURE 12-3 A client's presence during euthanasia of a companion animal helps say goodbye. Allow the client, with guidance, to make as many decisions as possible about the site, time, and tempo of the euthanasia process; this makes the event more personal and meaningful. (From Bassert JM, McCurnin DM: *McCurnin's clinical textbook for veterinary technicians*, ed 7, St Louis, 2010, Saunders Elsevier.)

in a nice blanket. This will be a lasting memory for the owner; practices do not want to leave negative impressions in the minds of clients.

> **PRACTICE POINT**   Animals should be presented to clients without catheters or bandages once the process has ended.

If owners decide to take the body home, it should be placed in a waterproof bag. Trash bags are not visually appealing, but they may be placed in another bag or box if needed. "Body bags" are visually appealing and waterproof. Several companies offer a variety of sizes that will usually accommodate even the largest pet (Figure 12-4).

If owners do not take the body, it must be placed in a strong, waterproof bag. Bags must be clearly marked with the patient's name, the client's name, the date, and the name of the practice. The tag must also identify whether the body is to go for mass cremation or private cremation.

PET MEMORIALS

It is nice to take steps to help clients remember a pet. Many practices will send bereaved clients the poem "Rainbow Bridge." Other practices may make a paw print with paint (Figures 12-5 and 12-6). (To do this, simply clip the hair around the pads and place paint on the pads. Position a nice piece of paper on a clipboard and press the pad firmly against the board. Allow the paint to dry.) Clay paw print kits are available as well.

It is customary to send the client a sympathy card with the team members' signatures within a week of the pet's passing. Some practices may also send flowers to clients; however, this can become expensive. Clients appreciate the extra steps practices take to remember their pets (Figures 12-7 and 12-8).

> **PRACTICE POINT** Clients appreciate any pet memorials received from practices. Cards, paw prints, and flowers can be sent to clients.

CREMATIONS

Cremations are available in most places in the United States. Clients can elect to have the pet's remains returned to them (private cremation) or to have the pet be part of a mass cremation (remains are not returned). Mass cremations are generally cheaper and may be the only option if the client does not want the ashes returned. Many cities and counties have enacted regulations that prevent pets from being buried on

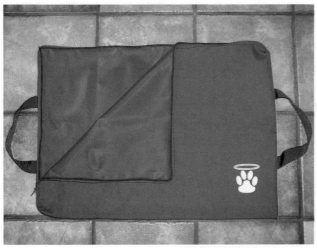

FIGURE 12-4 A waterproof body bag.

private property. City and county regulations should be verified before allowing owners to take the body for private burial. Pet cemeteries are available for burying pets in many cities. The local Humane Society chapter may have more information regarding the maintenance and upkeep of such places.

Owners Picking up Remains

Owners must return to pick up the ashes of their beloved pet when they have chosen a private cremation. Team members should call the client to state the ashes are ready. A simple and to-the-point statement of, "Taylor's ashes have been returned and are available for you to pick up when you are ready," can be made to the client. It is very hard for clients to return to the practice to pick up remains. Team members must make sure the ashes are easily accessible and that cremation containers and cards are labeled correctly. It is also important for the reception team to be familiar with the names of cremations that are ready for pick up. Often a client will come in to the practice and simply say that he is here "to pick up Taylor." The team members automatically assume Taylor is a patient and start looking for an active record. When the client is questioned further (since the file cannot be located), the client must state a request for the ashes. This is a painful statement for the client to make; therefore being prepared and knowing which ashes are ready can eliminate this painful situation.

> **PRACTICE POINT** Ashes should be clearly marked to prevent the wrong ashes from going home with the owner.

UNDERSTANDING AND DEALING WITH GRIEF

The loss of a pet can be as traumatic to some clients as losing a human family member. An animal is often a person's best friend. They are companions and guardians;

What Would You Do/Not Do?

A long-term client, Mrs. Walsh, has made the difficult decision to euthanize her dog of 15 years. She and her husband have chosen to have a private cremation, and then return to the practice to pick up the remains. The practice receives several private cremation containers at once, along with certificates of official cremation; the names of the pets have been placed on the bottom of the containers as well as on the cards.

A team member calls the Walshes informing them of Maggie's return; they arrive at the practice and take her home. The following day, Mr. Malcolm calls the practice to

see whether Jeff, his cat that was also cremated, is ready to be picked up. The receptionist comes across a horrible discovery; Jeff had been sent home with the Walshes, and Maggie was still at the practice.

What Should the Reception Team Do?

The most appropriate, albeit painful, task is to call the Walshes and inform them of the mix-up. A team member should deliver the appropriate remains and pick up Jeff immediately. The team members must sincerely apologize for this awful mistake. The owners will be very upset at first, but in time perhaps will become grateful for the honesty of the practice.

they are loyal, huggable, and touchable. People can be themselves with their pets; no pretense is needed to gain a pet's trust and love. Pets have many benefits; they decrease stress, tension, and blood pressure and can improve the heart rate of elderly and sick clients. Pets help induce exercise routines for elderly patients as well as provide protection. For children, pets can be their best friends, confidantes, and playmates (Figure 12-9). Pets may help children survive traumatic situations, such as divorce, a move or change in schools, or the loss of a parent or sibling. Pets provide unconditional love and support and live each day with abandon.

> **PRACTICE POINT** The five stages of grief include denial, anger, bargaining, depression, and acceptance.

With this human-animal bond, it is easy to see why clients can be so affected by the loss of a pet. Grieving is an individual process, and each person responds differently. Some social milieus do not allow people to

openly grieve for pets; therefore family and friends may not understand the loss and heartbreak a client may be experiencing. Other clients may immediately be able to show emotions and grieve openly. It should be shared with clients that grieving is acceptable and that it is a normal process.

There are five stages of grief that should be understood. *Denial, anger, bargaining,* and *depression* are normal steps a grieving person takes before *acceptance* of the loss.

Some clients may be in shock, denial, or disbelief regarding the loss of their pet, especially if it was a sudden death. Traumatic injuries resulting in death, particularly in young animals, may induce client anger. The client may place blame on the staff for not doing a better job or for not having the appropriate equipment to perform life-saving procedures. The owner may be angry at a family member for leaving a gate open, allowing the pet to escape and be hit by a car. The denial stage generally occurs during the first 24 hours, either after a pet's death or after a terminal illness has been diagnosed. Denial is a coping mechanism to help the

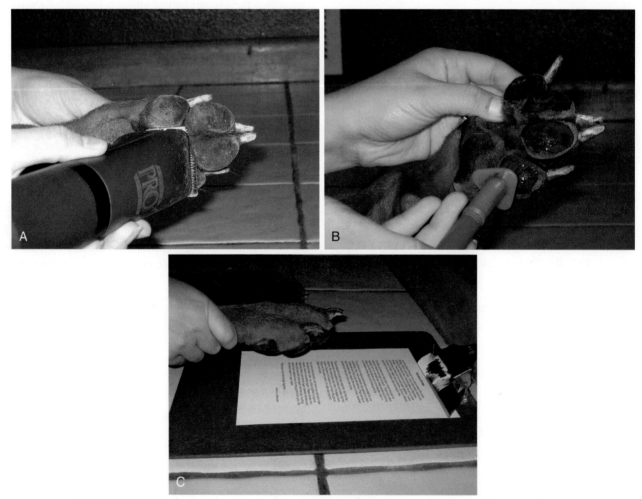

FIGURE 12-5 A, Clipping the paw for the paint. **B,** Applying paint to the paw. **C,** Preparing to stamp the paw.

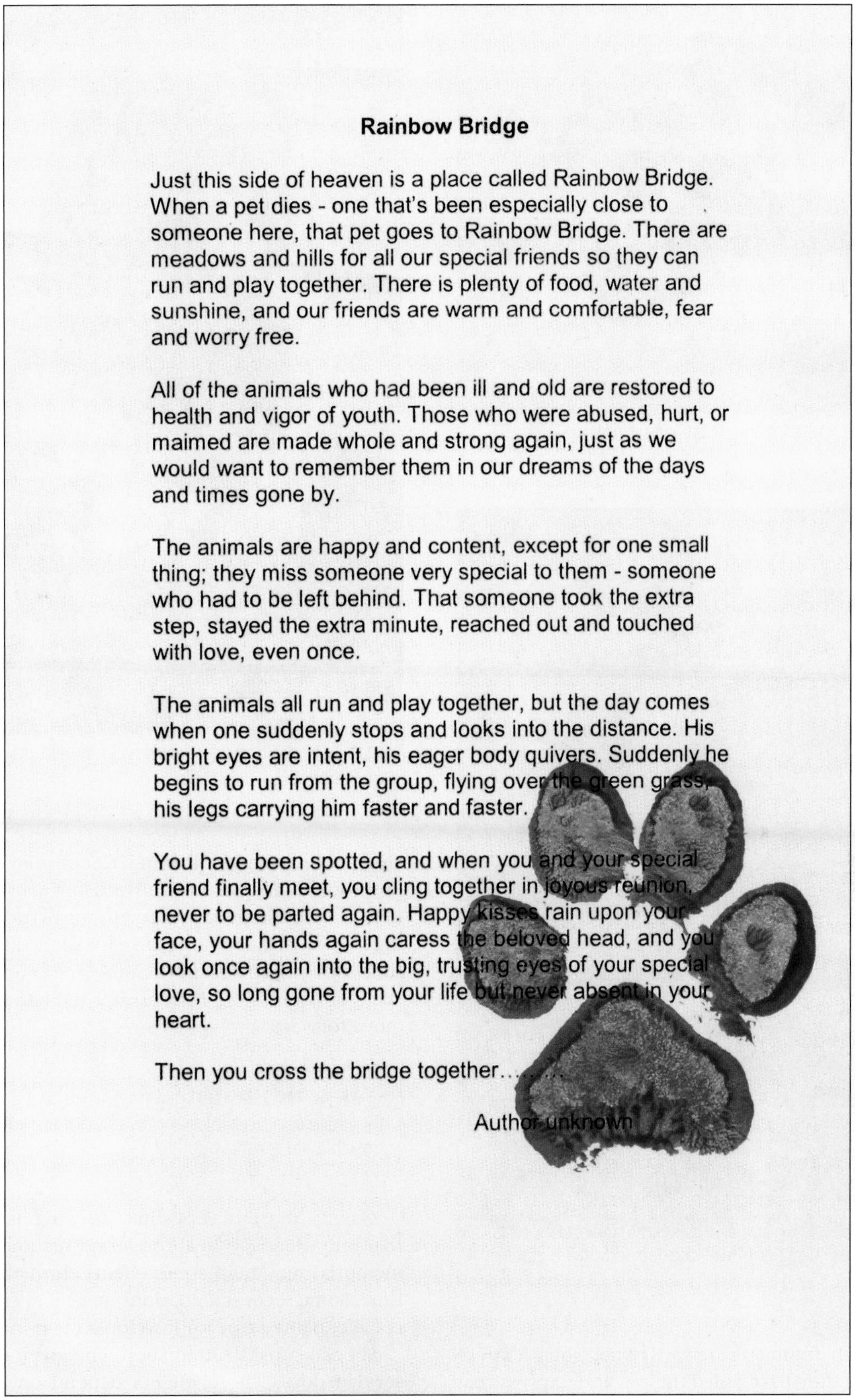

Rainbow Bridge

Just this side of heaven is a place called Rainbow Bridge. When a pet dies - one that's been especially close to someone here, that pet goes to Rainbow Bridge. There are meadows and hills for all our special friends so they can run and play together. There is plenty of food, water and sunshine, and our friends are warm and comfortable, fear and worry free.

All of the animals who had been ill and old are restored to health and vigor of youth. Those who were abused, hurt, or maimed are made whole and strong again, just as we would want to remember them in our dreams of the days and times gone by.

The animals are happy and content, except for one small thing; they miss someone very special to them - someone who had to be left behind. That someone took the extra step, stayed the extra minute, reached out and touched with love, even once.

The animals all run and play together, but the day comes when one suddenly stops and looks into the distance. His bright eyes are intent, his eager body quivers. Suddenly he begins to run from the group, flying over the green grass, his legs carrying him faster and faster.

You have been spotted, and when you and your special friend finally meet, you cling together in joyous reunion, never to be parted again. Happy kisses rain upon your face, your hands again caress the beloved head, and you look once again into the big, trusting eyes of your special love, so long gone from your life but never absent in your heart.

Then you cross the bridge together...........

Author unknown

FIGURE 12-6 The Rainbow Bridge poem with a pet's paw print is a nice way to honor a pet.

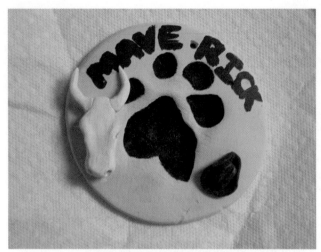

FIGURE 12-7 Clay paw print.

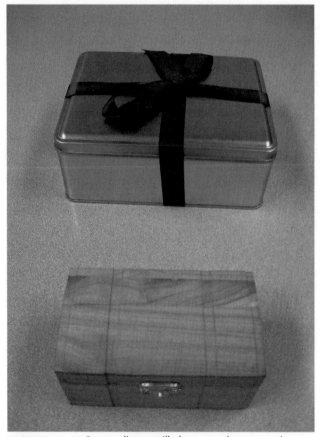

FIGURE 12-8 Some clients will choose to keep a pet's ashes in an urn.

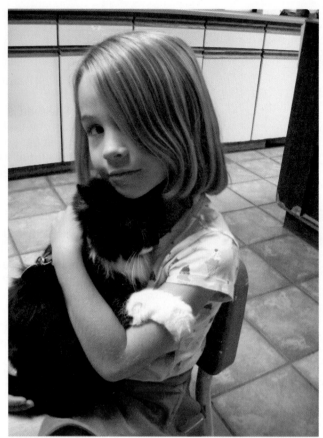

FIGURE 12-9 The bond between a child and a pet is often very strong.

Guilt is the enemy of healing. Clients may try to bargain or reason to keep the pet alive. They may offer vitamins or extra-special food to bargain for extra time. Bargaining is a way to keep hope alive for some clients, allowing time for them to accept the outcome. Many will suffer a stage of depression, then accept the loss and be able to move forward.

> **PRACTICE POINT** Many clients feel guilty when they lose a pet: guilty that they did not provide the best possible life for the pet.

Clients must accept that grieving is normal, and that only time can heal the loss. Creation of a personal memorial may help some clients through this difficult time. Some recommendations may be to create a picture collage, plant a tree, or develop a memorial garden.

Special consideration should be given to clients with service dogs. These clients depend on their pets for independence and freedom. The service dog has guided them and provided safety, and suddenly that security is gone. They will have to learn to trust another animal, and only time can build and replace that trust. Another special consideration is for a client who owns a dog

mind deal with traumatic news. Owners may experience guilt that they have failed the pet and express that guilt in anger toward the staff. If a pet has been sick for a longer time, they may be in disbelief that their pet is so sick and may be holding on for some reason. The client may feel guilty for not having done what the doctor had recommended years ago to help the pet live longer.

involved in law enforcement. This may include a drug-sniffing and/or bomb-sniffing dog or a police dog used for protection. These officers depend on their dogs for their livelihood. The dogs are their daily companions and protectors. Many times, the social circle of law enforcement does not allow grieving and prevents these clients from psychologically accepting the loss. Many officers are unable to continue their duties with replacement dogs and ultimately change positions within the law enforcement department.

> **PRACTICE POINT** Children can have a difficult time with the loss of a pet.

Children can have intense emotions and often deal with grief in different ways. Some children may be able to understand the process of euthanasia, whereas it confuses others. Children should be told the truth about euthanasia, and explaining the process will help children comprehend the situation. The child's age should be used to gauge the amount of explanation and detail needed. Words like "put to sleep" should be avoided, as many children associate this phrase with going to sleep at night. It should be explained that euthanasia is not a procedure done to sick and suffering people, that it is only available for animals. It may also help the child to reassure that the pet will no longer feel pain.

To help clients work through the grief process, team members may recommend that they change their daily routine until the pain from the loss subsides. Clients may go to dinner with friends or go for a walk after work instead of immediately rushing home. Clients should understand that they will never be able to replace a pet, but that a new relationship with another pet is possible, and each relationship is unique (Figure 12-10). Clients should not be pressured to get another pet. The grieving process can take months, and they should never be surprised with a new pet.

Pets experience depression associated with death as well, regardless of whether they have lost a human or animal companion. Pets may show decreased activity and diminished appetite and may pace. Some may whimper or simply curl up in the corner. Clients can help pets recover from the loss as well. Just as with humans, changing the daily routine can lessen the pain. Owners may take the pet for a walk or go for a ride in the car to the dog park; any new adventure will change

the routine. Pets should be shown extra love and attention as well. It must be remembered that both the client and pet are grieving, and any tools that team members can provide will help alleviate the pain associated with the loss of a pet.

> **PRACTICE POINT** Pets experience depression just as humans do with a loss of a companion animal. Their routines should also be adjusted to help them cope with the loss.

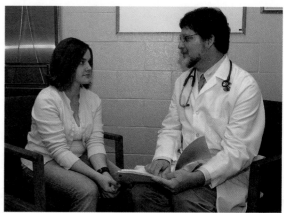

FIGURE 12-10 The diagnosis of a disease can be a difficult time for both clients and veterinary professionals. It is important to respond to both the pet's and the owner's needs. (From Bassert JM, McCurnin DM: *McCurnin's clinical textbook for veterinary technicians*, ed 7, St Louis, 2010, Saunders Elsevier.)

⚖ VETERINARY PRACTICE and the LAW

The emotions that a person feels with the loss of a pet are intense. Frequently clients do not understand the severity of a disease or injury; they may deny the importance of diagnostic studies and medical care until it is too late. They often feel that it is the practice's poor medicine that caused the pet's condition.

Clients must receive education on the disease, injury, or condition that the pet is experiencing as well as understand the prognosis of the case. Recommendations, whether accepted or declined, must be clearly noted in the record. With the information, communication, listening, and understanding that the team provides the client, the less likely clients will become angry with the practice.

Self-Evaluation Questions

1. What is euthanasia?
2. Why is quality of life important?
3. What are the five stages of grief? Describe each.
4. Why is the human-animal bond so strong?
5. In what ways can a pet be memorialized?
6. How should a pet be presented to an owner after it has been euthanized?
7. What drug is in a euthanasia solution?
8. How does this drug affect the body?
9. How can a team prevent the wrong ashes from being sent home with an owner?
10. Why must a euthanasia release form be signed by the owner?

Recommended Reading

Guntzelman J, Reiger M: Helping pet owners with the euthanasia decision, *Vet Med* 88:26–34, 1993.

Kay WJ, Cohen SP, Kutscher AH: *Euthanasia of the companion animal: the impact on owners, veterinarians and society*, Philadelphia, 1988, Charles Press.

Lagoni L: *The practical guide to client grief: support techniques for 15 common situations*, Denver, 1997, AAHA Press.

McCulloch WF: The veterinarian's education about the human-animal bond and animal-facilitated therapy, *Vet Clin North Am* 15: 1985.

Veterinary Practice Systems

Appointments and appointment management are critical factors in practices that use an appointment system; a system that keeps appointments on schedule is essential. A client's time is just as valuable as a veterinarian's time; if the practice cannot keep appointments on time, it cannot expect clients to run on time either. A number of factors contribute to the development of an appointment system, including the length of appointment, what the appointment is for, and which doctor is scheduled to see patients. A scheduler can be overwhelming for new employees; it is important to list the details for a new employee becoming familiar with the system.

Medical records are considered legal documents and also allow the team to follow cases as they progress. If paper records are used they must be legible, complete, and initialed by every author who enters information. If they are illegible, steps must be taken to correct the action because incorrect information and medication may be obtained from the record. Because it is a legal document, a judge or layperson should also be able to read the record in case a client chooses to sue the practice. It is imperative that legible medical records follow a SOAP (*s*ubjective, *o*bjective, *a*ssessment, *p*lan) format, allowing team members and referring veterinarians to follow the case.

Management of the practice inventory is a critical factor. Inventory is the second highest cost in a veterinary practice as well as the second highest revenue center. Successful management is essential to prevent shrinkage and product expiration. A practice cannot purchase many products that treat the same problem; a choice should be made to maintain one product. If a client or doctor chooses another product, a prescription can be written. The practice cannot afford to have multiple products that do not sell sitting on the shelf. Holding and ordering costs are accumulated with those products as well as cost absorption once the product expires. Along with inventory management is the markup of products once they are received. Product pricing must include holding, ordering, and receiving costs and recovering the hidden costs associated with the veterinary hospital. Most products are marked up 150% to 200% for the practice to profit from the pharmacy center.

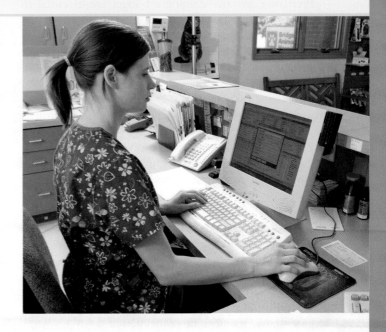

Controlled substances are drugs that the Drug Enforcement Agency (DEA) has classified as having the potential to be abused. Therefore it is imperative that they are maintained according to law. Every controlled substance that is dispensed must be recorded, and each drug must be balanced yearly or biannually depending on the state. Losses greater than 3% must be reported as a loss to the state board of veterinary medicine and the DEA. Expired medications must be disposed of properly, and a report must be generated stating that they were expired and incinerated. Logs associated with these medications must be maintained for several years. Logs can also be maintained for equipment and other products within the practice, including a radiology check-out log. This allows radiographs to be tracked in case they were never returned to the practice.

Accounts receivable must be managed just as strictly as inventory management because this is another area associated with loss in a veterinary practice. Accounts receivable should never reach more than a specified percentage of the monthly income. Once these outstanding accounts reach 90 days past due, they can be impossible to collect and must be sent to a collections agency. Team members responsible for collection of money must be familiar with

251

the Fair Debt Collections Practices Act, which ultimately protects the consumer from harassment. If clients are consistently asking to charge, a third-party payment plan may be recommended, such as Care Credit. This credit card is used exclusively for veterinary services and can provide clients an alternative to charging at the practice. Pet health insurance should also be recommended because many procedures and products are covered for pets. Premiums, copays, and deductibles are required just as in human medicine; however, practices do not file claims.

Preparing and maintaining a budget are essential to practice survival. Practices must plan budgets to prevent overspending of cash, especially during the hospital's slowest months. Preplanning allows the estimation of production, payroll, and taxes. Budgeting allows the practice to set aside money for team raises, bonuses, and the purchase of equipment. Excellent planning allows greater practice reinvestment and a return on investment for the owner.

Zoonotic disease is a real risk in veterinary medicine. Often, veterinary assistants, technicians, and doctors are the first to notice symptoms and come in direct contact with disease. Exceptional personal hygiene must be practiced at all times; team members must be familiar with diseases that are common to the area and practice transmission prevention on all levels. Zoonotic disease prevention should be included in any safety program. Safety programs should cover all aspects of team member safety, including those highlighted by the Occupational Safety and Health Administration (OSHA). To satisfy OSHA requirements, practices must maintain a safety program, create a hazards safety manual, and inform team members of the hazards associated with their jobs. A safety manger can be appointed who is responsible for training all team members, documenting the training procedures, and enforcing the use of personal protection equipment. Chemicals should all be listed in a hazards program and include a Material Safety Data Sheet informing team members of the properties of the products and measures to take in case ingestion, contamination, or inappropriate use has occurred.

Safety programs for the staff go beyond OSHA recommendations. Every practice is susceptible to crime and must take all precautions necessary to prevent harm to clients, patients, and team members. Perimeter lighting is very important to deter criminal activity against both clients and team members. Staff must be prepared for a robbery attempt during business hours or after hours. Security should also encompass the computer systems. Backup methods must be used if a computer is stolen or a hacker interrupts the system's functions. All computer systems should be password protected, adding a second level of security.

Practice and office management go far beyond client and patient care. Behind the scenes work must be completed and maintained on a daily basis, allowing the practice to function fully and prevent disasters from occurring. Preventing problems is much more efficient than resolving problems when they do occur. Veterinary assistants and technicians play an active role in troubleshooting, problem prevention, and problem solving. Skills gained from school, previous employment, and life experiences contribute to the success of the practice as well as each individual on the team.

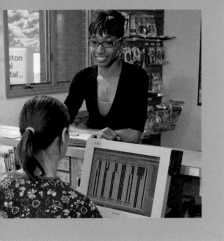

Appointment Management Systems

Learning Objectives

Mastery of the content in this chapter will enable the reader to:
- List factors that affect appointment scheduling.
- Effectively make appointments.
- Identify appointment cards.
- Discuss the importance of reminding clients of upcoming appointments.
- List methods used to increase the production and efficiency of the team by managing appointments.
- List methods used to manage clients who walk into the practice with minor emergencies.

Key Terms

Appointment Book Template
Appointment Cards

Appointment Scheduler
Appointment Units

Preoperative Instructions

Veterinary practices can use an appointment system or accept clients on a walk-in basis; most veterinary practices prefer appointments. A variation of both may work best for some hospitals. Appointments can help control the amount of traffic flow through the veterinary clinic at a given time. All team members should be available on days that the appointments are fully booked, whereas slower times require less staff. It is important to create a schedule that is going to keep the practice running on schedule for appointments; a client's time is just as

> **PRACTICE POINT** Appointments can help control the amount of client traffic in a hospital at any one time.

valuable as the doctor's time, and finding a medium between the two will contribute to a successful practice.

Walk-in practices allow clients to come into the clinic when it is convenient for them. However, this can decrease the efficiency of the team and prevents the

We are now accepting appointments!
Please speak with our receptionist to schedule your next appointment.

FIGURE 13-1 Hanging a "Now Accepting Appointments" sign in the practice encourages clients to adapt to the change in the practice.

regulation of traffic flow. Client wait times will increase, and team burnout will occur quickly. It is important to look at both the advantages and disadvantages of walk-ins versus appointments and decide what is best for the practice, considering both the team and the clients. The goals of an appointment system should be to maximize productivity, reduce staff tension, and control traffic flow through the veterinary hospital, all while maintaining concern for client and patient needs.

For those practices wishing to convert from a walk-in structure to appointment structure, the transition can be relatively easy. Clients are easy to train and will adapt to the new structure. A client newsletter or brochure can be sent to all clients indicating the change. The information contained in this newsletter or brochure can state the advantages to the client of the transition (Figures 13-1 and 13-2). Attractively framed posters in the reception area and exam rooms can also educate clients of the change. Once clients realize that this a better option for them, they will gladly embrace the transition.

> **PRACTICE POINT**   Clients can be informed of implementation of an appointment schedule by newsletters and postcards.

Some clinics prefer a slow transition, whereas others prefer to change immediately. Appointments can start slowly; they can be made in the mornings while walk-ins can be seen in the afternoons. This can continue for several months until appointments can be integrated into the entire day. Once appointments are scheduled throughout the day, slots can be left available for those walk-ins that have not adjusted to the change. When these clients return, they will know to make an appointment.

Those practices that integrate appointments immediately must schedule and allow for a large number of walk-ins for a short period of time. Once the clients have become trained, the amount of time set aside for walk-ins can be reduced. Walk-ins should never be turned away. If it appears that the wait time will be lengthy, team members can offer the client the opportunity to drop off the pet; the owner will be called when the patient is ready.

During the transition, team members will make mistakes; this can be a positive learning experience for all members. Teamwork, communication, and training among staff and clients will minimize the effect of these mistakes and will prevent errors from occurring in the future.

PAPER VERSUS SOFTWARE APPOINTMENT SCHEDULE

Some smaller veterinary practices have used a paper appointment schedule book with success and continue to do so. A book may work well with a one-doctor practice, but as practices continue to grow in the number of veterinarians on staff, appointment books can become difficult to manage and share when multiple clients are waiting to make appointments (Figure 13-3).

If a paper appointment book is preferred, studies indicate that a week-at-a-glance style works best. It will depend on the size of the veterinary practice as to what size of book to purchase, the number of columns, and appropriate appointment time slots. For example, a smaller one-doctor practice may use three columns per day. One column can be designated for the doctor's appointments, one column for technician appointments, and another for surgery. A larger number of veterinarians would require more columns.

Software appointment schedulers can be accessed from any computer in the clinic, thereby allowing multiple users to make appointments. This can increase the efficiency of the staff; one team member can make a surgery appointment while another can make an appointment for a yearly exam (Figures 13-4 and 13-5). Access from multiple computers can have one disadvantage. Multiple team members may be viewing one appointment slot available, and when they click on the appointment to secure it, another team member may have already booked it. This is only a minor disadvantage compared with the number of benefits that appointment software can provide.

Software appointment schedulers have far more features than just scheduling appointments. When a team

> **PRACTICE POINT**   Veterinary appointment software has several advantages that will help increase team efficiency and organization.

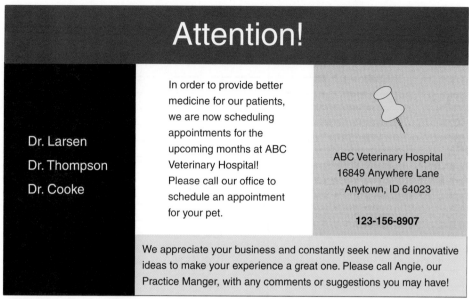

Attention!

Dr. Larsen

Dr. Thompson

Dr. Cooke

In order to provide better medicine for our patients, we are now scheduling appointments for the upcoming months at ABC Veterinary Hospital! Please call our office to schedule an appointment for your pet.

ABC Veterinary Hospital
16849 Anywhere Lane
Anytown, ID 64023

123-156-8907

We appreciate your business and constantly seek new and innovative ideas to make your experience a great one. Please call Angie, our Practice Manger, with any comments or suggestions you may have!

FIGURE 13-2 A postcard is a great way to let clients know about changes in the practice.

member fills an appointment slot with a current client, the software can show alerts reminding the team of overdue vaccinations, tests, previous no-show appointments, or a poor credit status. When the client account is accessed, all pets owned by that client will be available, and all overdue reminders will show. This allows the reception team to either schedule an appointment for multiple patients owned by the same client or remind the owner of the overdue condition (Figure 13-6).

If a client chooses to cancel or move an appointment, software allows the receptionist to cut and paste, keeping all pertinent information together. The receptionist will not have to retype or misinterpret information.

Software allows the veterinary practice to become proactive, instead of reactive, to client needs. Proactive service begins before the client walks in the door. The client is satisfied with the ability to make an appointment, the time available, and the ability to make an appointment with the veterinarian he or she wanted to see. Reactive service is taking care of the client *after* he or she is upset. Perhaps the client had to wait too long, was dissatisfied with the service, or did not get to make an appointment. Appointment scheduling software can only enhance the experience of a client and make it a more pleasant experience. If the practice is technology proficient and is able to use online Web portals, clients can make their own appointments. New trends show that clients take care of personal business online and prefer to shop, search for information, and make appointments online when possible.

> **PRACTICE POINT**   Many factors affect appointment scheduling, and all must be considered to keep appointments running as scheduled.

Every veterinary practice software program has an appointment scheduler available, which should be used to its maximum potential. Systems provided by different software companies will have both advantages and disadvantages and vary in their efficiency. Each version of software should be demonstrated before purchase. This will allow the practice to determine which software will integrate best with the practice. User friendliness and compatibility of the programs should top the list of items when looking for software. Refer to Chapter 8 for more information and guidelines on software selection for a veterinary practice.

DESIGNING THE APPOINTMENT BOOK TEMPLATE

The template is the outline of the appointment book and must be established before using a new system. Next, factors that affect appointment scheduling must be considered. The hours the clinic is open should be entered into the template first. This includes when the practice opens, closes for lunch, and closes in the evenings as well as any weekend hours. If the practice closes for weekly staff meetings, that should also be entered into the template. Holidays must be added into the system because most systems do not automatically recognize closed holidays. Permanent flex time should also be added so that employees cannot accidentally remove or book an appointment in a slot that has extra time built in. Generally, a practice manager or owner creates the template and is the only one who has access to modify it.

There are many factors that come into play when developing an appointment schedule. There is no written rule stating how many appointments should be seen or how long appointments should last. Schedules

Monday December 29, 2009

	Dr. C	Surgery	Drop Off
8:00			
8:15			
8:30			
8:45			
9:00			
9:15			
9:30			
9:45			
10:00			
10:15			
10:30			
10:45			
11:00			
11:15			
11:30			
11:45			
12:00			
12:15			
12:30			
12:45			
1:00			
1:15			
1:30			
1:45			
2:00			
2:15			
2:30			
2:45			
3:00			
3:15			
3:30			
3:45			
4:00			
4:15			
4:30			
4:45			
5:00			
5:15			
5:30			
5:45			
6:00			
6:15			
6:30			
6:45			
7:00			

FIGURE 13-3 Sample paper schedule.

vary with each practice, and the team determines what is best for both clients and staff. Appointment layout can change as the practice grows and team members identify problems with the current schedule. Once an appointment system has been integrated, it must be aggressively managed. Appointment times, availability, length of time, and available team members should be monitored and revised on a regular basis. When developing a scheduling system, the following factors should be taken into consideration.

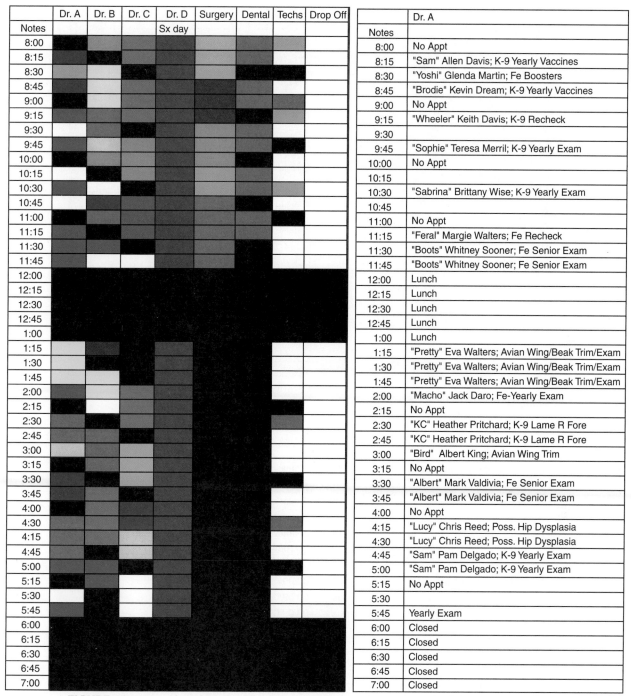

	Dr. A	Dr. B	Dr. C	Dr. D	Surgery	Dental	Techs	Drop Off
Notes				Sx day				
8:00								
8:15								
8:30								
8:45								
9:00								
9:15								
9:30								
9:45								
10:00								
10:15								
10:30								
10:45								
11:00								
11:15								
11:30								
11:45								
12:00								
12:15								
12:30								
12:45								
1:00								
1:15								
1:30								
1:45								
2:00								
2:15								
2:30								
2:45								
3:00								
3:15								
3:30								
3:45								
4:00								
4:30								
4:15								
4:45								
5:00								
5:15								
5:30								
5:45								
6:00								
6:15								
6:30								
6:45								
7:00								

	Dr. A
Notes	
8:00	No Appt
8:15	"Sam" Allen Davis; K-9 Yearly Vaccines
8:30	"Yoshi" Glenda Martin; Fe Boosters
8:45	"Brodie" Kevin Dream; K-9 Yearly Vaccines
9:00	No Appt
9:15	"Wheeler" Keith Davis; K-9 Recheck
9:30	
9:45	"Sophie" Teresa Merril; K-9 Yearly Exam
10:00	No Appt
10:15	
10:30	"Sabrina" Brittany Wise; K-9 Yearly Exam
10:45	
11:00	No Appt
11:15	"Feral" Margie Walters; Fe Recheck
11:30	"Boots" Whitney Sooner; Fe Senior Exam
11:45	"Boots" Whitney Sooner; Fe Senior Exam
12:00	Lunch
12:15	Lunch
12:30	Lunch
12:45	Lunch
1:00	Lunch
1:15	"Pretty" Eva Walters; Avian Wing/Beak Trim/Exam
1:30	"Pretty" Eva Walters; Avian Wing/Beak Trim/Exam
1:45	"Pretty" Eva Walters; Avian Wing/Beak Trim/Exam
2:00	"Macho" Jack Daro; Fe-Yearly Exam
2:15	No Appt
2:30	"KC" Heather Pritchard; K-9 Lame R Fore
2:45	"KC" Heather Pritchard; K-9 Lame R Fore
3:00	"Bird" Albert King; Avian Wing Trim
3:15	No Appt
3:30	"Albert" Mark Valdivia; Fe Senior Exam
3:45	"Albert" Mark Valdivia; Fe Senior Exam
4:00	No Appt
4:15	"Lucy" Chris Reed; Poss. Hip Dysplasia
4:30	"Lucy" Chris Reed; Poss. Hip Dysplasia
4:45	"Sam" Pam Delgado; K-9 Yearly Exam
5:00	"Sam" Pam Delgado; K-9 Yearly Exam
5:15	No Appt
5:30	
5:45	Yearly Exam
6:00	Closed
6:15	Closed
6:30	Closed
6:45	Closed
7:00	Closed

FIGURE 13-4 Sample software schedule. An appointment summary schedule appears on the *left,* along with a detailed view of Dr. A's appointments *(right).*

Number of Veterinarians

The number of veterinarians seeing appointments on a daily basis may vary. For example, if three veterinarians are seeing appointments on Monday morning, those times may be staggered so that three appointments do not show up at 9 AM and overwhelm the front reception team. One appointment may be scheduled for 9 AM, the second for 9:05 AM, and the third for 9:10 AM, for Dr. A, Dr. B, and Dr. C, respectively. If appointments are 15

minutes each, Dr. A's next appointment will be scheduled for 9:15 AM, Dr. B's next appointment will be scheduled for 9:20 AM, and Dr. C's next appointment will be scheduled for 9:25 AM (Figure 13-7).

Veterinary Technician Appointments

Some appointments can be scheduled for a technician alone, thereby leaving an appointment slot available for a producing doctor. Nail trims, suture removals,

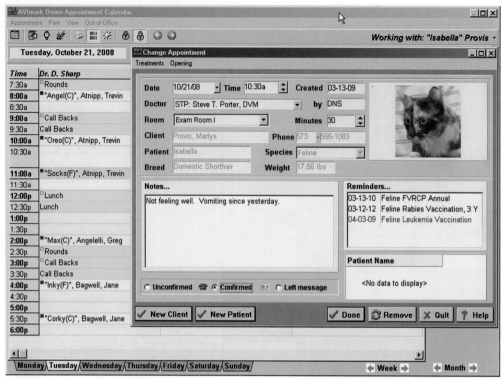

FIGURE 13-5 Sample screen from Avimark's appointment calendar. (Courtesy McAllister Software Systems, Piedmont, Mo.)

Patient Medical History		ABC Veterinary Clinic
Teresa Longmower	**Patient:** Jack	**DOB:** 10/01/02
123 Anystreet	**Species:** Canine	**Age:** 6y
Anytown, MI 89892	**Breed:** Boxer	**Sex:** MN
	Color: Brown/White	**Tag:** 123
Acct No: 1234	**Doctor:** Nancy Dreamer	**Weight:** 48.2#
Phone: (555) 555-5555	**As of:** 10/10/09	

Reminders:

3710	Heartworm Test	Overdue	03/09/09
0690	Canine Yearly Exam	Overdue	03/09/09
0602	DHPP 3 year	Overdue	03/09/09
0601	Rabies 3 year	Overdue	03/09/09

FIGURE 13-6 Sample overdue reminders in a software system.

weight-management rechecks, and anal gland expressions (among many other tasks) can be scheduled with a credentialed or skilled veterinary technician (Figure 13-8). This allows veterinarians to continue to see clients who need to have a diagnosis made. Technicians can always ask a veterinarian for help if they have a question about the case.

> ◎ **PRACTICE POINT**   Veterinary technician appointments can increase the efficiency of the veterinarian by allowing the doctor to diagnose, treat, and perform surgery. Technicians can trim nails, express anal sacs, and educate clients about a variety of diseases.

Length of Time of Appointments

Team members must decide what length of time an appointment should be to accommodate their clients' needs in the best way possible. Some teams feel that 10-minute slots are too short but have found them successful in increasing the overall practice profit. Thirty to forty percent of small animal practices use 15-minute slots. Time and motion studies indicate that it takes approximately 12 minutes to check in a patient, obtain a thorough history, perform a physical exam, prepare the necessary medications and client education materials, and write in the medical record. That leaves only 3 minutes

Appt Time	Dr. A	Dr. B	Dr. C
8:00	Angela Jones	Block	Eva Marsch "Pat" NT
8:05	"Cassidy" K-9	Sabrina Patterson	Block
8:10	Yearly Exam	"Sheba" Feline	Brittany Wilson
8:15	242-5678	Ear Infection	"Danny" K-9
8:20	Block	876-3334	New Puppy/vaccines
8:25	Nikki Ewing	Block	444-3834
8:30	"Sundance" Hamster	Julie Denamarin	Block
8:35	Vomiting	"Oscar" K-9	Nancy Dallop
8:40	Block	Lame, Left Fore	"Wheeler" K-9
8:45	Sue Biel	889-9098	Growth check 575-9808
9:00	"King" Avian		Block
9:05	Wing/Nail Trim/Exam		Jamie Dunlap
9:10	454-9084	Valarie Goodwill	"Cameron" Feline
9:15		"Sasha" K-9	Senior Wellness Exam/BW
9:30		Consult w/Dr. B	897-3938
9:45	Block	999-8987	
10:00	Denzel Marrow		Block
10:15	"Joy" K-9		Sarah Michael
10:30	Poss. Diabetic	Block	"Enzo" Booster
10:45	242-9098	Linda Block	876-0969
11:00		"Jackie"	Block
11:15		Check Eyes 466-8740	
11:30	Block	Frances Reed	
11:45		"Mike" K9	
12:00		Recheck 575-3493	

FIGURE 13-7 Staggered appointment blocks keep multiple clients from walking in at the same time.

> **◎ PRACTICE POINT**   Most practices use 15-minute appointment slots.

to educate the client about health issues that may be of concern. Some practitioners feel this is an inadequate amount of time to spend with their clients; however, a well-trained staff can educate the client while the veterinarian continues to the next appointment.

Other practices prefer 20-minute appointments. Some practitioners feel that they need to spend the time with the client and educate them personally, not delegate to the staff. By increasing the appointment slot to 20 minutes, the veterinarian has additional 5 minutes to educate the client. The disadvantage to 20-minute appointments is the reduction in the number of clients seen per day. On the other hand, the average client transaction can rise with the increased amount of time spent with the client. Decreased client volume per day can have a significant impact on the staff and prevent team burnout. The use of 20-minute appointment slots can also improve the practice's on-time performance.

A 10-minute flex system is also another option for staff members scheduling appointments. Team members can analyze the client's situation and estimate the length of time an appointment is likely to take. Staff can schedule several 10-minute blocks together to create the perfect appointment time. Each practice must decide what will benefit both the client and the team the best. Team members who schedule appointments must be knowledgeable about diseases, procedures, and clients to schedule effectively. If any question should arise regarding proper time allotment, an informed team member should be consulted; it is better to verify before making the appointment instead of overscheduling the team at a later time.

Length of Time for Client Education

Some practices schedule time for client education alone. Client education does not necessarily need to be given by a veterinarian, but should be scheduled so that clients do not have to wait. A pet may have just been diagnosed with a serious disease and the client will need to receive lengthy education regarding the patient's disease and health. Scheduling client education can significantly increase client compliance and understanding

> **◎ PRACTICE POINT**   Client education time can be reserved on the technician's appointment schedule, allowing the veterinarian to see other appointments.

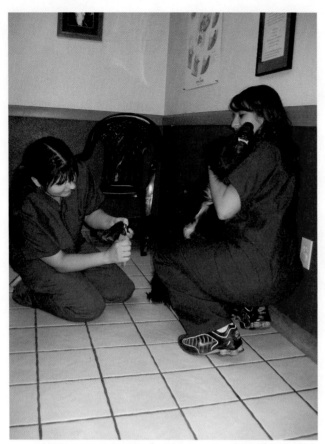

FIGURE 13-8 Two technicians perform a nail trim.

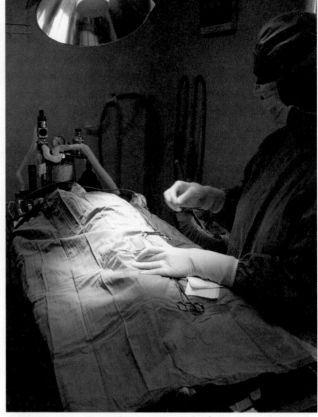

FIGURE 13-9 Operations may require longer appointment times.

while establishing a lasting client-practice bond. Client education can be scheduled with a veterinary technician, allowing the veterinarian to continue seeing appointments.

Surgery

The number of operations to schedule in a day depends on the team, the length of time it takes the veterinarian to complete a procedure, and the amount of time available to complete the procedures. One veterinarian may be faster at a particular procedure and therefore able to complete more operations in a day than another. Larger practices may have two surgical tables and are therefore able to accommodate a larger number of surgical patients at a time, increasing the efficiency of the team (Figure 13-9).

Dental Procedures

Some teams may have either one or two dental tables and units available, increasing the number of dental procedures a practice can accommodate in one day (Figure 13-10). Practices can have several credentialed technicians performing dental procedures concurrently while nonsterile or sterile procedures are being completed on another table.

Nonsterile Procedures

Abscess debridement, anal sac expression, ear flushes, and patients that need to be sedated for radiographs all take time of the treatment team (Figure 13-11). Time should be allotted to complete these procedures; this will help prevent the team from backing up and running late for appointments. Clients do not see the procedures being completed in the treatment area and therefore do not perceive that the hospital is busy. They will not understand why their appointments are late. An excessive number of nonsterile procedures can increase stress on the team, preventing lunches or breaks from being taken. Proper scheduling can prevent this situation, which can ultimately lead to team burnout when it occurs on a daily basis.

Holidays

The owners and manager can decide what holidays to close for and allow the scheduler to accommodate that time off. Team members should remember that business days after a holiday closure are generally very busy and should add flex time into the appointment scheduler to accommodate minor emergencies and walk-ins that will occur.

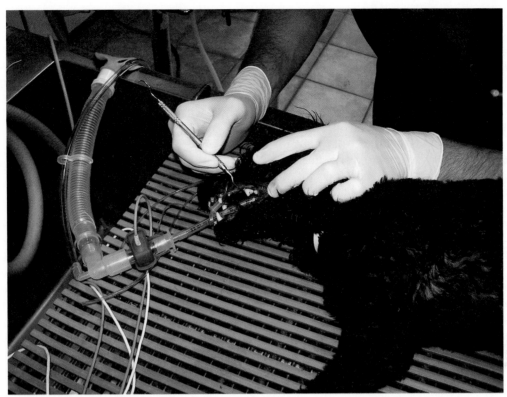

FIGURE 13-10 Being able to handle multiple dental procedures a day increases revenue.

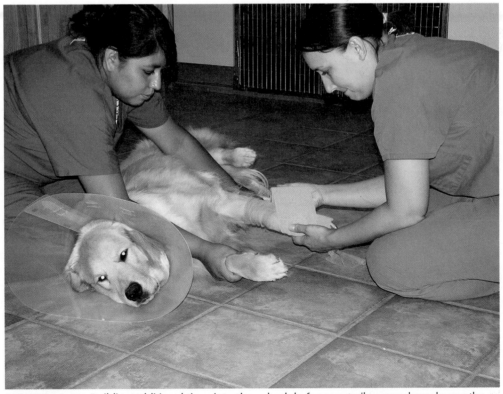

FIGURE 13-11 Building additional time into the schedule for nonsterile procedures keeps the practice from running behind schedule for the day.

> **PRACTICE POINT** The day after a holiday is always busy and needs to be factored into an appointment schedule. Clients will have minor emergencies that happened over the holiday.

Vacation and Continuing Education

Any time doctors or technicians take time off, it must be built into the schedule months in advance. It can be difficult and irritating to clients to have to reschedule their appointments. When the practice is short a doctor, the remaining team members must accommodate the veterinary shortage and increased traffic flow. Adjustments can be made to prevent appointments from running behind.

Type of Appointment

Appointment times can vary depending on what they are for. A yearly examination may only take 15 minutes, whereas a limping patient that requires an orthopedic exam can take 30 minutes. Team members should be aware of what types of problems are going to take longer to examine and diagnose and make adjustments when scheduling those appointments. (See Figure 13-14 for examples of appointment units and length of time.)

> **PRACTICE POINT** Certain clients always take more time, and this should be accounted for when making appointments for them.

Appointments for new patients may take more time than appointments for existing patients; new clients may take 30 minutes instead of the usual 15 minutes allotted for existing clients.

Clients

Certain clients will always take longer than others simply because of who they are. Team members should be able to identify these clients right away and add extra time for their appointments. These clients may be in the top 10% of the practice's producing clients, or they may like to chat. Whatever the reason, by accommodating these clients, team members can prevent appointments from running behind.

The benefit of appointment software is the ability to create an individual appointment setting for each doctor. If Dr. A prefers 20-minute appointment slots and can complete surgical procedures at a moderately quick pace, then the schedule can accommodate that change. If Dr. B prefers 15-minute appointments but is slower at completing surgical procedures, the software should be able to adjust for that.

A clinic will learn what works best for that individual practice and can make changes along the way. Word of mouth spreads quickly as clients say, "Oh, I have to go to the vet today; you know they will be running late." It is better to hear, "My veterinarian is always on time.

It is rare that I have to wait more than 5 or 10 minutes for my appointment." However, all practices should be able to accommodate the possibility of emergencies and walk-ins. Clients may feel their pets have an emergency regardless of whether it is only an ear infection. It is important to remember client perception; they do not know what is and is not an emergency.

> **PRACTICE POINT** Most clients feel that when their pet is sick, it is an emergency. Team members must realize that this is client perception and embrace it.

SCHEDULING FOR PRODUCTIVITY

Doctors should be able to delegate tasks to a well-trained staff member to continue seeing appointments and increase their productivity. If diagnostic work has been advised, the patient should be turned over to the lead technician, who can then complete the tests that the veterinarian has advised. Once results are available, the doctor can be notified and a treatment plan instituted. To keep appointments running as scheduled, the team may ask clients to wait in the reception area while laboratory work is being performed. This allows the exam room to be freed for the next appointment, preventing a 20- or 30-minute delay.

ADAPTING THE SCHEDULE FOR EMERGENCIES

Emergencies will always occur. If appointments are scheduled and emergencies arrive, it must be communicated to clients that there has been an emergency. Most clients understand the need to attend to the emergency and do not mind the wait. However, clients should be updated every 5 minutes to let them know they have not been forgotten. The team can offer the waiting client water, coffee, and/or a magazine to try to offset the wait. Remember, 5 minutes seems like 10 minutes to a client!

If an emergency arrives and it is apparent it is going to take more than a few minutes (e.g., the patient needs to go to surgery), reception members can call appointments scheduled for the day and explain that there has been an emergency causing appointments to fall behind. Team members can politely ask to reschedule appointments for a later time in the day or for another day if that does not work with the client's schedule. Yearly exams should always be asked first to reschedule because that appointment has less priority over a client who has a sick pet.

HABITUALLY LATE CLIENTS

There will always be clients who are late. Practices may post a sign indicating that any client who is more than 15 minutes late will be considered a walk-in; they can either be rescheduled or treated as a walk-in and seen as time

What Would You Do/Not Do?

Mrs. Morris calls the practice at 2 PM on a Friday and would like to come to the office as a walk-in in to see if her dog is pregnant. The reception team advises her that all the appointments are booked for the day and several emergencies have arrived, placing the team behind schedule. They advise Mrs. Morris to please schedule an appointment for the following week when her wait would not have to be so long. Mrs. Morris schedules her appointment for the following Tuesday, but shows up 15 minutes before closing anyway.

What Does the Reception Team Do?

The reception team must ask Mrs. Morris if something serious has happened causing her to come in early for her appointment; the client may have a valid concern for her pet's health. If she insists that the pet is feeling fine and she "just can't wait until Tuesday," then the team must inform her of her wait time. Because the practice has had numerous emergencies, the team is still approximately an hour behind schedule and she will be the last client seen. Communication with the client is essential, to make sure she understands the wait for a nonemergency. The client should also be advised once in the exam room that appointments are preferred, especially instead of arriving 15 minutes before closing.

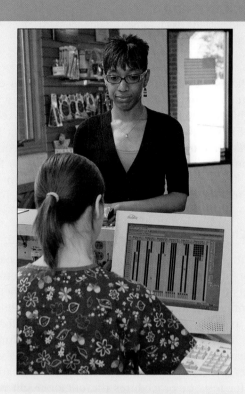

permits. To enforce this policy, however, practice appointments should run on time or clients will become irate.

Once a client has been denied an appointment because of tardiness, it is unlikely he or she will be late for the following appointment. Clients can be politely addressed regarding their constant tardiness. When Mr. Derk, a habitually late client, calls to make an appointment, team members may say "Mr. Derk, the nature of Fluffy's appointment requires the full time allotted for your appointment. Please remember your appointment is set for Tuesday, June 5, at 3 PM." This lets the client know that your practice has recognized his tardiness in the past and will be expecting him to arrive on time.

> **PRACTICE POINT**   Habitually late clients should be frequently reminded of their appointment times.

If a client calls ahead and lets the team know he or she will be late, the receptionist should check the schedule to make sure the client can still be accommodated without delaying the rest of the appointments. If it will be a tight squeeze, the appointment can be rescheduled.

MANAGEMENT DURING BUSY TIMES

Managers can determine the busiest time of a practice. This may be in the morning as patients scheduled for surgery are being checked in along with appointments that are to be seen by associate doctors. The busy time for another practice may be in the afternoon as clients are picking up patients, walk-ins arrive, and appointments are scheduled. Whichever the case may be, the appointment schedule can be modified to alleviate the busy time.

> **PRACTICE POINT**   Practice managers and owners must determine the busiest time for a hospital and schedule adequate staff at that time to manage the clientele.

MANAGEMENT OF WALK-INS

A veterinary practice is always going to have walk-ins regardless of an appointment policy. The client perception must be recognized as a part of good customer service. Therefore planning for these walk-ins can alleviate the stress associated with them. Time should be allotted in the scheduler for one or two walk-ins per hour, per veterinarian. Appointments should always be assured that they will be seen first, and walk-in clients must be advised that there will be a wait, but the team will do their best to get them in as efficiently as possible.

Practices can also hold appointments until the "day of." Appointments that were previously blocked off are made available that day. This allows clients with minor emergencies and walk-ins to be accommodated without having a significant impact on appointments.

Walk-ins set the appointments behind because they are often not routine exams. Practices certainly want to train their clientele that appointments are preferred, but should never give the impression that their pet is not important enough to be seen. If a client has a concern, the staff must recommend bringing the pet in for an exam. Team members can give the client the option to make an appointment, walk in, or drop the patient off.

PATIENT DROP-OFF

Depending on the veterinary team, accepting patients as drop-offs can eliminate the backlog of appointments. Patients that have been dropped off can be fit between appointments, and if bloodwork or radiographs need to be performed, they can be completed before the owner returns (with owner permission). Technicians must gather a complete history of the patient before the owner leaves and, if possible, provide a preliminary estimate for tests or procedures the doctor might recommend. After the doctor has been able to examine the pet, the owner can be called and decisions can be made regarding the patient's case. Once the case is completed, the owner can be called. This satisfies clients because they do not have to wait for a prolonged amount of time. Certain clients will never leave their "babies" at the clinic, and those clients must always be seen. Some team members may object to drop-offs, but with a well-trained staff this can free up a large amount of time.

NO-SHOW APPOINTMENTS

All practices have clients who do not show up for appointments. Emergencies may occur, a client may forget, or a pet may disappear for a few hours (cats especially!). Team members should call clients the day before their appointments to remind them of their scheduled appointment times. This can eliminate client forgetfulness; if the client knows making the appointment will be impossible, the appointment can be rescheduled during the phone call. If a client does not show up, a team member should call and attempt to reschedule the appointment. It should be noted in the record that the client did not show for the appointment and that a team member attempted to reschedule the appointment. Specific clients may frequently be no-shows. This should be documented in the record. These clients can be nicely advised that they will need to come as walk-ins and will be seen as appointments permit. Veterinary software allows alerts to be entered, informing team members as they access the account to make the appointment.

CLIENTS WHO ARRIVE ON THE WRONG DAY

Every veterinary practice has clients who arrive to the practice on the wrong day but still want to be seen. First, make sure the appointment card was written correctly. A team member may have incorrectly written the date, in which case every effort must be taken to correct the problem. The client should still be seen at the scheduled appointment time, and sincere apologies given to the client regarding the mistake. If a client has made an error, team members may ask the client if he or she wants to keep the original time scheduled (if it has not already passed) or prefers to reschedule the appointment. Otherwise, team members should make every effort to work the client into the schedule. Remember, excellent customer service is the goal, and being able to satisfy a client is very important.

APPOINTMENT CARDS

Clients should always be given appointment cards when they have made an appointment while they are in the clinic. Appointment cards may have a business card with the veterinary practice name, address, phone number, and veterinarian on the front and an open slot for the appointment in the back. The date, day, and time of the appointment should be written in along with the patient's name. It is a good idea to include the office policy regarding no-show appointments on the back of the card. This reminds clients that the veterinary practice time is valuable (Figure 13-12).

If a surgical procedure has been scheduled, instructions for the pet should be given to the owner. These patients are generally held off food and water before surgery, are dropped off at a specific time, and may be picked up at a specific time. Clients should be given this

has an appointment

on

☐ MON. ☐ TUES. ☐ WED. ☐ THURS. ☐ FRI. ☐ SAT.

_____ AT _____ A.M. / P.M.

If unable to keep appointment, kindly give 24 hrs. notice.

FIGURE 13-12 Appointment cards remind clients of their scheduled appointment times and prevent no-shows.

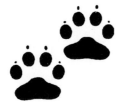

ABC Veterinary Clinic

Pre-operative Instructions for Healthy Dogs and Cats:
- No food after 6 pm
- No water after 10 pm

If your pet is over 7 years of age, please remove water first thing in the morning.

Please drop off your pet between 8 and 9 am
Please allow 10-15 minutes for a technician to ask you questions regarding your pet's health.

Your pet may be ready at 3 pm; please call before arrival to be sure your pet is ready.

- Pre-anesthetic bloodwork is available for each pet. Bloodwork is recommended the day of surgery to minimize the risk of anesthesia.
- Postoperative pain medication is available for each pet. Please inform us if you do not want pain medication for your pet.
- Bloodwork and pain medication are available for an additional cost and are highly recommended.

What can I expect after surgery?
- Your pet may be groggy from the anesthesia. Each pet may react differently to the medication. Each pet's health is evaluated before anesthesia administration.
- Provide your pet with a clean, quiet bed for recovery.
- Restrict exercise for 7 days.
- Check the incision daily. Do not allow your pet to lick the incision. If it is red and irritated, please return for a recheck.

Please call our clinic with any questions or concerns.
We are here to provide your pet with the best possible care.
123 Inspiration Lane
Anytown, MI
555-555-5555
Please give 24 hour advance notice of cancellations.

FIGURE 13-13 Preoperative instructions should be sent home with clients so they have all the information they need before their pet's procedure.

information in writing to take home; this allows them to review the information in a quiet place (Figure 13-13).

ENTERING APPOINTMENTS

Specific information is needed when making appointments for clients. Obviously, the client's first and last names are essential. The patient's name and the reason for the appointment come next, along with a phone number where the client can be reached. Veterinary appointment software automatically populates all the information except for the reason for the appointment when the client's name is entered. When using a manual appointment

book, it may benefit the team to add species, age, and breed of pet. Having all the above information allows the veterinary health care team to prepare for the appointment. Team members know which client will be arriving, what procedure to expect, and what equipment or lab work may be required. This increases the overall efficiency of the team, ultimately leading to a satisfied client.

> **PRACTICE POINT** Current phone numbers must be verified when making appointments; this allows the client to be called and reminded of the appointment or rescheduled if an emergency rises.

Training New Employees Appointment Unit List

1 Unit = 15 Minutes

Surgeries

Canine Neuter	2 Units
Canine Spay	3 Units
Feline Neuter	1 Unit
Feline Spay	2 Units
Growth Removal – Ask DVM performing surgery	
Dental	2 Units

Nonsterile Procedures

Radiographs	2 Units
Ear Flush	1 Unit
Anal Sac Flush	1 Unit

Exams

New Client	2 Units
Booster Exam	1 Unit
Yearly Exam	1 Unit
Senior Exam	2 Units
Orthopedic Exam	2 Units
Avian/Exotic Exam	2 Units

FIGURE 13-14 Appointment units make scheduling appointments easier.

It is important to have a phone number where the client can be reached on the day of the appointment (as well as a cell phone or pager) in case of an emergency or if questions arise. Veterinarians or team members may get sick or have family emergencies that must be taken care of. Clients will appreciate the phone call notifying them of the delay and may be happy to reschedule their appointment.

Once the appointment information has been completely entered, the team member should read the appointment back to the client, ensuring no miscommunication has occurred. "Mr. Lockridge, we have Rosie scheduled for her yearly exam on Monday, January 21, at 9 AM with Dr. Dreamer. Is there anything else I can help you with until we see you on the twenty-first?" is an excellent phrase to use because the date is repeated twice for the client.

UNITS FOR APPOINTMENT SCHEDULE

Many veterinary software applications name time increments as *units*. When the schedule is set up, the manager assigns a specific time to equal 1 unit. For example, 15 minutes may be classified as one unit. If a regular appointment will only take 15 minutes, then one unit is allotted for that patient. Orthopedic procedures can take 30 minutes and possibly more if radiographs are needed. Therefore this particular appointment would be given 2 units (30 minutes total). This can apply to surgical procedures as well. If a canine neuter takes a team 30 minutes from time of injection to time of extubation, then 2 units would be given for that particular operation. Tumor removals that may require extensive time are given more units. The veterinarian performing the surgery can be asked for a time estimate for the surgery. If the doctor requests 1 hour, then 4 units would be allotted for that operation. By giving time a unit, it is easier to schedule appointments and the efficiency of the staff is increased. It is imperative that the system that is being implemented be easy to understand and user friendly. Figure 13-14 gives examples of units assigned to specific procedures.

CALLING AND REMINDING CLIENTS OF APPOINTMENTS

All clients must be called and reminded of their appointments, regardless of whether it is a surgical or general appointment. Missed appointments represent lost income. Therefore the team should do everything possible to keep missed appointments to a minimum. Many veterinary practices can now send out reminders and updates by email or to pagers and cell phones. Clients appreciate the extra effort that team members are willing to put forth regarding their pets. If a procedure or lab work has been scheduled, this is a perfect time to remind clients of their instructions. Clients who don't follow instructions fall in the same category as missed appointments; a canceled surgical procedure is lost revenue.

> **PRACTICE POINT** Calling and reminding clients of appointments will reduce the number of no-shows, resulting in increased production.

TRAINING NEW EMPLOYEES HOW TO USE THE APPOINTMENT SYSTEM

Once team members have experience at scheduling appointments, making appointments becomes an easy, efficient task. However, scheduling appointments can cause anxiety for new employees. A training program should be implemented to ease this stress and decrease the chance of mistakes. Software systems generally have the usual amount of time allotted for appointments built into the template of the system. However, a list of conditions or diseases and the length of time preferred for related appointments should be made available. A list similar to Figure 13-14 can be created to assist new employees.

A list of clients who need extra time should also be made available to new employees if alerts have not already been added to these clients' accounts. This will increase the efficiency of the team and add another element to preventing appointments from running behind.

Selecting, managing, and revising an appointment schedule is an intricate but integral part of the veterinary practice. The schedule must be able to meet the needs of the practice, team members, and clients, while balancing productivity and profitability. Studies indicate that clients regard on-time performance to be a more important factor than the practice fee structure. If a patient is going to need further workup, including radiographs or diagnostic tests, it may be advised to leave the patient at the hospital while the workup is being completed. This prevents the client from waiting in the exam room for a prolonged period of time, thereby making other clients wait in the reception area. Clients may also choose to make another appointment for their pets when a workup needs to be completed if they do not wish to leave their pet. It is a common misconception that by meeting the needs of the one client in the exam room and satisfying that client the practice is providing good customer service. Unfortunately, the multiple clients who are waiting are not receiving good customer service. A balance between the two must be developed.

VETERINARY PRACTICE and the LAW

Client education time slots should be allotted for clients who have hospitalized pets that are to be released. Intense cases require owner communication; they must be informed about the disease or condition and how to treat it as well as the pet's prognosis. If owners are not provided with this information, the practitioner may be held liable.

If a diabetic patient is released to the owner without client education, the animal could die of hypoglycemia induced by the owner. Owners must be informed of how and when to give insulin injections, the care of insulin, symptoms of hypoglycemia, and the role of the diet in diabetes.

If a time slot is not held for client education, the team member or veterinarian may be rushed and not thoroughly explain the disease or condition. Clients should be provided with written materials that should be verbally reviewed, allowing the client to ask any questions.

Self-Evaluation Questions

1. Why should a veterinary practice implement an appointment system if one is not already in place?
2. How can clients be informed of the changes when practices want to implement an appointment system? Why create a positive atmosphere when making these changes?
3. What is the benefit of clients dropping off patients?
4. Why should veterinary clinics strive for a proactive environment?
5. Why should an appointment be established for client education?
6. Explain how to handle clients who are always late for their appointments.
7. What factors affect appointment scheduling?
8. Specific clients always take longer for appointments. Why allot those specific clients more time than other clients?
9. Why should walk-in clients be seen?
10. What information is vital when scheduling appointments?

Recommended Reading

Ackerman L: *Business basics for veterinarians*, New York, 2002, ASJA Press.

Ackerman L, Oster K: *Blackwell's five minute veterinary practice management consult*, Ames, IA, 2007, Blackwell Publishing.

Heinke MM: *Practice made perfect: a guide to veterinary practice management*, Lakewood, CO, 2001, AAHA Press.

McCurnin D: *Veterinary practice management*, Philadelphia, 1988, JB Lippincott.

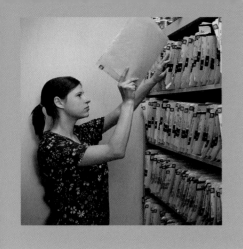

Medical Records Management

Learning Objectives

Mastery of the content in this chapter will enable the reader to:
- Explain methods used to file records.
- Identify a completed medical record.
- List the benefits of using labels for medical records.
- Explain how to purge medical records when needed.
- Define the advantages and disadvantages of computerized medical records.

- Develop and provide patient discharge instructions.
- Identify common abbreviations.
- Describe methods used to file radiographs.
- Clarify the importance of backing up computer systems on a daily basis.

Key Terms

Client Discharge Instructions
Computerized Medical Records
Herd Health Records
Legibility

Master Problem List
Paper Medical Records
Primary Complaint
Problem-Oriented Medical Record (POMR)

Prognosis
Purging Records
SOAP Medical Record
System Backup

Medical records are some of the most important documents in veterinary medicine, and medical record management is one of the most important management tasks. A medical record is a permanent written account of the professional interaction and services rendered in a valid patient-client relationship. The purpose of a medical record is to provide an accurate historical account for the veterinary health care team and owner, to alert staff to a patient's special needs, and serve as documentation for referrals. Records must be complete, legible, and easily accessible at all times. Clinics may choose to have paper records or computerized medical records (often referred to as *paperless medical records*); both have advantages and disadvantages. Inactive records must be kept on the premises for a certain length of time, regardless of whether they are paper or computerized, and can be purged after a

set period. A copy of any written communication with the owner must be in the medical record; the fact that these documents may become evidence in a malpractice suit warrants caution in writing and retaining them.

The office or practice manager should make it a daily task to pull random records and check for completeness. Practices get busy. The reception team takes the record to invoice the client, and occasionally it does not get returned to the original doctor or team member to be completed (Figure 14-1). Complete records must include the date of entry, initials of all team members writing in the record, a complete SOAP format, and all authorization forms a client has signed. If any charts have been referenced, those must also be in the record. The more information that is available in the medical record, the less the legal risk will be.

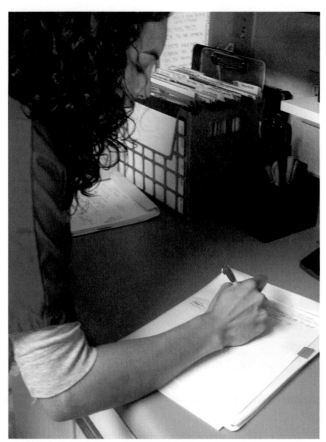

FIGURE 14-1 All medical records must be accurate and complete.

> **PRACTICE POINT** Failure to document any procedure or communication with a client in the medical record may prove costly in a lawsuit.

How medical records are maintained depends on each individual clinic. Some medical record systems have evolved with the practice; others may need updating to allow the veterinary practice to become more efficient and provide better patient and client care. The number of veterinarians and team members on staff, along with practice maturity, can affect a medical records system. There can be remarkable differences in medical records between team members, which can decrease the efficiency of the staff. It should be the goal of the team, office, and practice managers to develop a medical records system that allows maximum efficiency as well as excellent client communication and patient care.

LEGIBILITY OF MEDICAL RECORDS

Records must be legible and able to be read by anyone. Many team members become proficient at being able to read records written by another team member, but once those records are released to another clinic, specialty hospital, or court, the intended audience may not be able to read them. This can render a record incomplete. If a record was sent to court, a judge may return a decision based on the opinion that a treatment did not occur because he or she could not read the record. A veterinary specialist may not be able to determine if a specific treatment was done since it was not legible. An incomplete, illegible record can be considered an admission of professional incompetence and imply that the service provided was substandard. If records are illegible, changing to paperless records can be a good idea.

> **PRACTICE POINT** Records must be legible to be legal!

If legibility is problem within a veterinary practice, the use of labels or stamps may be suggested for routine procedures. Physical exams, urinalyses, routine dentals, and alterations are just a few labels that can be generated in a fill-in-the-blank form to accommodate details. Size of suture material can be easily added on surgical stickers, normal findings can be easily marked on physical exam stickers, and abnormal findings can be clearly defined below the label or stamp (Figure 14-2).

Blank labels can be purchased at a local office supply store relatively inexpensively. A label can be created within Microsoft Publisher and can be changed at any time to fit the needs of the practice.

A medical record is a legal document. Correction fluid cannot be used on any medical record, release, or authorization form at any time. If a mistake needs to be corrected, a one-line strike-through can be written, with the author's initials indicating the correction (Box 14-1).

CHOOSING A FILE SYSTEM

Practices that use paper records may file records according to different methods. One method is to file alphabetically. All records are filed by the owner's last name, then the first name. Other practices may file by client number. All pets are kept in the same file because many owners have more than one pet. Also included is a client/patient form (see Figure 2-8, *A*; Client Patient Information Sheet). Consent forms, patient check-in sheets, discharge sheets, and any other forms must be kept in this file as well.

PAPER RECORDS

Paper records can either be classified as full paper records or index card records. Paper records are written on 8.5 × 11-inch paper and usually fastened into a file folder with a two-hole fastener (Figure 14-3).

All lab work results, invoices, consent forms, and miscellaneous documents are kept in this folder. Pets can be separated by colored paper. Some clinics may use either blue or pink paper to draw attention to the sex of the patient. Names can be listed on the colored paper

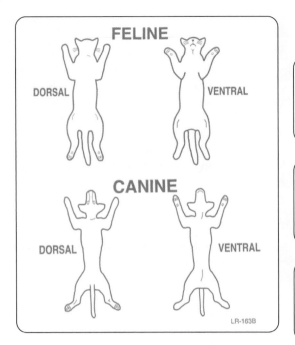

FELINE

DORSAL   VENTRAL

CANINE

DORSAL   VENTRAL

LR-163B

Feline Castration:

Using autoligation technique. No skin closure.
Surgery and recovery uneventful.

Canine and Feline OVH:

Ventral midline incision; _____Polysorb Double ligatures ovarian pedicles; _____Polysorb Double ligature encircling uterine body; _____ Polysorb Simple continuous body wall; _____Polysorb Simple cont. double layer; SubQ / subcut. closure. Surgery and recovery uneventful.

Canine Neuter:

Open/closed technique. Pre-scrotal incision, double ligate testicular artery, vein, and vas deferns with_____Polysorb. Subcutaneous and subcuticular layers closed simple continuous with _____Polysorb. Surgery/recovery uneventful.

Feline Declaw:

Using Roscoe blades, P3 was amputated and sealed with tissue adhesive.

Urinalysis		
Source_____		Crystals_____
S.G._____	Glu_____	Casts_____
pH_____	Ket_____	WBC_____
Leuk_____	Uro_____	RBC_____
Nit_____	Bili_____	Epith_____
Protein_____	Blood_____	Bact_____

DENTAL   Name _____   Date _____

Canine Upper

Feline Upper

MAXILLA

KEY: **O** = Displaced Tooth
X = Missing Tooth
= Caries, Injury, FX

a _____
b _____
c _____
d _____
Gingiva: _____
Occlusion: _____
Salivation: _____
Halitosis: Y   N
Periodontal Disease: _____
Other: _____

MANDIBLE

Feline Lower

Canine Lower

FIGURE 14-2 Examples of labels.

Box 14-1	**Single Line Correction**

> *stopped* (N.S.)
> Owner ~~started~~ antibiotics 5 days ago.

with tabs for quick access. The medical record may also be either blue or pink, indicating the sex of the patient. Some practices maintain one file per pet even when they come from the same household.

Index card files are usually kept in plastic holders and filed by the client's last name. Medical records are written on 5 × 8-inch index cards. All forms, charts, and lab work results are stored in the plastic holder.

Clinics that use full paper records generally have more complete records than those that use index cards. It is not unusual for a sick patient to have one full page of history on a full paper record, whereas those with index cards will have only a few words. Team members seem to write less on index cards. State board investigators do not recommend index card records for this reason; records are often incomplete and illegible.

PRACTICE POINT   Full 8.5 × 11-inch paper records are recommended over index cards.

FIGURE 14-3 An 8.5 × 11-inch paper record with patient separators.

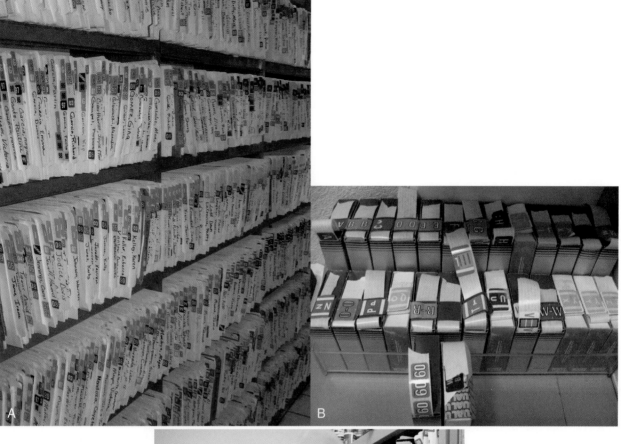

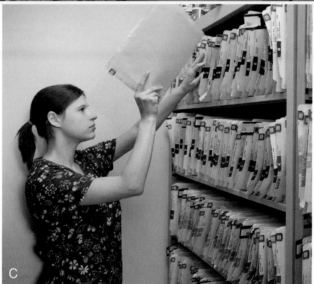

FIGURE 14-4 Examples of colored letters and numbers for files.

Either file folders or index card holders can be alphabetized by client name or filed by client number, and colored letters and/or numbered labels can help identify those that are misfiled (Figure 14-4). Color coding the exterior of files can help identify misfiled charts from either the front or the back. Numbers indicating the year on the outside of the file can also help identify the last time a client has been into the practice, making it easier for team members to purge files efficiently. Alphabetical filing is the most common method used in practice. The last name, then first, along with a client identification number, are generally listed on the exterior of a file; the file is then alphabetized by the client's last name.

Colored warning stickers attached to patient medical records may draw attention to special medical needs. Sample stickers may include: "Will Bite!" "Anesthetic Alert!" or "Vaccine Reaction!" Figure 14-5 shows a variety if stickers that a practice may use in a paper

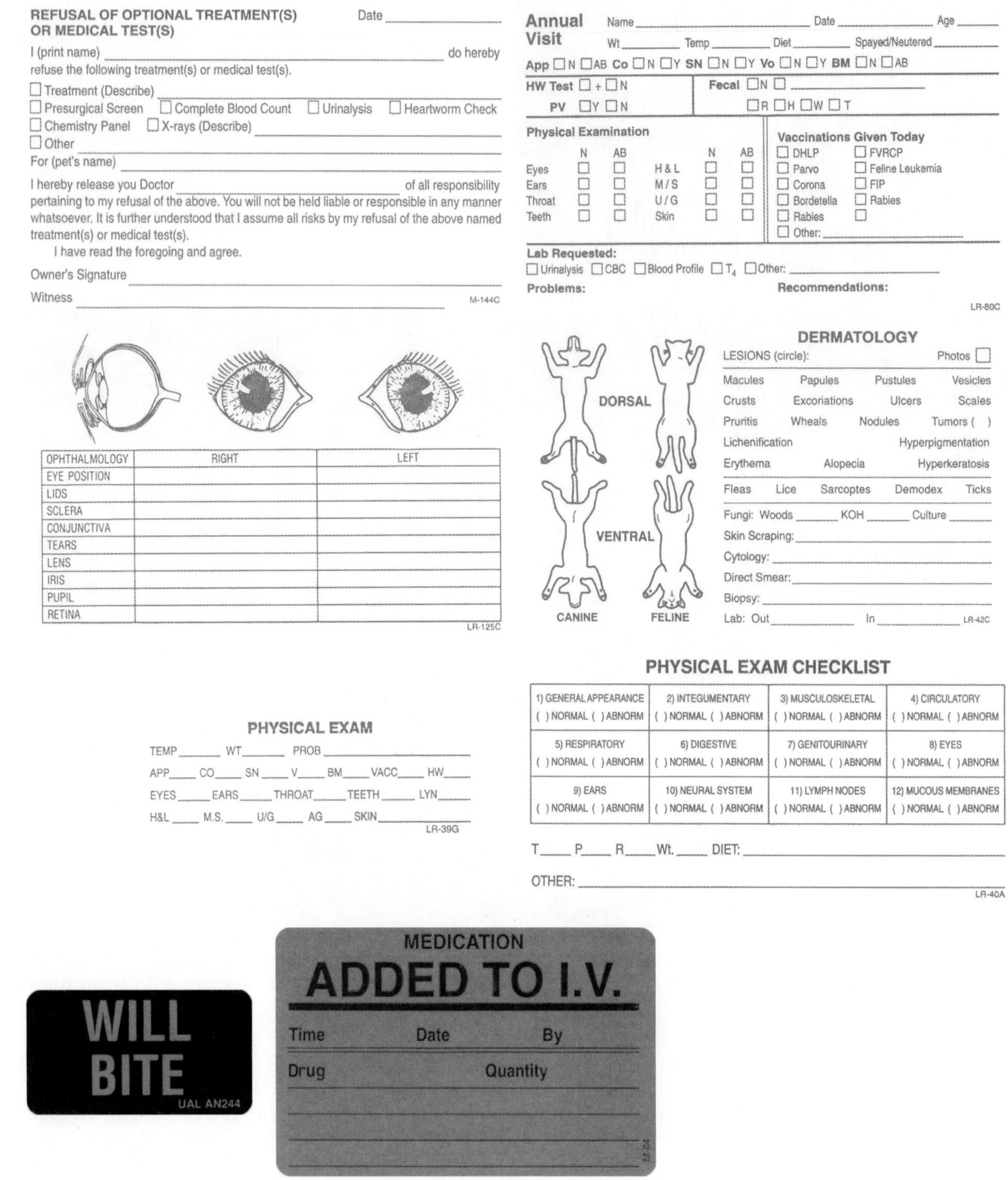

REFUSAL OF OPTIONAL TREATMENT(S) OR MEDICAL TEST(S)   Date _____

I (print name) _____ do hereby refuse the following treatment(s) or medical test(s).

☐ Treatment (Describe) _____
☐ Presurgical Screen   ☐ Complete Blood Count   ☐ Urinalysis   ☐ Heartworm Check
☐ Chemistry Panel   ☐ X-rays (Describe) _____
☐ Other _____

For (pet's name) _____

I hereby release you Doctor _____ of all responsibility pertaining to my refusal of the above. You will not be held liable or responsible in any manner whatsoever. It is further understood that I assume all risks by my refusal of the above named treatment(s) or medical test(s).

   I have read the foregoing and agree.

Owner's Signature _____

Witness _____   M-144C

Annual Visit   Name _____ Date _____ Age _____
Wt _____ Temp _____ Diet _____ Spayed/Neutered _____

App ☐N ☐AB Co ☐N ☐Y SN ☐N ☐Y Vo ☐N ☐Y BM ☐N ☐AB

| HW Test ☐ + ☐ N | Fecal ☐ N ☐ |
| PV ☐Y ☐N | ☐R ☐H ☐W ☐T |

Physical Examination

	N	AB		N	AB
Eyes	☐	☐	H & L	☐	☐
Ears	☐	☐	M / S	☐	☐
Throat	☐	☐	U / G	☐	☐
Teeth	☐	☐	Skin	☐	☐

Vaccinations Given Today
☐ DHLP   ☐ FVRCP
☐ Parvo   ☐ Feline Leukemia
☐ Corona   ☐ FIP
☐ Bordetella ☐ Rabies
☐ Rabies
☐ Other: _____

Lab Requested:
☐ Urinalysis ☐ CBC ☐ Blood Profile ☐ T₄ ☐ Other: _____

Problems: Recommendations:

                                              LR-80C

OPHTHALMOLOGY	RIGHT	LEFT
EYE POSITION		
LIDS		
SCLERA		
CONJUNCTIVA		
TEARS		
LENS		
IRIS		
PUPIL		
RETINA		

LR-125C

DERMATOLOGY

LESIONS (circle):   Photos ☐

Macules   Papules   Pustules   Vesicles
Crusts   Excoriations   Ulcers   Scales
Pruritis   Wheals   Nodules   Tumors ( )
Lichenification   Hyperpigmentation
Erythema   Alopecia   Hyperkeratosis

Fleas   Lice   Sarcoptes   Demodex   Ticks

Fungi: Woods _____ KOH _____ Culture _____
Skin Scraping: _____
Cytology: _____
Direct Smear: _____
Biopsy: _____
Lab: Out _____ In _____   LR-42C

DORSAL   VENTRAL   CANINE   FELINE

PHYSICAL EXAM

TEMP _____ WT _____ PROB _____
APP _____ CO _____ SN _____ V _____ BM _____ VACC _____ HW _____
EYES _____ EARS _____ THROAT _____ TEETH _____ LYN _____
H&L _____ M.S. _____ U/G _____ AG _____ SKIN _____

                                              LR-39G

PHYSICAL EXAM CHECKLIST

1) GENERAL APPEARANCE	2) INTEGUMENTARY	3) MUSCULOSKELETAL	4) CIRCULATORY
( ) NORMAL ( ) ABNORM	( ) NORMAL ( ) ABNORM	( ) NORMAL ( ) ABNORM	( ) NORMAL ( ) ABNORM
5) RESPIRATORY	6) DIGESTIVE	7) GENITOURINARY	8) EYES
( ) NORMAL ( ) ABNORM	( ) NORMAL ( ) ABNORM	( ) NORMAL ( ) ABNORM	( ) NORMAL ( ) ABNORM
9) EARS	10) NEURAL SYSTEM	11) LYMPH NODES	12) MUCOUS MEMBRANES
( ) NORMAL ( ) ABNORM	( ) NORMAL ( ) ABNORM	( ) NORMAL ( ) ABNORM	( ) NORMAL ( ) ABNORM

T _____ P _____ R _____ Wt. _____ DIET: _____

OTHER: _____

                                              LR-40A

WILL BITE   UAL AN244

MEDICATION ADDED TO I.V.
Time   Date   By
Drug   Quantity

FIGURE 14-5 Examples of colored warning labels. (Courtesy Para-Medical Labels of Cooo... kamonga, Inc., Diamond Springs, Calif.)

record system. Bright-colored stickers can also be used on cage identification cards to alert team members of a patient's special needs. A "Will Bite" sticker is beneficial for alerting team members to animals with which they must use special precautions.

Although patient medical alerts should be obvious, team members can get busy and overlook a handwritten alert. A sticker that is big, bright, and bold will catch the attention of staff members. This is a cheap method for preventing a potential disaster.

PRACTICE POINT Colored warning stickers can prevent an accident from occurring by drawing attention to the record.

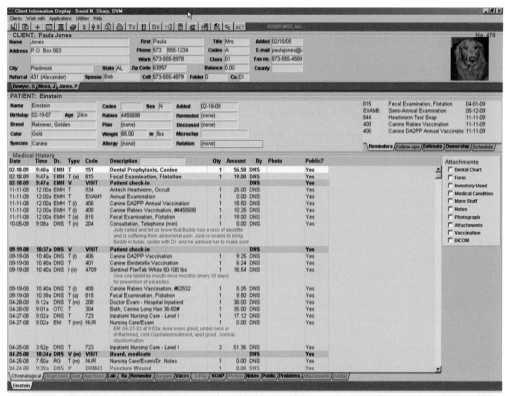

FIGURE 14-6 Sample medical history in a computerized medical record. (Courtesy McAllister Software Systems, Piedmont, Mo.)

COMPUTERIZED MEDICAL RECORDS

Computerized medical records, also referred to as *paperless records,* are filed in the computer by both client number and last name (Figure 14-6). Any record can be accessed from any computer. Lab work, radiographs, and ultrasound results are stored within the record. All charts, consent forms, and miscellaneous documents must be stored within the record. A practice that is truly paperless does not have any additional client files or folders that store release forms, lab work, or radiographs. Forms and lab work are scanned into the client's record, or the client must sign the forms electronically, which are then stored in the computer. Radiographs are either in digital form or they are scanned into the record. Most lab work machines will enter results into the client's file once the machine has completed the work. Client identification numbers must be verified before entering lab work to ensure the results will be populated into the correct records. When outside laboratory results are received, they can be electronically filed within the patient's chart. An onscreen notice pops up for the veterinarian or staff when those results have become available.

> ◎ **PRACTICE POINT** Computer medical records are never lost!

Computer medical records must be secure, with access limited to authorized individuals only. Computers must be backed up daily and monthly, preferably off site for the best security. Software should have an automatic lockout time period, preventing records from being changed after a backup has been completed. Late entries can be added, but a new date will appear with the updates.

Patient information can be added to computerized records in several ways. Doctors may enter information while they are examining the patient, a veterinary technician or transcriptionist can enter notes written by the doctor to complete the record, or a doctor may use a template that has been generated by the computer to compete the record.

Paper records and paperless records each have their advantages and disadvantages, all of which must be weighed when determining what is best for an individual practice (Box 14-2).

The greatest advantage of paperless records is being able to access them from any computer. Most paperless practices have a computer available in every exam room, office, and laboratory area. Records are never lost, misplaced, or misfiled. However, computer systems can fail; therefore records may be inaccessible until the system has been repaired. A "plan B" should be developed in case a system does crash to prevent a major catastrophe from occurring. This may include having a few laptops that serve as backups if a computer becomes unusable. The laptops should have software preloaded, allowing

Box 14-2	Advantages and Disadvantages of Computerized Medical Records

ADVANTAGES

- Easy to capture missing charges
- Easy to access medical records at any computer station
- Can target specific clients quickly and efficiently when promoting specific services
- Takes less time to enter information into the computer than to write it out
- Legible
- Client perceives progressive, higher quality medicine
- Computers take up less space
- Eco-friendly; saves paper

DISADVANTAGES

- Possibility of server crashing
- Records can be lost or altered through computer corruption
- Computer-generated records can lack medical details

them to be plugged into the server and available for use immediately. If the main server becomes unusable, a second unit should be available, and the CD with data from the last daily backup can be loaded. This will keep the practice flowing until the main server has been repaired.

A major disadvantage of computerized medical records is the lack of security to prevent alteration. If a record can be altered, it may be questioned in a court of law. The practice attorney should be consulted regarding the likelihood of problems if a malpractice claim arises. Backing up information onto CDs that can only be written on once may satisfy the court.

Some software companies are excellent at providing medical record lockout periods; these lockout periods prevent medical record alteration after 24 hours. Others do not have a lockout period, allowing records to be altered days, or even months, later. This disadvantage must be considered when choosing software for the practice.

The advantages and disadvantages of computerized software change annually as new technology is introduced. Computers and software initially can be costly, but the efficiency they make possible far outweighs the cost. Updates are made available for current software users and should be used to maximum potential.

CHOOSING MEDICAL RECORD SOFTWARE

Veterinary software can have a variety of applications. Some software may be management based, helping maintain inventory and create client invoices, whereas other software may be based on medical record management. Some companies have tried to integrate the two; however, computer-generated records are not as flexible as paper records.

PRACTICE POINT Choose software that protects medical records from being altered.

Many practices use a combination of both computerized and paper medical records. The computerized medical records can efficiently generate reminders, patient/client alerts, and invoices. Once the patient has been established in the computer system, a paper record is generated for the medical portion of the record. The invoicing system generates a patient history (assuming every procedure was charged for) but lacks the medical details needed to complete a medical record.

Efficiency of Computerized Laboratory Requisition Forms

Some laboratories work with veterinary practices to generate requisition forms online, creating a unique form and barcode. For example, IDEXX (Westbrook, Maine) LabREXX software (www.idexx.com/labrexx) works with existing veterinary practice software, allowing charges to be captured while ensuring no mistakes are made when submitting the client and patient name and doctor. To help increase efficiency, a quick guide of the most common tests the practice selects is available, allowing results to be emailed directly to clients and results to be downloaded to patient records. This prevents lost and/or misfiled results. Records are flagged, allowing the team to know that results have arrived in a patient's file.

Chapter 8 gives a brief overview of software that is available in today's market, along with a worksheet to help determine which software will work best for a veterinary practice.

MEDICAL RECORDS RELEASE

Records are confidential and can only be released when the owner has given permission to do so. Clients must sign a records release form that must be kept in the medical record (see Figure 2-14). This includes release to any other veterinary hospital, any boarding or grooming facility, or a new owner of the pet. Any practice can be held liable for the release of records without the owner's consent. It is important to understand the Privacy Act and not release any records without the client's authorization. The Privacy Act of 1974 states in part:

> *No agency shall disclose any record which is contained in a system of records by any means of communication to any person, or to another agency, except pursuant to a written request by, or with the prior written consent of, the individual to whom the record pertains.*

A client is entitled to a copy of his or her record. The original record is the property of the hospital, along with any diagnostic images and laboratory results; however, a client may request copies. Any time a client is referred to a specialist, a copy of the record should be sent, along with relevant images that have been taken (if not in digital form, radiographs should be checked out in a log book). If a digital radiograph has been taken, a CD can be generated and sent with the owner or the image can be emailed to the specialist with a consult form.

> **PRACTICE POINT** Clients may request copies of their records at anytime.

All cases should be kept confidential as well. Cases cannot be discussed by name with clients; the privacy of both the client and the pet must be respected.

ESTABLISHING A MEDICAL RECORD

Regardless of the software chosen or whether the records are on paper or computerized, every medical record must follow specific criteria.

- Each patient must have its own medical record. Multiple animals cannot be listed on the same index card in an index card file system. Multiple animals cannot be listed on one sheet of 8.5 × 11-inch paper. It is acceptable for multiple pets to be in one file folder under the name of one owner, but they must be separated with dividers.
- Records must be easy to retrieve. Lost records increase staff and client frustration, time, and labor costs.
- Medical records must be complete and well organized. Each entry should follow a standard SOAP format that allows the staff to easily follow the progress of the patient.
- Records should be composed as legal documents that can be admissible in court if needed.
- Legibility of records is a must! Illegible records can lead to incorrect dosing of medication and protocols.

WHAT IS INCLUDED IN A MEDICAL RECORD?

Each medical record must have the same information, regardless of the type of pet, client, or veterinary software used. The organization of the medical record depends on practice preference, but most hospitals use a reverse chronological order system.

> **PRACTICE POINT** Records must be initialed by the author after each entry.

The most recent records are placed on top of the file for easy access. Laboratory results, consultation reports, and estimates are placed after the written medical record.

The most current laboratory results are placed on top in this section. However a hospital chooses to organize the record, it should be consistent with all medical records throughout the medical record database. The following is required information for each patient record:

- **Client/Patient Information Sheet:** Some clinics separate these two forms and others combine them. It is critical that the owner complete the client information in as much detail as possible (see Chapter 2). Client information must be verified at each visit to ensure that the most current information, including the phone number, is kept on file.
- **Previous Medical History:** If a patient has been seen by another veterinarian and received prior medical treatment, the history should be recorded here.
- **Vaccination History:** Each patient should have some type of vaccine history unless it is a young puppy or kitten. Dates and types of vaccines administered should be documented. Once the patient has established a history with the practice, vaccine history can be reviewed and updated with each visit. It is important to document where vaccines have been administered on the pet's body for future reference.
- **The Primary Complaint:** This will accurately summarize the client's complaint and the history of the presenting problem. Team members must listen well to clients and determine the appropriate questions to ask.
- **Physical Examination:** A description of the pet's physical examination must be documented for each visit. If the animal is hospitalized, the patient must receive progress exams on a daily basis. These, too, must also be written in the record. Temperature, weight, mucous membrane color, auscultation of the chest, palpation of the abdomen, and the examination of the lymph nodes and musculoskeletal system must be documented. Many team members abbreviate terms, descriptions, and abnormalities. Please see the appendixes for common abbreviations used in veterinary medicine. The American Animal Hospital Association (AAHA) also produces an excellent booklet summarizing abbreviations.
- **Diagnosis and/or Possible Diagnosis:** Diagnosis is the identification of disease by analysis and examination. The patient may have one or several diseases, and they should all be documented.
- **Laboratory Reports:** All laboratory results (normal and abnormal), including radiographs, ultrasounds, and electrocardiograms, must be documented. If a consult was completed with a specialty veterinarian, that also must be documented in the record.
- **Treatment:** Any treatment recommendation and/or medications must be written in the medical record.
- **Prognosis:** A prognosis is the prediction of the outcome of the disease. The prognosis must be communicated to the client and documented in the record. The prognosis may help the client decide what medical

route to take when treating a pet. The prognosis can change with treatment, laboratory results, and surgery. If it does change, the record must be updated.

- **Surgical Report:** Any surgical procedure must be described in detail and include complications that might be expected postoperatively.
- **Estimates and Consent Forms:** Each client must give consent to treat a pet. If a treatment protocol has been recommended, clients should also receive an estimate. Both the consent to treat form and the client estimate should be signed and placed in the medical record.

A master problem sheet is an excellent summary sheet to include as the top sheet to all patient files. A master problem list should include the patient name, gender, species, breed, age, diet, allergies (including any to medications, vaccines, or anesthetics), current medications that the pet is receiving, and any vaccinations the pet has received. Although the master problem list is not required to complete the medical record, it helps increase the team's efficiency when refilling medications and determining vaccines for which the patient may be due. Figure 2-12 gives excellent examples of master problem sheets.

Another suggestion for increasing efficiency, although not required, is a laboratory diagnostic flow sheet for patients that return on a regular basis for lab work. The diagnostic flow sheet is a compilation of laboratory data from a patient that shows results in chronological order. These sheets can be of value when monitoring patients with ongoing or chronic diseases, such as diabetes, Cushing disease, renal failure, hyperthyroidism, or hypothyroidism.

> **PRACTICE POINT** Diagnostic flow sheets allow easy comparison of laboratory data.

TAKING A HISTORY

An accurate history is one of the most important aspects of a medical record. All the information the owner has presented must be summarized in the medical record. This allows the veterinary team to look at the presenting facts and may help the veterinarian diagnose the case more rapidly and more accurately. Many clients will chat with team members and give valuable information that neither the client nor the team member realized was pertinent. For example, a client may indicate he or she was on vacation in Florida. Fluffy has diarrhea now. Did the pet go on vacation with the owners? Was the pet exposed to a new environment? Did the pet have a new diet? Did the pet drink any beach water? Did Fluffy eat bird droppings on the beach? Were any special treats given? If the pet did not go on the trip, who stayed home with Fluffy? Did the house sitter stay at the house with Fluffy or did Fluffy go to a boarding kennel? These are all important questions that should be asked during a conversation about a client's recent vacation (Box 14-3).

SOAP AND POMR MEDICAL RECORDS

The problem-oriented medical record (POMR) is the medical record format most commonly used by veterinary health care teams. Each entry follows a distinct format: the defined database, the problem list (also referred to as *master list*), the plan, and the progress section. Within the progress section, a standard SOAP format (*s*ubjective, *o*bjective, *a*ssessment, and *p*lan) is followed. **Subjective** is the most important element for the reception staff, veterinary technicians, and assistants. Subjective information includes the reason for the office visit, the history, and observations made by the client. The opinions and perceptions of the client represent the most subjective information (Figure 14-7).

What Would You Do/Not Do?

Mrs. Carwell calls the practice because her dog has developed a case of diarrhea. She is advised to bring Domino in, along with a fresh fecal sample to check for intestinal parasites. When she arrives, she advises the veterinarian that she just brought home a new puppy from the shelter that also has diarrhea; however, she attributed the puppy's diarrhea to stress and diet change. The veterinarian diagnoses Domino with giardiasis and dispenses albendazole to treat the parasite. Teresa, the veterinary technician, advises the owner that the puppy probably also has the parasite and needs to be seen to receive the correct dose of medication. The owner calls Teresa 4 days later stating that the diarrhea in Domino cleared within 2 days, so she gave the rest of the medication to the new puppy. Now the puppy is vomiting, and she knows it is from the medication; she needs another medicine to treat the *Giardia*.

What Does Teresa Do?
The owner must be advised that many parasites and viruses can cause diarrhea, and the puppy must be examined before any medication can be dispensed. Not only could the puppy have vomiting and diarrhea associated with parvovirus, it may also be having an overdose reaction to the medication because the albendazole was dosed for a 45-lb dog. Teresa must inform the owner of the possible side effects of the medication and note the discussion in the record. She should also make an appointment for Mrs. Carwell as soon as possible.

Box 14-3	List of Questions to Ask During History Taking

IS THE PATIENT EATING NORMALLY?
- What is the patient fed?
- When was the last meal?
- How much did the patient eat?
- How often does the patient eat?
- Any treats? If yes, what treats? How often?

DRINKING
- Is the patient drinking the same amount of water as usual?
- How often?

VOMITING
- How often is the pet vomiting?
- What color is the vomit?
- What does the vomit consist of?
- Has the pet eaten any toys, blankets, or towels?

BOWEL MOVEMENTS
- Is the patient defecating normally?
- What does the stool look like (color and consistency)?
- How often is the patient defecating?
- Any straining to defecate?
- If the patient has abnormal bowel movements, when did the abnormal signs start?

URINATION
- How often does the patient urinate?
- Is the patient urinating the same amount as always?
- Is the urine a clear, steady stream?
- Any straining to urinate?
- If the patient is having abnormal urination, when did the abnormal signs start?

COUGHING
- Does the patient cough or gag?
- If so, how often?

- When did the coughing start?
- How often does the patient cough?
- How long does the episode last?

SNEEZING
- When did the patient begin sneezing?
- Does the patient have any discharge from the eyes and nose with the sneezing?
- If yes, what color is the discharge?

WALKING
- Is the patient walking normally?
- If not, when did the abnormal signs begin?
- Is the pet limping or not bearing weight on an extremity?
- If yes, which one?
- Did the owner see any trauma happen to the pet?

GROWTH(S)
- What is the location of the growth?
- How long has the growth been present?
- Has any previous diagnostic work been completed before?
- Has it increased in size? How much?
- Has the growth changed color? How much?

MISCELLANEOUS
- Swelling: Where is the location of the swelling? When did the client notice the swelling?
- Discharge from the eyes: When did the client notice the discharge? What color is it? Is the pet squinting the eye(s)?

This is not a complete list of questions to ask during history taking but gives some examples of different topics that should be addressed.

PRACTICE POINT   POMR = Problem-Oriented Medical Record
SOAP = Subjective, Objective, Assessment, Plan

Objective information is gathered directly from the patient; the physical exam, diagnostic workup, and interpretation are included in this section of the medical record. Objective information is factual information (Figures 14-8 and 14-9).

The **assessment** section includes any conclusions reached from the subjective and objective sections and includes a definitive diagnosis. If there are multiple or tentative diagnoses, they can all be documented here along with a list of "rule-ins" (R/I) or "rule-outs" (R/O). R/Is can be classified as any disease the patient could possibly have as well as diagnostic work that

must be done to rule out those particular diseases (Figure 14-10).

A **plan** is developed according to the assessment and includes any treatment, surgery, medication, intended diagnostics, or intended communications with the owner. This can also be a list of options that will be presented to the client (Figure 14-11).

Diligent team members can often catch common errors and omissions in a medical record before the record is filed. Some of the most common incomplete errors include lab work interpretation, progress notes while the patient is hospitalized, preoperative physical exams, anesthetic drugs, and initials of the author(s) writing in the record. Laboratory results must be documented along with any comments on abnormalities (Box 14-4).

If previous lab work is being compared with present results, this is also an excellent place to write the

Patient Medical Record

Client Name _Nancy Riley_ _____ Telephone Number _555-5555_ _____

Address _928 Sally Road, Anytown, MN 89890_ _____ Client Number _15641_ _____

Pet Name _Fred_ _____ Breed _Bassett_ _____ Color _Brown/Wh/Bl_ _____

Sex ___M___ Altered ___Y___ DOB _2/15/09_ _____ Age _12 weeks_ Species _K9_ _____

Date		Charges
5/15/09	Puppy shots	
	S: Owner states pt has had diarrhea for the past 3 days.	
	Very foul odor. Decreased appetite. Had 1 prev. vacc.	
	Had a puppy that died 1 mo ago. Unknown cause.	

FIGURE 14-7 Example of Subjective notes in a medical record.

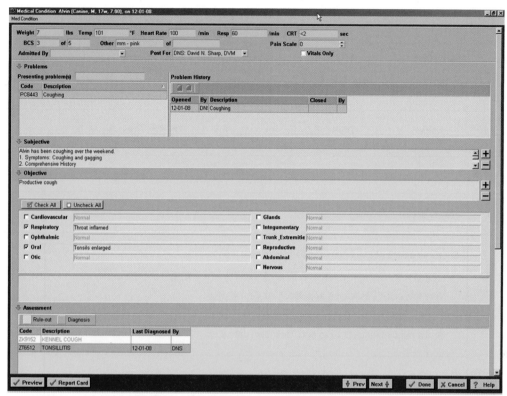

FIGURE 14-8 Example of Avimark's medical record SOAP format. (Courtesy McAllister Software Systems, Piedmont, Mo.)

comparison. Veterinarians must interpret the results, not just document them! Interpretation is defined as analyzing the results and explaining why those abnormalities may be present. The list of R/Is and R/Os can be completed with the analysis of pending lab work. Animals should have a daily physical exam while they are hospitalized and receive medications as recommended by the doctor. Results of the physical exam, any medications administered, and any urination, bowel movements, or vomiting must also be documented in the progress notes. Hospitalization sheets should be used to help keep track of patient status while patients are hospitalized (Figure 14-12).

Surgical patients must be examined within 12 hours of anesthesia, and the exam must be documented in the medical record. Anesthetic drugs, details of the procedure, the patient's response, and any complications of the procedure must also be documented in the record. The most common error made is not documenting the communication with the owner regarding the prognosis of the patient. The medical record must clearly state if the prognosis is poor, guarded, fair, or excellent.

◎ PRACTICE POINT   Any medication that is administered must be documented with notations of the drug, route, strength, and person administering the medication.

Medication names, strength, and route given must be accurately written in the medical records. For example,

"0.2 mL cefazolin IV" is an incorrect notation. This description does not indicate how many milligrams were given. The entry should read, "0.2 mL cefazolin (100 mg/mL) given IV," or it may read "20 mg cefazolin, given IV." Many drugs come in different strengths, and it is important to identify and document the correct strength of medication. The same drug can also be administered by different routes (some drugs will have a different dose depending on the route administered); it is therefore important to document by which route the medication was administered (Box 14-5).

If fluids are to be administered to patients, records must clearly indicate the name of the fluids, the amount the pet is receiving, and the route given (IV or SC). If a pet is simply receiving Normosol under the skin, the attending veterinarian or technician can indicate the number of milliliters administered. However, if a patient is receiving a drip intravenously, the rate must be indicated. "Normosol, 66 mL/kg/24 hours = 100 mL/hr IV" would be an accurate entry.

HERD HEALTH RECORDS

It is impossible for large animal veterinarians to have individual records for each food animal they examine. Herd health records refer to the practice of recording information for an entire herd, including medications and vaccinations on one record. Individual records may be kept if surgical procedures or special treatments are completed on one animal.

Patient Medical Record

Client Name _Nancy Riley_   Telephone Number _555-5555_

Address _928 Sally Road, Anytown, MN 89890_   Client Number _15641_

Pet Name _Fred_   Breed _Bassett_   Color _Brown/Wh/Bl_

Sex _M_   Altered _Y_   DOB _2/15/09_   Age _12 weeks_   Species _K9_

Date		Charges
5/15/09	Puppy shots	
	S: Owner states pt has had diarrhea for the past 3 days.	
	Very foul odor. Decreased appetite. Had 1 prev. vacc.	
	Had a puppy that died 1 mo ago. Unknown cause.	
	O: PE: General appearance: thin; 5% dehydrated.	
	Lethargic. EENT, LN, MS, NS, all WNL. Abd: tender when palpated.	
	MM = pale and tacky. T - 102.4, Wt - 9.9#	
	HR = 100/min, RR = 20/min, Thermom reveals bloody, loose stool.	

FIGURE 14-9 Example of Objective notes in a medical record.

Patient Medical Record

Client Name _Nancy Riley_   Telephone Number _555-5555_

Address _928 Sally Road, Anytown, MN 89890_   Client Number _15641_

Pet Name _Fred_   Breed _Bassett_   Color _Brown/Wh/Bl_

Sex __M__   Altered __Y__   DOB _2/15/09_   Age _12 weeks_ Species _K9_

Date		Charges
5/15/09	Puppy shots	
	S: Owner states pt has had diarrhea for the past 3 days.	
	Very foul odor. Decreased appetite. Had 1 prev. vacc.	
	Had a puppy that died 1 mo ago. Unknown cause.	
	O: PE: General appearance: thin; 5% dehydrated.	
	Lethargic. EENT, LN, MS, NS, all WNL. Abd: tender when palpated.	
	MM = pale and tacky. T - 102.4, Wt - 9.9#	
	HR = 100/min, RR = 20/min, Thermom reveals bloody, loose stool.	
	A: Gastroenteritis	
	R/O Parvo, Giardia, Garbage Gut	

FIGURE 14-10 Example of Assessment notes in a medical record.

Patient Medical Record

Client Name _Nancy Riley_ _____ Telephone Number _555-5555_ _____

Address _928 Sally Road, Anytown, MN 89890_ _____ Client Number _15641_ _____

Pet Name _Fred_ _____ Breed _Bassett_ _____ Color _Brown/Wh/Bl_

Sex ___M___ Altered ___Y___ DOB _2/15/09_ ____ Age _12 weeks_ Species _K9_ _____

Date		Charges
5/15/09	Puppy shots	
	S: Owner states pt has had diarrhea for the past 3 days.	
	Very foul odor. Decreased appetite. Had 1 prev. vacc.	
	Had a puppy that died 1 mo ago. Unknown cause.	
	O: PE: General appearance: thin; 5% dehydrated.	
	Lethargic. EENT, LN, MS, NS, all WNL. Abd: tender when palpated.	
	MM = pale and tacky. T - 102.4, Wt - 9.9#	
	HR = 100/min, RR = 20/min, Thermom reveals bloody, loose stool.	
	A: Gastroenteritis	
	R/O Parvo, Giardia, Garbage Gut	
	P: Fecal Exam, Parvo Test	ND
5/15/09	O: Parvo Test (+), Fecal (−)	
	P: Discuss Tx plan with owner. 1. Hosp vs home care	
	2. Abx;	
	3. Fluid care: SQ vs IV	
	Owner chooses home care	ND

FIGURE 14-11 Example of Plan notes in a medical record.

Box 14-4	**Rules for Medical Records**

- Records must be written in blue or black ink only; no color, no pencils.
- The author of the entry must date and initial each time an entry is made.
- No correction fluid!
- When scratching out a mistake, make a single line through the mistake and make the correction. The mistake must be initialed.
- Use standard and approved abbreviations only.
- Write in records immediately to prevent the loss of details.
- Records must be legible!
- Each continuation sheet must have all the patient information documented on it, including the owner's name and the pet's gender, breed, and age.

PURGING MEDICAL RECORDS

The length of time a practice must keep an inactive medical record varies from state to state. An inactive medical record is defined as a client who has not been seen by that practice for a year or more. Most states require medical records to be held for at least 3 years; many practices keep records much longer. Because some vaccine protocols have changed to every 3 years, some clients only return when vaccinations are due. Therefore it is more cost effective for veterinary practices maintaining paper records to keep inactive files in a storage room on premises where records can be easily accessed for a minimum of 3 years.

Many practices have limited space. Purging records on a yearly basis and moving the inactive records to another area of the practice frees up space for current records. By reducing the number of records in the active area, the possibility of lost records is decreased. Records can be lost from misfiling, misspelling, and misplacement, which can be irritating to both clients and team members.

> **PRACTICE POINT**   Do not yell out, "I can't find the file!" Imagine how this makes a client feel!

Long-term storage can be arranged at an off-site storage facility until state law allows purging. Those records that are purged must be shredded so that confidential information is not available to the public. This includes all lab work results, client informational sheets, and any authorization or release sheets that were signed by the client. The disadvantage of off-site storage is that when a record is needed, it can take 1 to 2 days to retrieve it. This may be too long a wait for the veterinarian who needs the patient's history.

CLIENT DISCHARGE INSTRUCTIONS

Client discharge instructions are very important (Figure 14-13). Clients will not remember everything that was advised while they were in the practice. Team members should print out materials for the owner to take home. These instructions and materials must be reviewed verbally with the owner before discharging the patient. It is also a good idea to keep a copy of all materials given to the owner in the record. It may also be of benefit to have the owners sign the bottom of the material to acknowledge receipt of the printed materials. Some clinics will use a carbonless copy set for discharge instructions. This way, the practice is covered when clients state they never received the instructions.

> **PRACTICE POINT**   All clients should receive written discharge instructions.

Different types of information may be required for various patient discharges. A patient that is returning home after a normal canine neuter will have different release instructions than a patient that has just a fractured bone repaired. A patient that has been hospitalized may have a different feeding protocol than that of a surgical patient. Computer software programs can print detailed release information when the appropriate information has been added to the system. For practices that do not have this ability, sheets can be created with options for team members to highlight for the client. Box 14-6 gives ideas for what to include on discharge sheets for a variety of patient discharges.

Charts, labels, and stamps can help a veterinary team become more efficient at writing in medical records correctly, legibly, and completely. Veterinary team members can place a label or stamp in the record for the veterinarian, who can then chart his or her notes accurately. Some examples of labels and stamps are listed in Figure 14-2; others can be found at various medical and office supply houses. Practices can also design the labels or stamps that will best increase efficiency in their hospital and have them commercially printed or print them with an office laser printer.

> **PRACTICE POINT**   Labels increase the efficiency of the team and can be ordered or made by the practice.

COMMON ABBREVIATIONS

Abbreviations are used in veterinary practices to help teams become more efficient. It is important to memorize these abbreviations because they are used in everyday practice. Examples of abbreviations are located in the appendixes of this book.

Client's last name: _____   Working diagnosis: _____

Pet's name: _____   Primary doctor: _____

Date:	8am	9	10	11	12	1	2	3	4	5	6	7	8
Feed													
Water													
Walk/litter													
Temperature													
Weight													
Appetite?													
Attitude?													
Urine?													
BM or diarrhea													
Vomit?													

Date:	8am	9	10	11	12	1	2	3	4	5	6	7	8
Feed													
Water													
Walk/litter													
Temperature													
Weight													
Appetite?													
Attitude?													
Urine?													
BM or diarrhea													
Vomit?													

FIGURE 14-12 Example of a hospital sheet.

Box 14-5   Routes of Medication Administration

- PO—*Per os,* or by mouth
- SC—*Subcutaneously,* or under the skin
- IV—*Intravenously,* or into the vein
- IM—*Intramuscular,* or into the muscle

For example, the following instructions have been written for a patient:

IV Normosol fluids maintenance rate; NPO ×12 hrs: sx in AM: 12 mg cefazolin IV pre/post sx; increase fluids to sx rate; 3 mg buprenorphine SQ pre/post op.

This can be interpreted as meaning that the patient will be receiving intravenous (IV) fluids with Normosol at the maintenance rate of 66 mL/kg/24 hours. The pet will receive nothing by mouth (NPO) for 12 hours before surgery (sx) and will have a surgical procedure in the morning. The patient will receive 12 milligrams (mg) of cefazolin intravenously (IV) both before and after surgery. The patient will also receive 3 mg of buprenorphine before and after surgery.

> **PRACTICE POINT**   All team members must be familiar with abbreviations.

Abbreviations greatly increase the efficiency of team members by saving time and space in the medical record.

RADIOGRAPHS

Patient radiographs are an integral part of the medical record. Radiographs must be correctly labeled with the veterinary hospital name and address, client's last name, patient's name, date, and a right or left indicator.

If a veterinary practice is paperless, these radiographs can be electronically filed in the patient record. A paper practice will have these radiographs stored in another location on the premises. It is important to be able to locate these radiographs quickly and efficiently when needed; therefore a filing system must be developed. Some practices may use colored letters (as indicated above for file folders) to help file radiographs (Figure 14-14). Practices can also purchase a radiograph scanner that scans films into a computer database, allowing clinics to pull up the images on a computer monitor. It must be

remembered that these are not digital radiographs; it is simply a storage system for films. This allows clinics to use that storage room for other items and prevents the loss or misfile of films. Images can easily be copied for owners or specialty veterinarians onto a CD; the radiographs will never be lost.

Radiographs are the property of the veterinary practice; therefore practices that do not have a scanner or digital radiographs may provide clients with copies of them. Copies of radiographs can be made at a local imaging center that has radiographic copying capabilities. If clients are taking radiographs to have them copied or films are being sent to another veterinary clinic, a log should be kept indicating where the radiographs went. This log should include who received the films, the date, and the reason the films have left the practice. Once they have been returned, a single strike line can be made through the entry indicating their return, along with the date and initials of the team member returning the radiographs to radiology. Figure 14-15 is an example of a completed radiograph checkout log. It can be frustrating and time consuming for veterinary team members when films have become lost or misfiled. Developing an effective file system is as important for radiographs as it is for medical records. Being able to refer to the log is important because films often have not been returned by owners or other hospitals.

> **PRACTICE POINT**   Radiographs are the property of the practice; however, copies can be made at the client's request.

BACKING UP THE COMPUTER SYSTEM DAILY

The importance of backing up systems on a daily basis cannot be stressed enough. It is best if the system is backed up to a system both on site and off site, which increases the safety of the protected information. If a fire or burglary occurs, all records will still be available to reinstall on a new computer. If a computer system fails in the middle of the day, the only information that will need to be reentered is the information from earlier that day. It would be impossible to locate all information that was lost if only a weekly or monthly backup were performed.

ABC Veterinary Clinic 555-555-5555
Dr. Roe, Dr. Morton, Dr. Larsen
Post-anesthesia Release Sheet

Please provide clean, dry bedding and a quiet place for your pet to recuperate. Please notify the hospital with any concerns.

DIET:

( ) Wait a few hours after arriving home to offer your pet water. Please give only a small amount. If no vomiting occurs, you may offer more water about an hour later. You may feed a small amount (1/4 normal amount) if water stays down.

( ) You may continue to feed your pet normally.

( ) Special diet instructions _____

ACTIVITY:

( ) Restrict exercise for 1 day. NO RUNNING, JUMPING, CLIMBING OR BATHING.

( ) Restrict exercise for 7 days. NO RUNNING, JUMPING, CLIMBING OR BATHING.

( ) Other _____

OTHER:

( ) Please use paper strips or pinto beans in place of litter for 7 days.

( ) Please booster vaccines in 3-4 weeks.

( ) Your pet's metabolism may permanently decrease after surgery. You may need to decrease the amount of food you feed to prevent obesity.

INCISION:

( ) Watch for swelling, redness, or drainage. Prevent scratching, rubbing, and licking of the incision. Please ask for an E-collar if you think your pet will lick the site.

( ) Ice incision for 5 minutes, 3 to 4 times daily for the first 72 hours.

MEDICATION:

( ) Give pain medication _____

( ) Give antibiotics _____

( ) Give other medication _____

_____

( ) Start medication _____

FOLLOW-UP VISITS:

( ) Recheck in _____ days.

( ) There is no need to return for suture removal; the skin was closed with absorbable suture or tissue adhesive.

( ) Not necessary unless you feel there is a problem.

Comments:

Doctor _____ Tech _____ Client _____ Date _____

A

FIGURE 14-13 **A** to **C**, Examples of discharge instructions.

Discharge Instructions

ABC Veterinary Clinic
1001 Any Circle
Boston, MA 88012

Owner _____ Patient _____ Date _____

Diagnosis: _____
_____
_____

Medication: _____
_____
_____
_____

Start Medication: _____
_____

Diet: ( ) Normal ( ) Other _____
_____
_____

Exercise: ( ) No restriction ( ) Other _____
_____
_____

Special Instructions: _____
_____
_____
_____

Recheck _____ Dr. _____

B

FIGURE 14-13, cont'd **B,** Example of discharge instructions.

POSTSURGICAL/ANESTHETIC INSTRUCTIONS

Pet's name _____ Date _____ Procedure _____

_____ First offer your pet water in small quantities. Too much water at one time may cause vomiting.

_____ If there is no vomiting with water, feed 1/2 the normal amount of food the evening after anesthesia. The next morning, feed the normal amount.

_____ Keep you pet confined INDOORS the first evening after anesthesia.

_____ Your pet should be kept QUIET until all sutures/staples are removed. This includes no jumping or running.

_____ Give all medication(s) as directed:
Antibiotics:

Pain medication:

Other:

_____ Prevent your pet from irritating the incision site. ANY licking, rubbing, or scratching of the incision MUST be discouraged. We suggest using a T-shirt, ace bandage, buster collar, or even a tube sock for cats and small dogs.

_____ The incision site must be kept CLEAN and DRY. DO NOT apply anything to the incision without consulting us first. Watch for any bleeding, discharge, redness, and/or swelling.

_____ There are no stitches externally; they are located under the skin and will be absorbed by you pet's body.

_____ There are stitches/staples present. They must be removed in _____ days.

_____ A recheck appointment is needed in _____ days. The stitches/staples may be removed at this time.

Your pet's appointment time is: _____

_____ Your pet was spayed during her heat cycle. Spaying her has eliminated any possibility of a pregnancy, but she will remain attractive to males. Be careful that she is not in contact with any males during her recovery to prevent any injury.

_____ Your pet's gums may be painful after the dentistry. Softening the dry food with water may help so it can eat. Do NOT feed canned food unless it is the normal diet because it may cause diarrhea. To decrease further plaque buildup, brush the teeth, give rawhides to chew, or choose a food that can help; please ask which would be best for your pet.

_____ Use newspaper, shredded paper, or packing peanuts INSTEAD of you cat's regular litter until the incision site(s) are healed to prevent infection.

_____ Tape a plastic bag around the splint or bandage temporarily to keep the leg dry when going outside. Keep the area clean and dry. Discourage chewing by keeping the buster collar on at all times. Please call us if ANY swelling, odor, or discharge occurs.

DO NOT GIVE YOUR PET Advil, Nuprin, Motrin (ibuprofen), Tylenol (acetaminophen), or Aleve (naproxen)

C

FIGURE 14-13, cont'd C, Example of discharge instructions.

Radiology Checkout Log							
Date	**Owner's Name**	**Patient's Name**	**Check out by?**	**Going to?**	**Initials**	**Return Date**	**Initials**
10/6/09	Pacheco	Cherry	Owner	Crossroads A.H.	LP	12/8/09	MV
10/8/09	Ziehl	Bud	UPS	SW Specialty	CS		
11/1/09	Soules	Blackie	Owner	Arroyo V.C.	SP	12/1/09	DC
12/15/09	Miale	Twinkle	Mail	Tuscon	CS		

FIGURE 14-15 Radiology checkout log.

Box 14-6   Discharge Sheet Ideas

FOOD
- Normal or special diet?
- Restricted-time feedings or feeding intervals, or feed ad lib?
- For what length of time?

ACTIVITY
- Restricted or unrestricted?
- For what length of time?
- Physical therapy such as range of motion or pool swimming?

MEDICATIONS
- What kind? (Antibiotic, antiinflammatory, etc.)
- Name of the drug and strength
- How much? (How many pills, capsules, or liquid will be given at once?)
- How often will the medication be given?
- What are the side effects?
- When should client start medications?

MISCELLANEOUS INFORMATION
- Bandage care
- Vaccine boosters
- Icing the incision area
- Prevent licking (Elizabethan collars if needed)

RECHECKS
- When is a recheck needed?
- Do sutures need to be removed? When?
- Any detailed specific patient instructions can be added here.

All hospital contact information (including an emergency phone number) should be clearly indicated on the discharge sheet, along with the veterinarian and team member who have discharged the patient.

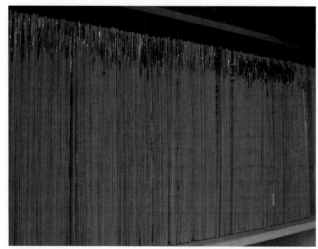

FIGURE 14-14 Example of alphabetized, color-coded radiographs.

VETERINARY PRACTICE and the LAW

Medications have the potential to treat conditions or induce harm. Many lawsuits are medication related, so the veterinary assistant and technician have a tremendous responsibility to carefully follow all procedures when administering medications to avoid doing harm.

Many patients are prescribed various medications at different stages in their lives. For example, a dog may receive a thyroid supplement as well as a nonsteroidal antiinflammatory (NSAID) for arthritis. If the dog were to develop an immune-related disorder, a veterinarian might prescribe a steroid. The dog should not receive the steroid and NSAID together. Owners also add medications and herbs to their pets' diets, hoping to improve the pets' quality of life. Clients should be asked if any additional vitamins, minerals, or herbs are being supplemented to prevent the possibility of a toxic interaction.

When administering and dispensing medications, review the record, checking for all medications that have been dispensed. The assistant or technician should verify the medications with the veterinarian to ensure that the new medication is not contraindicated with the other medications.

Before administering the medication, the drug, dose, and route of administration must be verified. Labels should be verified for correct information and the client should be read the instructions.

Self-Evaluation Questions

1. Why is legibility so important in medical records?
2. How often are medical records purged?
3. What is the earliest that records can be shredded?
4. Why is history taking critical for a medical record?
5. What is a SOAP progress note? Give an example of each part.
6. What items are mandatory in a medical record? Why?
7. Why are discharge sheets vital?
8. Does a client record belong to the client? Why or why not?
9. Who owns the radiographs of a pet?
10. What is the most common method for filing paper medical records?

Recommended Reading

Heinke MM: *Practice made perfect: a guide to veterinary practice management*, Lakewood, CO, 2001, AAHA Press.

McCurnin D: *Veterinary practice management*, Philadelphia, 1988, JB Lippincott.

McCurnin D, Bassert JA: *Clinical textbook for veterinary technicians*, ed 7, St Louis, 2010, Saunders Elsevier.

Sheridan JP, McCafferty O: *The business of veterinary practice*, Tarrytown, NY, 1993, Pergamon Press.

Wilson JF: *Law and ethics of the veterinary profession*, Yardley, PA, 1988, Priority Press.

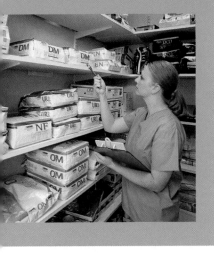

CHAPTER 15

Inventory Management

Chapter Outline

Fundamentals of Inventory
Distributors and Manufacturer Representatives
Designing an Inventory System
    Central Inventory Location
    Developing Reorder Points and Quantities
    Developing a Want List
    Order Book
    Receiving an Order

Handling Expired Medications
Returning Products to Distributor
Developing an Effective Product
    Markup
Material Safety Data Sheets
Capital Inventory
Decreasing Loss

Learning Objectives

Mastery of the content in this chapter will enable the reader to:
• Develop an effective inventory system.
• List methods used to maintain an appropriate amount of
  inventory on hand.
• Define and create a central inventory location.

• Define capital inventory.
• Identify and use Material Safety Data Sheets.
• Calculate an effective price markup for products.
• Describe methods used to handle expired medications.

Key Terms

Capital
Central Inventory Location
Distributor Representative
Food and Drug Administration
    (FDA)

Inventory
Inventory Turns per Year
Just-in-Time Ordering
Manufacturer Representative
Markup

Material Safety Data Sheet (MSDS)
Order Book
Reorder Point
Reorder Quantity
Want List

Effective inventory controls are an important part of the overall profit of a veterinary practice. Creating and maintaining an inventory system takes continuous planning and monitoring. Without proper organization, inventory can become a full-time duty. Inventory is the balance between having enough products on the shelves to meet client needs and not running out of product or supplies. Outdated products decrease the practice's profits, as does not having enough product. Managing inventory requires knowledge of what product is used, how much is used, how often it is sold, as well as how long it takes to reorder and replace the product. A combination of all the above will make it possible to implement an effective inventory management system that takes little time to control (Box 15-1).

It is an advantage to have one team member in charge of inventory. By having one person in control of this task, mistakes are decreased, overordering is prevented, and other team members know whom to contact if an item is in short supply. One person can easily organize an inventory system, which will streamline the process. By decreasing the steps and time required to maintain inventory, profits are increased, time is saved, and clients are satisfied.

FUNDAMENTALS OF INVENTORY

Although one person should be in charge of inventory, a second team member or manager should be able to fill in as needed. If an emergency happens to the inventory manager, another team member should be able to effectively step up without creating a glitch in the system. Distributor and manufacturer phone numbers, account numbers, and order histories should be readily available.

Box 15-1	Losses Associated With Poor Inventory Management

- Practice billed for product never received
- Practice double-billed
- Practice billed for damaged goods
- Practice billed for items different than what were received
- Backorders
- Expired items
- Wrong items shipped
- High costs of overnight shipment for products needed ASAP
- Account not credited for returned goods

Box 15-2	Keys to a Successful Inventory Management System

- Buy in volume from one distributor to reduce shipping costs.
- Minimize the number of times ordered per week or month.
- Evaluate expired drugs monthly. Can they be returned for credit or replaced?
- Evaluate payment plans. If companies offer a discount if the bill is paid by the tenth of each month, make sure the payment is made!
- Make a goal of having an inventory turnover rate of at least four to six times per year—10 to 12 turns per year for pet food.
- Limit the duplication of drugs (package size and brand).
- Maintain inventory costs between 12% and 15% of gross revenue of the practice.

The front of an order book or Rolodex is an excellent place to keep a summary of all distributors and manufacturers. Small orders may need to be placed with specialty companies, and if there is easy access to their information, orders can be placed quickly and efficiently (Box 15-2).

PRACTICE POINT Putting one person in charge of inventory reduces mistakes such as placing double orders for products.

This information is only the beginning of establishing a successful inventory system. Excellent books are available through the American Animal Hospital Association and the American Veterinary Medicine Association to help improve existing systems and build a more profitable practice through inventory management.

An organized manager must determine which technique is most effective to maintain inventory. A variety of techniques are discussed in this chapter; however, the combination of several techniques may work better. Each practice is different and each manager must be flexible in determining the best technique.

Drugs might be arranged in a pharmacy area in such a way as to help improve the efficiency of a team (Figure 15-1). Drugs may be arranged by category, such as oral solids, oral liquids, injectable, ophthalmic, otic, and/or external topical medications. Other pharmacies may be arranged by type of drug, such as tranquilizers, analgesics, cardiac, diuretics, and so forth.

DISTRIBUTORS AND MANUFACTURER REPRESENTATIVES

Distributor representatives generally work for a company that carries a full line of manufactured products ranging from equipment to pet foods. *Manufacturer* representatives sell products to distributors or, in some cases, distribute products themselves. Manufacturer and distributor representatives may discuss specials with the inventory manager and educate the veterinarians when new products are launched.

PRACTICE POINT Distributors and manufacturer representatives can provide valuable knowledge and continuing education for the staff along with sales and product information.

Manufacturer and distributor representatives can provide team members with valuable information regarding products and how they may increase sales for the practice. They can provide a sales history, allowing a prediction for the use of product for the next year (this is an excellent tool when preparing a budget for the following fiscal year). They can be an excellent source of continuing education for team members and can provide brochures to increase the level of client education. (Box 15-3).

Caution should be used when companies have sales promotions. Many practices cannot sell the minimum amount of product, and product should not be purchased for the reason of a good friendship. Product should only be ordered when it has been determined that it can sell within a 3-month period.

Working with a limited number of distributors and manufacturers allows larger orders to be placed at one location, usually allowing shipping and handling fees to be waived by the company. These fees are generally imposed on smaller orders and can add up quickly. Many distributors will guarantee the best price to their top clients, eliminating the need to "shop around" on a weekly basis looking for the best price available. These representatives work for the practice; they want the business and will find the product or equipment requested in a reasonable amount of time.

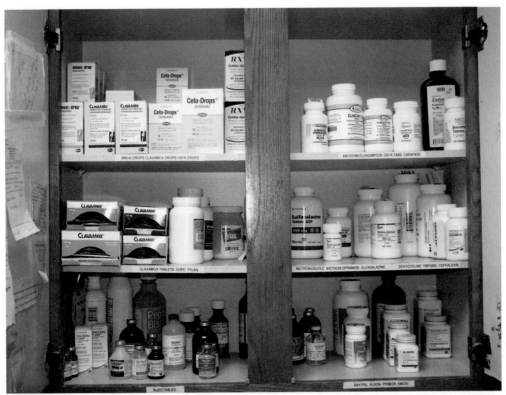

FIGURE 15-1 This pharmacy is organized by drug function, allowing the team to be more efficient.

Box 15-3	Examples of Manufacturers and Distributors

MANUFACTURERS	**DISTRIBUTORS**
Merial	Butler Schein Animal
Pfizer Animal Health	Health
Novartis Animal Health	DVM Resources
Intervet/Schering Plough	MWI Veterinary Supply
Animal Health	Columbus Serum
Purina Veterinary Diets	Webster Veterinary
Royal Canin Veterinary Diets	
Hills	

This list is not exhaustive.

DESIGNING AN INVENTORY SYSTEM

Two methods exist to create and maintain an inventory system. Computer software generally integrates inventory management into the system and is easily accessible from any computer (Figures 15-2 to 15-4). A manual method takes time to maintain but is almost always accurate.

Categories must be refined when entering products into the computer. By refining these categories, reports can be generated regarding product order and sales history as well as a client usage report. Categories may include antibiotics, injectables, pet foods, shampoos, radiographs, surgical supplies, or laboratory services.

Reorder points and quantities can be established when entering these products into the computer. A physical inventory must be taken at the same time so the amount on the shelf is the same as that entered into the computer. A weekly reorder report can be produced and checked against the shelf items to ensure the report is accurate. Once the product arrives, the invoices can be entered into the computer. The date, distributor, product, and price are entered into the computer from the invoice. The software will pick up any price changes from previous orders, verify the change with the operator, and amend the price if cleared to do so. This allows the practice to prevent the loss of any profit from the changing price of products. These advantages of the computer software system far outweigh any disadvantages.

> **PRACTICE POINT** Received orders must be checked against the invoices, ensuring that the correct product was shipped.

The disadvantages to computer inventory software are minimal. Human error does occur; therefore reports must be verified. Without verifying product inventory, incorrect quantities may be ordered. It can be difficult to effectively trace bandage material, suture material, surgical or exam gloves, or any other items used to complete services. For a computerized system to be effective, all items must be entered each time they are used. It can be more labor intensive to add a pair of exam

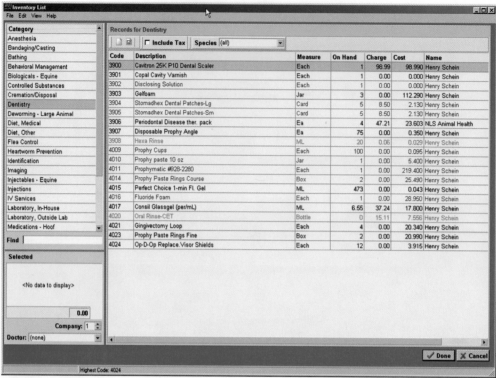

FIGURE 15-2 Example of Avimark's inventory list. (Courtesy McAllister Software Systems, Piedmont, Mo.)

gloves to each ear cleaning or anal sac expression than to check the inventory levels each order period.

Manual inventory systems are time consuming; however, they are generally quite accurate. When products are received, invoices are reviewed and entered onto individual alphabetized index cards. The date, distributor, product, strength, quantity, and price are entered on the card. Any changes in price should be observed by the person making the entries, and a price change should take effect immediately.

A complete review of all products is made weekly or bimonthly to create an order. The inventory manager should have a listing of reorder points and quantities on the index cards to help facilitate the correct order. To help the inventory manager maintain a successful system, a red flag system may be developed (Figure 15-5). Once the reorder point has been established, the manager can place a red flag on the product bottle, with the date the product was received. When a team member takes that bottle, the red flag is removed and placed in a designated area. The inventory manager can review the flag, look at the date of purchase, and determine if, when, and how much product should be ordered.

A combination of both methods may be effective for veterinary practices. No one method works better than another; it takes a team to make a system succeed. Double-checking the inventory is the easiest and fastest way to ensure reorder points and quantities are correct. A report helps prevent the manager from missing items.

A complete physical inventory must be completed each year and the system updated with correct quantities. It cannot be emphasized enough that the system needs continuous monitoring and that changes may have to be made to maintain the implemented inventory system.

> **PRACTICE POINT** Visual examination of inventoried products is the quickest and most accurate method to prevent running out of products.

Central Inventory Location

It is ideal to have a central location to store all excess inventory products (Figure 15-6). Items can be checked in when they are received and checked out when a bottle is needed in the pharmacy. New items should be placed behind old items, allowing the older items to be sold first. In smaller practices with limited space, this system may not work. Therefore placing items on the shelf in the correct location may be the next best method. Practices may have one cabinet that can be used for excess product. When a bottle is emptied, the new bottle can be pulled and placed in the correct location. This can help prevent overcrowding of products in one area. Overcrowding loses items in the clutter; they may be displaced or overlooked (Box 15-4).

> **PRACTICE POINT** A central inventory location is a place within the practice that has limited access and stores excess quantities of product.

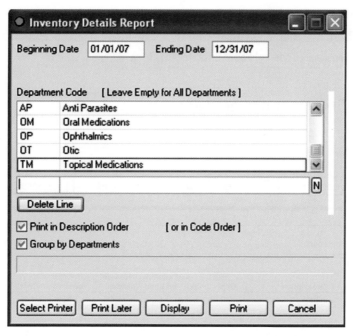

Code	Description	Purchases Amount	Qty	Sales Qty	On hand Amount	Qty	Cost	Percent Markup	Price
Topical medications (TM)									
TM050	Allermyl Shampoo	131.16	12.00	8.00	78.05	7.00	11.1500	10	12.26
TM055	Allermyl Spray	84.56	8.00	3.00	21.58	2.00	10.7900	10	11.87
TM073	Animax Cream 15 ml	177.24	30.00	29.00	99.00	20.00	4.9500	33	6.60
TM075	Animax Ointment 15 ml	156.75	31.00	26.00	80.75	19.00	4.2500	88	8.00
TM125	Corti Sooth Shampoo	24.18	2.00	0.00	24.66	2.00	12.3300	8	13.30
TM220	Doxirobe Gel 8.5%	74.90	3.00	1.00	49.93	2.00	24.9667	0	0.00
TM350	Gentocin Topical Spray	27.25	5.00	4.00	16.35	3.00	5.4500	50	8.18
TM450	Hetacin K	18.72	12.00	7.00	8.15	5.00	1.6300	50	2.45
TM600	Medicated Shampoo	260.11	39.00	43.00	33.68	4.00	8.4200	10	9.26
TM610	Miconazole Lotion 1%	67.30	10.00	11.00	30.55	5.00	6.1100	65	10.10
TM675	Oatmeal Shampoo	115.80	20.00	16.00	77.87	13.00	5.9900	0	5.99
TM690	OxyDex Shampoo	5.57	1.00	1.00	0.00	0.00	5.5700	10	6.13
TM700	Resicort Conditioner	73.68	6.00	10.00	12.52	1.00	12.5200	17	14.61
Vaccinations (VA)									
VA106	Imrab 3 Rabies Vaccine	1216.22	900.00	594.00	743.51	499.00	1.4900	1108	18.00
VA116	Intra-Track-3 Bordetella Vaccine	9193.70	425.00	458.00	301.29	121.00	2.4900	623	18.00
VA118	Merial Corna Vaccine	175.51	50.00	6.00	89.30	25.00	3.5720	404	18.00
VA119	Merial DA2PP Vaccine	3442.32	1200.00	1171.00	702.00	216.00	3.2500	854	31.00
VA138	Merial Leptospira	75.76	25.00	0.00	78.20	23.00	3.4000	429	18.00
VA152	Merial RCP Vaccine	1019.90	450.00	381.00	589.68	216.00	2.7300	559	18.00
VA158	Merial PUREVAX FeLV Vaccine	3621.22	500.00	353.00	1828.34	226.00	8.0900	160	21.00
VA114	Progard DPV Vaccine	59.75	25.00	1.00	57.36	24.00	2.3900	1197	31.00
VA112	Purevax Rabies/RCP	189.53	25.00	0.00	213.50	25.00	8.5400	298	34.00
VA111	Purevax Feline Rabies Vaccine	2912.43	525.00	328.00	1570.80	255.00	6.1600	192	18.00
VA141	Recombitek Lyme Vaccine	185.25	20.00	2.00	194.58	18.00	10.8100	113	23.00
		149843.44			**48829.95**				

An onhand quantity marked with an asterisk (*) indicates that one or more warehouses has a negative quantity and was not added into the onhand quantity for that code.

FIGURE 15-3 Example of IntraVet's inventory details report. (Courtesy IntraVet, Dublin, Ohio.)

Developing Reorder Points and Quantities

A reorder point is defined as the point a stock level reaches before reordering. A reorder quantity is the amount of product to be reordered. The shelf life of a product is the amount of time from when it is received in the practice until it is sold. The average shelf life an item should not exceed 3 months. Anything greater than 3 months decreases the profits of the veterinary hospital and increases the risk of the product expiring as well as the risk of theft or breakage of the product. A sales history of a product should be examined when determining a reorder point and quantity. As stated, the quantity

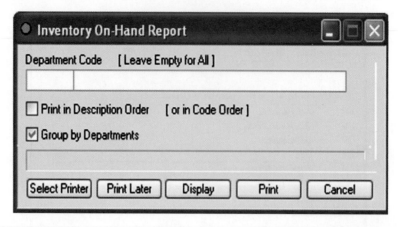

Inventory On-hand Report　　　　　　　　　　　　　　　　**INTRAVET VETERINARY CARE**

Ophthalmics (OP)

Code	Description	Dept	Tax	Quantity on hand	Reorder level	Reorder quantity	Cost	Percent mark-up	Price
OP100	Atropine Sulfate 1% Ophth Sol.	OP	N	5.00	2.00	4.00	1.05	319	4.40
OP101	Atropine Sulfate 1% Ophth Oint.	OP	N	28.00	2.00	3.00	0.95	387	4.63
OP200	Dexamethasone Drops	OP	N	24.00	2.00	4.00	3.13	468	17.81
OP405	Gentocin Ophth Solution	OP	N	29.00	12.00	24.00	31.00	0	6.40
OP500	BNP Ophth Oint 1/8 oz	OP	N	19.00	2.00	4.00	19.00	0	5.74
OP510	BNP-H Ophth Oint 1/8 oz	OP	N	27.00	2.00	4.00	17.64	0	7.01
OP550	NPS w/Dex Ophth Sol	OP	N	40.00	12.00	24.00	1.73	137	4.09
OP552	*Neo Poly Dex Ophth Ointment	OP	N	24.00	0.00	0.00	1.60	240	5.42
OP600	Optimmune Ophth Oint	OP	N	14.00	3.00	6.00	8.78	184	24.90
OP800	Terak Ophth Oint	OP	N	12.00	0.00	0.00	2.50	190	7.24
OP850	Terramycin Ophth Oint 3.5 gm	OP	N	3.00	3.00	2.00	7.84	62	12.71

Otic (OT)

Code	Description	Dept	Tax	Quantity on hand	Reorder level	Reorder quantity	Cost	Percent mark-up	Price
OT050	Acarexx Otic Solution	OT	N	24.00	2.00	6.00	7.64	102	15.43
OT150	Baytril Otic	OT	N	20.00	2.00	6.00	9.16	100	18.31
OT160	Baytril/Conofite/Dex SP	OT	N	53.00	0.00	0.00	8.40	138	20.00
OT670	Otomax 15 gr	OT	N	32.00	12.00	12.00	8.92	18	10.50
OT830	Synotic	OT	N	8.00	1.00	3.00	8.40	100	16.80
OT832	Synotic w/Banamine	OT	N	8.00	0.00	0.00	19.30	0	4.19
OT834	Synotic w/Gentocin	OT	N	12.00	0.00	0.00	22.30	0	6.19
OT850	Tresaderm	OT	N	62.00	12.00	36.00	8.38	67	13.97
OT855	Trizedta Flush	OT	N	16.00	1.00	2.00	0.61	128	1.39
OT910	Vet Sol Ear Cleaner	OT	N	44.00	12.00	24.00	6.00	50	9.01

Vaccinations (VA)

Code	Description	Dept	Tax	Quantity on hand	Reorder level	Reorder quantity	Cost	Percent mark-up	Price
VA106	Imrab 3 Rabies Vaccine	VA	N	261.00	50.00	200.00	1.56	1054	18.00
VA111	Purevax Feline Rabies Vaccine	VA	N	230.00	50.00	100.00	6.16	192	18.00
VA112	PurevaxRabies/RCP	VA	N	97.00	12.00	25.00	8.72	290	34.00

FIGURE 15-4 Example of IntraVet's inventory on-hand report. (Courtesy IntraVet, Dublin, Ohio.)

ordered should not exceed a product sitting on the shelf for more than 3 months. A reorder point can then be determined. Factors affecting reorder points may include:

- **Seasonal products:** Flea and tick products are seasonal in many parts of the country and sales will increase during the summer months. Higher quantities of product can be ordered during the summer and less in the winter.
- **Packaging of product:** Some products are only sold in boxes of 10, 1000-count bottles, or in case quantities.
- **Lead time:** Amount of time it takes to receive a product after placing order.

Practices may wish to keep as little inventory on hand as possible. This can be an advantage because it can lower holding costs (costs associated with holding product on the shelf, such as taxes and insurance) and prevent shrinkage (unexplained loss of inventory). However, it can contribute to product shortage (losing clients and money from not having the product available for resale). Therefore practices may wish to have a cushion, which allows enough product to be on the shelf until the next order arrives. This can increase the holding cost but decreases shortage, which ultimately increases client satisfaction.

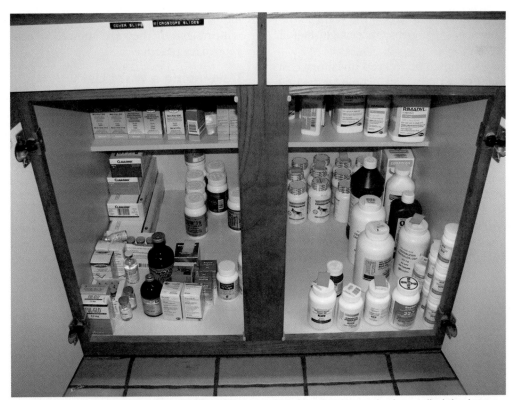

FIGURE 15-5 A red flag system notifies the team member that he or she has pulled the last bottle and the product must be placed on the want list.

> ◎ **PRACTICE POINT** Reorder quantity is the amount of product to reorder that will be sold within a 3-month period.

Just-in-time ordering is defined as ordering a product when it is needed but before running out. This can work for some practices, but it does not account for manufacturer or distributor backorders. If a product is backordered, the inventory manager must find the product with another distributor or find a product that is equivalent. If a match is not available, other team members and veterinarians must be made aware of the backorder.

Inventory turns per year is a goal every inventory manager should set. *Turns per year* is defined as the number of times inventory turns over in a practice. This helps determine correct reorder quantities and points. Each practice should set a goal of eight to 12 turns per year. This increases the profits of the practice and decreases expired product, shrinkage, holding, and ordering costs. To determine the inventory turns per year, the beginning inventory is added to the ending inventory and divided by two. This results in the average inventory per year. The total amount of product purchased during that period divided by the average yields the number of turns per year for that product. Taking the equation one step

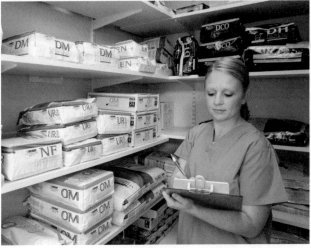

FIGURE 15-6 Managing inventory in an organized manner keeps products from being overlooked or lost.

Box 15-4	Disadvantages of a Large Inventory

- Items missing in action (e.g., employee theft)
- Bottles breaking
- Items expiring
- Doctors wanting to change to another product and being unable to do so because of large quantity of previous product

further, dividing the number of days in the year (365) by the number of turns per year gives the average shelf life of the item (Box 15-5).

The ultimate goal should be to keep inventory costs between 12% and 15% of the overall income for the practice. If a practice generates $1 million, 12% is $120,000. Costs of products should not exceed $120,000 for the year. This contributes to successfully implementing a budget. (See Chapter 20, "Preparing and Maintaining Budgets," for more information. Chapter 24, "Calculations and Conversions," also has more examples of how to determine inventory turns per year.)

A clinic may decide to purchase a large amount of product at one time due to a greatly discounted price. Regardless of the terms, a large purchase should ONLY be made if the practice is saving at least 40% of the original cost AND the product can be sold within a 6-month period. If both of those conditions cannot be met, the "deal" is not a good deal.

A few solutions exist for a doctor or a team of doctors who want to carry or dispense a product that has a short expiration date, or where the minimum quantity that can be ordered is larger than what the practice can sell. First, a practice may script the drug out to a local pharmacy. Products that are expensive and do not sell fast can be obtained or compounded at many local pharmacies. Second, several practices in a community may wish to share the product and split the order equally. One practice can be responsible for purchasing the product; the other practices can either purchase the product or trade with other products in lieu of dollars. Third, a local human hospital may have the drug and allow the clinic to purchase the product from them in a smaller quantity, sometimes at a cheaper price. An inquiring phone call to the human hospital pharmacy will indicate if they are allowed to sell products to a veterinary practice.

Developing a Want List

A want list may be developed for team members who recognize that a specific product is running low. A dry erase board works well for a want list because products can be erased as soon as they arrive. A special order board may established for those medications that need to be custom-ordered for clients; this may include compounded and/or flavored medication (Figure 15-7). This special order board can provide a quick reference for team members preparing the medication once it has arrived to the practice because it will have the client and pet name listed.

> **PRACTICE POINT** A "want list" can be written on a dry-erase board placed in a central location of the practice. It allows team members to write down products that need to be reordered. Want lists assist the inventory manager and decrease the chance of missing low-quantity products.

A spreadsheet of items may be developed for the inventory manager to follow as an order is being made (Figure 15-8). Many times, items are removed from the shelves and team members forget to write the product on the board or place the red tag in the designated place. This spreadsheet allows a third check of the inventoried items. It may not be noticed that a product is missing until a doctor needs it. If a spreadsheet is used, the need can be detected and the product ordered. A spreadsheet may simply contain the name and size of the product. It is useful to have it as a simple reminder of all products that should be on the shelf at all times.

Figure 15-8 is an example of a spreadsheet of inventoried products for a veterinary practice. This specific practice has a pharmacy that is first organized by location (refrigerator, controlled substance, shelf); then the product is alphabetized. The quantity in which the product is supplied is listed in column B; distributor or manufacturer in column C, the quantity to reorder in column D, and the shelf life of that particular product in column E.

Order Book

All orders should be kept together, listed chronologically in a book. This allows the inventory manager to see what products were ordered, how many, from which distributor or manufacturer, the date the order was placed, and the name of the representative who took the order. This is also a great history resource. As a key to decreasing order confusion, the same representative should be called each time. Inside sales representatives become familiar with

---

Box 15-5	**Example of Inventory Turns per Year**

Beginning inventory + Ending inventory/2
= Average inventory for the year

Total number of product purchased/
Average invertory for the year = Number of turns per year

365/# of turns per year = Average shelf life of product

For example, inventory for eye drops at the beginning of the year was two. Ending inventory was two. Total purchased for the year was 36.

$$2+2=4.\ 4/2=2.\ 36/2=18$$

The product turned 18 times. This is an excellent value!

$$365/18 = 20$$

Average shelf life is 20 days.

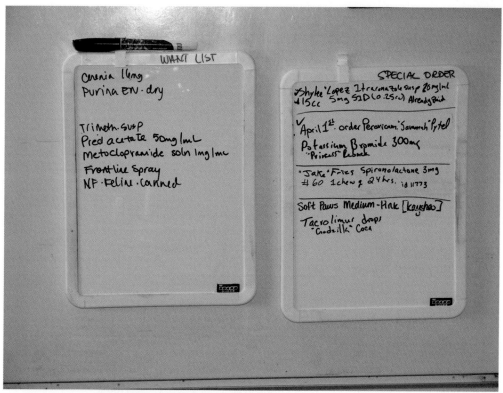

FIGURE 15-7 A want list and special order list are placed on two separate dry erase boards.

products the practice prefers and make every effort to ensure the order is 100% satisfactory. If an item is on backorder, the representative should notify the manager at that time, and a decision can be made to order an alternative product or to search for the product through another company. The backorder should be noted in the book at this time and a notice posted for all team members.

> **PRACTICE POINT** An order book is an excellent place to keep a summary of all distributors and manufacturer phone numbers as well as account numbers.

Receiving an Order

When a shipment is received, the inventory manager should, ideally, inspect the order before it is put away. Items should be inspected for damage and compared to the invoice and order book (Figure 15-9). Quantity (e.g., number of bottles), strength of product (e.g., in milligrams or grams), and size of product (e.g., number of tablets, capsules, milliliters) should be double-checked. Once it has been determined that the products match the invoice and book, products can be placed in the appropriate location. These invoices also need to be matched to the monthly statement to guarantee that no other charges were added to the account. An example would be to create an open order file. Once packing slips have been checked against the product received, the slip can be placed in an open file; this indicates that

the packing slip needs to be matched to the invoices received at the end of each month. Once the match has been completed, the packing slip can be placed in a closed file (Figure 15-10).

HANDLING EXPIRED MEDICATIONS

The Federal Drug Administration (FDA) requires that all drugs that it has tested and approved have an expiration date (Figure 15-11). Drug manufacturers determine this date by performing efficacy tests on the product. Once the efficacy of a drug has dropped below a certain percentage, it is no longer effective. Products must be removed from the shelves once they have expired and they cannot be sold. Not only is it unethical to dispense expired drugs, it is illegal. Also, the medication being dispensed for a pet may not work as well as it should. Many practices do not want to lose money associated with expired products; therefore an effective inventory management system must be implemented to prevent medications from expiring. Inventory managers may keep a running list of products and expiration dates that can be completed each time an order is received. If a product bottle is opened that is getting close to expiring, a note should be made for the doctors, allowing them to increase the dispensing of the product. If the bottle is not opened, the distributor or manufacturer may exchange the product at no charge. Return policies should be verified and kept on file for referencing.

Product	Quantity	Distributor	Reorder #	Shelf Life	Notes
FELV/FIV	30/bx	Butler	1	30d	
General Health Profile	2/bx	Butler	6	1d	
Heartworm 3DX	30/bx	Butler	2	15d	
Parvo	5/box	Butler	2	10d	
Plasma	1	ABB	1	30d	
Pre-op Profile	4/bx	Butler	6	1d	
Apomorphine	1	VPA	5	3 mo	
Buprinex	1 ml x 10 vials	DVM	2	7d	
Butorpehnol Inj	50 mg	DVM	1	6 mo	
Butorphenol Tabs	100	DVM	1	6 mo	
Diazepam	10 ml; 5 vials	DVM	1	6 mo	
Ketamine	10 ml; 5 vials	DVM	1	2 mo	
Hycodan	100 tabs	DVM	1	6 mo	
Telazol	5 ml	DVM	5	7 d	
Activated Charcoal	1	Butler	5	30d	
Albon	100	Pfizer	1	30d	
Amoxi Clavulanate	210	Pfizer	1	30d	
Amoxicillin	100	Butler	1	30d	
Antirobe	100 and drops	Pfizer	1	30d	
Artifical Tears	1	Butler	5	7 d	
Atropine Ophth	1	Butler	2	10 d	
Barium Sulfate	1	DVM	1	30 d	
Baytril oral	100	Bayer	1	60 d	
Benedryl Capsules	500, 1000	DVM	1	3 mo	
Benedryl Susp	473 ml	DVM	1	6 mo	
Carafate	473 ml	DVM	1	6 mo	
Cefa Drops	15 ml	DVM	6	10 d	
Cephalexin Caps	100, 500	Butler	1	7 d	
Chlorpheniramine	1000	DVM	1	30 d	
Deramax	90	Novartis	1	60d	
Doxycycline	100, 500	Butler	1	7 d	
Droncit	50	Butler	1	4 mo	
Fenbendazole	Liquid or powder	DVM	1	5 mo	
Genesis	1	Butler	6	30 d	

FIGURE 15-8 Example of spreadsheet for inventoried products.

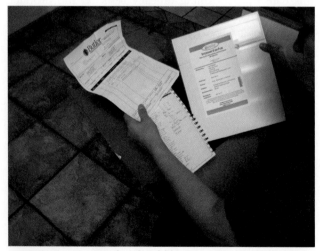

FIGURE 15-9 An order should be compared to the invoice and want list, ensuring that the correct product and quantity were received.

When medications have expired, they should not be discarded in the trash or flushed down a drain. Pills can be added to a small amount of water and mixed until dissolved. A small amount of cat litter can then be added, and the mixture can then be thrown away. Solutions and injectable medications can also be added to cat litter and then thrown away. The Environmental Protection Agency advises against pouring medications into the toilet to discard them.

Expired controlled substances must be submitted to a facility certified to dispose of controlled substances. A receipt for the controlled substances submitted will then be returned to the clinic and should be kept with the current controlled substance log indicating they were disposed of. State veterinary boards should have a current list of manufacturers certified to accept controlled substances. Disposing of controlled substances is described in greater detail in Chapter 16.

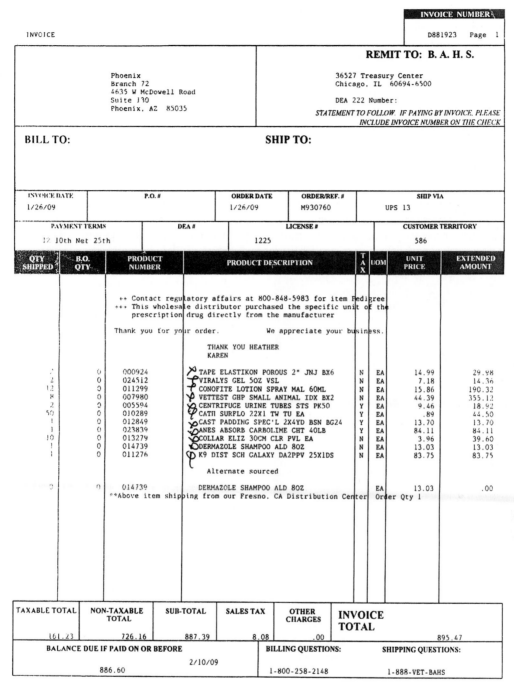

FIGURE 15-10 Sample packing slip.

RETURNING PRODUCTS TO THE DISTRIBUTOR

Products may need to be returned to the distributor for a variety of reasons, including damage, the wrong product being sent, or the wrong product being ordered. Most distributors are happy to return the products, although some may institute a restocking or shipping fee. A call should be placed to the sales representative who handled the order to notify that person of the problem. The representative may ask whether a replacement product or credit is requested. A call tag will be sent for the return of the item. A call tag is an address label produced by the company to be placed on the outside of the shipment box. This label has a special reference number on it so that the returned product can be credited to the appropriate account. Once the tag has been received, it is important to document on the original invoice when the product was returned. A credit should be given to the practice upon receipt of the product, and a credit invoice will be generated. The credit may take a few weeks to be received. Distributors and manufacturers may also take unopened bottles of recently expired product. However, instead of a credit, the product will be replaced. Each company has different policies regarding the expired product, and options should be researched before ordering new product.

DEVELOPING AN EFFECTIVE PRODUCT MARKUP

The *markup* of a product is defined as the cost (of the product) multiplied by a percentage to recover hidden costs associated with inventory management. Many

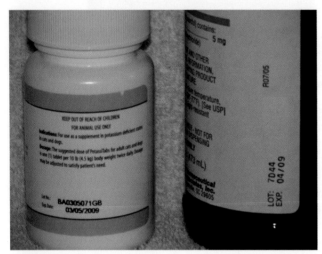

FIGURE 15-11 Expired drugs cannot be sold. Inventory managers must watch expiration dates of products and dispose of expired drugs appropriately.

practices mark products up by 100% to 200%. Shopped items, such as vaccines and routine surgeries, should be kept competitive with other local or regional veterinary practices. Non-shopped items must be increased to accommodate the lower priced shopped items. Special services and supplies must be marked up appropriately, covering the extra charges that generally accommodate the special services.

> ◎ **PRACTICE POINT** Products must be marked up at least 40% to break even.

Practices may also add a product dispensing fee as well as a minimum prescription charge. The average dispensing fee ranges from $8 to $14 to cover the cost of the label, the pill vial, and the time used to count the medication. If a bottle of shampoo or a full bottle of medication is dispensed, the average dispensing fee ranges from $3 to $5. Many practices initiate a minimum prescription fee of $14 to $18 to help recover hidden pharmacy costs.

Hidden pharmacy costs include costs associated with expired medications, ordering and shipping costs, and insurance and taxes on products and supplies. These costs can increase rapidly and must be covered.

Examples of inventory turnover and markup calculations, along with dispensing fees and recovering hidden costs, are covered more extensively discussed in Chapter 24.

MATERIAL SAFETY DATA SHEETS

Material Safety Data Sheets (MSDSs) are required for all chemical products that are sold or used within a veterinary practice. The Occupational Safety and Health Administration (OSHA) set forth standards for current practice

What Would You Do/Not Do?

Ms. Eoff's cat, Harvey, was recently diagnosed with hyperthyroidism. The veterinarian prescribed 1 month of methimazole tablets. The owner was advised to return in 3 to 4 weeks to recheck the thyroid values. Ms. Eoff called 2 weeks after therapy started and stated she could not get Harvey to take the pills and that she wanted another option for treatment. Dr. Dreamer advised her that radioactive iodine was an option at the specialty center; however, the owner declined. Dr. Dreamer offered to special order a transdermal medication that could be applied to the tip of the ear. Ms. Eoff was greatly appreciative of the solution and authorized the ordering of the medication.

Upon arrival of the special order, Alex, a veterinary technician, calls to inform Ms. Eoff that the medication has arrived. He advises Ms. Eoff that he would like to schedule an appointment with Harvey, which will allow him to review

the medication and show her how to apply it. She informs Alex at that time that she has learned how to give Harvey the tablets and that she will no longer need the specially ordered medication. Alex knows that the inventory manager ordered this medication specifically for the dose that Harvey requires and that the medication cannot be returned to the company that produces methimazole gel.

What Should Alex Do?

Alex must inform Ms. Eoff that this medication was specially ordered for Harvey, which she approved when she last spoke with Dr. Dreamer. Alex can advise Ms. Eoff that she should try the medication because it may ultimately be easier for her to administer once she tries it. If it does not work, she can return to the use of tablets at the end of the month. Ms. Eoff must understand that the medication cannot be returned and the product cannot be sold to another client because this particular dose was for Harvey.

relations. The OSHA Act of 1970 was enacted to ensure safe work environments for all employees. The law is based on the simple concept that all employees have the right to know about any potential hazard to which they may be exposed. Each MSDS lists the potential hazards related to that substance and what protective measures can be taken if any hazard occurs (Figure 15-12). Chapter 21 includes more information regarding the use of MSDSs.

Distributors are reliable about sending MSDSs when a product has been ordered from that company for the first time; however, it is the ultimate responsibility of the veterinary practice to ensure they are available for any team member when needed. The inventory manager should know when a new product arrives and ensure the new sheet is added to the current MSDS notebook.

```
------------------------ MATERIAL SAFETY DATA SHEET ------------------------
                               LASIX(R) (FUROSEMIDE) INJECTION
----------------------------------------------------------------------------

------------------------ SECTION I ------------------------   ------------------------ SECTION VII - SPILL OR LEAK PROCEDURES ------------------------

MANUFACTURER'S NAME: HOECHST-ROUSSEL AGRI-VET COMPANY          STEPS TO BE TAKEN IN CASE MATERIAL IS RELEASED OR SPILLED:
   ROUTE 202-206                                                 Using protective equipment as stated in Section VIII,
   P.O. BOX 2500                                                 large spillage for salvage or waste disposal is to be
   SOMERVILLE, NEW JERSEY 08876-1258                             collected in a waste container.
EMERGENCY TELEPHONE NO.: HUMAN, FIRE, SPILL OR                 WASTE DISPOSAL METHOD: Avoid flushing large amounts into
   ENVIRONMENTAL: 1-800-228-5635, Ext. 132                       sewer; minor spillage may be flushed away with water.
   ANIMAL: 1-800-345-4835, Ext. 104                              Review all Federal/State regulations concerning health
TRADE NAME: Lasix(R) (Furosemide) Injection                      and pollution standards to determine an approved disposal
PRODUCT CLASS: Veterinary diuretic-saluretic                     procedure.
MANUFACTURING IDENTIFICATION:                                 ------------------------------------------------------------
DATE OF PREPARATION: June 23, 1992                            SECTION VIII - SPECIAL PROTECTION INFORMATION
------------------ SECTION II - HAZARDOUS INGREDIENTS ------   RESPIRATORY PROTECTION:
                                                              VENTILATION:
              NATURE OF          TLV                          PROTECTIVE GLOVES: Yes
INGREDIENTS   HAZARD       PERCENT PPM MG/M3 MPPCF            EYE PROTECTION: Yes
                                                              OTHER PROTECTIVE EQUIPMENT: None
Furosemide         Non-hazardous   5%                        ------------------ SECTION IX - SPECIAL PRECAUTIONS ------------------
  (CAS #54-31-9)
  LEL:                                                        PRECAUTIONS TO BE TAKEN IN HANDLING AND STORING: Store at
  UEL:                                                           room temperature.
  LD50:
------------------ SECTION III - PHYSICAL DATA ------------   N/A = Not applicable
                                                              NM = Not measured
BOILING POINT: N/A                                            DNA = Does not apply
VAPOR DENSITY (AIR = 1): N/A
DENSITY (BULK): N/A                                           DISCLAIMER OF EXPRESSED AND IMPLIED WARRANTIES: Although
MELTING POINT: 206 deg C                                      reasonable care has been taken in the preparation of this
PERCENT VOLATILE:                                             document, we extend no warranties and make no
EVAPORATION RATE:                                             representation as to the accuracy or completeness of the
------------------ SECTION IV - FIRE AND EXPLOSION HAZARD DATA   information contained therein, and assume no responsibility
                                                              regarding the suitability of this information for the
DOT CATEGORY:                                                 user's intended purposes or for the consequences of its
FLASH POINT: N/A                                              use. Each individual should make a determination as to the
  LEL:                                                        suitability of the information for their particular
  UEL:                                                        purpose(s). A request has been made to the manufacturer to
EXTINGUISHING MEDIA: All                                      approve the contents of this material safety data sheet.
UNUSUAL FIRE AND EXPLOSION HAZARDS: None                      Upon receipt a new MSDS will be made available.
SPECIAL FIRE FIGHTING PROCEDURES: None                       ------------------------------------------------------------
------------------ SECTION V - HEALTH HAZARD DATA ---------   COMPAS Code: 33200050        NAC Approved Date:  / / .

THRESHOLD LIMIT VALUE:
TOXICITY: Oral LD50 4600 mg/kg Rat; 1050 mg/kg Mouse; 1000
   mg/kg Dog; 720 mg/kg Rabbit.
EFFECTS OF OVEREXPOSURE: In animals signs of acute toxicity
   include lethargy, prostration, diuresis and weight loss.
   In humans diuresis should be the first sign of exposure.
   Excessive diuresis may result in dehydration,
   hypokalemia, hypocalcemia & orthostatic hypotention.
   Other symptoms include weakness, fatigue, and malaise.
EMERGENCY AND FIRST AID PROCEDURES: Treatment is
   symptomatic and includes replacement of fluid and
   electrolytes.
------------------ SECTION VI - REACTIVITY DATA -----------

STABILITY: Stable
INCOMPATIBILITY (Materials to avoid):
CONDITIONS TO AVOID:
HAZARDOUS POLYMERIZATION: Will Not Occur
CONDITIONS TO AVOID:




4/06/98--------------------------------------------------------------------------------
MWI VETERINARY SUPPLY            3952003    JORNADA VET CL              Page 1 of 1
```

FIGURE 15-12 Sample Material Safety Data Sheet.

CAPITAL INVENTORY

Capital inventory includes any equipment purchased throughout the life of the practice. Equipment includes items used to provide veterinary services, along with office printers, credit card machines, and copy machines. A running capital inventory list should be kept in a safe place and added to each time a piece of equipment is received. A spreadsheet can be created that includes the equipment name, manufacturer, model number, serial number, purchase date, where it was purchased from, and the purchase amount. If the building is vandalized or the equipment stolen, this information will be invaluable for the police report and insurance claims. Equipment purchase information is also important for tax purposes. This list is also handy when needing to look up dates for warranty expiration. Figure 15-13 is an example of an inventory list that has equipment purchased before the inventory manager's hire date. The cost and manufacturer of several pieces of equipment are unknown, but the fact that they are listed completes the inventory sheet.

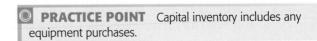

PRACTICE POINT Capital inventory includes any equipment purchases.

DECREASING LOSS

Inventory is the second largest liability to a practice, next to payroll. A large amount of money is invested in this segment, and all areas must be managed well, making changes when necessary to decrease loss. Chapter 3 discusses at length means of decreasing loss. Four ways that teams can contribute to decreasing the loss of inventoried items is to use a travel sheet, appropriately set fees, have a structured inventory system, and ensure team member accountability. Travel sheets must be used by each team member and double-checked by others that all charges have been circled. A good policy to instill into team members is that the one who performs the procedure should circle the code. For example, when the veterinarian does the exam, the veterinarian should circle the exam code. If a technician performs a heartworm test, the technician should circle the heartworm

Product	Name	Manufacturer	Purchase Date/Price	Model Number	Serial Number
Anal Gland Excision Kit		Jorgenson		J-101	
Anesthesia Machine #1	Anesthesia Machine #1	Matrix		VMS	6380
Anesthesia Vaporizer #1	Anesthesia Vaporizer #1	Cyprane LTD			300437
Anesthesia Machine #2	Anesthesia Machine #2	Matrix	12/24/2003		SN14989
Anesthesia Vaporizer #2	Anesthesia Vaporizer #2	Vet Tech 4	12/24/03, $400 for both	100F	SN BASPOX7
Aspirator	Schuco Vac	Schuco		130	49500008498
Autoclave	Tuttanauer Autoclave	Tuttanauer	04/02/02, $2600	2340M	2110582
Bird Scale		Pelouze		PE5	
Camera	Digital Camera	HP	Aug 2003, $177.52	Photosmart 320	CN318111DG
Cast Cutter		Stryker		9002-210	8H8
Cautery Unit	AA Cautery	Jorgenson		J313	
Centrifuge	MS Centrifuge MicroHCT	Damon/IEC Division		MB	2513
Centrifuge	Sta-o-Spin	Stat-o-Spin	3/14/06, $1026.83 Butler	V0901.22	607V90111962
Centrifuge (lab)	Cinaseal	Vulcon Tech		C56C	6840
Clippers	Speed Feed	DVM	12/15/04, $91		
Clippers Cordless	Oaster	Butler		78400-01A	
Clippers Cordless	Oaster	Butler		78400-01A	
Clippers Cordless	Oaster	Butler		78400-01A	
Credit Card Terminal					
Credit Card Terminal	Care Credit				SN 207-397-407
Copier	Cannon			PC 940	NVX37080
Dental Machine	Ultrasonic Scaler/Motor Pack	Delmarva			C028-647
Doppler, BP	Mini Dop ES 100VX	Hadeco	11/2000, $800		SN-00090054
Doppler Probe		Jorgenson			
Doppler Ultrasound	Grafco Mini Doppler			4070	
Dremel Unit		Craftsman		5 Speed	
ECG PAM	VM8000PAM Cardiac Monitor	Technology Transfer	12/10/00, $2775	VM8000	SN V04408
ECG Printer PAM		Technology Transfer	12/10/2000	930	1029
ECG Biolog		QRS Diagnostic	9/2006 DVM Solutions $2735		2004-054237
ECG Printer Biolog			Came with Biolog	Brother HL-207	U61230M5J5
Glucometer	One Touch Ultra	Walgreens			RHW4E23Ft
Home Again Scanner		Schering Plough			SN 070535
Hair Dryer					
ECG Surgery	KENZ ECG 103	KENZ	GW Gift		9509-2815
IDEXX Electrolytes	VET LYTE	IDEXX	Aug. 2000		U15.9976
IDEXX Lasercyte	Lasercyte	IDEXX	Jun. 2006	93-30002-01	DXBP005586
IDEXX Vet Test	Vet Test 8000	IDEXX	08/01/00, $2700		OA26949
IDEXX Server				PCNE	H1BFQ91
IDEXX Printer				HP Deskjet 565(	MY45F4NOHI

FIGURE 15-13 Sample capital inventory spreadsheet.

test code. If an assistant gets medication ready, the assistant should circle the medication on the travel sheet. Once the receptionist team receives the record and travel sheet, they compare the travel sheet to the record, looking for any missed charges.

Team members should also be held accountable for their actions. If a silly mistake occurs while running a test and a second test must be run, then the team member should be held accountable for the wasted test.

As previously mentioned, fees for both products and services must be appropriately set to cover all of the overhead costs associated with a veterinary practice. This can have a severe effect on the bottom line of a veterinary practice. Last, but not least, effective inventory systems have the greatest impact on decreasing loss of products. Several methods have been discussed in this chapter, which must be used to create and maintain a profitable practice (Box 15-6).

Box 15-6   What NOT to Do With Inventory
• Order large quantities of products that will expire before they are sold.
• Order multiple brands of the same product.
• Order multiple products that provide the same service.
• Order more than twice weekly.
• Order on an as-needed basis.
• Run out of inventory.
• Store large amounts of products in full view of customers and staff.

VETERINARY PRACTICE and the LAW

Many people do not think about medications having an expiration date, but the fact is that medications expire much in the same way that food expires. There are people who would not consider drinking milk 1 day after the expiration date, but the same people are often unaware that their medicine cabinets contain expired products. All medications, both prescription and over-the-counter, have expiration dates and should be discarded when expired.

Expired medications are not always dangerous, but they can become weak and possibly ineffective after the "use by" date. Expired medicine in pill and liquid form often changes in color and consistency. Liquids can separate and pills deteriorate over time. These changes are sometimes obvious, but in other cases medication appears to be fresh when in fact it has been compromised by time and improper storage.

Self-Evaluation Questions

1. Why should distributor and manufacturer representatives be seen by the inventory manager?
2. What is the goal of an inventory system?
3. Why should a "want list" be developed?
4. What is an order book?
5. What is an MSDS?
6. What is capital inventory?
7. What does an inventory manager do with expired medications?
8. What minimum percentage should products be marked up to break even?
9. What are some losses associated with poor inventory control?
10. How many times should inventory be turned over per year?

Recommended Reading

Ackerman LJ: *Business basics for the veterinarian*, New York, 2002, ASJA.

Heinke MM: *Practice made perfect: a guide to veterinary practice management*, Lakewood, CO, 2001, AAHA Press.

Lukens RL, Landon P: *Guide to inventory management for veterinary practice*, West Chester, PA, 1993, SmithKline Beecham.

McCurnin D, Bassert JA: *Clinical textbook for veterinary technicians*, ed 7, St Louis, 2010, Saunders Elsevier.

Opperman M: *The art of veterinary practice management*, Lenexa, KS, 1999, Veterinary Publishing Group.

Sheridan JP, McCafferty O: *The business of veterinary practice*, Tarrytown, NY, 1993, Pergamon Press.

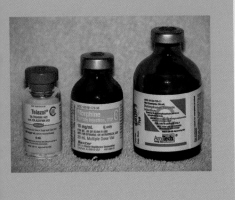

Controlled Substances

Chapter Outline

Schedule of Drugs
Management of Controlled Substances

Learning Objectives

Mastery of the content in this chapter will enable the reader to:
- Define controlled substances.
- Identify drugs available for use in the veterinary practice.
- Explain the importance of logging all drugs used.
- Discuss the importance of managing controlled substances.
- Discuss methods used to inventory controlled substances.

- Describe methods used to order controlled substances for a veterinary practice.
- Identify appropriate documents to order Schedule II drugs.
- List the process used to report the loss of controlled substances.

Key Terms

Controlled Substance
Controlled Substance Act of 1970
Drug Enforcement Agency (DEA)

Controlled substances are drugs that have a high abuse potential and that must be regulated to help prevent those abuses (Figure 16-1). The Controlled Substance Act of 1970 was passed to reduce drug abuse by restricting certain substances with a high abuse potential. The act was established, and is controlled by, the Drug Enforcement Agency (DEA) and provides approved means for proper manufacturing, distribution, dispensing, and use through licensed handlers.

> **◉ PRACTICE POINT** Drugs with abuse potential are labeled as controlled substances.

All veterinarians are required to have a DEA license to purchase or dispense controlled substances. DEA licenses must be posted within the facility and available for inspection at any time. All controlled substances that are kept on the facility property must be kept in a securely locked, substantially constructed cabinet or safe. The cabinet or safe must be irremovable from the wall or floor (therefore bolted to the wall or floor). Drugs must be placed in a secure lock box

within this cabinet or safe. Therefore controlled substances must be kept behind two locks, and access to them should be limited—granted to only one or two individuals.

SCHEDULE OF DRUGS

A controlled substance will have a "C" written in red on the bottle, with a notation next to it indicating what schedule that particular drug is. Drugs are classified into five schedules according to their abuse potential. Controlled substances include opiates (narcotics), barbiturates, hallucinogens (e.g., ketamine), amphetamines, and other addictive and habituating drugs. Class I drugs have the highest abuse potential; therefore medical use of these substances is not allowed in the United States. Drugs such as LSD and heroin are examples of controlled substances in Class I and are illegal. Class II drugs

> **◉ PRACTICE POINT** All records, logs, and invoices must be kept on premises for 2 years and must be available at any time for inspection.

produce severe psychic and physical dependencies and include drugs such as morphine, oxymorphone, and pentobarbital. Table 16-1 lists drugs and their schedules.

The DEA can inspect records, invoices, inventory, and facilities that house controlled substances at any time. State agencies, such as the board of veterinary medicine or the board of pharmacy, may also inspect at any time and may have stricter rules and regulations than the DEA. The agency that has more stringent regulations takes precedence. Records and invoices must be kept for a minimum of 2 years for any agency to inspect.

MANAGEMENT OF CONTROLLED SUBSTANCES

An initial inventory must be taken, then taken again biennially thereafter (be sure to verify state requirements, which may supersede biennial inventory). Drugs must

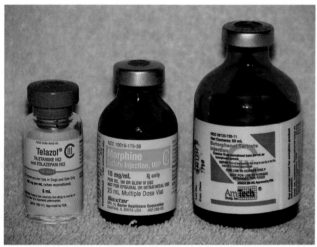

FIGURE 16-1 Controlled substances are labeled with a "C" and a roman numeral.

be balanced on a perpetual inventory balance system; this provides a running balance that can be compared with the physical inventory at any time. The American Animal Hospital Association produces an excellent bound controlled substance log book that can be used in any veterinary practice.

A folder should be kept separate from the controlled substance log book to house all invoices that list controlled drugs that have been received by the clinic. Drug listings should be highlighted on the invoice, along with the assigned bottle numbers. A stock supply sheet, or closed bottle sheet, can help keep track of bottle numbers.

Figure 16-2 shows that 12 bottles of Telazol were received on August 4, 2000. Initially, there were no bottles available for use. Once the 12 bottles were added, the initial amount became 12 bottles. The bottles were assigned the numbers 100 through 112; these were the next numbers in sequence (99 bottles had been previously used). The stock supply list states that bottles were checked out to the surgical plain on August 5, 8, and 10 by two team members. Each time bottles are checked out, they must be recorded on this list and initialed by the team member removing the bottle.

Figure 16-3 is an example of a running drug log. Notice the bottle number, date, time, client name, patient name, initial amount, amount used, and balance are all required entries. Each bottle should be fully accounted for before opening another bottle.

Ketamine is the drug being logged in Figure 16-3. The initial amount and bottle number are on line 1, along with the owner's information and the amount of drug used. Each milliliter is accounted for before opening the next bottle. Bottles 1 and 3 balance well. Obviously, bottle 2 is missing 0.7 mL, which is almost 10% of a bottle. This amount of drug must be searched for; surgical records should be examined and team

Table 16-1	Controlled Substance Schedule			
Schedule	Abuse Potential	Dispensing Limits	Restrictions	Examples
I	Highest	Research only	DEA 222 required	LSD, heroin
II	High	Written prescription, no refills	DEA 222 required	Oxymorphone, morphine, pentobarbital, fentanyl
III	Less than II	Written prescription; can refill five times	DEA number	Hycodan, codeine, buprenorphine, hydrocodone, ketamine, Telazol, anabolic steroids
IV	Low	Written prescription; can refill five times	DEA number	Diazepam, phenobarbital, alprazolam, butorphanol, midazolam
V	Low	No DEA limits	DEA number	Lomotil, Robitussin AC

Date	Time	To/From	Bottle #	Initial Amount	Amount Change	Balance	Initials
4-Aug	2:00 pm	DVM Res	100-112	0 Bottles	12 Bottles	12 Bottles	CS
5-Aug	8:00 am	SX Plain	100	12	1	11	NS
8-Aug	10:40 am	SX Plain	101	11	1	10	CS
10-Aug	2:00 pm	SX Plain	102	10	1	9	CS
					9		

Year 2007

Name of Drug: Telazol 100 mg/mL, 5 mL

FIGURE 16-2 Sample stock supply sheet.

Bottle #	Date	Time	Owner's Name	Animal's Name	Initial Amount	Amount Used	Balance	Initials
1	4-Aug	8:00 am	Slatery	Waldo	10 mL	3	7	CS
	4-Aug	8:00 am	Garcia	Baby	7	0.5	6.5	NS
	4-Aug	8:15 am	Jones	Prancer	6.5	1	5.5	CS
	4-Aug	8:15 am	Loving	Tootsie	5.5	0.8	4.7	CS
	5-Aug	8:15 am	Pinto	Wonder	4.7	0.4	4.3	NS
	5-Aug	9:15 am	Adams	Wendy	4.3	2	2.3	NS
	5-Aug	9:30 am	Howard	Bobo	2.3	0.3	2	NS
	6-Aug	8:15 am	Bush	Tristen	2	2	0	CS
2	7-Aug	8:00 am	Evans	Ashley	10	0.6	9.4	NS
	7-Aug	8:00 am	Langford	Bobby	9.4	0.7	8.7	CS
	7-Aug	8:15 am	Smith	Casper	8.7	6	2.7	CS
	8-Aug	8:15 am	Howard	Wimpy	2.7	2	0.7	NS
			MIA	MIA		0.7	0	CS
3	8-Aug	9:30 am	Brown	Blackie	10	1	9	NS
	9-Aug	8:15 am	Hyatt	Lawrence	9	2	7	CS
	9-Aug	8:30 am	Ralph	Ariel	7	2.5	4.5	CS
	9-Aug	9:00 am	Jameson	Taylor	4.5	0.5	4	HP
	9-Aug	10:15 am	Lee	Wheeler	4	1	3	HP
	9-Aug	10:30 am	West	Katie	3	3	0	SM

Year 2007

Ketamine 100 mg/mL, 10 mL

FIGURE 16-3 Sample running drug log.

members questioned regarding who may have pulled the drug without writing the information down. If the missing drug cannot be found, management must consider inside theft. This information must be logged and highlighted so that it may be reported as a discrepancy on the annual controlled substance physical inventory list.

Each drug must have an individual log for the year. Each log must be balanced to ensure all drugs that were purchased are accounted for. An annual controlled substance physical inventory should be performed, allowing inspectors to quickly review use within the practice. Ideally, practices should inventory controlled substances on a monthly basis. Human error occurs, and team members will forget to write down substances used to treat patients in emergency situations or drugs dispensed to clients for their pets. If practices perform monthly inventories and balances of their drugs, discrepancies can be located more easily in a month as opposed to a year.

> **PRACTICE POINT**   Controlled substance invoices and stock supply sheets should be kept in a separate file from log sheets.

To complete an annual controlled substance physical inventory, each drug log must be finished, and a physical count of the drug must be completed. The discrepancy is the physical count minus the running balance. The percentage of annual use should be calculated by dividing the discrepancy by the total number of milliliters or tablets (whichever form the drug comes in) and multiplied by 100 to obtain a percentage. If the discrepancy is greater than 3% for the year, the loss must be reported. Figure 16-4 uses Figure 16-3 to calculate the annual use of ketamine. The running balance (the total

in milliliters that the practice has received for the year) minus the physical count (inventory performed) gives a discrepancy of −0.7 mL. Therefore 0.7 mL divided by 30 mL (the total use for the year) equals 0.02. To obtain the percentage, 0.02 is multiplied by 100. This gives an annual percentage use of 2.3%. If this number equaled 3% or higher, it would have to be reported to the DEA, the police department, and the state board of pharmacy.

> **PRACTICE POINT**   If more than 3% of a drug is missing, the loss must be reported to the local police department, the DEA, and the state board of pharmacy. Some states may also require a report to the state board of veterinary medicine.

It is expected that there will be a small amount of hub loss associated with each draw. It is advisable to ask the state veterinary inspector or the local DEA office for the best way to account for hub loss. Some departments may allow a small percentage of the total use to be written off as hub loss. If a bottle is broken, two people must initial the log indicating the broken bottle.

Theft or drug loss must be reported to the police and DEA immediately. Ongoing losses can result in loss of license and strict fines. DEA Form 106 should be filled out and forwarded to the local DEA office; another copy may have to be forwarded to the state board of pharmacy. One copy should be maintained for the controlled substance file (Figure 16-5).

If veterinarians write controlled substance prescriptions for clients, a pharmacy can only fill a 30-day supply for classes III, IV, or V. Those prescriptions can have five refills available for 6 months, at which time a new prescription must be submitted to the pharmacy. Class

What Would You Do/Not Do?

Amber is in charge of controlled substances at a veterinary practice but does not have time to balance controlled drugs on a monthly basis. Therefore once a year she sits down and tries to balance the drugs. However, large discrepancies usually exist. Instead of researching records and looking for lost drugs, she creates pets in employee files and falsifies medical records. She creates procedures that were never completed and logs controlled substances that were never given. She completes enough records to meet the maximum 3% loss for the year.

The new practice manager reviews employee medical records and notes that medical records are not complete in several cases and reviews the procedures with the veterinarians who oversaw the cases. Several veterinarians did not recall completing procedures on those pets, and

therefore question the employees. They inform the new practice manager that this is how Amber often balances lost drugs and compensates for those that were not recorded.

What Should the New Practice Manager Do?

First, Amber must be called into the practice and informed that falsifying medical records is a crime and unethical. Controlled substances are controlled for a reason and must be accounted for. The practice manager must implement new controlled substance inventory procedures, ensuring drugs are logged on a daily basis. Inventory must be performed on a monthly basis, ensuring all drugs are accounted for. Amber must find all drugs for the previous year and document them correctly. If she does not, she should be terminated immediately for lying and jeopardizing the loss of the veterinarians' controlled substance licenses.

Year 2007

Drug and Strength	Physical Count	Running Balance	Discrepancy ±	Percentage of Annual Use
Diazepam 5 mg Tabs	152 Tabs	155 Tabs	−3	3/225 = 0.013 × 100 = 1%
Torbutrol 1 mg Tabs	112 Tabs	112 Tabs	0	0
Ketamine Inj 100 mg/mL	29.3 mL	30 mL	−0.7 mL	0.7/30 = 0.02 × 100 =2.3%
Sleepaway 100 mg/mL	157 mL	150 mL	+7 mL	N/A

FIGURE 16-4 Annual controlled substance physical inventory.

II drugs can only be filled for 30 days and must have a new prescription submitted every 30 days; no refills are allowed on the original script.

DEA Form 222 must be filled out and sent to distributors or manufacturers that wish to purchase Schedule II drugs. Morphine, oxymorphone, and Sleepaway are examples of drugs that require DEA Form 222 (Figure 16-6 and Box 16-1).

These forms must be filled out without error. Any errors will void the form and the distributor or manufacturer will be unable to fulfill the order. The name of the company, address, drug name, strength, and quantity must all be correct. The signature and license must match those on file or the order will be denied. Just as the DEA and state board of pharmacy are strict with veterinarians, they are just as strict (if not more) with distributors and manufacturers. The DEA supplies veterinarians with forms to order Class II drugs.

VETERINARY PRACTICE and the LAW

Controlled drugs have specific laws that regulate their ordering, storage, and dispensing. Failure to adhere to these regulations may cause a veterinarian to lose his or her license. Veterinary team members must be aware of any drug-seeking behavior from clients and the physical symptoms of addiction. Many clients will create a story to get a prescription for their pet, and then take the medication themselves. They will frequently call for refills, often with excuses of spilling the medication, losing the pill vial, or leaving it out of town at a relative's home.

Team members should also be aware of co-workers' behavior and report any abnormal behavior to the owner or practice manager. Many co-workers will divert medication for their own use; a tablet here and a tablet there add up, and substance abusers consistently need more chemical to achieve the high they desire.

U.S. Department of Justice
Drug Enforcement Administration

REPORT OF THEFT OR LOSS OF CONTROLLED SUBSTANCES

Federal Regulations require registrants to submit a detailed report of any theft or loss of Controlled Substances to the Drug Enforcement Administration. Complete the front and back of this form in triplicate. Forward the original and duplicate copies to the nearest DEA Office. Retain the triplicate copy for your records. Some states may also require a copy of this report.	OMB APPROVAL No. 1117-0001

1. Name and Address of Registrant (Include ZIP Code)   ZIP CODE

2. Phone No. (Include Area Code)

3. DEA Registration Number 2 ltr. prefix 7 digit suffix	4. Date of Theft or Loss	5. Principal Business of Registrant (Check one) 1 ☐ Pharmacy 5 ☐ Distributor 2 ☐ Practitioner 6 ☐ Methadone Program 3 ☐ Manufacturer 7 ☐ Other (Specify) 4 ☐ Hospital/Clinic

6. County in which Registrant is located	7. Was Theft reported to Police? ☐ Yes ☐ No	8. Name and Telephone Number of Police Department (Include Area Code)

9. Number of Thefts or Losses Registrant has experienced in the past 24 months	10. Type of Theft or Loss (Check one and complete items below as appropriate) 1 ☐ Night break-in 3 ☐ Employee pilferage 5 ☐ Other (Explain) 2 ☐ Armed robbery 4 ☐ Customer theft 6 ☐ Lost in transit (Complete Item 14)

11. If Armed Robbery, was anyone: Killed? ☐ No ☐ Yes (How many) _____ Injured? ☐ No ☐ Yes (How many)_____	12. Purchase value to registrant of Controlled Substances taken? $	13. Were any pharmaceuticals or merchandise taken? ☐ No ☐ Yes (Est. Value) $

14. IF LOST IN TRANSIT, COMPLETE THE FOLLOWING:

A. Name of Common Carrier	B. Name of Consignee	C. Consignee's DEA Registration Number
D. Was the carton received by the customer? ☐ Yes ☐ No	E. If received, did it appear to be tampered with? ☐ Yes ☐ No	F. Have you experienced losses in transit from this same carrier in the past? ☐ No ☐ Yes (How many) _____

15. What identifying marks, symbols, or price codes were on the labels of these containers that would assist in identifying the products?

16. If Official Controlled Substance Order Forms (DEA-222) were stolen, give numbers.

17. What security measures have been taken to prevent future thefts or losses?

PRIVACY ACT INFORMATION

AUTHORITY: Section 301 of the Controlled Substances Act of 1970 (PL 91-513).
PURPOSE: Report theft or loss of Controlled Substances.
ROUTINE USES: The Controlled Substances Act authorizes the production of special reports required for statistical and analytical purposes. Disclosures of information from this system are made to the following categories of users for the purposes stated:
  A. Other Federal law enforcement and regulatory agencies for law enforcement and regulatory purposes.
  B. State and local law enforcement and regulatory agencies for law enforcement and regulatory purposes.
EFFECT: Failure to report theft or loss of controlled substances may result in penalties under Section 402 and 403 of the Controlled Substances Act.

In accordance with the Paperwork Reduction Act of 1995, no person is required to respond to a collection of information unless it displays a ly valid OMB control number. The valid OMB control number for this collection of information is 1117-0001. Public reporting burden for this collection of information is estimated to average 30 minutes per response, including the time for reviewing instructions, searching existing data sources, gathering and maintaining the data needed, and completing and reviewing the collection of information.

FORM DEA-106 (11-00) *Previous editions obsolete*   **CONTINUE ON REVERSE**
Electronic Form Version Designed in JetForm 5.2 Version

FIGURE 16-5 DEA Form 106. (Courtesy U.S. Department of Justice, Drug Enforcement Administration, Washington, DC.)

FORM DEA-106 (Nov. 2000) Pg. 2

LIST OF CONTROLLED SUBSTANCES LOST

Trade Name of Substance or Preparation	Name of Controlled Substance in Preparation	Dosage Strength and Form	Quantity
Examples: Desoxyn	Methamphetamine Hydrochloride	5 mg Tablets	3 x 100
Demerol	Meperidine Hydrochloride	50 mg/ml Vial	5 x 30 ml
Robitussin A-C	Codeine Phosphate	2 mg/cc Liquid	12 Pints
1.			
2.			
3.			
4.			
5.			
6.			
7.			
8.			
9.			
10.			
11.			
12.			
13.			
14.			
15.			
16.			
17.			
18.			
19.			
20.			
21.			
22.			
23.			
24.			
25.			
26.			
27.			
28.			
29.			
30.			
31.			
32.			
33.			
34.			
35.			
36.			
37.			
38.			
39.			
40.			
41.			
42.			
43.			
44.			
45.			
46.			
47.			
48.			
49.			
50.			

I certify that the foregoing information is correct to the best of my knowledge and belief.

Signature   Title   Date

FIGURE 16-5, cont'd DEA Form 106. (Courtesy U.S. Department of Justice, Drug Enforcement Administration, Washington, DC.)

See Reverse of PURCHASER'S Copy for Instructions | No order form may be issued for Schedule I and II substances unless a completed application form has been received, (21 CFR 1305.04). | **OMB APPROVAL No. 1117-0010**

TO: *(Name of Supplier)* | STREET ADDRESS

CITY and STATE | DATE | **TO BE FILLED IN BY SUPPLIER** — SUPPLIERS DEA REGISTRATION No.

LINE No.	TO BE FILLED IN BY PURCHASER					
	No. of Packages	Size of Package	Name of Item	National Drug Code	Packages Shipped	Date Shipped
1						
2						
3						
4						
5						
6						
7						
8						
9						
10						

◀ LAST LINE COMPLETED *(MUST BE 10 OR LESS)* | SIGNATURE OF PURCHASER OR ATTORNEY OR AGENT

Date Issued | DEA Registration No. | Name and Address of Registrant

Schedules

Registered as a PRACTITIONER | No. of this Order Form

DEA Form -222 (Oct. 1992)

U.S. OFFICIAL ORDER FORMS - SCHEDULES I & II
DRUG ENFORCEMENT ADMINISTRATION
SUPPLIER'S Copy 1

104586067

FIGURE 16-6 DEA Form 222. (Courtesy U.S. Department of Justice, Drug Enforcement Administration, Washington, DC.)

Box 16-1 Common Questions and Answers Regarding DEA Form 222

Question: How do I obtain additional official copies of DEA Form 222?

Answer: Official order forms may be ordered by calling the DEA Headquarters Registration Unit toll free at 800-882-9539 or the nearest DEA Registration Field Office. The forms will be mailed within 10 working days. Official order forms may also be obtained by submitting a completed requisition form, DEA Form 222a, to DEA, Registration Unit, PO Box 28083, Washington, DC 20038-8083. There is no charge for official order forms.

Question: Can a distributor accept a DEA Form 222 that contains minor misspellings in the registrant's name, address, or drug name?

Answer: Yes, the DEA Form 222 is acceptable if the registrant's name or address contains minor misspellings. The registrant should request corrected official order forms and, if necessary, a corrected registration certificate from DEA. If the drug name has been misspelled and there is no question as to what product has been ordered then the DEA Form 222 is acceptable.

Question: Can a distributor fill in sections omitted by a registrant on a DEA Form 222?

Answer: *Date of the form:* The distributor may place the date on the form. When possible, the date ascertained from the delivery document should be used as the issue date. The form is acceptable unless the ascertained date of issue is greater than 60 days from the date of receipt.

Size of the package: The size of the package must be completed by the purchaser unless the product is only manufactured in one size. If more than one package size is manufactured and no package size is indicated, then the package size may **not** be added by the supplier. The line item with the missing package size must be voided by the supplier and the purchaser notified.

Strength of the drug: If the product is only manufactured in one strength, then it is not necessary to indicate the strength in the section "Name of Drug." If the product is available in more than one strength, then the strength may **not** be added by the distributor. The line should be voided on the DEA Form 222 by the supplier and the purchaser notified.

Last line completed: A distributor may **not** fill in the "Last Line Completed" area of the DEA Form 222. This section must be completed by the purchaser. If the purchaser enters an incorrect number, such as the total number of packages ordered instead of the last line completed, then the DEA Form 222 is **not** valid.

Question: Can a distributor accept a DEA Form 222 if the size and strength of a product have been placed incorrectly on the form?

Answer: Yes, the DEA Form 222 is acceptable as long as there is no question as to what product has been ordered.

Self-Evaluation Questions

1. What are controlled substances?
2. What is the abuse potential of ketamine?
3. Why are controlled substance log sheets required?
4. What is the purpose of a year-end physical inventory?
5. What is DEA Form 106 used for?

Recommended Reading

United States Department of Justice, Drug Enforcement Agency: *Physicians manual: an information outline of the controlled substance act of 1970*, rev ed, Washington, DC, 1990, GPO.

http://www.deadiversion.usdoj.gov/

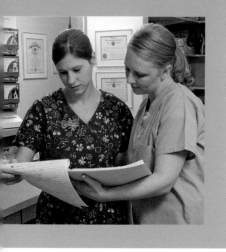

CHAPTER 17

Logs

Chapter Outline

Controlled Substances Log
Radiology Log
Surgical Log

Laboratory Log
Miscellaneous Logs

Learning Objectives

Mastery of the content in this chapter will enable the reader to:
• Define the importance of logs in the veterinary practice.
• Develop a practical log for each area of the practice.

Key Terms

Controlled Substance Log
Laboratory Log

Radiology Log
Surgical Log

Veterinary practices use many log books to help keep items organized, and to some extent these are required by law. Log books should be easy to use and maintain; the more difficult they are to use, the less likely it is that the staff will use them. Log books can be created by team members to include information the team may need as well as that information required by law. State laws should be reviewed to determine what logs are required in each state as well as the length of time logs are required to be kept on premises. Logs can be kept in binders in each area identified as having a log book.

CONTROLLED SUBSTANCES LOG

Controlled substances are reviewed in Chapter 16, with an example of a drug log in Figure 16-3. This log is required by the Drug Enforcement Agency and the state board of pharmacy. It may also be required by the state board of veterinary medicine in some states. These logs must be kept for 2 years and should be easily retrievable for inspection. Individual controlled drugs must include the date, owner's name, pet's name, the amount used, and the initials of the person responsible for the drug. All drugs must be accounted for, and a running drug log must be kept to indicate the balance of each drug at any time.

> **PRACTICE POINT** Controlled substance logs are required by federal law and must be kept current and accurate at all times. Failure to do so can result in fines.

RADIOLOGY LOG

Some states may require a radiology log; all hospitals should maintain a radiology log regardless of any requirement. Logs are excellent references when taking radiographs or looking up the history of a radiograph. Technicians taking the radiographs can record the information needed as they prepare for the x-ray (Figure 17-1). Radiology logs should include the owner's name, pet's name, the body part being radiographed, position, kilovolts, milliamperes, and the initials of the technician. If a radiograph needs to be repeated several days later, team members can review the log and use the same setting (if comparison radiographs are being taken, it is extremely important to have the same settings).

If radiographs are checked out to owners or are sent out for referral, a log needs to be in place to document the removal of the radiographs from the premises (Figure 17-2). Radiographs are the property of the practice and should remain on the premises at all times.

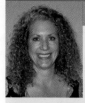

What Would You Do/Not Do?

Sarah, a practice manager, balances the controlled drugs on a monthly basis. She finds that drugs are often not recorded when they are taken from the lock box and has recently become very frustrated with the team for not being responsible enough to write down the drugs. She has talked to each team member individually but the situation has not improved. Sarah tried to implement a protocol that only she could remove drugs from the box. However, the system was ineffective when Sarah was not at the practice.

members often are so busy they forget to write down the controlled substances. Sarah could place one log sheet on the outside of the lock box; all drugs could be written on one sheet at the time of removal instead of having to locate the controlled substance binder and recording the drug on the appropriate sheet. Sarah can then record the drugs on the appropriate log sheet on a monthly basis. This keeps team members from walking away from the box before the drugs are recorded, and the log sheet serves as a simple reminder to log the substances.

What should Sarah Do?

Each team member must be responsible for writing down drugs as they are taken from the box; however, team

Date	Owner's Name	Patient's Name	Study	Position	kVp	mA	Initials
5/4/09	Patterson	Riley	Abdomen	Lat/VD	78/85	300	HP
5/4/09	Burns	Ariel	Chest	Lat x 2, VD	65/69	300	DB
5/5/09	Montoya	Blue	Right foreleg	Lat, ap	69	300	DB
5/5/09	Valdivia	Twinkle	Cat-o-gram	Lat, dv	72	300	HP

FIGURE 17-1 Sample radiology log.

Date	Owner's Name	Patient's Name	Check out by?	Going to?	Initials	Return Date	Initials
10/6/09	Pacheco	Cherry	Owner	Crossroads A.H.	LP	12/8/09	MV
10/8/09	Ziehl	Bud	UPS	SW Specialty	CS		
11/1/09	Soules	Blackie	Owner	Arroyo V.C.	SP	12/1/09	DC
12/15/09	Miale	Twinkle	Mail	Tuscon	CS		

FIGURE 17-2 Sample radiology checkout log.

It is acceptable to lend them out for referrals or second opinions, but it should be documented that the radiographs were removed. This also helps when team members are looking for radiographs and cannot find them. Instead of assuming they are misfiled, the log can be consulted to see that they were removed. Checkout logs should include the date, owner's name, pet's name, who took the radiographs (whether the owners checked out the radiographs or they were sent by mail), where they went, and the team member's initials. The last column should be left blank to indicate their date of return, with another area for team member initials indicting that they were returned to the files. Practices that are digitized do not have to use radiograph logs. Digital radiographs are automatically loaded into a patient's file with all the setting information attached to them. If radiographs need to be sent out for a second opinion, they can be copied to a CD. The film is never lost or misfiled. The log can be printed when needed if required by the state.

> **PRACTICE POINT** Radiology logs may not be required by the state but should be required by practices using nondigital systems. Logs allow repeat radiographs to be taken at the same exposure, as indicated by the log.

SURGICAL LOG

Some states may require a surgery log listing all patients that have received anesthesia within the practice. The surgery log can also be a great reference when looking for a lost controlled substance, when estimating the time an anesthetic machine has been in use, or for reviewing surgical cases (Figure 17-3). Surgical logs should contain the date, time, owner's name, patient's name, the surgical procedure, drugs used, and the initials of the team member overseeing the surgical case. Surgical logs are often referred to as *anesthesia logs* because this is where all anesthetics are recorded.

Date	Time	Owner's Name	Patient's Name	Procedure	Pre-Anesthetic	Anesthetic	Gas	Initials
12/2/09	8:15 am	Berry	Vicky	K-9 OVH	0.1 mL Morph, 0.03 mL Ace	0.03 mL Tel	Iso	CS
12/2/09	8:45 am	Congleton	Flower	K-9 Neuter	1.0 mL Morph, 0.1 mL Ace	0.2 mL Tel	Iso	CS
12/2/09	9:15 am	Larsen	Sadie	K-9 OVH	0.5 mL Ket, 0.5 mL Diaz	0	Iso	NS
12/3/09	8:20 am	Davis	Blue	Fe Neuter	0.01 mL Ace, 0.04 mL Torb	0.05 mL Tel	Iso	MB
12/3/09	2:00 pm	Lockridge	Brooke	Laceration	0.3 mL Morph, 0.1 mL Ace	0.1 mL Tel	Iso	CS
12/4/09	8:30 am	Patterson	Gia	Growth Removal	2.0 mL Morph, 0.1 mL Ace	0.2 mL Tel	Iso	MB
12/4/09	10:15 am	Verda	Kile	Dental	1.0 mL Ket, 1.0 mL Diaz	0	Iso	CS
12/4/09	10:45 am	Saete	Looney	Fe OVH	0.01 mL Ace, 0.04 mL Torb	0.05 mL Tel	Iso	NS

FIGURE 17-3 Sample surgery log.

LABORATORY LOG

Some practices may find it helpful to record laboratory tests and results on a sheet for referencing if needed. In-house testing such as fecal examinations, urinalyses, heartworm tests, parvovirus tests, and feline leukemia/AIDS tests can be recorded. Occasionally, authors of the medical record will forget to record test results in the record. A log allows the team to locate the sample result without having to run another sample (Figure 17-4). Samples sent to outside laboratories can also be recorded and easily referenced if needed. An outside laboratory log can be used to compare with monthly statements to ensure the practice was billed correctly. If any questions arise, the record can be pulled to verify the charges.

MISCELLANEOUS LOGS

Other logs that may be useful in practice but are not required by state or federal agencies include maintenance logs. Radiograph developers, anesthetic machines, and autoclaves must be cleaned on a regular basis, and a maintenance log indicates the history of each piece of equipment. If repairs are needed for the equipment, notes can be added to the maintenance log. Quality control samples should be run on in-house laboratory equipment on a regular basis as well; a log is occasionally required by the company as evidence that regular quality control and maintenance procedures have been completed on machines.

Logs may be kept for incoming telephone calls for a veterinary practice. Notes from telephone calls and conversations with current clients should be kept in those clients' files so that all team members can be familiar with the conversation that occurred. Calls from potential clients can be logged in a telephone log book; if the client arrives for an appointment, the conversation can be added to the medical record at that time.

PRACTICE POINT Miscellaneous logs can increase the efficiency of the team.

Date	Owner's Name	Patient's Name	Test	Result	Initials
5/4/09	Dasher	Rambo	HW/E/L/A	(−) (−) (−) (−)	HP
5/4/09	Biel	Whitney	Parvo	(−)	DB
5/5/09	Venzie	Kim	Felv/FIV	(+) (−)	DB
5/5/09	Bates	Sadie	HW/E/L/A	(−) (+) (−) (−)	HP

FIGURE 17-4 Sample laboratory log.

VETERINARY PRACTICE and the LAW

Although some logs are required by state veterinary boards to be kept and maintained, other logs that the practice implements may provide more of a protection for the practice. Surgery logs may be required, whereas radiology checkout logs may not be required. Often, radiographs are given to owners to take with them for a specialty consultation, or the practice may send them to a radiologist for review. Frequently, these radiographs are not returned, and the staff spends hours looking for the lost items. Not only is the practice liable because the radiographs are unaccounted for, but the owner may become frustrated.

Radiology checkout logs can prevent a lawsuit by accounting for the radiographs and showing that they were released either to the owner or another practice. Efficiency of these logs can show an investigator or judge that the practice behaves responsibly with the radiographs that are taken in the practice and can prove their checkout status.

Self-Evaluation Questions

1. What log is required by the Drug Enforcement Agency?
2. Why would a radiograph log benefit the team?

Recommended Reading

Heinke MM: *Practice made perfect: a guide to veterinary practice management*, Lakewood, CO, 2001, AAHA Press.

McCurnin D, Bassert JA: *Clinical textbook for veterinary technicians*, ed 7, St Louis, 2010, Saunders Elsevier.

U.S. Department of Justice, Drug Enforcement Agency: *Physicians manual: an information outline of the controlled substance act of 1970*, rev ed, Washington, DC, 1990, GPO.

http://www.deadiversion.usdoj.gov/

CHAPTER 18

Accounts Receivable

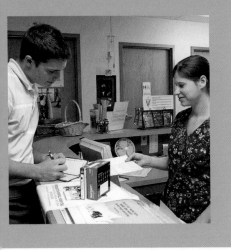

Chapter Outline

Accepting Payment on Accounts Receivable
Instituting a No-Charge Policy
Monthly Statements
   Calculating Finance Charges
Collection Procedures for Outstanding Accounts

Fair Debt Collection Practices Act
Telephone Calls to Collect Outstanding Accounts
Collection Letters
Collections Agency
Employee Accounts Receivable

Learning Objectives

Mastery of the content in this chapter will enable the reader to:
- Explain insufficient funds charges.
- Describe the process used to accept payments on client accounts.
- Define and enforce a no-charge policy.
- Calculate finance charges.

- Describe the process used to collect outstanding accounts receivable effectively.
- Define the Fair Debt Collection Practices Act.
- Develop effective collections letters.

Key Terms

Accounts Receivable
Better Business Bureau
Billing Cycle
Collections Agency
Embezzlement

Fair Debt Collection Practices Act
Finance Charge
Interest
Ledger Cards
Monthly Statement

Postdated Checks
Returned Checks
Statement

Accounts receivable is defined as the money owed to a business for services rendered or products that are sold and not paid for at the time of service. Each time clients are allowed to charge a service, profit for the veterinary practice decreases; essentially the practice has paid for the entire visit, receiving nothing in return. Every practice should institute a goal of not allowing accounts receivable to exceed 1% of the yearly gross revenue. Amounts over 3% deserve the full attention of the entire team. A practice policy can be instituted, and all members of the team must follow the policy to *begin* to control the accounts receivable. If a client becomes upset that he or she cannot charge the services rendered, the team should discuss how valuable that client is. A bigger loss occurs to the practice from the collection process. Valuable time should be spent on clients who will pay for, and who value, the service they receive.

Discussing finances with a client can be emotional. It is important to discuss this sensitive issue in an exam room, away from other clients and staff members. Clients may be embarrassed that they cannot afford the best care or are in a financial bind that is beyond their control. They can express anger, sadness, or fear toward the staff; team members should know not to take the expression personally. It is simply the responsibility of the team to offer the best medicine to every client regardless of finances. Conservative options can be presented as alternatives and should be documented in the record. This may alleviate some of the emotions of the client.

Compassion is an important aspect of the veterinary profession. The veterinary health care team loves animals, which is what makes team members enjoy their jobs. There will always be a charity case that a team member wants to help. Many veterinary practices have instituted a flex or indigent account. Some practices have given this account a special name and determine as a team which clients can use funds in this account. At times, wealthy clients want to donate money to help clients that cannot help their pets, and this is the perfect account to receive such donations. It allows the books to balance at the end of the day and generates a receipt for those who have donated. Clients must meet requirements for team members to consider the use of this account. Team members can develop guidelines, which may include such items as owner compassion, decreased finances, exceptional pet(s), and an intense owner-patient bond. These clients will truly appreciate the services and may eventually donate back to the fund once they are economically stable.

> **PRACTICE POINT**   Create a flex, indigent, or charity account to help special clients in need of financial assistance.

Checks returned for insufficient funds are a common problem for practices that do not use a check machine. Practices may try to collect these balances themselves or hire an outside collection agency to collect the funds. Returned check fees must be applied to the client account to recoup bank charges, lost time, and money (Figure 18-1). If a collection agency collects the delinquent amount, service fees will be deducted from the check total once it has been collected. Most companies add a $30 service fee for returned checks. A notice that is clearly visible to clients must be posted indicating all fees that will be added to a client's account if a check is returned.

> **PRACTICE POINT**   Automatic check machines prevent returned checks.

ACCEPTING PAYMENT ON ACCOUNTS RECEIVABLE

Two methods are available to record transactions when clients have paid on their account. Some clinics use a manual method of recording and tracking transactions, and others may use veterinary practice software.

Manual accounts receivable must be managed well to prevent internal embezzlement. All charges, statements, billing cycles, interest, account aging, and payments are calculated and recorded separately, generally on individual ledger cards. Aged accounts can be flagged with different colored flags, and appropriate notices can be sent to clients. When a payment is received, a receipt should be given to the client, and a copy should be given to the accounts receivable manager, who will then update the ledger manually. This allows record keeping and payment handling to be separated.

A computerized accounts receivable management program has a large advantage over manual management. All calculations, interest, and statement fees are automatically calculated and added to the client's account. This eliminates errors associated with calculations and can decrease employee embezzlement. Clients simply pay on their accounts, a receipt is produced, and a new balance is listed.

INSTITUTING A NO-CHARGE POLICY

Signs should be clearly posted for clients to see throughout the clinic regarding a no-charge policy. Signs should say, "Full payment is required at time of service" (Figure 18-2). Although some practice owners believe this message is simple and to the point, it is unfortunately not adequate. Estimates must be given to all clients, regardless of client "status," for all services that are expected to be rendered for that patient. Team members can print out an estimate, verbally review it with owners, and explain all procedures and medications the pet will be receiving. The client should sign the estimate; this gives

---

Notice: By providing your check
   as payment, you authorize us to
use information from your check
to make a one-time electronic
fund transfer from your account.

Funds may be drawn from your
account the same day, and you
will not receive your check back
from your bank.

If payment is returned unpaid, you
authorize ABC Veterinary Clinic to
debit from your account a one-time
electronic transfer fee of $30.00.

FIGURE 18-1 Sample insufficient funds notice.

NOTICE!

Due to the high number of
outstanding accounts, credit
will no longer be available.
All accounts must be paid
in full at the time of service.

FIGURE 18-2 Sample "no charge" sign.

the practice legal documentation that the client accepted the services that the veterinarian has recommended. Clients need to clearly understand that a deposit of at least half of the estimate is required before procedures are performed, and the remainder is due when the animal is released from the hospital.

> **PRACTICE POINT** Providing estimates for clients helps decrease the amount of outstanding accounts.

Every team member must understand and accept this policy, and it must be enforced consistently to be effective. A good policy can be both fair and compassionate. Remember, a goal of less than 3% must be set. A practice that produces $100,000.00 a month should have a total of only $3000.00 in accounts receivable each month. It should be the goal of every clinic to have the lowest accounts receivable possible.

> **PRACTICE POINT** A goal should be set that the total of the accounts receivable will not exceed 3% of the monthly gross revenue.

Holding checks for clients is not recommended. A held check is defined as accepting a check with the current date that the check is written, but holding it for deposit until the client agrees on a date for it to be deposited. This adds another level of difficulty for the receptionist because held checks must be kept in a safe and secure place and deposited on the correct date. There is no guarantee that the funds will be available the day of deposit or that the client will not close the checking account. If a team member accidentally deposits the check early, the client will be unhappy with the practice and may try to collect returned check fees from the practice negligence. This creates a no-win situation, although the practice was trying to help the client.

Accepting postdated checks is against the law in some states. A postdated check can be defined as a check that is written but dated at some point in the future. Some prosecutors will not prosecute cases when a postdated check has been accepted. Check authorizing companies will not authorize or accept postdated checks.

Driver's license numbers should be documented for every client in case of nonpayment or a returned check. This allows practices to refer nonpaying clients to collections agencies to continue trying to collect the balance. The driver's license numbers can be collected from clients when they fill out the client/patient form. If a check machine is used, a driver's license number will be required to accept the check. If local district attorney's offices prosecute stolen check writers, a driver's license may be required for prosecution.

MONTHLY STATEMENTS

If clients are allowed to charge, there will be an accounts receivable collection. These clients have an outstanding balance and will have a statement generated monthly. A statement advises clients of their balance and indicates charges, payments, and the balance of their account for the month that has just concluded (Figure 18-3). Statements are also a request for money. Outstanding accounts can be difficult and time consuming. Practice managers must remember to institute monthly statement fees. State laws vary regarding the amount of interest (if any) that can be added to an account. Laws should be verified before determining an interest rate. Adding interest fees to client accounts encourages quicker payoff because clients do not wish to pay additional fees.

Statement fees include time, paper, and postage along with any finance charges or interest rates the clinic feels are appropriate. Veterinary software systems allow a standard percentage to be added to each invoice, or a set dollar amount can be selected (Figure 18-4). One or two dollars is no longer an acceptable fee. Postage, paper, and the time it takes an employee to run statements far exceeds two dollars!

Calculating Finance Charges

If a practice continues to use a manual accounts receivable system, staff must learn how to calculate finance charges. The cost of the stamp, paper, and envelope is a set cost. For example, consider $0.42 for the cost of postage; envelopes are approximately $0.02 each, and paper and ink are about $0.05 per invoice. Labor includes the time it takes to produce the monthly statements (from the initial calculations until the final stamp is applied). Six hours may be standard for some practices, when statements are completed without interruption. An office manager may be paid $12 per hour, and it must be remembered to add 20% to account for payroll taxes. The interest rate determined by the practice is 6.25%. Therefore, according to this example, the monthly fee must be at least $1.35 to break even. To encourage the clients to pay off their balances quicker, the interest rate can be 6.25% on a monthly basis. The client's balance in this example is $98.45. Once this balance has been multiplied by 6.25%, the new balance is $104.60 (Box 18-1).

Statements should be printed on approximately the same day each month. Having one person in charge of accounts receivable will decrease mistakes and increase the efficiency of printing statements. This team member should indicate in the client's medical record the date, statement fee, new balance, and the team member's initials. This allows other team members to easily follow the billing fees if the client has any questions regarding the account (Figure 18-5).

ABC Animal Clinic
555 Uptown Circle
Anytown, MN 89000
555-555-5555

STATEMENT

Date 05/28/09

Page 1

Maria Rogers
6454 Downtown Circle
Anytown, MN 89001

Account # 21312

Date	Description/Patient	Invoice No.	Charges	Payments
04/28/09	Scruffy	1090	$398.34	$0.00

Current	30 Days	60 Days	90 Days	**Amount Due**
$398.34	0.00	0.00	0.00	**$398.34**

Payment is due upon receipt. For your convenience, we accept Visa, MasterCard, and Discover. PLEASE NOTE THAT A $5.00 MONTHLY STATEMENT FEE WILL BE ASSESSED TO ALL BALANCES OVER 30 DAYS PAST DUE.

FIGURE 18-3 Sample statement.

COLLECTION PROCEDURES FOR OUTSTANDING ACCOUNTS

Although collection procedures can seem fairly simple, there are laws that protect the client. Accounts should be paid by clients within 30 days of charging. However, particular clients may have higher bills that will require longer collection times. Some veterinary software systems allow the practice to choose whether a statement fee and/or percentage of the balance should be added to those accounts less than 30 days old. The software will age accounts, generally 0 to 30 days, 31 to 60 days, 61 to 90 days, and over 90 days (Figure 18-6). This allows a practice manager to look at the status of

accounts receivable with a more accurate prediction of payment. Accounts that are greater than 90 days are very difficult to collect (Figure 18-7).

Clients should be sent a statement immediately after the service has been performed and medications have been dispensed. Clients are more willing to pay a balance while the treatment and procedures are still fresh in their minds.

If a client is making monthly payments, it is advisable to continue working with the client before turning accounts to a credit agency. Clients not making payments by 60 days should be notified of the overdue account. A handwritten note on the statement or sticker may grab the client's attention (Figure 18-8). Clients not

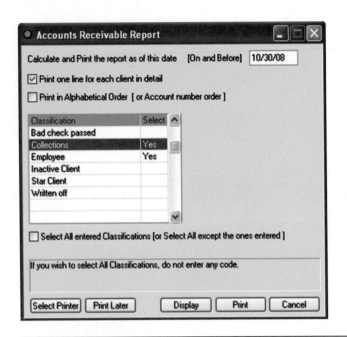

Total 30 days past due:			2626.99
Total 60 days past due:			1581.40
Total 90 days past due:			2229.62
Total past due:			**6438.01**
Total current balances:			1003.07
Acc# 1 (OCS) balance:			0.00
Total balance due:			**7441.08**
Credit balances:			−641.21
Total net receivables:			**6799.87**

Accounts Receivable Report   INTRAVET VETERINARY CARE

As of 10/30/2008

Exclude the following client classifications: COL, EMPL

Acc#	Client	Phones	Current	30 days	60 days	90 days	Total	YTD
25	Gregory Beck	(614)555-5262 (614)555-9398	99.56				99.56	99.56
28	Tim Brokaw	(614)555-4422 (614)555-7975		4.81		130.53	135.34	130.53
59	Marley Johnson	(614)555-3537 (614)555-9311	496.67				496.67	616.67
69	Chloe Sartin	(614)555-1915 (614)555-0053	0.15				0.15	1229.15
71	Keenen Carson	(614)555-3457 (614)555-1823	199.12				199.12	199.12
85	Andrew Ross	(614)555-3250 (614)555-9384		5.84	5.23	228.46	239.53	348.46
92	Doug Zinn	(614)555-8765 (614)555-8755	10.27	5.00	524.50	2.75	542.52	707.25
100	Irwin Hilton	(614)555-1103 (614)555-7470		360.00			360.00	375.00
104	Veronica Casper	(614)555-2798 (614)555-2717			24.71		24.71	44.71
243	Kirk Matthews	(614)555-3783 (614)555-1869		21.00			201.00	201.00
265	Chris Matthews	(614)555-8872		4.00		49.78	53.78	49.78
280	Taylor Pennington	(614)555-7616 (614)555-0184		35.00			35.00	

FIGURE 18-4 Sample accounts receivable report. (Courtesy IntraVet, Dublin, Ohio.)

Box 18-1   Example of Finance Charges

- 100 statements to run
- 6.25% interest
- Set cost per invoice: $0.49

Labor : $12.00 × 6 hours = $72.00 × $\dfrac{20\%(0.20)}{\$14.40}$

Total Labor: $86.40 ($72.00 + $14.40)
Labor per invoice: $0.86 ($86.40/100)
Labor + set costs: $1.35

An invoice has a balance of $98.45. The interest rate is 6.25%.
    $98.45 × 6.25% (0.0625) = $6.15
    $98.45 + $6.15 = New balance: $104.60

---

making payments within 90 days can be notified that arrangements need to be made or the account will be turned over to a credit collection agency. Team members should try to call owners to discuss the account, and try to make payment arrangements with the client. If contact has been made with the client, a summary of the conversation must be documented in the record. Once team members have exhausted all opportunities to collect the outstanding balance, accounts must be turned over to a collections agent. If the agent is unable to collect, the outstanding amount will be reported to the credit bureau or the consumer reporting agency. A credit bureau reports specific information about a person's previous payment history and provides information of

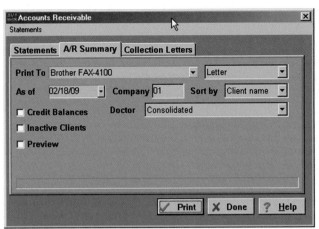

FIGURE 18-5 Sample accounts receivable summary. (Courtesy McAllister Software Systems, Piedmont, Mo.)

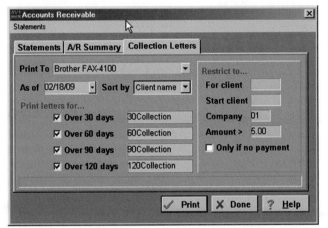

FIGURE 18-6 Sample accounts receivable collection letters. (Courtesy McAllister Software Systems, Piedmont, Mo.)

> **PRACTICE POINT**   Clients paying their accounts on a monthly basis cannot be turned over to a collections agency.

public interest. A client's credit will be affected for the following 7 years.

Clients that have been turned over to a collections agent should have their account flagged so that they do not return to the practice and expect service. Veterinary software programs allow alerts to be entered into the computer, and when a nonpaying account is opened, the computer alerts the team member of the delinquent account. Noncomputerized practices should have a special color file folder to indicate uncollected accounts, or the file may be kept in a separate area. Some clients will return to a clinic years later, hoping that the staff will not remember the bad debt they once had. It is fair to ask the clients to pay the previous balance before any new services being rendered.

If a clinic decides not to turn an outstanding account over to a collection agent and is unable to collect the balance, it may be worthwhile to simply write off the

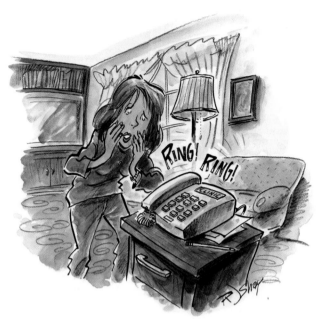

FIGURE 18-7 "Oh no! The vet's office is calling again!"

account as bad debt. Again, the client record must be flagged so that all team members know of the account status. At the end of the day, time, money, and the effort spent collecting accounts receivable could be better spent on other areas of the practice.

FAIR DEBT COLLECTION PRACTICES ACT

Collection procedures are regulated by the Fair Debt Collection Practices Act of 1996. The act was passed to protect the public from unethical collection procedures and mainly applies to collection agencies. Debtors cannot be subjected to harassment, oppressive tactics, or abusive treatment. The law prohibits the collector from making any false statements to the client, such as claiming to be a lawyer or government agency. Clients may not be called at work if the employer or client objects or be called at inconvenient times or places, such as before 9 AM and after 9 PM. Delinquent payments can only be discussed with the clients themselves. These same regulations must be considered as the veterinary health care team attempts to collect outstanding accounts.

> **PRACTICE POINT**   The Fair Debt Collection Practices Act was established to protect consumers.

TELEPHONE CALLS TO COLLECT OUTSTANDING ACCOUNTS

Contact with clients can be made with a telephone call to try to determine the client's financial status. Team members may find it difficult to try to collect delinquent accounts over the phone and often find the client has a negative attitude once the phone call has been made. It

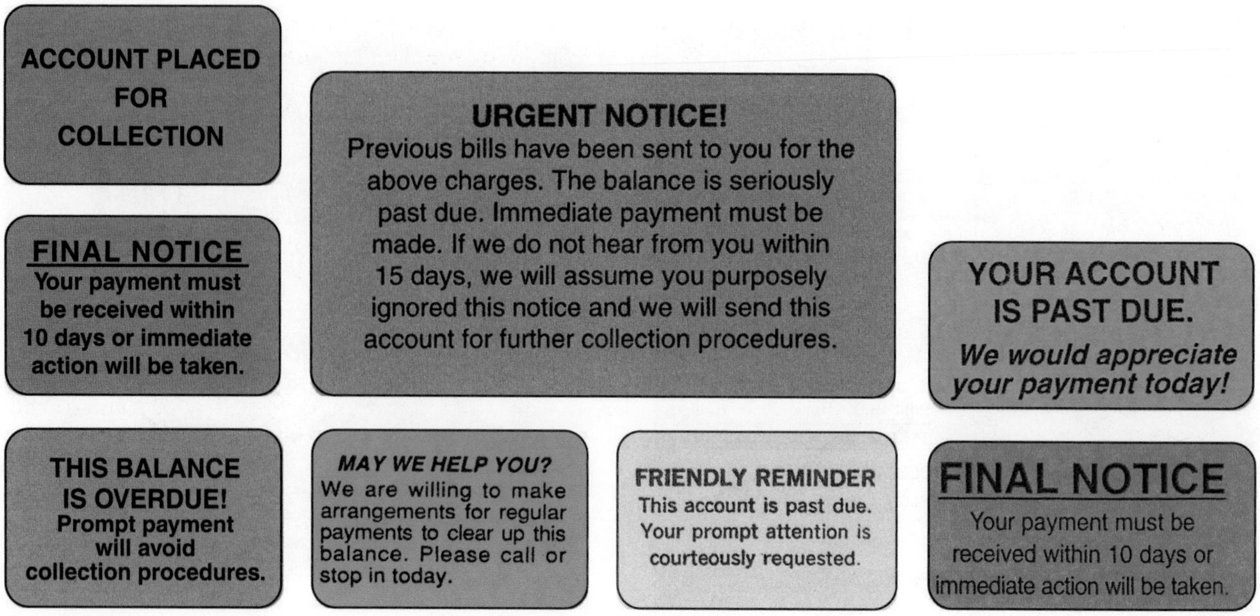

FIGURE 18-8 Examples of late payment stickers.

should be remembered not to take the negative words personally; it is frustrating to everyone to be under financial strain. Team members should keep a friendly, helpful, and positive tone in their voices. Discussion of the animal should be avoided, keeping the conversation focused on the account collection. Clearly state the hospital policy regarding charging and set a date for when the account will be paid in full. Be prepared to offer the client a payment plan, and advise the client that interest charges will accrue each month.

Team members should remember not to call clients before 9 AM or after 9 PM, as stated by the Fair Debt Collection Practices Act. Team members must verify who they are speaking with, then identify themselves. "Hello, is this Mr. Stone?" Once the client has verified himself, the team member can continue, "This is Teresa with ABC Animal Clinic." The purpose of the phone call can then be established. Team members may act as if the client is going to pay the balance and that payment arrangements are simply being made. A specific date and amount of payment can be established and documented in the record. A written letter to follow up the details of the conversation can be sent to the client as a simple reminder. Clients should never be threatened, and the account should never be discussed with anyone other than the client. Messages should not be left regarding the delinquent balance; simply state the team member's name and a phone number where he or she can be reached.

PRACTICE POINT Team members cannot call clients with outstanding balances before 9 AM or after 9 PM.

Many clients have caller ID and will not answer the phone when an outstanding account or collections agent is calling. If possible, calls should be made on a blocked line eliminating the identification. Some clients still may not answer the phone, especially if they are in debt and have several businesses calling. All attempts to make contact with the client must be documented in the record. After several attempts have been made, a certified letter may have to be mailed. A certified letter requires that the recipient sign a card indicating receipt of the letter, and the card is then returned to the sender.

COLLECTION LETTERS

A collection letter may be sent at the discretion of the veterinary practice along with a monthly statement. Veterinary software can generate a collection letter at any time management has specified in the setup program. A series of computer-generated letters can be sent at 30, 60, and/or 90 days after the account has become past due. Specified messages can be printed on each letter informing the client of the past due status of the account. Clients should be reminded that unpaid accounts will be sent to a collections agency and reported to the credit bureau. The last letter should include a deadline date of when the account will be turned over to collections if the recipient has not responded. Box 18-2 can be used as a guideline for developing a collection letter. Letters should be kept short and simple. Long, rambling letters will be ignored by the client and may inadvertently have words or phrases that will offend the client, ultimately delaying payment (Figure 18-9).

Studies show that clients pay outstanding balances for health care last, after paying rent, mortgage, and utilities, because of the fear of losing their homes. Team members can send a simple reminder to clients that a

| Box 18-2 | Guidelines for Developing an Effective Collection Letter |

- Keep the letter short and brief.
- Make sure the date, amount, and client information are correct.
- Use simple words and phrases.
- Provide a specific date by which the client must respond.
- Provide a date for when a specific action will take place. For example, give the date when the account will be turned over to a collection agent.
- Be firm and polite.
- Include "thank you" at the end of the letter; this is a valuable tool in public relations.

small payment each month will prevent the account from being sent to a collections agency.

COLLECTIONS AGENCY

After every attempt has been made to collect the account, it may be necessary to appoint the services of a collection agency. The longer an account is delinquent, the less likely it is the account will be collected on, regardless of whether it is by the practice or a collection agent. Agencies will generally charge between 40% and 60% of the total balance that is being collected or may only charge the practice if they are able to collect (some agencies may charge an up-front, nonreturnable

---

ABC Animal Clinic
555 Uptown Circle
Anytown, MN 89000
555-555-5555

05/28/09

Maria Rogers
6454 Downtown Circle
Anytown, MN 89001

Dear Mrs. Rogers,

On April 28, 2009, you brought Scruffy into ABC Animal Clinic to be spayed. At the time of Scruffy's release, you notified the receptionist that you left your purse at home and asked if you could send a payment in the mail. The receptionist kindly extended credit to you, which was a rare circumstance.

It is against our policy at ABC Animal Clinic to extend credit. We have sent you several overdue notices but have received no response from you.

We have enclosed the original receipt with the total amount due of $398.94. If we do not hear from you by 06/15/09, we will be forced to turn your account over to our collections agency.

Please contact us immediately. Your prompt attention is greatly appreciated.

Thank you,

Melva Flowers
Practice Manager, ABC Animal Clinic

FIGURE 18-9 Sample collection letter.

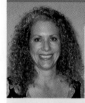

What Would You Do/Not Do?

Linda, the office manager, is in charge of accounts receivable and runs statements on a monthly basis. She notices that the employee accounts receivable is quite high: almost 20% of the accounts receivable total. On closer examination, she sees that several employees have not made a payment for several months. She realizes that the economy has been difficult for many, but does not know whether she should speak with the employees about their account balances.

What Should Linda Do?

Instead of Linda speaking to team members herself and thereby increasing tensions among the staff, she should discuss the situation with the owner and practice manager, allowing them to handle employees when they become frustrated. Employees, like clients, can be embarrassed by their financial situations and become upset when addressed for lack of payments on their account.

Box 18-3　Vital Information to Provide to a Collection Agent

- Client's full name, address, and all telephone numbers (including cell phone and work phone)
- Total balance due on account, including finance charges
- Client's occupation, if known
- Client's employment address, if known
- Driver's license number
- Copy of client information sheet and signature of client guaranteeing payment for services rendered

fee, even if they are unable to collect). A check for the remainder of the balance will be sent to the veterinary practice with a notice that account has been paid. It is important that all staff members know when an account has been sent to collections; nonpaying clients should not be seen.

A collection agency should be chosen based on its professionalism, ethics, and reliability. References can be obtained from the Better Business Bureau (BBB), the local Chamber of Commerce, or the Associated Credit Bureaus of America. Make sure the agency will generate reports and updates on accounts that will be turned over to them, and that legal action will not be pursued until the veterinary practice has been contacted. Agents should be asked how they want the account handled if the client comes into the veterinary clinic to pay the balance. Some agencies prefer to simply refer the client to the agent; others may advise the clinic to accept payment and notify the credit agent of any payment activity.

Information that should be made available to the collection agent is summarized in Box 18-3. The most up-to-date and accurate information will aid in the collection of accounts. Information collected from the client at the initial visit is vital at this point. If a clinic does not have accurate information, including a driver's license number, the agency cannot report the delinquent's history to the credit bureau.

Once the account has been sent to collections, the client should not be sent any more statements. The medical record and computer record must indicate the account has been turned over to an agent. An opinion from a tax professional should be sought as the best way to handle the lost money from a nonpaying account. Some states may allow a tax write-off due to bad debt.

EMPLOYEE ACCOUNTS RECEIVABLE

Employees will accumulate a balance with a veterinary clinic as procedures and products are added to their accounts. It is important that each employee be mandated to make monthly payments. Practices generally give employee discounts on services and may allow products to be sold to employees at cost. Therefore the veterinary practice is losing money by allowing employees to accumulate large balances; practices may be unable to collect on an account if the employee leaves. It can then be extremely difficult for the team to make phone calls and/or send the former employee to collections if he or she left the practice on good terms. It is in the best interest of the clinic to prevent employee balances from accumulating by mandating monthly payments.

VETERINARY PRACTICE and the LAW

Collecting outstanding accounts can be a difficult and time-consuming task. Team members must abide by the Fair Debt Collection Practices Act, an act that was passed to protect the public from unethical collection procedures. Those that do not follow the Fair Debt Collection Practices Act can be sued by clients, and any damages sustained by the client can be collected. A judge may determine the actual amount of damages, which cannot exceed $500,000 or a percentage of the total net worth of the debt collector. Collection procedures must be followed to prevent a lawsuit from being initiated.

Self-Evaluation Questions

1. What is the Fair Debt Collection Practices Act and why was it established?
2. What characteristics should be considered when choosing a collections agent?
3. What is an insufficient funds charge?
4. Why should a percentage of interest be added to outstanding client accounts?
5. What information is needed when reporting delinquent accounts to the credit bureau?
6. Why should postdated checks not be accepted?
7. What is a held check?
8. How often should statements be sent?
9. What percentage of gross profits should be allowed as accounts receivable?
10. If a practice generates a yearly gross income of $1,123,598.68, and accounts receivable is 1%, what is the total accounts receivable balance?

Recommended Reading

Heinke MM: *Practice made perfect: a guide to veterinary practice management*, Lakewood, CO, 2001, AAHA Press.

Opperman M: *The art of veterinary practice management*, Lenexa, KS, 1999, Veterinary Medicine Publishing Group.

Wilson J: Managing your credit policy. In Chubb D, editor: *Business management for the veterinary practitioner*, Denver, 1995, Chubb Communications.

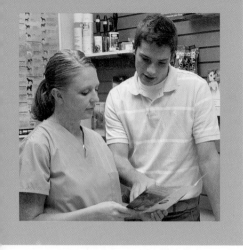

Pet Health Insurance

Learning Objectives

Mastery of the content in this chapter will enable the reader to:

- Define and explain insurance policies to fellow team members and clients.
- Identify the differences between hereditary and congenital conditions.

- Clarify insurance claim forms.
- Explain the disadvantages of third-party payment systems.
- Define insurance plans to clients.

Key Terms

Allowance
Annual Deductible
Annual Payout Limit
Benefit
Chronic Conditions
Claim
Congenital Conditions
Copay
Deductible

Exclusion
Hereditary Conditions
Incident
Indemnity Insurance
Lifetime Limit
Managed Care
National Commission on Veterinary
    Economic Issues (NCVEI)
Per-Incident Deductible

Per-Incident Limit
Preexisting Condition
Premium
Rider
Waiting Period

Pet health insurance has been available for more than 20 years but has not been a popular choice among owners until recently. Insurance is a method by which pet owners can manage the risks of expensive health care. Accidents and diseases are unexpected costs for owners, and insurance allows them to provide the best treatment available. Many pet owners are forced to make treatment decisions based on cost alone. Insurance allows owners the financial resources they may need to provide life-saving treatments they would otherwise not consider.

The National Commission on Veterinary Economic Issues (NCVEI) released a landmark study in 1999 indicating that the increased use of veterinary pet health insurance could increase the demand for service, thereby decreasing the euthanasia rate in the United States. Studies indicate that pet owners look to their veterinarians for education regarding pet health and insurance for their pets. It is imperative that the entire staff understand the concept of pet insurance and offer it to all clients.

Pets are now living longer due both to improved veterinary health care and to clients' willingness to spend additional money to treat medical conditions. Veterinary medicine has benefited from the progression of human medicine with regard to new pharmaceuticals, disease treatments, and diagnostic equipment such as computer-based imaging. These advancements have increased the quality, quantity, and cost of veterinary care; with that, clients have also come to expect a higher level of service.

The human-animal bond has dramatically strengthened over the past 25 years. Along with the increased use of diagnostic tools, specialists, and treatments, clients are willing to spend a large amount to save a pet's life. Veterinary Pet Insurance completed a study in 2006 indicating that clients with insurance visited their veterinarian 40% more often than those without insurance. They were also willing to spend twice as much on products and services over the lifetime of their pets (Figure 19-1).

Clients should be made aware of the various companies that offer pet health insurance. Terms that should be considered include whether hereditary conditions are covered and if benefit schedules or exclusions are listed in the policy. Some benefit schedules only cover a small percentage of what would be considered a reasonable expense for a condition. Some companies may not use a benefit schedule and set payout limits instead, regardless of illness or condition (Box 19-1). Most pet insurance companies set high dollar amounts "for reasonable expenses"; they do not want to set prices for veterinary practices, nor do they want to dissuade owners from purchasing packages.

> **PRACTICE POINT**   Insurance policies vary by state; each plan must be read carefully to allow accurate comparison of policies.

INDEMNITY INSURANCE

Indemnity insurance offers compensation for treatment of injured and sick pets. Owners purchase a policy directly from a pet health insurance company and are eligible for compensation based on the care provided and policy terms. Policies are available for comprehensive illness, standard care, and accident coverage and may cover species ranging from dogs and cats to exotics and birds.

Indemnity insurance is different from insurance available for people. Insurance on the human side is generally offered through health management organizations (HMOs) or preferred provider organizations (PPOs), which are managed organizations. Physicians are contracted to provide medical service at a set price and are then reimbursed directly by the insurance company. Indemnity insurance is not managed care; indemnity insurance policies provide compensation for accidents and illnesses and are paid directly to the client. This leaves the veterinary practice out of the process because the client pays the veterinary practice when the service is rendered.

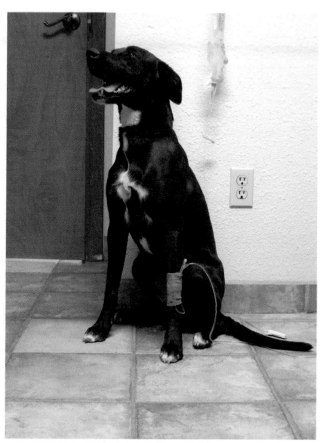

FIGURE 19-1 Black Labrador with intravenous catheter.

Box 19-1	Most Common Reasons Pets Visit a Veterinarian

DOGS
1. Ear infection
2. Skin allergies
3. Hot spots
4. Gastritis
5. Urinary tract infections
6. Skin tumors
7. Eye inflammation
8. Osteoarthritis
9. Hypothyroidism

CATS
1. Urinary tract infections
2. Gastritis
3. Renal failure
4. Diabetes
5. Skin allergies
6. Ear infections
7. Respiratory infections
8. Hyperthyroidism

Premiums

A premium is defined as the amount an owner pays monthly or annually to maintain an insurance policy for a pet. Premium amounts are affected by a number of factors, including the deductible; the copay; and the per-incident, annual, or lifetime payout limit. The species and breed of the animal also affect the cost of the premium as well as whether the pet is spayed or neutered, the age of the pet, and the geographic location of the owner in the United States (Figure 19-2). Cats tend to have lower premiums than dogs, and a Border Collie will have a lower premium than a Shar-Pei. Altered pets tend to have fewer behavioral issues and hormone-driven instincts and may have a decreased chance of developing hormone-related cancers; therefore a lower premium is likely. Owners living in rural Arizona will also have a lower premium than those who live in Los Angeles because the price of veterinary care is drastically different in these two locations.

> **PRACTICE POINT** Premiums are affected by a number of factors, including the breed and age of the pet.

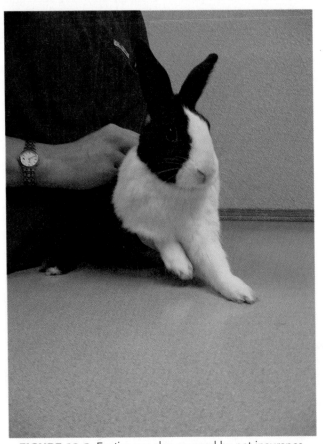

FIGURE 19-2 Exotics are also covered by pet insurance.

Deductibles

A deductible is the amount an owner must pay before the insurance company will offer compensation. Insurance companies vary, offering either a per-incident deductible or an annual deductible. Per-incident deductibles refer to the owner paying the chosen deductible amount each time an incident occurs with the pet. An annual deductible refers to an owner paying the chosen deductible one time each year. Once the annual deductible amount has been met, the owner does not have to pay a deductible until the following year. For example, if a dog has an ear infection in March, a foreign body in June, and a fractured leg in November, and the owner chose a policy that was per-incident based, the owner would pay a deductible for each of the three claims. If the owner chose an annual deductible, he would pay the deductible amount once and would no longer be subject to a deductible for the rest of the year. Lower deductibles increase the cost of the premium, just as higher deductibles lower the premium.

> **PRACTICE POINT** Annual deductibles are more advantageous than per-incident deductibles, especially for the treatment of complex diseases and conditions.

Copay

A copay is the percentage that the owner is responsible for after the deductible has been met. Lower copays increase the amount of the premium and generally range from 10% to 20%. As an example, if a client's policy includes a $100 deductible and a 10% copay and the invoice balance is $4500, the owner is responsible for $540. This is calculated as follows:

$$\$4500 - \$100 \, \text{deductible} = \$4400 \times 10\% \, \text{copay} = \$440$$

$$\$440 + \$100 = \$540 \, (\text{client responsibility})$$

$$\$4500 - \$540 = \$3960 \, (\text{insurance responsibility})$$

Annual Policy, per-Incident, or Lifetime Limits

Some insurance companies offer clients a choice of an annual policy or a per-incident limit; others offer one or the other. Annual limits refer to the maximum amount that the insurance company will pay for a condition or illness during the policy term. Per-incident limits refer to the maximum amount an insurance company will pay each time a new problem or disease occurs. Lifetime limits refer to the maximum amount an insurance company will pay during the pet's life.

Per-incident limits can range from $1500 to $6000, but some companies do not have a per-incident limit. Annual limits range from $8000 to $20,000, allowing a larger amount for serious conditions. If a pet has been diagnosed with cancer and must undergo surgery, chemotherapy, and radiation, the invoice will likely exceed the $6000 per-incident limit. Because the cancer is classified as one incident, the maximum amount paid to the client will be the per-incident limit established in the policy. If an annual limit was chosen, the total amount paid to the client will be higher, based on the annual maximum amount established in the insurance policy. Few companies offer a lifetime limit, but if they do, it may be as high as $100,000. Policies should be examined carefully to determine which limit will meet the client's needs.

> **PRACTICE POINT** Per-incident payout limits can be a disadvantage if a pet has been diagnosed with cancer.

Preexisting Health Conditions

A preexisting heath condition is defined as any accident or illness contracted, manifested, or incurred before the policy effective date. The pet may be enrolled; however, any preexisting condition will be excluded from coverage. It is highly recommended to enroll puppies and kittens in an insurance plan before any medical conditions arise (Box 19-2).

Waiting Period

A waiting period is a period of time when coverage is not available and generally applies to the time between submission of the application and the date the policy becomes effective. Each company varies in the length of time between application acceptance and activation. Some companies may have a 48-hour waiting period for accidents and a 2- to 4-week waiting period for a condition or illness. Any condition that occurs during the waiting period is usually considered a preexisting condition.

Hereditary and Congenital Conditions

Purebred pets that are known to have congenital and hereditary conditions may, based on company policy, also be excluded from an insurance plan (Figure 19-3). Recent veterinary books, including *Current Veterinary Therapy, Medical and Genetic Aspects of Purebred Dogs,* and the *Textbook of Small Animal Internal Medicine* reference common congenital and hereditary conditions. A congenital condition is generally defined as an abnormality present at birth, whether apparent or not, that can cause illness or disease.

Congenital defects may be caused by medications administered to the mother in utero. Examples of congenital defects may include an umbilical hernia, a cleft palate, or a portosystemic shunt. Presence of a shunt may not be known until the dog matures, whereas a

---

| **Box 19-2** | Helpful Terms |

Allowance: The maximum amount available for a specific diagnosis.

Annual Deductible: The dollar amount the client chooses when signing up for an insurance plan. The client pays this amount before payout.

Annual Payout Limit: The maximum amount an insurance company will pay out on one policy, per year.

Benefit: The payment made for a specific diagnosis in accordance with an insurance plan.

Claim: A submission for a request for payment.

Copay: A specified dollar amount of covered services that is the policyholder's responsibility.

Deductible: The dollar amount an individual must pay for services before the insurance company's payment. Clients may have a choice of per-incident deductible or annual deductible.

Exclusion: A condition that is excluded from the coverage of a medical plan.

Incident: An individual accident, illness, or injury, including those that may require continual treatment until resolution.

Indemnity Insurance: A system of pet health insurance in which the client is reimbursed for services after they have been provided.

Lifetime Limit: The maximum dollar amount a company will pay out on one policy for the lifetime of the pet.

Per-Incident Deductible: The dollar amount that the policyholder is responsible for before the company will begin to pay out for each incident for which a claim form is submitted.

Per-Incident Limit: The maximum dollar amount an insurance company will pay out per incident filed.

Preexisting condition: Injury or illness contracted, manifested, or incurred before the policy effective date.

Premium: The amount paid annually or monthly for a policyholder to maintain an insurance policy.

Rider: An extension of coverage that can be purchased and added to a base medical policy.

---

cleft palate is obvious immediately after birth. A hereditary condition is an abnormality that is transmitted genetically from the parent to the offspring. Examples include hip dysplasia, luxating patella, or cardiomyopathy. Some companies may also argue that some congenital defects are hereditary, thereby excluding coverage of such conditions. A portosystemic shunt is an example of a condition that may be subject to such argument. Policies must be reviewed carefully for such exemptions.

Coverage of diseases may vary among insurance companies; therefore a list of excluded diseases and conditions should be requested. Some companies will cover congenital conditions if they have not been previously diagnosed; others will not cover them at all. Companies that offer coverage of hereditarily diseases will have higher premiums.

What Would You Do/Not Do?

Ms. Luke, a longtime client, has recently acquired a Great Dane puppy. Upon examination, Dr. Abbey tentatively diagnoses osteochondritis dissecans (OCD), a common skeletal growth abnormality in large-breed puppies. However, to make a true diagnosis, Dr. Abbey recommends radiographs. Ms. Luke declines radiographs at this time because of the cost. Team members advise her that pet health insurance may be an option for her new puppy and hand her a brochure discussing the benefits of health insurance.

The following month, Ms. Luke returns to the practice stating she has pet health insurance now and would like the radiographs that were recommended last month. Alex, a longtime veterinary technician, knows that preexisting health conditions are not covered by insurance, and because the pet had previously been seen for this condition, that the policy will most likely not cover the costs of the radiographs. Alex advises the owner of this, who claims, "They won't know the difference; they are only office workers!"

What Should Alex do?

Alex should continue with the case and take radiographs at the veterinarian's request. However, it is not his place to call the insurance company; this may foster client disloyalty. He can, however, offer to fill out the pet health insurance claim form for the owner, copy the medical records, and send the claim for Ms. Luke. The insurance company will then be able to read the medical record and make a judgment based on the copies provided.

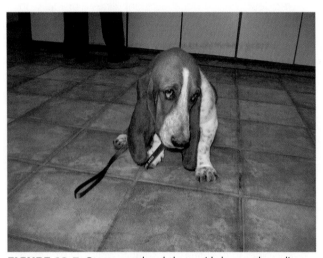

FIGURE 19-3 Some purebred dogs with known hereditary conditions may not be eligible for pet health insurance with certain companies.

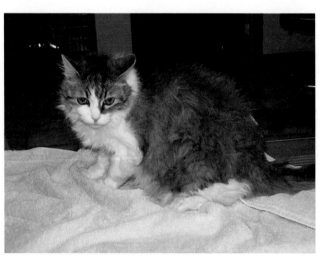

FIGURE 19-4 Some pet health insurance companies may cover chronic health conditions such as diabetes or renal failure.

Chronic Conditions

Many diseases or conditions that are diagnosed will require years of care. Diabetes, Cushing disease, and Addison disease are just a few conditions that require care beyond the initial diagnosis and treatment (Figure 19-4). These conditions are known as *chronic conditions,* and some companies will only cover the initial diagnosis and treatment for the first year. Once it is time to reenroll the pet for the upcoming year, some insurance companies may consider the condition as a preexisting condition and exclude it from the policy.

> **PRACTICE POINT** Some companies do not offer continued coverage of chronic conditions such as diabetes or Cushing disease.

Exclusions

Many companies have a list of exclusions: diseases, conditions, or treatments that are excluded from policies. Frequently, behavior counseling and medications are not covered, nor are compounded medications, nutraceuticals, or diets. Exclusions should be carefully reviewed before choosing a policy.

WELLNESS PLANS

Policies that include wellness plans will have higher premiums. Traditionally, indemnity insurance covers accidents and illnesses; therefore wellness plans are considered supplementary. Preventative care may include vaccinations, worming medication, heartworm preventative, spays or neuters, and dental prophylaxis. Plans should be carefully considered because a puppy or kitten

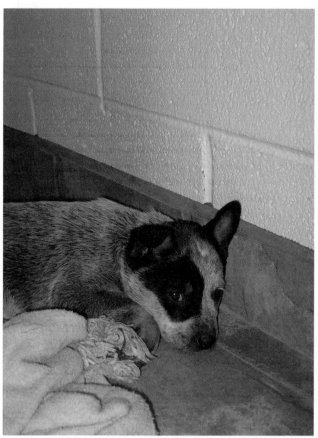

FIGURE 19-5 Pet owners should evaluate insurance options as the needs of their pet change.

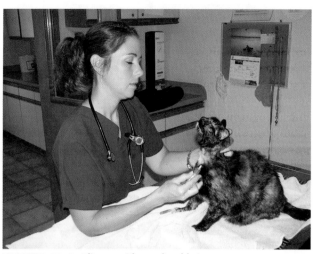

FIGURE 19-6 Clients with pet health insurance are more likely to have diagnostics performed as recommended by the veterinary health care team.

may benefit from the first year of coverage that includes vaccines and surgery; however, during the second year, coverage for surgery is not needed (Figure 19-5). A policy should be reevaluated annually to determine whether the pet's needs will be met if insurance is required. Most wellness plans are prepaid medical care rather than insurance and are paid out by a benefits schedule.

BENEFITS OF PET HEALTH INSURANCE

Pets can receive superior care with pet health insurance and can visit any hospital of the client's choice. If a client has an emergency at night, the client can visit the emergency hospital and have peace of mind that the expenses will be covered. If clients are traveling and need to see a veterinarian in another state, the insurance will still cover the cost of the veterinary service. Clients who choose wellness plans will elect to have preventive procedures completed more often, keeping pets healthier longer (Figure 19-6).

> **PRACTICE POINT** Pet health insurance has many benefits, including allowing clients to visit veterinarians of their choice.

Most pet insurance companies have streamlined the claims process, making it simple and hassle free. Clients simply fill out the pet and client information, and practices fill out the form indicating the diagnosis. The veterinarian signs the claim form and the client submits it to the company by fax or mail. Clients receive reimbursement within a short period. Veterinarians can practice the medicine they want; clients can choose the best options available to them. The insurance companies do not make decisions for the doctor or client; medical decisions are made between the practice and client.

Many companies are beginning to offer pet insurance to their employees as a part of a benefits program. Office Depot, eBay, Amazon.com, and Blockbuster are just a few of more than 2000 companies nationwide that offer pet health insurance to their employees.

FILING A CLAIM

First and foremost, clients should understand that they pay the practice when the service is rendered. Insurance companies then reimburse the client. Policyholders will receive several claims forms with their packet, or they can print forms from the insurance company's Web site (Figure 19-7). Clients simply fill out their information, policy number, and pet's information and sign the form. It is imperative that the team member helping the client with the claim form be knowledgeable about the pet's diagnosis. Incorrect wording and incomplete forms are the most common reason for claim payment delay. Some carriers offer a comprehensive list of diagnoses for team members to use when filling out forms. If a diagnosis has not been determined, some companies allow team members to include symptoms on the claim form; forms should be read for correct wording. If multiple diagnoses are made, then all diagnoses should be listed. For

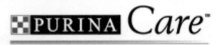
Pet Health Insurance

Claim Form

Policy Number: _____

Name: _____

Address: _____

City: _____ State: _____ Zip Code _____

Section 1: To be completed by the Policyholder

Pet's Name:	Date of Birth:
BEST phone number:	E-mail:

By my signature below, I authorize PurinaCare to request any medical records necessary to process this claim.

POLICYHOLDER SIGNATURE: _____

Section 2: To be completed by Veterinarian providing care

If this claim includes **PREVENTIVE CARE SERVICES,** check this box   ☐

If this claim includes **MEDICAL or ACCIDENT SERVICES** complete the table section below

Diagnosis	Date	Check One	
		Initial Visit	Recheck
1)			
2)			
3)			
4)			
5)			

If you are unable to provide a diagnosis or tentative diagnosis, please list the major presenting symptoms in the space below, or please attach a printed copy of the medical history for the problem being presented.

1)

2)

3)

Hospital

Stamp

Here

CLAIMS SUBMISSION CHECKLIST

To facilitate a short claim turnaround time, please make sure you have done the following:

➢ Policyholder has filled out and signed Section 1
➢ The veterinarian or hospital representative has filled out and stamped Section 2
➢ Mail or Fax all original receipt(s) for all visits noted on the claim form to

Mail: P.O. Box 599500, San Antonio, Texas 78258   Fax: 314-982-3312

FIGURE 19-7 Sample claim form from PurinaCare Pet Health Insurance. Claim forms will vary for different companies and policies. (Courtesy Nestle Purina, St. Louis, Mo.)

example, a dental prophylaxis may also find an abscessed tooth and periodontal disease; these must be written on the claim form so that the client is reimbursed for all three diseases, not just the dental procedure. Attaching a copy of the invoice and medical record will help insurance companies review the case more efficiently and will likely result in higher benefits payout. If a claim is denied, a request for review should be submitted as soon as possible. The request should provide additional information or clarification of a claim.

THIRD-PARTY PAYMENT SYSTEMS

Third-party payment systems may help owners cover unexpected costs associated with providing health care for their pet. Several systems are available, and team members should be familiar with all systems before making recommendations to clients.

> **PRACTICE POINT** Third-party systems should be fully evaluated before making recommendations to clients or accepting plans at a veterinary practice.

Discount Clubs

Discount clubs are member-driven organizations. Pet owners pay for a membership that allows access to a member veterinary practice. The practice agrees to provide discounted veterinary services and/or products to members. This may increase the awareness for veterinary services but decreases practice profitability because service relies mainly on discounts. Members are only allowed to visit a member veterinary practice, thereby limiting the discount to one hospital in a given area. These organizations may also offer discount plans. Clients should be warned against discount plans because these companies are not actual insurance companies; instead, pet owners pay a fee to receive a discounted service from participating veterinarians. These companies are not regulated as strictly as are insurance companies and can, at times, be fraudulent. Caution should be taken when dealing with companies of this sort. It should also be warned that veterinary clinics do not receive any benefit from these membership clubs, except a promise that it will bring more clients into the practice. Basically, the veterinarian is giving away services in exchange for the hope of receiving new clients.

Managed Care

Managed care allows veterinarians to join a network that may set fees for veterinarians. Veterinarians are then reimbursed in exchange for seeing patients that are part of the network. If patients go out of the network, they are penalized by fees. Managed veterinary care is similar to managed health care programs in human medicine, such as PPO and HMO organizations, and medical decisions tend to be made by the company instead of the veterinarian. Managed health care will probably never penetrate the pet health insurance industry because the market is too small.

RECOMMENDATIONS TO CLIENTS

In a recent study completed by Brakke Consulting in January 2008, 41% of owners surveyed said they would purchase insurance if it was recommended by their veterinary practice. A majority of the responders were younger, well educated, and more affluent urban/suburban pet owners. Veterinary practices may target owners of this class with materials for pet health insurance and explain the benefits associated with policies.

Having brochures for recommended insurance companies at the counter for clients to see is an easy introduction to pet health insurance. Clients can ask questions about the insurance available, and team members can give them an estimate of how much they would receive if their pet was covered with insurance. Placing brochures in puppy and kitten kits will also increase the awareness of insurance as well as placing posters throughout the clinic in high traffic areas. Team members should remember the most important tip when discussing pet insurance: pet health insurance helps pay for unexpected accidents and/or illnesses. It is best for clients to enroll pets when they are young, before the manifestation of disease or illness. Once the pet ages and diagnoses are made, coverage may be limited.

It should be remembered that 15% to 20% of the practice's active clientele account for 75% of the practice revenue. If clients with pet health insurance spend twice the amount as the noninsured, the practice volume, production, revenue, and quality of medicine will dramatically increase (Figure 19-8). More active clients will spend more money and opt for specialized services.

To successfully implement insurance into a practice, one person may be placed in charge of the program. This person can select one or two companies that the practice chooses to represent and be trained by the representatives of those companies. Training programs can then be implemented for the staff.

The training coordinator may place educational posters throughout the practice, brochures at the receptionist desk, and brochures in puppy and kitten kits. When clients call for appointments, team members may ask if they have pet health insurance. Although the majority will respond no, the point is for the client to become familiar with the phrase "pet health insurance." Once clients become comfortable with the phrase, they may have interest in it and be ready to purchase a policy for their pets. They will look to the team for advice and recommendations, and because the team is well educated on the benefits of pet health insurance, any team member can make a helpful recommendation.

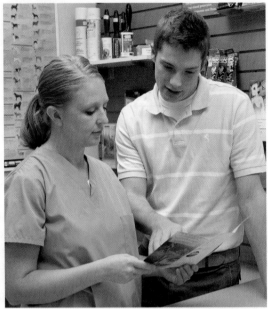

FIGURE 19-8 Staff should be trained to discuss pet health insurance policies with clients. Clients who purchase policies can be quite profitable to the veterinary practice.

Once polices are in use in the practice, a team member can fill out the diagnosis and simply have the veterinarian sign the claim form. The team member may want to copy the medical record for claim purposes to ensure that the client receives the largest benefit possible. The team member may want to continue to provide "wow" service to the client and place the claim form in the mail for the client. Clients appreciate this level of service.

In the future, claim forms may be available through computer software. Once team members click on a claim form, the client and patient information will be automatically populated onto the form. If the practice uses computerized medical records, the medical record will also be automatically uploaded with the form and sent electronically to the pet health insurance company. This will allow rapid claim processing, reimbursement of the client within a short time and, ultimately, an increase in client satisfaction.

Many insurance companies exist, and they should be examined carefully. Box 19-3 lists some references practices can look into regarding reputable pet health insurance.

Box 19-3	References Regarding Reputable Pet Health Insurance

- Pets Best: www.petsbest.com
- PurinaCare Pet Health Insurance: www.purinacare.com
- Veterinary Pet Insurance (VPI): www.petinsurance.com
- www.thebestpetinsurance.com

This is not an exhaustive list.

VETERINARY PRACTICE and the LAW

Because veterinary practices do not file insurance claims, they are rarely implicated in insurance fraud schemes. However, some clients try to defraud the system. Some clients will purchase an insurance policy and declare that there are no preexisting conditions; once the policy has been accepted, they will immediately file a claim for a preexisting lameness or abnormal bloodwork. Once this occurs, many insurance companies will call the practice and ask for a copy of the medical records. The medical records from practices indicate the true dates of the examinations and claim information, allowing insurance companies to determine fraudulent cases.

Self-Evaluation Questions

1. What is an annual deductible?
2. What is a copay?
3. What is an annual premium?
4. What are the three most common canine conditions?
5. What are the three most common feline conditions?
6. What is the benefit of an annual deductible versus a per-incident deductible?
7. What is considered a hereditary condition?
8. What is considered a congenital condition?
9. What is a lifetime limit?
10. Why should wellness plans be reevaluated yearly?

Recommended Reading

Ackerman LJ: *Business basics for veterinarians*, New York, 2002, ASLA.

Ackerman LJ: *Blackwell's 5 minute veterinary practice management consult*, Ames, IA, 2007, Blackwell Publishing.

Kenney D: *The complete guide to understanding pet health insurance*, 2008, Doug Kenney.

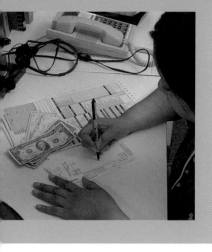

 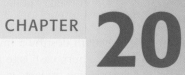

Preparing and Maintaining a Budget

The quickest way to destroy a business is to burn cash; the easiest way to burn cash is to not have a budget. Creating and maintaining budgets is one of the most useful tools in team management, yet it is underutilized. Budgets can be created for 2 to 3 years in advance, allowing for the planning and purchasing of equipment, the planning and implementation of an increased number of team members and/or veterinarians, and the implementation of raises for long-term employees. Created budgets can be changed at any time to account for market fluctuations and the economic conditions of the surrounding environment.

If budgets have not been previously used in a practice, one must be created and maintained for the current fiscal year. Once this has been completed, the following year's budget can be created, followed by goals to achieve for the future. Previous years' financial statements can be looked at to help create a budget. The initial setup will be time consuming; however, once data have been meticulously added, creating and maintaining budgets in the future will be simple and worthwhile.

ACCOUNTING AND BOOKKEEPING

Accounting and bookkeeping are closely related activities. The accounting process depends on the information produced by bookkeepers. A bookkeeper may be responsible for accounts payable, accounts receivable, and payroll. One or more team members may actually share the duties of a bookkeeper yet never be defined as one. An accountant is a professional that specializes in producing and interpreting financial statements, tax planning, cash flow projections, and estate planning. Bookkeepers may be employed by an accounting firm to aid in the practice's tax preparation, payroll, or benefit plans. The use of an accounting firm may depend on the size of the practice and the experience of the managers. Some practices may use an accountant only once a year to help prepare year-end statements and tax documents; others may use an accountant on a monthly basis.

Certified Public Accountant

A certified public accountant (CPA) should be the first choice of a practice when looking to hire a professional accountant. CPAs have extensive experience and have passed a comprehensive exam that tests their knowledge of accounting and tax principles, auditing standards, and business law. They must attend yearly classes to maintain continuing education requirements and comply with a strict code of ethics. Bookkeepers may give themselves the self-designation as accountants, although they may not have attended college. Public accountants (PAs) may have attended college and completed a degree in accounting but have not taken the CPA exam. CPAs are held to the highest standard; a CPA should be a practice's chosen accountant.

PRACTICE POINT   Bookkeepers often learn by trade, whereas accountants and CPAs have graduated from a 4-year program.

ACCOUNTING BASICS

To understand budgeting, a few accounting terms must first be reviewed. This will help in the understanding of creating and maintaining budgets. Box 20-1 lists helpful terms.

A variety of basic information is needed when compiling reports for a veterinary hospital. These statistics are also known as *key performance indicators*. These reports help monitor the practice on a monthly, quarterly, and yearly basis. Key performance indicators can help explain changes in financial statements, and all contribute to the success of the hospital. Practices should take time to develop their own set of key performance indicators, determining what reports are needed and what aspects of the practice that management wants to focus on (Figures 20-1 and 20-2). Following are some examples of reports:
- Accounts payable, total of owed amount and due dates
- Accounts receivable summary
- Average client transaction
- Cash available for investment
- Client survey results
- Compliance rate
- Inventory of equipment owned with original purchase date and price
- Inventory on hand
- Inventory sold within a given period
- Number of active clients
- Number of employees and the total number of hours worked per payroll period
- Number of new clients
- Taxes owed; payroll, sales, and other
- Team member survey results

Accounts Payable

Accounts payable should be monitored on a monthly basis to ensure that there is not more spending than receiving. If the practice spends more money than it takes in, the practice will be in serious financial deficit in the upcoming months. Small practices that are relatively new may experience months that produce less than others, and a plan should be implemented in case this occurs. Spending must decrease, and the practice employees should be held accountable for wastage. The fee structure may be reevaluated, and practice managers should ensure charges are not being missed. If a line of credit is needed to keep the practice floating during the slow months, then a plan must be implemented to pay back the loan as soon as possible.

Box 20-1	Accounting Terms

Accrual basis method: A system that recognizes income as it is earned and expenses as they are incurred rather than when the actual cash transaction occurs.

Asset: Any property owned by a business or individual. Cash, accounts receivable, inventory, land, building, leasehold improvements, and tangible property are examples of assets.

Balance sheet: A financial report detailing practice assets, liabilities, and owner's equity.

Budget: An estimate of revenues and expenses for a given period.

Cash basis method: A system that recognizes income as it is received and expenses as they are paid, rather than when the income was earned or the expense was acquired.

Cash flow statement: Report on the sources and uses of cash during a given period of time.

Direct expense: An expense that can be directly related to a patient, client, or revenue center.

Equity: The rights or claims to properties; Assets = Equities + Liabilities.

Fixed cost: A cost that does not change with the variation in business. Rent, mortgage, and utility costs remain the same regardless of how busy the practice is.

Income statement: Report on financial performance that covers a period of time and reports incomes and expenses during that period. Income statements are also known as *profit and loss statements.*

Indirect expense: An expense that contributes to the delivery of patient care, but that cannot be tied directly to a patient, client, or revenue center.

Intangible property: Nonphysical property that has value; franchises, copyrights, client lists, goodwill, and noncompete agreements are examples of intangible property.

Key performance indicators: Statistics that can be generated from client transaction data and reviewed for performance data.

Liabilities: Obligations resulting from past transactions that require the practice to pay money or provide service. Accounts payable and taxes are examples of current liabilities.

Owner's equity: Owner's interest or claim in the practice assets.

Principal cost: Initial cost of equipment when purchased.

Profit and loss statement: Summary of the practice's income, expenses, and resulting profit or loss for a specified period of time (also known as the *income statement*).

Tangible property: Physical property, such as desks, chairs, equipment, computers, software, and vehicles, that has value.

Transaction: A purchase that must be recorded.

Variable cost: Any cost that varies with the volume of business for the practice. Medical supplies and drugs increase or decrease depending on the volume of business.

PRACTICE POINT Accounts payable must not exceed monthly income.

PRACTICE POINT Accounts receivable should never exceed 1% of the gross income.

An accounts payable ledger will help monitor expenses on a monthly basis (Figure 20-3). A team member can add invoices as they arrive as well as enter a due date and the amount of the payable. This ensures bills will not be overlooked and gives a running balance of those accounts with revolving credit lines. It also allows easy access to retrieve information if the payment of a specific bill comes into question.

Accounts Receivable Summary

Accounts receivable (AR) must be monitored on a monthly basis. A large AR can be detrimental to the practice. AR reports should list the amounts due in 30-, 60-, and 90-day increments. Clients who owe practices money after 90 days not only are unlikely to pay, but also prevent practices from being able to pay their own accounts and employees. The practice must implement a no-charge policy to prevent AR from growing rapidly and hurting the practice's gross revenue. AR should never be more than 1% of the gross revenue in 1 year.

Figure 20-4 is an AR report that shows that the largest balance of the accounts receivable is the current

amount due, followed by 90 days past due. The sum of $3661.32 is unlikely to be collected, and the AR manager must determine appropriate strategies to collect these funds as soon as possible. The current balance must also be monitored; if this balance does not decrease within 30 days, strategies must be implemented to prevent past due amounts from rolling over to 60 and 90 days past due. Chapter 18 discusses AR in more detail.

Average Client Transaction

The average client transaction should be monitored to ensure that team members are making recommendations and clients are accepting them. If the average client transaction is consistently low, leaders must determine why and develop a solution to increase the low figure.

One reason for low client transactions may be lack of team member training. Assistants and technicians may not be educating the clients regarding the benefits of certain products. Veterinarians may not be educating clients regarding the benefits of recommended procedures or may not be recommending sufficient diagnostic workup on their cases. For a practice to offer high-quality medicine, diseases and conditions must be diagnosed

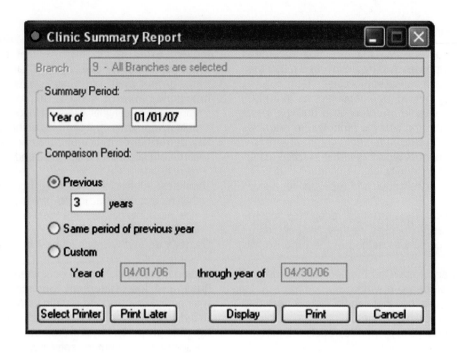

FIGURE 20-1 Sample clinic summary report. (Courtesy IntraVet, Dublin, Ohio.)

with tests, along with consideration of the presenting clinical symptoms. Whatever the reason, management must determine the cause of the low transactions and implement changes immediately.

PRACTICE POINT Low average client transactions can indicate a decrease in the number of diagnostics performed by the veterinarian.

Cash Availability

The cash available for reinvestment is very important to managers who are planning to purchase capital equipment. Practices may wish to purchase equipment through financing if cash is not available for reinvestment. Purchasing equipment outright is a better option because the interest that practices pay can accumulate to high amounts. Interest could be considered profit or cash for reinvestment with proper planning and budgeting.

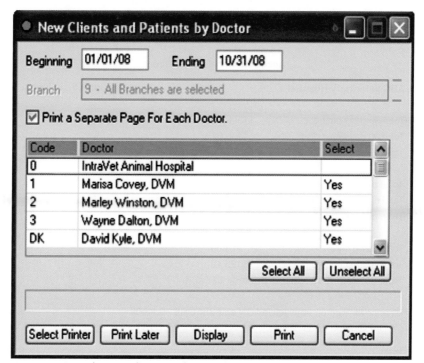

New Clients and Patients by Doctor   **INTRAVET VETERINARY CARE**

New Clients and patients with at least one visit between: 01/01/2008 - 10/31/2008

Doctor Code	Doctor Name	Number of New Clients With a Visit	Number of New Patients With a Visit
1	Marisa Covey, DVM	84	162
2	Marley Winston, DVM	60	92
3	Wayne Dalton, DVM	32	59
DK	David Kyle, DVM	12	35

NOTE: It is a possibility that a new client and/or patient can be seen by more than one doctor within this date range.

FIGURE 20-2 Sample new clients and patients report. (Courtesy IntraVet, Dublin, Ohio.)

Client Surveys

Client surveys are an easy monitoring solution to understand the satisfaction and level of client comfort with the services the practice provides (Figure 20-5). Clients maintain the business; therefore it is imperative to make sure they are satisfied and perceive the value of the service provided. If clients are unsatisfied, practices want to be notified and given the opportunity to address the problem. Hospitals do not want to lose clients or have negative comments made about them throughout the community. It is very important to strive for a high level of satisfaction from every client.

Compliance Rate

Monitoring client compliance rates is useful in many ways. If clients are accepting recommendations, then the staff is doing an excellent job of educating clients and clients perceive the value in the services that are advised. Second, client compliance drives profits. The client relationship has already been established, and it is essential to maintain that relationship. It is easier to maintain relationships than to build new ones. Compliance reports should include reminder compliance as well as the profit centers the practice has chosen to monitor (Figure 20-6).

Date	Due Date	Payee	Category	Amount Due	Balance	Check#
1/8/09	1/21/09	Merial	Drugs/Supplies	$4567.09	0	1225
1/8/09	1/27/09	Wells Fargo	Equip Payment	$423.00	$4567.98	1226
1/8/09	1/25/09	Citibank	Drugs/Supplies	$17,245.98	0	1227
1/8/09	1/29/09	Electric Co	Utilities	$678.98	0	1228
1/8/09	1/27/09	City Gas	Utilities	$69.07	0	1229
1/8/09	1/25/09	Qwest	Telephone	$457.97	0	1230
1/25/09	2/1/09	Ledger Fin	Mortgage	$2398.08	$255,789.78	1267
2/1/09	2/22/09	Verizon	Telephone	$237.98	0	1289
2/8/09	1/21/09	Merial	Drugs/Supplies	$234.98	0	1345
2/8/09	1/27/09	Wells Fargo	Equip Payment	$423.00	$4123.90	1346
2/8/09	1/25/09	Citibank	Drugs/Supplies	$16,715.54	0	1347
2/8/09	1/29/09	Electric Co	Utilities	$648.01	0	1348
2/8/09	1/27/09	City Gas	Utilities	$89.06	0	1349
2/8/09	1/25/09	Qwest	Telephone	$343.67	0	1350

FIGURE 20-3 Sample accounts payable ledger.

Accounts Receivable Report

ABC Veterinary Hospital   **Accounts Receivable**

Total 30 days past due:	$1896.51
Total 60 days past due:	$1455.07
Total 90 days past due:	$3661.32
Total past due:	**$7012.90**
Total current balance:	$4652.79
Total net receivables:	**$11,665.69**
Total billing fees:	$78.00
Total interest charges:	$125.49
Total number of statements printed: 52	

Balance forward on transactions ON and BEFORE: 9/23/09
Printed statements as of: 10/23/09

FIGURE 20-4 Sample accounts receivable report.

Inventory of Equipment

It is very important to keep a list of equipment owned by the practice along with the purchase date and original purchase price. This is excellent for taxation purposes and also aids the practice if the equipment is stolen or damaged by fire or other natural causes. Serial numbers and model numbers may also be added for security and act as a quick reference when looking up information for warranty purposes.

Figure 20-7 lists equipment that was purchased before and after the practice manager began a capital inventory list. Anesthesia machine #1 was purchased before the list was developed. However, the model number and serial number are available for reference in case a fire or theft ever occurs. Anesthesia machine #2 was purchased in December 2003 for $400 as one unit. This is valuable information, along with the name of the manufacturer, in case a machine malfunction occurs and warranty dates come into question. A column could be added for warranty expiration dates, which would also help the practice manager.

Inventory on Hand

Current inventory reports should be accessible at any time. Inventory is recorded as an asset and contributes to factors included on financial reports.

Client Survey

We appreciate your business at ABC Veterinary Clinic and value your suggestions for improvement. Please take a few moments to fill out our survey and return it to the hospital.

Please rate the following questions from 1 (superior) to 5 (unacceptable).

I received an appointment that was convenient for me.	1 2 3 4 5
The hospital was clean when I arrived.	1 2 3 4 5
The receptionist acknowledged me immediately.	1 2 3 4 5
The veterinary technician was friendly.	1 2 3 4 5
The veterinary technician was knowledgeable.	1 2 3 4 5
The veterinarian was friendly.	1 2 3 4 5
The veterinarian was knowledgeable.	1 2 3 4 5
I received materials to take home and review.	1 2 3 4 5
My pet received exceptional care.	1 2 3 4 5
The staff cares about my pet.	1 2 3 4 5
The services are reasonably priced.	1 2 3 4 5

What can we do to improve our services for you? _____

_____

_____

_____

If one of our team members provided exceptional care today, please let us know so that we may recognize that person: _____

_____

_____

_____

_____

FIGURE 20-5 Sample client survey.

Recommendation and Compliance Report   **ABC Animal Hospital**

For Period 1/1/09 - 12/31/09

Code	Description	# of Recommendations	# of Compliance	(%)
R0001	Vaccinations	1265	965	(76)
R002	Heartworm Test	1600	1500	(94)
R003	Heartworm Prevention	1600	1000	(63)
R004	Dental Prophylaxis	1456	920	(63)
R005	Pre-Anesthetic Profiles	1500	880	(59)

FIGURE 20-6 Sample compliance report.

Product	Name	Manufacturer	Purchase Date/Price	Model Number	Serial Number
Anal Gland Excision Kit		Jorgenson		J-101	
Anesthesia Machine #1	Anesthesia Machine #1	Matrix		VMS	6380
Anesthesia Vaporizer #1	Anesthesia Vaporizer #1	Cyprane LTD			300437
Anesthesia Machine #2	Anesthesia Machine #2	Matrix	12/24/2003		SN14989
Anesthesia Vaporizer #2	Anesthesia Vaporizer #2	Vet Tech 4	12/24/03, $400 for both	100F	SN BASPOX7
Aspirator	Schuco Vac	Schuco		130	49500008498
Autoclave	Tuttanauer Autoclave	Tuttanauer	04/02/02, $2600	2340M	2110582
Bird Scale		Pelouze		PE5	
Camera	Digital Camera	HP	Aug 2003, $177.52	Photosmart 320	CN318111DG
Cast Cutter		Stryker		9002-210	8H8
Cautery Unit	AA Cautery	Jorgenson		J313	
Centrifuge	MS Centrifuge MicroHCT	Damon/IEC Division		MB	2513
Centrifuge	Sta-o-Spin	Stat-o-Spin	3/14/06, $1026.83 Butler	V0901.22	607V90111962
Centrifuge (lab)	Cinaseal	Vulcon Tech		C56C	6840
Clippers	Speed Feed	DVM	12/15/04, $91		
Clippers Cordless	Oaster	Butler		78400-01A	
Clippers Cordless	Oaster	Butler		78400-01A	
Clippers Cordless	Oaster	Butler		78400-01A	
Credit Card Terminal					
Credit Card Terminal	Care Credit				SN 207-397-407
Copier	Cannon			PC 940	NVX37080
Dental Machine	Ultrasonic Scaler/Motor Pack	Delmarva			C028-647
Doppler, BP	Mini Dop ES 100VX	Hadeco	11/2000, $800		SN-00090054
Doppler Probe		Jorgenson			
Doppler Ultrasound	Grafco Mini Doppler			4070	
Dremel Unit		Craftsman		5 Speed	
ECG PAM	VM8000PAM Cardiac Monitor	Technology Transfer	12/10/00, $2775	VM8000	SN V04408
ECG Printer PAM		Technology Transfer	12/10/2000	930	1029
ECG Biolog		QRS Diagnostic	9/2006 DVM Solutions $2735		2004-054237
ECG Printer Biolog			Came with Biolog	Brother HL-207	U61230M5J5
Glucometer	One Touch Ultra	Walgreens			RHW4E23Ft
Home Again Scanner		Schering Plough			SN 070535
Hair Dryer					
ECG Surgery	KENZ ECG 103	KENZ	GW Gift		9509-2815
IDEXX Electrolytes	VET LYTE	IDEXX	Aug. 2000		U15.9976
IDEXX Lasercyte	Lasercyte	IDEXX	Jun. 2006	93-30002-01	DXBP005586
IDEXX Vet Test	Vet Test 8000	IDEXX	08/01/00, $2700		OA26949
IDEXX Server				PCNE	H1BFQ91
IDEXX Printer				HP Deskjet 5650	MY45F4NOHI

FIGURE 20-7 Sample capital inventory.

Inventory Sold Within a Given Period

Sales of products and services must be reported on a monthly basis for sales tax purposes.

Number of Active Clients

The number of active clients in a practice is a benchmark number and allows comparison with other practices in the region. The definition of *active* can vary from practice to practice; therefore it is much more effective to measure from year to year for the same practice. If the number of active clients is low, this may indicate the need for further internal and external marketing techniques. Internal techniques such as reminder systems should be evaluated for effectiveness, and external techniques may be developed. See Chapter 10 for more internal and external marketing tips.

PRACTICE POINT The number of active clients may indicate excellent internal marketing techniques.

Number of Employees and Total Number of Hours Worked per Payroll Period

Payroll is important to monitor because overtime can eat practice profits. A payroll budget should be created, allowing raises when needed with flexibility to add additional team members if needed (Figure 20-8). Payroll and payroll taxes are a large portion of expenses and must be monitored closely. Payroll budgets are discussed at length later in this chapter and include estimation for taxes. Overtime is not estimated; team member schedules and hours should be monitored closely to cut this undesirable expense.

Number of New Clients

Some practices want to monitor the growth of the practice in new clients and compare numbers on a month-to-year basis. The number of new clients per year can be affected by the type of service offered, species, demographics, and external marketing. If a marketing technique has been used, this is also an efficient way

Payroll Summary

Name	Average Hours per 2-week period
Clint Stover	80
Stoney Almarez	40
Katie Soules	30
Brooke Miale	30
Brittany Wilson	54
Sabrina Montoya	72
Cerelia Brice	80
Cat Valdivia	75
Jenny Larsen	74
Chris Vega	80
Tammy Smith	76
John Garcia	80

FIGURE 20-8 Sample payroll summary.

to monitor how effective the technique has been. If the number of new clients is low, an external marketing plan should be initiated to help increase the number.

> **PRACTICE POINT** The number of new clients may indicate an excellent external marketing technique as well.

Taxes Owed

Taxes must be paid on a monthly and/or quarterly basis, depending on what type of tax is due. Amounts should be calculated at the first of each month, with the scheduled dates of payment.

Tax ledgers can be beneficial when paying monthly bills, preventing overspending. Quarterly taxes can be shockingly high and must be budgeted for when paying current accounts payable. Figure 20-9 lists the history of tax payments as well as those due for the month of April 2009

Team Member Surveys

The team is the primary asset to the practice. It is essential to understand team members' thoughts and concerns and address them in a timely fashion. The team *is* the practice; every member contributes to the success of the practice. They relate to clients on a daily basis and have valuable input regarding clients' perceptions and values. Surveys should be conducted one to two times per year and should not coincide with employee evaluations.

Team member surveys should vary by position. Figure 20-10 gives examples for veterinary technician responsibilities. The survey could also include how team members value other positions within the practice as well as how they feel each department completes its tasks. Each department and/or position affects other departments or positions in a practice and must be considered.

CREATING A BUDGET

A budget is a critical management tool that can be used for strategic planning. The word *budget* has been given a bad name; many people feel that budgets are a number-crunching game. Instead, a budget should be considered a useful planning tool that helps ensure practice success. Budgets should be created for both revenue and expenses; revenue budgets are developed to reach strategically planned goals, whereas expense budgets are used to determine where the cash went and to create goals to reduce costs where possible. More information on revenue budgeting is given later in this chapter.

> **PRACTICE POINT** A budget is an excellent management tool that is underutilized in practice.

Expense budgets are also known as *cash flow budgets.* Budgets can be used to determine the practice's ability to produce cash flow strictly from operations, create internal resources necessary for expansion and growth, allow for the evaluation of equipment purchases, provide a return profit for the owners, and discover unfavorable trends that require intervention. To predict expenses, practices must also be able to predict revenue; therefore both revenue and expenses must be evaluated when creating a budget.

Two main categories exist when creating a cash flow budget. These categories are further broken down into subcategories to make comparisons, projections, and evaluations.

Cost of Goods Sold and Cost of Professional Services

Cost of goods sold (COGS) is also known as cost of professional services (COPS); these phrases can be used interchangeably. COGS or COPS represents the direct costs associated with producing a service or product. It covers the direct costs of patient care and product sales, drugs, supplies, and laboratory fees (Box 20-2 and Figure 20-11).

The second category, general administrative costs, covers all executive, organizational, and managerial expenses related to the management of the practice versus delivering patient care. General administrative costs are broken down into further subcategories to isolate discrepancies and develop a plan for repair. Payroll is placed in the general administrative category because it represents a common cost that is spread to all areas of the practice, not just patient care.

Fixed and Variable Costs

General administrative costs or expenses may be fixed or variable. Fixed expenses and/or costs are those that do not fluctuate with volume, whereas a variable expense

Date	Due Date	Payee	Category	Amount Due	Check#
1/7/09	1/15/08	IRS	Payroll	$4596.95	1567
1/15/09	1/25/09	NM Tax & Rev	Payroll	$1897.00	1599
1/15/09	1/25/09	NM Tax & Rev	Sales	$4567.98	1600
1/15/09	1/25/09	NM Dept of Lab	Unemployment	$56.98	1601
1/15/09	1/25/09	NM Tax & Rev	Work. Comp	$567.98	1602
2/7/09	2/15/08	IRS	Payroll	$3456.95	1631
2/15/09	2/25/09	NM Tax & Rev	Payroll	$1546.00	1632
2/15/09	2/25/09	NM Tax & Rev	Sales	$3245.90	1633
3/7/09	3/15/08	IRS	Payroll	$4876.35	1654
3/15/09	3/25/09	NM Tax & Rev	Payroll	$2245.85	1655
3/15/09	3/25/09	NM Tax & Rev	Sales	$4563.91	1656
4/7/09	4/15/08	IRS	Payroll	$4356.98	1689
4/15/09	4/25/09	NM Tax & Rev	Payroll	$2234.97	_____
4/15/09	4/25/09	NM Tax & Rev	Sales	$4456.98	_____
4/15/09	4/25/09	NM Dept of Lab	Unemployment	$68.97	_____
4/15/09	4/25/09	NM Tax & Rev	Work. Comp	$612.45	_____

FIGURE 20-9 Sample tax ledger.

What Would You Do/Not Do?

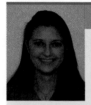

Shelly, a long-time office manager, has recently attended continuing education classes and has learned the importance of creating and maintaining a budget for the practice. She has never created a budget, as the owners of the practice (in business for 20 years) have never needed one. The practice has "functioned fine" without one, so why start now? After attending the continuing education, Shelly feels that she can make a drastic impact on the practice if a budget is created and maintained.

What Should Shelly Do?
First, Shelly should develop a proposal stating why she believes the budget could make a change for the practice and why it is worth her time to develop one. Shelly may need to attend further classes on the development of a budget before making the recommendation. She should not make the recommendation if she cannot follow through with the proposal. A practice budget may be developed, allowing her to discover her weaknesses and learn how to correct them before creating a permanent budget for the practice.

and/or cost fluctuates directly with volume. Accounting is a fixed cost that rarely changes. The accountant charges a set fee each month for maintaining payroll and taxes. Office supplies are a variable cost; the amount used may increase or decrease with the number of patients seen. Other operating expenses that may be fixed or variable are payroll, payroll taxes, utilities, rent, insurance, repairs, and maintenance. COGS is a variable expense because it increases or decreases with volume (Box 20-3).

PRACTICE POINT Fixed expenses include rent, mortgage, building insurance, and utilities.

Direct and Indirect Expenses
Direct costs or expenses are directly related to patient care and can be traced to a specific client or specific profit center. Direct costs may include drugs, supplies, and foods. Indirect costs are those that are associated with providing patient care but that cannot be traced to

a specific profit center. Indirect costs include uniforms, equipment depreciation, and holding and ordering costs associated with product orders. Indirect costs can be as high as 45% of direct costs, higher if internal theft is a problem.

PRACTICE POINT Indirect expenses include uniforms and holding and ordering costs.

Steps of a Budget
First, it is important to ensure that the practice has an adequate program to help with the budget process. QuickBooks and Peachtree are excellent programs that include a preestablished budgeting program. Microsoft Excel spreadsheets allow data to be exported into the tables to create a budget. Creating a budget by hand can be overwhelming because subcategories can fill as many as 30 to 40 line items; therefore an effective software program must be implemented. In a software spreadsheet

---

Team Member Survey

Please give your honest, most objective assessment of projects and ideas over the past 6 months.

Please rate the following from 1 (poor) to 5 (outstanding). Assign NA if not applicable.

1. Clients understand the importance of dentals.   1 2 3 4 5

2. Clients understand the importance of yearly exams   1 2 3 4 5

3. Clients appreciate the education the practice provides.   1 2 3 4 5

4. The practice appointments run on time.   1 2 3 4 5

5. Doctors value the clients' time.   1 2 3 4 5

6. Technicians value the clients' time.   1 2 3 4 5

7. Technicians are trained adequately.   1 2 3 4 5

8. Technicians share duties equally.   1 2 3 4 5

9. Doctors value the technicians.   1 2 3 4 5

10. Duties are delegated equally and adequately.   1 2 3 4 5

What areas of the practice need improvement? _____

_____

What areas of the practice are the strongest? Weakest? _____

_____

What is the most satisfying aspect of this job? _____

_____

What can you do to help increase client satisfaction and compliance? _____

_____

What can you do to help your team members improve themselves over the next 12 months?

_____

_____

List any suggestions, comments, or improvements that you feel would help benefit the practice.

_____

_____

_____

FIGURE 20-10 Sample team member survey.

model, a 1% increase projected to gross income can flow through the entire expense categories and change them automatically while providing a new calculation of the estimated net profit. This will take much less time in spreadsheet fashion as opposed to completing the calculations by hand. Although a basic budget could be prepared by hand, making adjustments to the budget or preparing a breakdown of a yearly projection into monthly or quarterly mini-budgets can become unreasonable. Computerized spreadsheets allow the visualization and results of countless changes, assumptions, and trials.

Second, take a closer look at the relation of specific expenses to gross income. By having a few years of data, what is normal for the practice can be compared with benchmark data. The previous year's complete financial statements plus any results from the current year of operations will be needed. If financial statements are

---

Box 20-2 | Budgets: The Big Picture

COGS/COPS
- Laboratory supplies
- Radiology supplies
- Treatment supplies
- Pharmacy supplies
- Medications
- Foods

GENERAL ADMINISTRATION
- Payroll
  - Payroll taxes
  - Health insurance for employees
- Occupancy expenses
  - Utilities
  - Rent/mortgage
  - Building maintenance
  - Insurance
  - Property tax
- Equipment
  - Repairs and maintenance
  - Vehicle

- Administration
  - Advertising
  - Bank and credit card fees
  - Dues/subscriptions
  - Office supplies
  - Meals/entertainment
  - Professional services
- Accountant
- Lawyer
- Telephone

REVENUE
- Professional fees
- Pharmacy center
- Laboratory center
- Vaccination center
- Dental center
- Radiology center
- Food/retail center
- Other

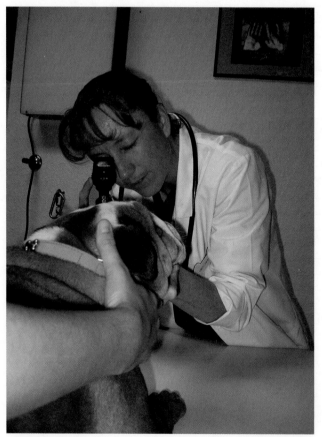

FIGURE 20-11 The cost of professional services applies to the direct costs associated with producing a service, such as a general health exam.

Box 20-3 | Fixed and Variable Expenses

FIXED
- Advertising
- Building maintenance
- Employee benefits
- Rent, mortgage
- Licenses, dues, and subscriptions
- Property tax
- Utilities

VARIABLE
- Drugs
- Laboratory fees
- Supplies
- Payroll

---

not available, reconciled checkbook registers will suffice for the expense portion of the budget. Reports will need to be generated from the practice management software to help create the revenue budget.

> **PRACTICE POINT** Expenses must be entered into the correct categories each time.

It is critical that expenses are listed in correct subcategories when they are entered. Occasionally there are inconsistencies as to how an expense is entered. Perhaps the purchase of computer-generated reminder cards were classified as office supplies one month, computer supplies another month, and nonmedical supplies in a third month. A decision should be made in cases such as this to allow each expense to be consistently classified into the same account.

Computerized check-writing programs help provide consistent classification of expenses since many of them retain the specific transaction. When a recurring payee is used, the computer automatically classifies that payee to a specific account based on the previous transaction. Such programs quickly and easily provide profit and loss reports, the underlying data for the budget, after the end-of-month and checkbook reconciliation. An in-house profit and loss report is more than adequate for providing the historical information that forms the basis of the budget. The annual financial statements provided by an accountant are also useful but will never be as quickly available and do not allow the monthly assessment needed to successfully manage a budget.

Third, budgeting requires the reassessment of the present fee structure, evaluation of the total gross practice income, and a plan of how to achieve the necessary growth to result in adequate profits.

There are many methods for establishing budgets. Budgets can be established for the entire practice or for small segments of the practice. For example, where staffing costs have historically been higher than normal in the practice, a budget for different segments of support staff, including receptionists, technicians, or veterinarians may be established. Likewise, mixed practices may benefit from budgeting for the different segments of the practice, which likely have different profit margins.

There are several budgeting methods that work in veterinary practice; the "top-down" method appears to be used the most. Expenses from the previous year's budget are forwarded to the following year's budget, allowing the input of changes needed to reach the goals established for the following year. For example, if the COGS in Figure 20-12 is 17.1% (column 4) of the gross revenue ($1 million) for 2008, 17.1% will then be forwarded to the projected 2009 budget. It is at this time that the percentage can be changed based on the goals established for the following year's budget. It should be remembered that gross revenue is the total money received before expenses or taxes.

> **PRACTICE POINT** Gross income is the amount of income received before expenses and taxes are paid.

The cost of supplies will increase in the new year; therefore the increase needs to be projected and budgeted. An average increase of 4.8% will cover the increase for most items. Figure 20-13 highlights the 4.8% projected increase in expenses for the 2008 fiscal year. If a payroll budget has been created, projected values for payroll, payroll tax, and benefit contributions may be added for a more accurate projection.

The green column in Figure 20-13 demonstrates actual expenses incurred in 2008. The yellow column adds 4.8% and calculates the new, predicted expense. The blue column gives the monthly projected value.

> **PRACTICE POINT** Profits must be budgeted for as well as expenses.

Last, but not least, profits must be budgeted as well. Remaining profits also use the top-down approach, using previous percentages in the future budget. If profits are inadequate to achieve goals, additional assessments are needed and a price increase for professional services may be warranted. The goal is to obtain the necessary profit to allow adequate return on investment and reinvestment to the practice. See the section "Analyzing Profits" later in this chapter for additional information.

The Spreadsheet

Creating a spreadsheet is easy and exciting. The first column should begin with the descriptions of each line item: gross revenue, costs of providing veterinary services (COGS or COPS), including drugs, anesthesia, surgery cost, dentistry, radiology, and so forth, and general and administrative expenses. The second column contains the numeric amount of each line item. Figure 20-12 shows columns 1 through 4.

In the third column, use the spreadsheet to create linked formulas, relating each revenue and expense item as a percentage of the total practice gross revenue. For example, the cost of drugs is shown as a percentage of gross revenue by creating a mathematical formula representing total dollars of drugs divided by total dollars of gross revenue. A similar formula is created for each revenue and expense item shown in the third column. For example, the cost of medical supplies is $69,829.93. This figure, divided by $1 million = 0.07 × 100 = 7%. Remember, to express a value as a percentage, it must be multiplied by 100.

The reason for this approach is to create a spreadsheet that will automatically update the percentages whenever changes are made to the absolute values for income and expense. Next year, when the budget spreadsheet is updated, new data will be added. All related percentages will be calculated by the spreadsheet because of the preestablished formulas.

> **PRACTICE POINT** Microsoft Excel, QuickBooks, and Peachtree are excellent software applications for budget creation.

The next step is to begin a projection forward to the next financial period. An expected rate of growth is projected for the hospital based on historical gross revenue increases. At the top of the revenue spreadsheet, enter

EXPENSES Jan-Dec 2008 ABC Animal Hospital			
Revenue Jan-Dec		**$1,000,000.00**	**%**
Column1	Column 2	Column 3	Col 4
COGS	Medical Supplies	$ 69,829.93	7.0
	Pharmacy	$ 79,034.84	7.9
	Radiology	$ 1,890.43	0.2
	Surgery	$ 1,984.54	0.2
	Dentals	$ 457.65	0.0
	Foods	$ 15,839.98	1.6
	Misc.	$ 1,674.87	0.2
		$ 170,712.24	**17.1**
Gen Admin	Accounting	$ 7,441.82	0.7
	Advertising	$ 9,874.09	1.0
	Bills		
	Cable/Satellite Television	$ 600.00	0.1
	Cell Phone	$ 2,456.87	0.2
	Electricity	$ 4,423.98	0.4
	Natural Gas/Water/Sewer	$ 3,657.98	0.4
	Online/Internet Service	$ 252.89	0.0
	Telephone	$ 4,897.09	0.5
	Building Maintenance	$ 2,398.09	0.2
	Business Expense	$ 1,427.88	0.1
	Check Machine Fees	$ 2,477.28	0.2
	Client Care (Flowers)	$ 1,698.05	0.2
	Continuing Education	$ 3,000.00	0.3
	Credit Card Fees	$ 5,600.00	0.6
	Donation	$ 1,500.00	0.2
	Equipment Maintenance	$ 1,529.88	0.2
	Equipment Purchase	$ 4,800.00	0.5
	Insurance-Health	$ 18,000.00	1.8
	Insurance-Liability	$ 3,000.00	0.3
	Insurance-Property	$ 769.00	0.1
	Insurace-Workers Comp	$ 2,341.76	0.2
	License	$ 1,096.00	0.1
	Loan	$ 6,720.97	0.7
	Mortgage	$ 16,560.76	1.7
	Office Supplies	$ 2,105.88	0.2
	Payroll-Non-DVM	$ 209,092.00	20.9
	Payroll-DVM	$ 227,990.00	22.8
	Refund-Client	$ 1,568.98	0.2
	Reimbursement-Staff	$ 691.87	0.1
	Shipping	$ 1,754.65	0.2
	SIRA	$ 13,112.46	1.3
	Staff Care (B-day cakes)	$ 450.00	0.0
	Taxes-Payroll	$ 55,727.93	5.6
	Taxes-Sales	$ 62,500.00	6.3
	Unemployment	$ 7,176.00	0.7
	Workers Comp-State	$ 924.00	0.1
	Total Expenses	$ 860,330.40	**69.0**
	Revenue − Expenses = PROFIT	**$ 139,669.60**	14.0

FIGURE 20-12 An example of expenses for 2008.

Projected Revenue $1,100,000.00
Jan-Dec 2009

		2008 Actual $	%		4.8% increase in COGS and GA			Per Month	
					Total	%		Total	
COGS	Medical Supplies	$ 69,829.93	6.3		$ 3,351.84	$ 73,181.77	6.7	$ 6,098.48	
	Pharmacy	$ 79,829.93	7.3		$ 3,831.84	$ 83,661.77	7.6	$ 6,971.81	
	Radiology	$ 1,890.43	0.2		$ 90.74	$ 1,981.17	0.2	$ 165.10	
	Surgery	$ 1,984.54	0.2		$ 95.26	$ 2,079.80	0.2	$ 173.32	
	Dentals	$ 457.65	0.0		$ 21.97	$ 479.62	0.0	$ 39.97	
	Foods	$ 15,839.98	1.4		$ 760.32	$ 16,600.30	1.5	$ 1,383.36	
	Misc.	$ 1,674.87	0.2		$ 80.39	$ 1,755.26	0.2	$ 146.27	
Gen Admin	Accountant	$ 7,441.82	0.7		$ 357.21	$ 7,799.03	0.7	$ 649.92	
	Advertising	$ 9,874.09	0.9		$ 473.96	$ 10,348.05	0.9	$ 862.34	
	Bills								
	Cable/Satellite TV	$ 600.00	0.1		$ 28.80	$ 628.80	0.1	$ 52.40	
	Cell Phone	$ 2,456.87	0.2		$ 117.93	$ 2,574.80	0.2	$ 214.57	
	Electricity	$ 4,423.98	0.4		$ 212.35	$ 4,636.33	0.4	$ 386.36	
	Natural Gas/Water/Sewer	$ 3,657.98	0.3		$ 175.58	$ 3,833.56	0.3	$ 319.46	
	Online/Internet Service	$ 252.89	0.0		$ 12.14	$ 265.03	0.0	$ 22.09	
	Telephone	$ 4,897.09	0.4		$ 235.06	$ 5,132.15	0.5	$ 427.68	
	Building Maintenance	$ 2,398.09	0.2		$ 115.11	$ 2,513.20	0.2	$ 209.43	
	Business Expense	$ 1,427.88	0.1		$ 68.54	$ 1,496.42	0.1	$ 124.70	
	Check Machine Fees	$ 2,477.28	0.2		$ 118.91	$ 2,596.19	0.2	$ 216.35	
	Client Care (Flowers)	$ 1,698.05	0.2		$ 81.51	$ 1,779.56	0.2	$ 148.30	
	Continuing Education	$ 3,000.00	0.3		$ 144.00	$ 3,144.00	0.3	$ 262.00	
	Credit Card Fees	$ 5,600.00	0.5		$ 268.80	$ 5,868.80	0.5	$ 489.07	
	Donation	$ 1,500.00	0.1		$ 72.00	$ 1,572.00	0.1	$ 131.00	
	Equipment Maintenance	$ 1,529.88	0.1		$ 73.43	$ 1,603.31	0.1	$ 133.61	
	Equipment Purchase	$ 4,800.00	0.4		$ 230.40	$ 5,030.40	0.5	$ 419.20	
	Insurance-Health	$ 18,000.00	1.6		$ 864.00	$ 24,000.00	2.2	$ 2,000.00	
	Insurance-Liability	$ 3,000.00	0.3		$ 144.00	$ 3,144.00	0.3	$ 262.00	
	Insurance-Property	$ 769.00	0.1		$ 36.91	$ 805.91	0.1	$ 67.16	
	Insurace-Workers Comp	$ 2,341.76	0.2		$ 112.40	$ 2,454.16	0.2	$ 204.51	
	License	$ 1,096.00	0.1		$ 52.61	$ 1,148.61	0.1	$ 95.72	
	Loan	$ 6,720.97	0.6		$ 322.61	$ 7,043.58	0.6	$ 586.96	
	Mortgage	$ 16,560.76	1.5		$ 794.92	$ 17,355.68	1.6	$ 1,446.31	
	Oxygen	$ 2,495.88	0.2		$ 119.80	$ 2,615.68	0.2	$ 217.97	
	Payroll-Non-DVM	$205,198.04	18.7		$ 9,849.51	$248,508.00	22.6	$20,709.00	
	Payroll-DVM	$227,908.71	20.7		$10,939.62	$238,000.00	21.6	$19,833.33	
	Refund-Client	$ 1,568.98	0.1		$ 75.31	$ 1,644.29	0.1	$ 137.02	
	Reimburement-Staff	$ 691.87	0.1		$ 33.21	$ 725.08	0.1	$ 60.42	
	Shipping	$ 1,754.65	0.2		$ 84.22	$ 1,838.87	0.2	$ 153.24	
	SIRA	$ 15,946.00	1.4		$ 765.41	$ 14,595.24	1.3	$ 1,216.27	
	Staff Care (B-day cakes)	$ 450.00	0.0		$ 21.60	$ 471.60	0.0	$ 39.30	
	Taxes-Payroll	$ 67,748.70	6.2		$ 3,251.94	$ 61,928.43	5.6	$ 5,160.70	
	Taxes-Sales	$ 62,500.00	5.7		$ 3,000.00	$ 68,750.00	6.3	$ 5,729.17	
	Unemployment	$ 7,176.00	0.7		$ 344.45	$ 7,520.45	0.7	$ 626.70	
	Workers Comp-State	$ 924.00	0.1		$ 44.35	$ 968.35	0.1	$ 80.70	
	Total Expenses	$872,394.55	79.3			$944,079.24	85.8	$78,673.27	
	Revenue − Expenses = PROFIT					$155,920.76	14.2		

FIGURE 20-13 An example of predicted 2009 expenses.

Revenue Centers 2008 ABC Animal Hospital			Projected Rate of Growth: 10% 10% = $1,100,000.00		2009	
Column 1	Column 2	Column 3	Column 4	Column 5	Column 6
Professional Fees	$ 200,000.00	20%		$ 20,000.00	$ 220,000.00	20%
Surgery Fees	$ 250,000.00	25%		$ 25,000.00	$ 275,000.00	25%
Pharmacy Fees	$ 250,000.00	25%		$ 25,000.00	$ 275,000.00	25%
Laboratory Fees	$ 200,000.00	20%		$ 20,000.00	$ 220,000.00	20%
Vaccination Fees	$ 15,000.00	1.50%		$ 1,500.00	$ 16,500.00	1.50%
Dental Fees	$ 20,000.00	2%		$ 2,000.00	$ 22,000.00	2%
Food Sales	$ 50,000.00	5%		$ 5,000.00	$ 55,000.00	5%
Retail Sales	$ 10,000.00	1%		$ 1,000.00	$ 11,000.00	1%
Other Income	$ 5,000.00	0.50%		$ 500.00	$ 5,500.00	0.50%
	$ 1,000,000.00	100%			$ 1,100,000.00	100%

FIGURE 20-14 An example of revenue centers for 2008.

a description, "Projected Rate of Growth." In the cell adjacent to the description, insert a percentage increase such as 5% or 10%. This number can be changed as assumptions are made regarding growth of the practice (see Figure 20-13).

In the fifth column, gross income is projected for the following year as a formula, multiplying the current gross income (column 2) by the projected rate of growth (10%). If the cells are referenced correctly, any change in the percentage growth rate changes the gross income projected for the upcoming year. Figure 20-14 lists the revenue centers for 2008, along with the practice's predicted 10% growth for the 2009 fiscal year. ABC Animal Hospital historically has a 10% increase each year. Each revenue center's income is multiplied by 10% to predict the 2009 revenue.

Areas of Expense

When creating budgets, practices may choose different categories in which to place expenses. The most important factor is to place the same expenses in the same category every time they are entered. Wrong placement of expenses can create a cash flow gap or an unexplained change. It is important to be consistent. Below are a few suggested categories; practices can add and change as needed to suit their needs.

- Accounting
- Advertising
  - Brochures, business cards, Yellow Pages ads
- Benefits
  - Health and liability insurance, dues, contributions to retirement fund
- Building maintenance
  - Roof repair, heating/cooling/plumbing repair
- Continuing education
- Cleaning supplies
  - Bleach, paper towels, toilet paper
- Donations
  - Nonprofit organizations

- Equipment
  - Maintenance of existing
  - Purchasing of new
- Gifts
- Insurance
  - Building
- Inventory
  - Pharmacy, supplies, therapeutic diets
- Lawyer
- Mortgage/rent
- Office supplies
  - Pens, paper
- Payroll
- Staff meetings
- Taxes
  - Payroll tax
  - Sales tax
- Uniforms
- Utilities
  - Water, sewer, gas, electricity, trash, cable

These categories allow for gross examination of all transactions made. Subcategories can then be placed into categories as needed for the financial reports. Payroll tax is an example that can be changed with practice preference. It can be placed in the payroll category or in the tax category.

EQUIPMENT BUDGET

When creating a budget for equipment, two topics need to be kept in mind: the maintenance of existing equipment and the purchase of new equipment. Existing equipment may need repairs or there may be maintenance agreements that must be kept. When purchasing new equipment, several issues must be addressed:

- Is the equipment completely new, or is it replacing an existing piece of equipment?
- Is the new piece of equipment going to provide improved, more accurate results compared with the piece it is replacing?

- Is the money used to purchase the new equipment being used in the most efficient manner?
- How will the equipment be paid for? Cash? Leasing? Financing?
- If the practice is going to finance the capital, what is the interest rate? Can a better rate be found elsewhere? How much are the doctors going to use this piece of equipment?
- What will the client charge be?
- How long will it take to achieve the payback period?
- How long will it take to make a profit on the equipment?

> **PRACTICE POINT** Equipment costs should be included in a budget.

If a budget has been created in advance, cash should be set aside for an equipment purchase. This is the smartest, most economical way to pay for equipment because practices will not accumulate application fees, finance charges, or late penalties if a late payment is sent.

Equipment leasing should be used with caution because tax is commonly built in to the payment. Interest rates tend to be higher for leases, and a balloon payment may be due at the end of the lease period if the practice wants to keep the equipment. Other options include returning the equipment at the end of the lease, which leaves the practice without any equipment. This may be of benefit to some practices if they want to purchase a new and updated piece of equipment at the end of the lease. If a piece of equipment has a short life and is replaced with an update quickly, leasing may be the best option. However, most pieces of equipment in veterinary medicine hold value and provide service for a long period, especially when correct maintenance and repair schedules are followed. Companies offer low payments that entice practices to lease equipment; however, all options should be examined before making a decision.

> **PRACTICE POINT** Equipment should be purchased with cash when possible, not financed.

When borrowing money, practices must consider the financing rate and the length of time the money will be borrowed. Cash flow projections of revenue and expenses should be developed as well as a payback plan. Credit lines should not be used for equipment purchases because they generally have to be fully paid within a year and are better to leave for emergency withdrawals if needed. Equipment loan lengths should not exceed the expected life of the piece of equipment, normally 5 to 7 years.

> **PRACTICE POINT** A break-even analysis will determine the point at which the equipment will pay for itself.

A break-even analysis should be completed before purchasing the equipment. The break-even point is the point at which the sales of the service will cover all costs related to the equipment, including maintenance, supplies, and the capital itself. A break-even point can be determined by dividing the total cost of the equipment by the cost to the client. The resulting number gives the number of times the service must be performed to break even. For example, a practice wants to purchase a digital dental radiograph unit. The unit originally costs $11,000. The practice will charge the client $88 for a set of radiographs. The cost associated with taking the radiographs is $22; this includes the technician's time to take the views and the veterinarian's time to interpret the views. $88 − $22 = $66. $11,000 divided by $66 equals 166.67 views; therefore 167 views must be taken to break even with a digital dental radiograph unit. If two dentals are completed on a daily basis, and both dentals have radiographs completed, it will take 83 business days to recover the cost of the equipment.

PAYROLL BUDGET

Payroll is the largest expense in the operating budget and, depending on the practice, can be considered a variable or fixed expense. Practices that are busy year-round and have a similar payroll each period can consider payroll a fixed expense. Practices that are busy in the summer and slow in the winter should consider payroll a variable expense because it changes with the revenue of the practice.

To help with budget estimations, a weighted hourly wage may be used for each employee. A weighted hourly wage takes the average of a team member's pay when a raise will be expected later in the fiscal year. The original pay plus the new pay divided by two gives the weighted hourly wage. For example, Clint currently makes $15 an hour and will receive a raise to $17 per hour in 6 months. Therefore his weighted hourly wage is $16. Table 20-1 lists the previous wages (gray columns) along with the weighted salary (yellow columns) to help establish a budget for the current fiscal year.

When developing a payroll budget, it should be remembered that not every employee will receive a raise every year. Raises should be based on team member skills and assets, not on length of employment. Some practices may give a cost-of-living raise; those who have achieved new skills and have proven competency should receive more.

Table 20-1   Sample Payroll Budget

						PAYROLL BUDGET 2008			
Col 1	Col 2	Col 3	Col 4	Col 5	Col 6	Col 7	Col 8	Col 9	Col 10
Position	Name	hr/wk	Curr. Wage	Weekly Payroll	Annual Payroll	Taxes W/held (6%)	Taxes Due From Employer ($56 + 6.2%)	Sum for Division	sIRA Cont./ Year (3%)
Tech	Clint S	40	$15	$600	$31,200	$1,979.64	$1,990.40	$89,700	$936.00
Tech	Katie S	15	$12	$180	$9,360	$593.89	$636.32		$280.80
Tech	Brooke M	15	$12	$180	$9,360	$593.89	$636.32		$280.80
Tech	Brittany W	15	$12	$180	$9,360	$593.89	$636.32		$280.80
Tech	Sabrina M	35	$11	$385	$20,020	$1,270.27	$1,297.24		$600.60
Tech	Fake	20	$10	$200	$10,400	$659.88	$700.80		$312.00
Recep	Cerelia B	40	$12	$480	$24,2960	$1,583.71	$1,603.52	$73,632	$748.80
Recep	Cat V	36	$11	$396	$20,592	$1,306.56	$1,332.70		$617.76
Recep	Jenny L	20	$10	$200	$10,400	$659.88	$700.80		$312.00
Recep	Chris V	34	$10	$340	$17,680	$1,121.80	$1,152.16		$530.40
Asst	Tammy S	20	$10	$200	$10,400	$659.88	$700.80	$45,760	$312.00
Asst	John G	40	$9	$360	$18,720	$1,187.78	$1,216.64		$561.60
Asst	Fake	40	$8	$320	$16,640	$1,055.81	$1,087.68		$499.20
DVM	Dr. M				$76,000	$4,822.20	$4,768.00	$227,990	$2,280.00
DVM	Dr. S				$81,000	$5,139.45	$5,078.00		$2,430.00
DVM	Dr. B				$70,990	$4,504.32	$4,457.38		$2,129.70
	Per year				$437,082	$27,732.85	27,995.08		$13,112.46
	Per mo				$36,423.50	$2,311.07	$2,332.92		$1,092.71

Tech, Technician; *Recep,* receptionist; *Asst,* Assistant; *Curr.,* current; *Cont.,* contribution; *Med/yr,* health insurance contribution per year; *Ann.,* annual; *Wt.,* Weighted.

> **PRACTICE POINT**   A payroll budget allows raises and bonuses for team members.

A maximum amount should be determined each year for payroll, allowing for raises, bonuses, and an allocation for new team members if needed. If the practice does not hire a new team member, the funds can be disbursed as a bonus to all employees. Team members can be ranked from most valuable to least valuable. Raises can be disbursed as management feels appropriate, reaching the amount set aside for the payroll budget. When estimating projected gross income increases, consider which individuals will help produce that gross and determine raises accordingly.

It should be remembered to review employees who receive minimum wage and keep abreast of the changes in minimum wage at both the federal and state levels. Both federal and state minimum wage amounts change frequently, and whichever is higher supersedes the other. Minimum wage employees may receive two raises per year and should be included in the payroll budget.

Overtime eats practice profits. Team members' schedules should be created with the intent to decrease the amount of overtime the practice has to pay. It is imperative to decrease labor costs by decreasing overtime. Team members must learn to work harder at completing tasks within a set amount of time, with the fewest team members needed to complete the tasks. Slow-moving, lazy team members are not an asset to the practice and should be replaced with fast-moving, motivated "10" employees.

To help create a payroll budget, the use of a Microsoft Excel spreadsheet is extremely beneficial (see

				PAYROLL BUDGET 2008					
Col 11	Col 12	Col 13	Col 14	Col 15	Col 16	Col 17	Col 18	Col 19	Col 20
Med/yr	Wt. Wage	Weekly Payoll	Ann. Payroll	Taxes W/held From Employee (6%)	Taxes W/held From Employer ($56 + 6.2%)	Sum for Division	sIRA Cont./yr (3%)	Med/yr	Liability
$3,600	$16	$640	$33,280	$2,111.62	$2,119.36	$101,660	$998.40	$4,800	
-	$13	$195	$10,140	$643.38	$684.68		$304.20	—	
-	$13	$195	$10,140	$643.38	$684.68		$304.20	—	
-	$13	$195	$10,140	$643.38	$684.68		$304.20	—	
$3,600	$14	$490	$25,480	$1,616.71	$1,635.76		$764.40	$4,800	
-	$12	$240	$12,480	$791.86	$829.76		$374.40	—	
-	$14	$560	$29,120	$1,847.66	$1,861.44	$91,728	873.60	—	
-	$13	$468	$24,336	$1,544.12	$1,564.83		$730.08	—	
-	$13	$260	$13,520	$857.84	$894.24		$405.60	—	
$3,600	$14	$476	$24,752	$1,570.51	$1,590.62		$742.56	$4,800	
-	$11	$220	$11,440	$725.87	$765.28	$55,120	$343.20	—	
$3,600	$11	$440	$22,880	$1,451.74	$1,474.56		$686.40	$4,800	
$3,600	$10	$400	$20,800	$1,319.76	$1,345.60		$624.00	$4,800	
			$79,000	$5,012.55	$4,954.00	$238,000	$2,370.00		$1,000
			$85,000	$5,393.25	$5,326.00		$2,550.00		$1,000
			$74,000	$4,$695.30	$4,644.00		$2,220.00		$1,000
$18,000			$486,508	$30,868.93	$31,059.50		$14,595.24	$24,000	$3,000
$1,500			$47,493	$3,013.43	$3033.23		$1,424.79	2000	$250

> **◎ PRACTICE POINT**　Management must control and prevent overtime.

Table 20-1). Employees should be listed (column 2) along with their start date, weighted hourly wage, and the projected number of work hours per week. By multiplying the weighted hourly wage (column 12) by the number of hours per week (column 3), a weekly budget is developed for that employee. Multiply the weekly dollar amount by 52 (the number of weeks per year) to determine an annual dollar amount (column 14). If employees are salaried, the above calculation can be skipped; simply list the annual salary. Benefits that have a dollar value can be listed, including retirement programs, health insurance, and liability insurance (columns 18, 19, and 20). Payroll taxes are listed (columns 15 and 16), and can easily be calculated as a percentage of the

employees' gross income. Columns can then be added, giving an annual total for each employee. The annual amount can be divided by 12 (12 months in a year), to determine the monthly payroll estimation and can be added into the monthly budget.

To create a payroll budget for a future team member, a fake name may be added to the payroll spreadsheet. Assumed weighted hourly wages can be added, along with benefits and taxes. This allows room in the budget if an additional team member must be added without exceeding the monthly payroll budget. Not all team members will have the same benefits or use health insurance provided by the practice. Veterinarians are the only team members with liability insurance; therefore several columns will be left blank.

If salary cost is more than anticipated, better staff utilization through improved scheduling may be an answer. Another solution is to increase revenues so that support staff cost, as a percentage of gross, stays in line with practice health.

Analyzing Profits

The bottom line should be the remaining profits after expenses have been subtracted from the revenue. If this profit number is not high enough, adjustments must be made to both revenue and expense categories.

> **PRACTICE POINT** Profits should be budgeted, allocating money to practice reinvestment, equipment, and/or team member incentives.

In Table 20-2, the profits for ABC Animal Hospital were $139,669.60, or 14% (see Figure 20-12). This is an excellent percentage and a goal that each practice should create and implement. This allows the implementation of equipment and practice reinvestment, building maintenance and upgrades, team incentives, and an owner's return on investment for the 2008 fiscal year. To maintain this profit for 2009, a budget must be determined, limiting expenses and increasing revenue as much as possible.

Increasing Profits

There are a number of ways to help increase profits, and all team members can assist in achieving that goal. First and foremost, services must be charged appropriately. Veterinarian and technician time is a valuable resource, and they must be compensated for the skills and productivity they provide to the profession and practice. Second, charges cannot be missed. Many practices lose profits due to a number of missed charges for both hospitalized patients and outpatients. Procedures should be implemented to decrease missed charges. Third, practices must instill goals in the staff to increase profits. Team members must be on board to help develop and implement goals. A leader can make suggestions and provide materials for the team, but the team makes the goals happen. Teams should try to decrease the costs of operating expenses as well. Once a budget has been created, teams can effectively look at subcategories, determine what areas are controllable, and make an impact

on those areas. It is essential to communicate the budget to the staff. Numbers, projections, and goals should be posted for the team to share. Goals should be celebrated when they have been achieved, and brainstorming sessions should be held when they have not been met. The team environment goes beyond working together and satisfying clients; it is also about helping and contributing to the success of the practice. Increased profits increase salaries for team members, allow greater reinvestment into the practice, and increase the owner's profits. These lead to a satisfied team that will work efficiently, intelligently, and happily because an exceptional place of employment has been created.

> **PRACTICE POINT** Team members should be involved in the creation of goals for increasing practice profits.

CREATING FINANCIAL REPORTS

The American Animal Hospital Association (AAHA) has an excellent chart of accounts that is highly recommended when creating financial reports. The chart of accounts requires detailed, accurate information that is flexible for every veterinary practice, regardless of size. A chart of accounts is an organized listing of all income, expense, asset, liability, and equity categories used in the business, leading to the ultimate goal of creating a picture of the practice's operations on a daily, monthly, and yearly basis.

Creating charts allows the comparison of the practice year to year, along with comparison with other practices industry-wide. Owners and practice managers can see the impact every decision has made throughout the year. The financial status of the practice is made clear.

Financial reports contribute to the understanding of the practice and allow a manager to recognize current problems and prevent further financial problems from occurring. By recognizing issues early, troubleshooting and repair can resolve problems before they become a financial nightmare for the practice. It is essential to develop a balance sheet and income statement yearly, if not quarterly, to keep the snapshot of the practice's finances in clear view.

Balance Sheet and Income Statement

A balance sheet is referred to as the *statement of financial condition of the practice*. It summarizes the assets, liabilities, and equities of the practice. The income statement is also referred to as the *profit and loss statement* and reports values that have accumulated between two set points of time. This report matches revenue to expenses between two selected dates.

> **PRACTICE POINT** The income statement is also referred to as the *profit and loss statement*.

Table 20-2	Profit Budget	
	ABC ANIMAL HOSPITAL	
PROFIT BUDGET	$ 139,669.60	
Building reinvestment	$ 27,933.92	20%
Equipment reinvestment	$ 27,933.92	20%
Staff incentive	$ 27,933.92	20%
Owner return on investment	$ 55,867.84	40%

Balance sheets represent the basic accounting equation: Assets = Liabilities + Owner Equity. Assets include all things of value that the practice owns, including property, equipment, inventory, building, land, and goodwill. Liabilities include accounts payable and loans. Balance sheets may require the assistance of an accountant to complete. Discrepancies in amounts and percentages should be investigated to determine if a problem or opportunity exists. Problems should be resolved and opportunities capitalized on.

The income statement is easy to understand and interpret because revenues, expenses, and profits for a given time period are listed. Most income statements are prepared on an accrual basis for practice review and cash basis for tax purposes and should be made available in a dollar amount and percentage. Income statements are more beneficial when practices are able to compare month to month, reviewing changes in trends. Once again, large discrepancies should be investigated, looking for problems to fix and opportunities to capitalize on.

Cash-Based and Accrual-Based Accounting

Income and expenses can be recorded in two different ways; the method a practice chooses is usually dictated by the need for federal income tax reporting. If income is measured when cash is received and expenses are measured when cash is spent, then a practice uses cash-based accounting. In practice, only fees paid by clients are recognized in cash-based accounting; therefore accounts receivable are not included. Those fees have yet to be paid by clients. Accounts payable transactions are only recorded when they have been paid, not when they occurred. If a practice is recording income and expenses as they occur, then the practice uses an accrual-based accounting system. Practices that use an accrual basis record fees as they are earned, therefore including accounts receivable. Accounts payable are recorded at the time of accrual, not at the time of payment.

> **PRACTICE POINT** Cash-based accounting is measured when payment is received, not when the service is rendered.

Historically, practices have used a cash-based method because it is easier to maintain and understand. However, reviewing the two reports gives two different pictures of the financial status of the hospital. Comparison of cash reports can provide varied results from month to month, especially when a practice has a large accounts receivable balance.

In 1998, the Internal Revenue Service (IRS) deemed many practices ineligible to use cash-based accounting for taxation purposes because of the mixed sales of products and services. Therefore many practices have switched accounting methods. Consultation with the practice CPA is essential for determining which method a practice should use to prevent any wrongdoing in the eyes of the IRS.

ANALYZING REVENUE

Key performance indicators can give indications of changes that are occurring in revenue centers. Revenue centers are defined as the areas of a practice that can be assessed for the revenue produced and the cost of expenses. Laboratory, pharmacy, and radiology are just a few examples of revenue centers (Box 20-4).

When revenue centers are established, changes can be identified, and it can be determined whether intervention is needed to prevent loss or if an area needs to be capitalized on. For example, dentistry is a common revenue center in veterinary practice. To determine the percentage of profit that the dental center is contributing to the overall gross revenue, a simple equation can be used. The total amount of the dental revenue divided by the total gross revenue and multiplied by 100 gives the percentage needed for comparison purposes.

> **PRACTICE POINT** Revenue centers should be evaluated yearly for potential increases.

Figure 20-14 lists dental services as producing $20,000 for the 2008 fiscal year. Gross revenue produced $1 million. The sum of $20,000 divided by $1 million equals 0.02. To express this number as a percentage, 0.02 × 100 = 2%. Therefore 2% of gross revenue is contributed by the dental revenue center. The practice can then set goals to increase this number the following year. If this number is lower than the previous year, management can implement changes to prevent this number from decreasing further. Figure 20-14 calculates a 10% increase in services for the 2009 year. Teams may want to create a goal of increasing this percentage for the following year because it falls far below benchmark numbers.

Box 20-4	Revenue Centers

- Anesthesia
- Boarding
- Dentals
- Diets
- Examinations
- Grooming
- Hospitalization
- Laboratory
- Pharmacy
- Radiology
- Retail
- Surgery

To help increase and promote revenue on all levels, teams should be dedicated to promoting excellent veterinary medicine. This includes diagnostics, treatments, and preventive medicine. A case should be completely worked up with diagnostic tests before a diagnosis is given. Assuming an animal has pancreatitis according to clinical signs is not working up a case. Bloodwork, such as the Spec cPL test, and radiographs may be indicated to complete the diagnosis. Complete treatment for pancreatitis should also be initiated; conservative treatment of sending the pet home on a bland diet is unacceptable. Pets should have the comprehensive care they deserve to improve their painful condition. Preventive medicine must be offered and encouraged to all clients, regardless of the perceived client economic factor. Excellent quality of care must be offered across the board.

> **PRACTICE POINT** Diagnostic workups promote high-quality medicine.

Many pieces of equipment are underutilized in practice. Radiograph machines, dental units, and ultrasound machines should be placed into a profit center, allowing management to determine and monitor the percentage that these centers produce on a monthly basis. If the numbers are lower than average benchmark numbers, leaders should ask teams why they believe those centers are used less than others. What can be done to increase revenue for those centers? Increased continuing education? Increased marketing to clientele? Increased recommendations? Are client education materials needed to help explain the benefits to clients? Leaders should ensure that all team members have appropriate training and are committed to recommending procedures using those profit centers.

Budgets generally run from year to year, using figures from a profit and loss statement or income statement. It is easier to create a realistic budget with 2 or 3 years of historical data to provide an excellent baseline and produce practical goals. The entire team should help determine realistic goals; each team member has valuable input and ideas. The team will also help ensure the goals are met when the budget is created as a team. Once all the goals and projections have been added into a spreadsheet, it should be determined whether the bottom line adds up; if not, a revision should be made. Numbers can then be added monthly to compare actual to projected numbers; if the actual numbers are favorable, the team can be congratulated. If the numbers fall short of projections, the team can create a strategy to obtain desired outcomes for the following month.

> **PRACTICE POINT** Teams that develop goals together will have a higher success rate.

Table 20-3	Year-End Budget Sheet
ABC Animal Hospital Year-End Budget Sheet December 2009	
Cash available 1/1/08	$ 48,567.98
Inflow	1,000,000.00
Outflow	860,330.40
Ending balance 12/31/08	188,237.58
Cash available 1/1/09	188,237.58
Building reinvestment from 2008	27,933.92
Equipment reinvestment 2008	27,933.92
Team incentive 2008	27,933.92
Owner return on investment 2008	55,867.84
Projected inflow	1,100,000.00
Projected outflow	985,166.36
Projected ending balance	$ 163,401.62

Goals

The end result of a budget sheet is the amount of cash currently available plus the projected cash, minus projected outflows. This creates the ending cash balance. The ending cash balance then becomes the following year's budget sheet's beginning cash value. A positive cash flow indicates the practice produced well during the set period, a negative cash flow reflects a cash flow gap. Causes and discrepancies of the cash flow gap must be determined. To help decrease gaps, practices may temporarily need to decrease inventory purchases and nonessential operating expenses, decrease accounts receivable totals, borrow from a line of credit, or increase professional service fees.

> **PRACTICE POINT** Cash flow gaps must be investigated and repaired immediately.

Table 20-3 displays a 2008 year-end budget along with predictions for the 2009 fiscal year. The 2008 budget started with $48,567.98 in cash and ended with a $188,237.58 cash balance. Due to the profit of 2008, building and equipment reinvestment, team incentives, and the owner's return on investment can be implemented during 2009. The ending balance for 2009 is projected to be $163,401.62 if all the inflows and outflows follow predicted amounts.

Industry standards have created percentages for budgets that are ideal for a well-managed practice. The goal is to achieve these percentages; it is important to remember that many factors contribute to budgets, and not all practices may be able to meet these percentages (Box 20-5).

Creating budgets is a trial and error process. It is based on assumption, and mistakes will occur. Future, unpredictable events can occur and will affect projections in ways beyond the practice's control. Natural

Box 20-5 Budget Percentages

- Non-DVM labor: 20%
  - Tech labor: 9.5%
  - Receptionist: 3.5%
  - Payroll overhead: 6.5%
- DVM: 20% to 25%
  - (25% to 30% with benefits package included)
- Direct expenses: 20%
  - Drugs/supplies/food
- Indirect expenses: 20%
  - Rent, marketing, utilities, accounting, legal, continuing education
  - 8%: Overhead
  - 4%: Office supplies
  - 8%: Facility and equipment maintenance
  - 2% to 3%: Marketing/public relations
  - 2%: Legal/accounting
- Profit: 15% to 20%

disasters such as hurricanes or tornados can affect the practice as well as the economy surrounding the practice. Therefore it can be detrimental to project more than 3 years in advance.

Keep it simple to start with. Having a simple budget projection is better than having none at all. Creating a budget requires a definite commitment. Take small steps first, perhaps starting with a payroll budget first, then adding an inventory and supplies budget. With experience, a budgeting system becomes easier and the practice will reap the benefits.

PRACTICE POINT Keep budgets simple by starting small.

BENCHMARKING

Benchmarking is the process by which a practice compares its data to others in the industry: locally, statewide, regionally, or nationally. Benchmarking can also be taken from the practice's historical financial information. Both types of benchmarking must be considered when analyzing and making decisions for the practice. Benchmarking can be beneficial when determining what steps need to be taken to take the practice to the next level.

Areas of desired improvement must be determined before steps can be taken. Common areas to analyze may include customer service, productivity, and profitability. In this case, profitability is going to be discussed. Information should be collected regarding the practice's financial history, current practice data, and benchmark numbers, which are available from American Veterinary

Medical Association (AVMA), Veterinary Hospital Managers Association (VHMA), or AAHA. Comparison by numbers can be completed, analyzing deviations along with a cause and effect relation. National benchmarking numbers may not be in line with current practice figures due to differences in the economic status of the city or state, or it may be simply that the practice is not charging enough. Other factors affecting differences may include the size of the practice, type of practice, services offered, length of time the practice has been in business, and the location of the practice.

Team members can then develop a plan to determine which factors they can affect and what changes can be implemented. A target date should be set by the team in which a follow-up analysis can occur to determine whether the changes have been successful. Once the issue has been resolved, another area can be targeted.

Benchmarking is a continuous process that increases the practice's success while maintaining a high level of commitment and care to the clients and patients. Clients expect premier service, and they deserve to have the best available.

 VETERINARY PRACTICE and the LAW

Tax evasion is illegal; taxes cannot be avoided. Sales tax must be paid on a monthly basis, and payroll tax is paid either monthly or biweekly. Sometimes practices will underreport income and overreport expenses. This can alert the IRS to look for inconsistencies in the tax returns from year to year and may result in an audit for the practice.

Payments that are made 1 day late accrue penalty fees. The IRS accrues interest on the original tax due, and the penalties vary based on failure to pay or paying late. If payments are not received, the IRS will file a lien on the practice assets and garnish wages.

Self-Evaluation Questions

1. What is benchmarking?
2. What is the difference between a CPA and a bookkeeper?
3. What is the purpose of a client survey?
4. What is a key performance indicator?
5. Why should a budget be created?
6. What is a variable expense? Give some examples.
7. What is a fixed cost? Give some examples.
8. What is a direct expense? Give some examples.
9. What is an indirect expense? Give some examples.
10. What is COGS?

Recommended Reading

Ackerman L: *Business basics for veterinarians*, New York, 2002, ASJA.

Dickey T: *The basics of budgeting: a practical guide to better business planning*, Menlo Park, CA, 1992, Crisp Publications.

Heinke MM: Beyond compensation: what to discuss when hiring a new associate, *DVM Magazine* 3:51, 1997.

Heinke MM: *Practice made perfect: a guide to veterinary practice management*, Lakewood, CO, 2001, AAHA Press.

Pinkleton R: Staff leveraging—use your staff to build your practice, *Vet Forum* 6:32, 1995.

Williams J, et al: *Financial accounting*, New York, 2009, McGraw-Hill.

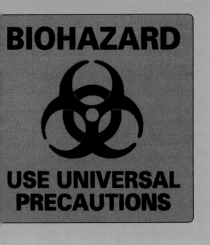

Occupational Hazards and Safety Issues

Learning Objectives

Mastery of the content in this chapter will enable the reader to:
- Identify zoonotic diseases.
- Describe methods used to prevent the transmission of zoonotic diseases.
- Identify the hazards associated with veterinary medicine.
- List methods used to lift equipment and animals appropriately.
- Define the role of the Occupational Health and Safety Administration.
- Develop safety protocols.
- Define the right to know.
- Develop a hospital safety manual.
- Discuss and implement a training program.
- Describe how to prevent fires.
- Discuss fire inspections.
- Discuss methods used to prevent the escape of animals.

Key Terms

Biohazard
Carcinogen
First Notice of Accident
Hospital Safety Manual
Material Safety Data Sheet (MSDS)

Occupational Health and Safety
    Administration (OSHA)
OSHA 300
OSHA 300A
Permissible Exposure Limits

Personal Protective Equipment (PPE)
Scavenger System
The Right to Know
Waste Anesthetic Gases
Zoonotic Disease

Many hazards exist in a veterinary practice, and each team member needs to be aware of all hazards. Every employee must be proactive and prevent hazards from occurring, keeping the facility safe for all team members, patients, and clients.

The Occupational Safety and Health Administration (OSHA) was developed in 1970 to ensure employee safety. Every employer must provide a safe working environment for all team members, and OSHA will severely penalize those that do not follow regulations. OSHA oversees all workplace hazards, including the safe use and disposal of chemicals. Each practice must have Material Safety Data Sheets (MSDSs) available for quick reference in case any team member is exposed to a chemical hazard. MSDS sheets give information regarding the chemical, specifications for cleanup and exposure, as well as any special properties the chemical possesses.

It is essential to prevent the transmission of zoonotic disease. Team members must be made aware of diseases that are transmissible to them and take all precautions necessary to prevent transmission. Zoonotic diseases can spread from animal to human and may spread by different methods depending on the disease. Some disease can be treated, whereas others may be fatal.

Safety plans must be developed in case of a fire or natural disaster, and all team members must be aware of the evacuation plans that have been developed. Team members, clients, and patients should all be accounted for when developing such plans. Fire inspections by the local fire department generally occur once a year, ensuring that businesses are in regulation with city ordinances regarding fire codes. Practices that are not up to code should make it a priority to ensure the safety of all involved with the practice.

ZOONOTIC DISEASES

Zoonoses are defined as diseases that may be directly or indirectly transmitted to humans from wild or domesticated animals. More than 1400 diseases are currently known to be zoonotic, of which 60% are caused by pathogens known to cross species lines. The need to educate the public and veterinary practice team members is imperative because veterinarians may be held liable for the transmission of such diseases. Veterinarians play a vital role in public health and control of zoonotic diseases (Table 21-1).

Veterinarians are ethically required to educate the public about zoonotic diseases. Because public health has been addressed in the American Veterinary Medicine Association (AVMA) Code of Ethics, many state boards and regulatory agencies have mandated such education, which can leave many veterinarians liable for a malpractice suit. To present a claim for malpractice, four elements must be proven: existence of a valid client-patient relationship, failure to practice the standard level of care, proximate cause, and harm that occurred to the patient as a result of substandard care. For more information on malpractice, see Chapter 4.

Once a patient has been presented to a practice for treatment, a client-patient relationship has been established. Because veterinarians have been trained in the risks and transmission of zoonotic diseases, it has become the standard of care for them to educate the public. Therefore if a patient with a zoonotic disease is presented for treatment, it is the obligation of the veterinary practice not only to diagnose and treat it, but also to educate the client regarding the disease and to recommend that the client visit a physician to seek medical attention. If a patient has not been diagnosed with a zoonotic disease, it is standard of care to educate clients about potential zoonotic diseases that are present in the area and advise methods of prevention if available.

It is recommended that any new puppy or kitten brought to the practice be dewormed on the first visit. Puppies and kittens can easily transmit intestinal parasites, and this is the best opportunity to educate clients about these potential risks. If the veterinary practice initiates deworming protocols, sends home material for clients to read, and documents the procedure in the record, it has protected itself from a potential liability lawsuit.

If a practice educates a client about the risk of contracting a zoonotic disease and advises a treatment protocol to reduce the risk of contracting that disease and the client refuses the treatment, it must be documented in the record.

Team members should receive extensive training on zoonotic diseases and the precautions to take to decrease the possibility of transmission. Employees should sign a statement indicating that they have received prevention training. General cleanliness, handwashing, and the use of disinfectants are essential and must be implemented in every practice's protocol to reduce transmission of disease.

DISEASE TRANSMISSION

The mode of disease transmission is important to understand when trying to prevent the spread of a disease. Reservoirs and hosts are also important to understand because these are necessary in the transmission of infectious diseases. A *reservoir* is a place where an infectious organism survives and replicates, such a within an animal or the soil. A *host* is a living organism that offers an environment for maintenance of the organism but that may not be required for the organism's survival. Depending on the disease, the organism may be transmitted to more than one host or reservoir. Programs are generally aimed at reservoirs and hosts of diseases when control methods are being implemented.

Direct transmission of diseases requires close contact between the reservoir of the disease and the susceptible host. Contact with infected skin, mucous membranes, or

Table 21-1   Zoonotic Diseases

	Causative Organism	Small-Animal Host	Livestock Host	Wildlife Host	Mode of Transmission
BACTERIAL INFECTION					
Anthrax	*Bacillus anthracis*	Dogs	Cattle, sheep, horses, goats	Most except primates	Contact
Brucellosis	*Brucella melitensis*	Dogs	Cattle, pigs, sheep, goats	All except primates	Contact, inhalation, ingestion
Campylobacteriosis	*Campylobacter fetus*	Dogs, cats	Cattle, poultry, sheep, pigs	Rodents, birds	Ingestion, contact
Capnocytophaga infection	*Capnocytophaga canimorsus*	Dogs, cats			Bite wound
Cat scratch disease	*Bartonella henselae*	Cats		Cats	Cat bite, scratch
Erysipelas	*Erysipelothrix rhusiopathiae*		Pigs, sheep, cattle, horses, poultry	Rodents	Contact
Leptospirosis	*Leptospira* spp.	All	All	Rats, raccoons	Contact with urine or birthing fluids
Lyme disease	*Borrelia burgdorferi*	Dogs, cats	Cattle, horses	Deer, birds, rodents	Tick bite
Pasteurellosis	*Pasteurella multocida*	Dogs, cats		Bite wound	
Plague	*Yersinia pestis*	Cats		Rodents, rabbits	Flea bite
Q fever	*Coxiella burnetii*		Cattle, sheep, goats	Birds, rabbits, rodents	Inhalation, milk ingestion, contact
Rat bite fever	*Streptobacillus moniliformis*			Rats	Rat bite
Salmonellosis	*Salmonella* spp.	All	All	Rodents, reptiles	Ingestion
Tetanus	*Clostridium tetani*		Horses	Reptiles	Wound
Tuberculosis	*Mycobacteria tuberculosis*	Dogs, cats	Cattle, pigs, sheep, goats, poultry	All except rodents and monkeys	Ingestion, inhalation
Tularemia	*Francisella tularensis*	All	All except horses	Rodents, rabbits	Tick bite, contact with tissue
FUNGAL DISEASES					
Cryptococcosis	*Cryptococcus neoformans*			Birds	Contact
Ringworm	*Trichophyton* spp.	Dogs, cats	Cattle, horses, pigs, sheep	Rodents	Contact
PARASITIC INFECTION					
Cryptosporidiosis	*Cryptosporidium parvum*		Cattle		Ingestion
Hydatid disease	Echinococcus	Dogs	Herbivores	Wolves	Ingestion
Larva migrans	*Toxocara, Ancylostoma, Strongyloides* spp.	Dogs, cats	Pigs, cattle	Raccoons	Ingestion
Scabies	*Sarcoptes scabiei*	Dogs, cats, rodents	Horses	Primates	Contact
Schistosomiasis	*Schistosoma*	Dogs, cats	Pigs, cattle, horses	Rodents	Contact

Continued

Table 21-1	Zoonotic Diseases—cont'd				
	Causative Organism	Small-Animal Host	Livestock Host	Wildlife Host	Mode of Transmission
Taeniasis cysticercosis	*Taenia*		Pigs, cattle	Boars	Ingestion
Toxoplasmosis	*Toxoplasma gondii*	Cats	Pigs, sheep, goats		Ingestion
Trichinosis	*Trichinella spiralis*		Pigs	Rats, bears, carnivores	Ingestion
RICKETTSIAL DISEASES					
Psittacosis	*Chlamydia psittaci*	Psittacine birds	Ducks, turkeys	Birds	Inhalation
Rocky Mountain spotted fever	*Rickettsia rickettsii*	Dogs		Rodents, rabbits	Tick bite
VIRAL DISEASES					
Contagious ecthyma (orf)	Poxvirus	Dogs	Sheep, goats		Contact
Encephalitis (EEE, WEE)	Togavirus		Horses, poultry	Birds, rodents	Mosquito bite
Hantavirus	Hantavirus			Rodents	Contact
Lymphocytic choriomeningitis	Arenavirus	Mice			Varied
Monkeypox	Orthopoxvirus			Rodents	Contact
Newcastle disease	Paramyxovirus	Domestic birds	Poultry	Wild fowl	Contact, inhalation
Rabies	Rhabdovirus togavirus	Almost all	Most	Most	Animal bite
Simian herpes	Herpesvirus simiae			Primates	Animal bite, direct contact
Yellow fever	Togavirus			Primates	Mosquito bite
PROTOZOAL INFECTION					
Balantidiasis	*Balantidium coli*		Pigs	Rats, primates	Ingestion
Cryptosporidiosis	*Cryptosporidium* spp.	Most	Calves, sheep	Birds	Ingestion
Giardiasis	*Giardia lamblia*	Dogs, cats	Pigs, cattle	Beavers, zoo monkeys	Ingestion
Sarcocystosis	Sarcocystis	Dogs, cats	Pigs, cattle		Ingestion
Toxoplasmosis	*Toxoplasma gondii*	Cats, rabbits, Guinea pigs	Pigs, sheep, cattle, horses	Cats	Ingestion

EEE, Eastern equine encephalitis; *WEE,* Western equine encephalitis.

droplets from the infected animal or human can cause disease. Soil or vegetation that is contaminated also serves as a method of direct transmission.

Indirect transmission of diseases is more complex and involves intermediaries that carry the agent of disease from one source to another. A *vector* is a living organism that transports infectious agents. A *vehicle* is a mode of transmission of an infectious agent from the reservoir to the host. Airborne transmission involves spread of the agent through dust particles or droplet particles over long distances.

Arthropods, such as fleas, ticks, and mosquitoes, are considered vectors. They can carry an infectious agent to a susceptible host as well as be involved in the multiplication of organisms. They can also assist in a specific stage of development of the organism.

Food and water are vehicles of indirect transmission of disease; both may be sources of bacterial, viral, and parasitic diseases. Foodborne diseases are acquired by the consumption of contaminated food or water and may be caused by toxins released by bacteria that are contained in the food. Parasites can also be transmitted through food, either through the ingestion of eggs or undercooked meat that contains cysts.

CONTROL OF ZOONOTIC DISEASES

Because of the contact veterinarians and veterinary technicians have with potentially infected pets, they may be the first to notice symptoms. It is important to recognize the most common diseases seen in a practice's local area and be knowledgeable about their symptoms, treatments, and prevention. Prevention programs require complete knowledge of the disease and how it is maintained to break the cycle of the disease. Prevention of disease may be aided by a vaccination for such diseases, water filtration, and excellent hygiene skills.

People at particular risk of zoonotic disease are those with compromised immune systems, such as those undergoing chemotherapy and/or treatment for HIV or AIDS. Pregnant women and individuals who have had their spleens removed are also immunocompromised and should use extra precaution when working with or around animals with zoonotic potential. Children may also be at a higher risk because they come into contact with contaminants in the outdoor environment.

Animal Bites

Animal bites can be a source of infection, trauma, and zoonotic diseases. An animal bite is defined as a bite wound that penetrates the skin, causing bleeding and swelling at the area. *Pasteurella* is present in more than 50% of dog bite wounds and 90% of cat bite wounds. Other bacteria that may present in animal bites include *Staphylococcus aureus*, *Staphylococcus epidermidis*, *Streptococcus* spp., *Bacteroides* spp., *Fusobacterium* spp., and other gram-negative bacteria. In people, these bacteria can cause fever, septicemia, meningitis, endocarditis, and septic arthritis. Any team member who is bitten by a patient should wash the area well with warm, soapy water for at least 5 minutes, apply a dilute Betadine solution, then rinse with a strong stream of water. The team member should consider seeking medical attention, taking into account the potential risk for infection.

SAFETY HAZARDS IN THE VETERINARY PRACTICE

Each team member must practice safety while working in the practice. Many hazards exist, and everyone must be responsible for his or her own safety and prevention of injury. Moving equipment, slips, and lifting are a few causes of injuries that can be prevented. Team members should become diligent about washing their hands to prevent accidental ingestion of toxic substances as well as the spread of zoonotic diseases. Safety protocols must be developed and enforced; fire prevention, response, and rescues should be discussed among team members. Each person contributes a significant amount of time and energy to each practice, and each practice must protect these valuable team members.

Moving Equipment

When moving equipment, multiple employees should be involved. If the equipment is heavy, more than one person must be responsible for the lifting. Another team member should ensure the entryway is clear of clutter and debris that would trip the team members. One team member should be allowed to lift up to 40 lb if he or she is able. Anything over 40 lb requires additional team members.

Wet Floors

When floors are being mopped, they can become extremely slippery. Signs that indicate a wet floor should be posted around the wet area, and team members should dry the wet area as soon as possible with a dry towel (Figure 21-1). Team members and clients should be encouraged to walk around the wet area. However, the sooner it is dry, the less likely it is that a slip or fall will occur. Team members are encouraged to wear nonskid shoes to help prevent slips in the veterinary practice.

> **PRACTICE POINT** Wet floors must have a large sign that indicates the floor is wet.

Running

Team members should not be allowed to run through the practice, regardless of how busy the practice is. Running increases the risk of slipping, especially on wet surfaces. An employee may have finished mopping the floor and just be setting the signs out; if a team member is running through the area at the same time, he or she will not know the floor is wet.

Lifting

Team members must learn how to lift properly to prevent back injury (Figure 21-2). Lifting must always be done with the legs rather than the back; women are especially prone to use their backs. Team members should watch out for each other and guide others when lifting objects to ensure the back is kept straight and the legs are used to the maximum potential. It should be instituted that animals over 40 lb must be lifted by two team members to prevent back injuries.

Many people believe that they can lift animals very easily; they are strong and would never injure their

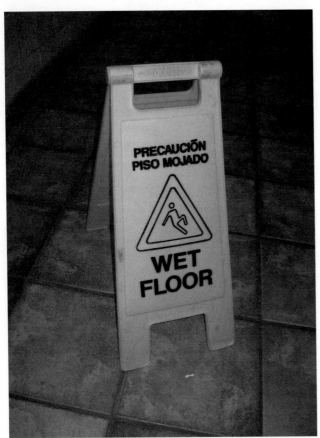

FIGURE 21-1 Any time the floor is wet, a sign should be posted for the safety of team members and clients.

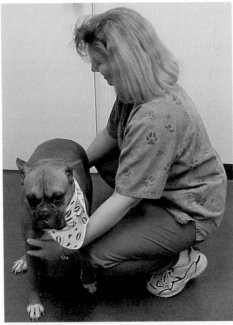

FIGURE 21-2 Proper lifting technique includes keeping the back straight and lifting with the legs. (From Bassert JM, McCurnin DM: *McCurnin's clinical textbook for veterinary technicians*, ed 7, St Louis, 2010, Saunders Elsevier.)

backs. This is untrue; the second most common workplace hazard in veterinary medicine is a back injury. Most injuries occur over time, and prevention methods must be instilled in all employees to prevent injury.

> **PRACTICE POINT**   Use your legs to lift, not your back!

Toxicities

There are many possibilities for toxic exposures in veterinary medicine. Chemical exposure can come in the form of cleaning supplies, chemotherapy, x-ray developer solutions, and medications that are dispensed or used in the hospital for patients.

The mixing of two or more chemicals can create caustic fumes that are harmful to both team members and patients. The fumes may not seem harmful, and at times may even smell good, such as combining bleach and a lemon disinfectant; however, prolonged exposure may be dangerous.

> **PRACTICE POINT**   Cleaning agents should never be mixed unless specified on the label.

Every team member is exposed to chemotherapy agents (discussed in further detail later in this chapter) if they are administered in the veterinary practice. Many chemotherapeutic agents are expelled in the urine and feces of pets; therefore each time the animal eliminates in the cage, some of the drug is left behind. Therefore team members may be exposed to the drug unknowingly.

Radiology developer rooms should be ventilated to the outdoors because the chemicals used to develop radiographs are strong and harmful. If the developer and fixative mix for some reason, the chemical released can be caustic. The chemical used to develop radiographs can be poured down the drain, but the fixing solution must be collected by a specialized company because it can be damaging to the environment. This applies to both used and unused fixative.

It is often forgotten that when handling medication, excess drug powder and residual collects on the hands. Various types of medications are handled as team members count and dispense medications for owners or pull medications to treat patients. If team members do not wash their hands immediately after handling medications, they may ingest the substance or wipe it onto their faces. Many drugs appear to be safe, but repeated ingestion may not be safe. Some drugs are known to have side effects. Chloramphenicol, for example, may suppress bone marrow production in individuals who have a reaction to it. Unfortunately, this reaction is not known for months, or even years, after the exposure to the drug. It is essential that all team members wash their hands immediately after handling medication, just as hands are washed immediately after handling an animal, to prevent the accidental ingestion of medications.

> **PRACTICE POINT** Hands must be thoroughly washed after handling medication.

Radiation

Radiation exposure in a practice must be taken seriously. Excess radiation causes birth defects, decreased fertility, and cancer; therefore every precaution must be taken when exposed. Team members must wear personal protective equipment (PPE) at all times when taking radiographs. Employers who do not provide proper PPE are in violation because they are not providing a safe work environment without it. Team members can be fired if they do not use PPE that is available (as provided by OSHA).

Lead gloves, gown, and thyroid collars comprise the minimum PPE that must be worn to take radiographs. If at all possible, team members should leave the room for best protection. If an animal is sedated, rice bags, sand bags, ties, and tape can be used to position the animal for the desired view, allowing the team members to leave.

> **PRACTICE POINT** ALL PPE MUST BE WORN WHEN TAKING RADIOGRAPHS!

Radiographs should be collimated to prevent excess radiation from being used and exposing the team member. Gloves should never be in the direct x-ray beam because radiation can penetrate lead that is cracked and/or broken. All PPE should be x-rayed on a yearly basis to look for cracks that may have occurred over the year. If any cracks or holes have developed, the PPE device must be replaced immediately. Radiographs should be kept for comparison from year to year.

Portable units are extremely dangerous because the beam can be pointed in any direction. A cassette-holding pole should be used to hold the cassette during the x-ray process. A gloved hand should never hold the cassette. Team members should also make sure there is not another person in the direct line of the beam, even at a distance.

A dosimeter, used to measure radiation exposure, must be worn every time an x-ray is taken. The badges should be stored outside the room to prevent scatter radiation from affecting the badges. Badges should be worn at collar level, and indicate the amount of exposure the team member is receiving. Badges should be sent to a monitoring company on a monthly or quarterly basis, where a report will be generated and returned to the practice. These reports must be monitored and reviewed upon their return to check for any significant change in exposure readings. If a badge reads high,

this could indicate that the x-ray machine is functioning improperly, sending out excess radiation. This is detrimental to employee safety and must be corrected immediately. Reports must be kept on hand indefinitely; team members should always have access to data on the amount of radiation that they have been exposed to while employed at the practice (Figure 21-3). Veterinary staff members are allowed a maximum exposure of 5 rem/year of radiation, whereas the general public is only allowed a maximum exposure of 0.5 rem/year.

> **PRACTICE POINT** A dosimetry badge must be worn by any team member taking a radiograph.

Machines must be registered with the appropriate state agencies on a yearly basis. Most state agencies will inspect the machines, ensure their paperwork matches in serial and model numbers, and conduct individual tests. These tests indicate the safety of the machine and that it is working properly and in an acceptable condition.

Appropriate signage must be posted outside radiology rooms (Figure 21-4). Some states also require rights and responsibilities of both employers and employees to be posted, along with a written protocol of how to take and process a radiograph.

Anesthesia

Prolonged and long-term exposure to anesthetic gases has been linked to congenital abnormalities in children, liver and kidney damage, and abortions. Every effort must be made to monitor and prevent exposure. Technicians and doctors who are in surgery every morning must ensure the anesthetic machine has a proper scavenging system and that no leak exists. Anesthetic exposure badges are available to help determine the amount of anesthesia team members are exposed to and, although not required, are advised as part of a safety plan. Team members who are pregnant and required to work around anesthetic gases should wear a badge for their own safety along with proper PPE (Box 21-1). OSHA's exposure limit for halogenated gases (e.g., halothane, isoflurane, sevoflurane) is 2 ppm/year. Nitrous oxide's maximum exposure limit is 25 ppm/year. Anesthetic dosimeter badges can be purchased from a variety of companies.

> **PRACTICE POINT** Excessive exposure to anesthesia can be detrimental to one's health.

To help decrease waste anesthetic gases, team members should turn off the anesthesia to the patient, allowing the continued flow and intake of oxygen. This allows the patient to breath off excess anesthetic gas, which circulates through the system, instead of in the operating room for team members to inhale. Once the patient

Account Number: 0000976
Report Date: 02/13/2009
Wear Period: 01/09/2009 to 02/07/2009

ANNUAL RADIATION EXPOSURE LIMITS:
Whole body, blood forming organs   5,000 mrem/yr
Lens of eye   15,000 mrem/yr
Extremeties and skin   50,000 mrem/yr
Fetal   500 mrem/gestation period
General public   100 mrem/yr

These limits are based on USNRC Regulation Title 10, Part 20.

DOSAGE LEGEND:

curr - current badge reading
ytd - year-to-date accumulated dosage
life - lifetime accumulated storage

View your dosage report online & provide feedback at http://myTLDaccount.PLMedical.com

	Name	Employee ID / DOB	Type	Badge #		Dose Equivalents (in millirem)			Comments
						Deep	Eye	Shallow	
1	Control	-----	T		curr				
					ytd				
					life				
2	Bevery Rains	001 -----	T	0049402	curr	18	18	18	
					ytd	18	18	18	
					life	421	421	409	
3	Bernice Kim	002 -----	T	0103557	curr	11	11	11	
					ytd	11	11	11	
					life	292	292	282	
4	Alice Lynch	003 -----	T	0104208	curr	25	32	21	
					ytd	25	32	21	
					life	264	264	258	
5	Nicole Allen	004 -----	T	0041925	curr	MR	MR	MR	
					ytd	MR	MR	MR	
					life	284	284	275	
6	Margaret Moss	005 -----	T	0052765	curr	45	43	45	
					ytd	45	43	45	
					life	280	280	270	
7	Mary Williams	006 -----	T	0042873	curr	MR	MR	MR	
					ytd	MR	MR	MR	
					life	315	315	301	
8	Jeffrey Dodson	007 -----	T	0034456	curr	MR	MR	MR	
					ytd	MR	MR	MR	
					life	252	252	245	
9	Roy Robinson	008 -----	T	0044819	curr	101	97	98	
					ytd	101	97	98	
					life	255	255	246	
10	Christopher Gagne	009 -----	T	0083207	curr	MR	MR	MR	
					ytd	MR	MR	MR	
					life	242	242	234	

OCCUPATIONAL RADIATION DOSE RECORD — Page 1 of 1

This report must not be used to claim product certification, approval, or endorsement by NVLAP, NIST, or any agency of the Federal Government. A copy of the PL Medical Co., LLC NVLAP certificate and scope of accreditation can be found on http://www.plmedical.com/public/Accreditation.htm.

FIGURE 21-3 Example of a dosimetry report.

has received approximately 5 minutes of oxygen, it can be moved to the recovery area of the practice. "Boxing-down" patients (placing in a sealed container with direct administration of oxygen and anesthesia) also creates waste anesthetic gases that the team inhales. Every effort should be made to use an injectable means of anesthetic induction until the patient is ready for an endotracheal tube. If the box or mask is needed, proper ventilation in the room should be mandatory.

PRACTICE POINT A procedure to decrease waste anesthetic gases must be implemented for team safety.

For the safety of both the patient and team members, anesthetic machines must have adequate scavenging systems. Several scavengers exist; the practice should use the one that works best in that individual practice. Active scavengers provide the best protection; however, passive exhaust and adsorption scavengers are also effective means of removing gases.

The active system has some means of energetic collection. This is usually a fan enclosed in a box that creates a vacuum through a series of tubes that are connected to the patient or machine. Active scavengers may also attach directly to the machine and push the waste anesthetic gases through the system instead of producing a vacuum. Active scavengers are best for practices with a large volume of anesthetic procedures and for anesthetic procedures that occur at various locations throughout the practice. The main disadvantage to an active scavenger system is cost. Systems can range in price from $400 to $4000, depending on the complexity of the system. Other lesser disadvantages include maintenance of the machine and manual activation. Team members must turn on a switch to active the scavenger; many forget until the patient's breathing bag fails to work properly.

The passive exhaust system channels waste anesthetic gases through a tube to an acceptable location for evacuation. This system is only good for short distances because the only means of expelling the gas is the patient's lung pressure and the flow rate of gas. Therefore small and weak animals may not be able to expel gases efficiently.

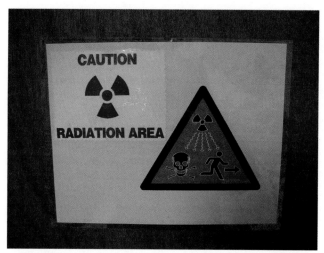

FIGURE 21-4 Radiation signs should be clearly posted.

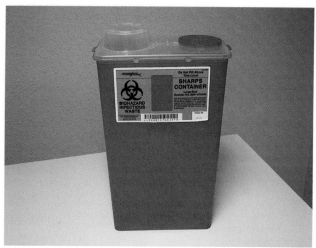

FIGURE 21-5 Biohazard containers are available in a variety of sizes.

Box 21-1	Anesthetic Monitoring Badge Suppliers

- Assay Technology: 800-833-1258
- Surgivet: 888-745-6562
- Vetamac Inc: 800-334-1583

This list is not exhaustive.

> **PRACTICE POINT** It is the practice owner's responsibility to ensure team member safety.

The adsorption scavenger uses charcoal to remove all halogenated gases. It does not adsorb nitrous oxide. Charcoal canisters must be replaced after 20 g of adsorption; therefore canisters must be monitored for replacement. If canisters are not replaced, waste anesthetic gases will overflow into the room.

Machines should be inspected daily for leaks. A pressure test should be performed indicating that the machine holds pressure without leaks, the vaporizer refill lid is secure, and all hoses are attached properly. Hoses and gaskets should be replaced yearly as part of an anesthetic maintenance plan, which helps prevent small, undetectable leaks. OSHA expects that practices will have a professional service maintain their anesthetic machines every 3 to 12 months.

When team members change soda lime granules on anesthetic machines, gloves should be worn. Used soda lime can be caustic to tissues.

If a spill of liquid anesthesia occurs, all other team members should be evacuated from the area. Windows should be opened and exhaust fans turned on. Cat litter can be poured over the spill. Once it has been absorbed, the litter can be swept up and disposed of. Spills may occur when the machine is being refilled or as bottles are being unpacked from a received order. All caution should be taken to prevent the inhalation of gases.

Anesthesia-related training topics should include:
- Depth and planes of anesthesia
- Proper anesthetic hose size
- Correct endotracheal tube size and proper inflation
- Anesthetic machine maintenance
- Scavenging systems
- Clean-up of liquid anesthesia spills
- Leak-checking machine

Anesthesia safety meetings should occur regularly to remind team members of the risks of anesthesia. New team members must be fully trained and made aware of the risks involved while working with anesthesia and anesthetized patients.

> **PRACTICE POINT** Spilled anesthesia should not be allowed to evaporate; it must be absorbed and cleaned up as soon as possible.

Biohazards

Needles, glass, slides, surgical blades, and coverslips are all considered sharps and must be discarded in a biohazard or sharps container. Containers must be puncture resistant and sealable once the container is full. Milk jugs are unacceptable. Biohazard containers are red and come in a variety of sizes depending on the needs of the practice (Figure 21-5). These containers should be picked up on a regular basis by a specialized company that incinerates the contents for a specified price. Team members must take every precaution when handling biohazard material so as not to poke themselves or expose themselves to unnecessary disease and injury. Containers cannot be opened once the cap has been applied unless the plastic tabs are broken. If this happens, the container is regarded as unusable and must be emptied and discarded.

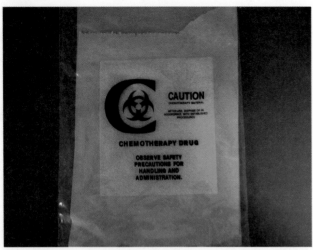

FIGURE 21-6 Chemotherapeutic agents must be identified with a bright yellow label.

Needles should not be cut off at the tip because this increases the risk for aerosolizing the contents of the needle and syringe. The entire needle must be discarded.

Chemotherapeutic Agents

Every team member is exposed to chemotherapeutic agents if they are administered in the practice. Chemotherapy is composed of chemicals used to kill tumor cells; these chemicals inadvertently affect healthy cells as well. Therefore all precautions must be taken when working with these drugs (Figure 21-6). Patients excrete both used and unused drug in their bodily secretions, including vomitus, urine, and feces.

When prepping such drugs for administration, PPE must be worn. This includes a mask, eye protection, a disposable gown, and thick, nonpowdered gloves. Chemicals can be easily inhaled, and a hood with a vent must be used during the mixing process. A mask can protect the team member to a minimal degree; a hood will remove the excess aerosolized chemical. Contact lenses should not be worn at any time during the mixing and or administration of chemotherapy, regardless of eye protection. A disposable gown should be used and disposed of when the mixing and administration process has been completed. Cuffs should be tucked inside gloves. Thick, nonpowdered gloves are the only acceptable glove type. Thin latex gloves protect the team member to a lesser degree; powdered gloves tend to attract

drug residue. Once the entire mixing and administration process has been completed, all gloves, gowns, needles, and items used must be disposed of in a yellow biohazard container. The yellow container indicates that chemotherapeutic agents are inside; these containers will be incinerated separately from other biohazard containers.

Bedding used for animals receiving chemotherapy should be handled with gloves; the team member should also wear a disposable gown for protection. Bedding must be washed separately from other bedding. It must also be washed twice with laundry detergent.

If a chemotherapeutic agent is spilled, team members should evacuate from the area both patients and other team members. The team members should double-glove and place an absorbable material over the spill. Once the agent has been completely absorbed, all material must be placed in a yellow container. The area must be washed with 70% alcohol twice before the area can be declared safe.

Zoonotic Diseases

All team members are at risk of being exposed to zoonotic diseases. If a zoonotic disease is suspected, protective equipment should be used to prevent transmission. Because diseases can be unique in their mode of transmission, each disease needs to be evaluated for the best means of prevention.

Special Chemicals

Chemicals that require special attention include ethylene oxide, formaldehyde, and glutaraldehyde. Ethylene oxide is a carcinogen that is used for gas sterilization procedures. It is extremely important to have a safe handling protocol when this product is used. Only approved sterilization devices must be used with ethylene oxide, and levels should be monitored to ensure team member safety. This chemical is very flammable and must be used with caution.

Formaldehyde, which is used to fix tissue samples, is also a carcinogen. Vapors can be extremely dangerous and are known to cause cancer and abortion. Practices should order biopsy jars that are prefilled with formalin. This prevents unnecessary exposure to team members. If gallon containers of formalin are used, the chemical should be poured into smaller containers under a hood that will capture the vapors. Goggles and gloves should also be worn when handling the chemical to prevent any contact.

Glutaraldehyde is a chemical used to disinfect instruments, generally in cold trays. It is an excellent fungicide and virucide but can be extremely traumatic to tissue. If glutaraldehyde is not diluted to the proper strength, it can cause tissue damage to both team members and patients. Many other disinfectants provide superior protection and are much safer to use in the veterinary practice.

OCCUPATIONAL SAFETY AND HEALTH ADMINISTRATION

It is the responsibility of every veterinary practice to remain in compliance with safety regulations at the local, state, and federal levels. OSHA enforces federal laws to ensure a safe workplace environment. These laws require employers to have a safety program that includes the training of employees. This training must inform employees about the inherent risks associated with their jobs. It must also include training on the proper use of PPE. OSHA requires employees to read the Workplace Rights Poster (#3165), comply with standards, use PPE that has been provided, report hazardous conditions to management, and report any injuries received and seek immediate treatment for them (Figure 21-7). Penalties and fines exist for those who break the law. For example, not displaying the Workforce Safety and Heath Poster is a $1000 fine. Other willful violations can exceed $70,000.

> **PRACTICE POINT** OSHA is overseen by the U.S. Department of Labor.

There are four sections to fulfilling OSHA's compliance and safety program:
1. Administrative tasks
2. Evaluation of the facility
3. PPE
4. Training program

Administrative tasks include the posting of signs and information. The Workplace Rights Poster must be displayed and all paths leading to exits must be clearly indicated with signs and arrows. The safety program should be in writing and documented.

> **PRACTICE POINT** OSHA poster #3165 is required to be displayed by employers.

OSHA requires a written plan for any practice with 10 or more employees. An evacuation plan must be displayed for clients and employees to see. A diagram of the practice should list potential hazards and safety equipment in each room. The diagram should include exits, circuit breakers, compressed gas cylinders, hazardous materials, and fire extinguishers. A hospital safety manual should be developed and be kept in a central location within the practice.

When evaluating the facility, all potential hazards should be analyzed. Doors should have one-way locks, which allow clients and team members to escape at any time. Emergency lighting must be available to help guide clients and team members to exits in the event of an emergency or a power outage. Areas that should not be overlooked when evaluating the practice include, but are not limited to:
- Air quality (Good flow? Even heating and cooling distribution?)
- Damaged equipment (broken rollers, exposed electrical wire, etc.)
- Distance between fire extinguishers
- Emergency lighting
- Fire alarms
- Lighting
- Proper lighting in all rooms
- Smoke alarms
- The use of extension cords
- Walking surfaces (smooth or uneven?)

Under OSHA guidelines, PPE must be used at all times. This includes protective equipment for radiology, surgery, and laboratory functions. Eyewear must be worn when performing tasks that could inflict injury to the eye, and eyewash stations must be available for team members and clients to use in case of emergency.

> **PRACTICE POINT** Employers must enforce the use of PPE at all required times.

Staff training is imperative; without training, safety programs are useless. It is advisable to videotape training sessions because these tapes can provide training as new team members are added to the practice. They also provide proof that a safety program exists if a complaint is filed against the practice. When safety meetings begin, it is wise to cover the most serious hazards first while team members are paying attention. Less severe hazards can follow. Several training topics are required by OSHA (Box 21-2).

OSHA has the right to inspect any veterinary practice. Every veterinary practice owner has the right to be present for an OSHA inspection. Therefore if the owner is not present and a representative has not been appointed, OSHA can be denied the opportunity to inspect the premises. If OSHA has a court order, however, it must be allowed in to inspect the premises.

> **PRACTICE POINT** Most OSHA inspections are triggered by complaints from employees.

The inspection notice must be posted on the staff bulletin board for all team members to see until the inspection has been completed. Copies of violations must be posted for at least 3 days or until the violation is corrected, whichever is longer.

OSHA does not endorse products. Many companies use marketing tactics to say that their product is "OSHA

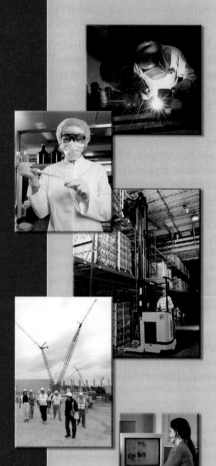

FIGURE 21-7 OSHA poster #3165 informs employees of their rights and must be visibly posted.

Box 21-2   OSHA Required Training Topics

- Animal handling
- Chemicals
- Chemotherapy agents
- Ethylene oxide
- Emergency and fire prevention plans
- Formaldehyde
- Ionizing radiation
- Medical services and first aid
- Medical waste and sharps
- Occupational noise exposure
- Personal safety, violence prevention
- Portable fire exit
- Personal protective equipment
- Signs and tags
- Waste anesthetic gases
- Workers' rights and responsibilities
- Zoonotic disease prevention

Courtesy Occupational Safety and Health Administration, Department of Labor, Washington, DC.

approved" when, in reality, the product only meets OSHA standards.

DEVELOPING SAFETY PROTOCOLS

Protocols should be developed in each practice to ensure employee safety. Plans must be instituted regarding how each employee will be notified in case of an emergency, where staff will meet in case of emergency, and how the safety plan will take effect. Protocols should be role played for all team members to be comfortable if an emergency situation ever arises. All common sense may be lost in the event of an emergency; the more the practice instills role playing, the safer the practice will be. Safety must be addressed at every meeting; it is taken for granted in many situations and needs to be discussed frequently. Common sense can be applied to many safety procedures and protocols.

Practices should have two separate refrigerators; one for human food and the other for biologics, laboratory tests, and drugs (Figure 21-8). This prevents the contamination and ingestion of products used to practice medicine. Team members should be encouraged to keep food, coffee, and drinks in break rooms or lounges instead of on hospital counters or exam tables. Bacteria, dirt, and residual medications reside on counters and can be easily ingested when food is placed on them.

Frequent handwashing with antiseptic soap must be done between patients and when counting medication, cleaning, or maintaining equipment.

Electrical outlets should not be overloaded with excessive plugs and extension cords (Figure 21-9). Extension cords should not be used on a permanent basis; they are for temporary use only (Figure 21-10). When an extension cord is in use, it should have a three-way conductor for better protection, and should never be run through doorways or windows that could damage the wire as they are opened or closed.

> **PRACTICE POINT**   Overloaded electrical circuits are the most common cause of fires in veterinary practices.

Symptoms of electrical problems include frequently tripping circuits and lights that dim when large pieces of equipment are used. If additional circuits are needed, a certified electrician should be asked to add them to the areas of need as soon as possible. This may prevent a fatal fire in the future.

An exit cannot be blocked regardless of whether it is the garage door, employee entrance, or client exit. If a fire occurred and employees or clients could not escape, severe liability would exist.

Common sense should be used when storing supplies. Heavy items must be placed on the lower shelves, along with chemicals and liquids. All chemicals must be stored in tightly sealed containers and be placed below eye level in case they are spilled. Shelves should never

What Would You Do/Not Do?

Mr. Yazzi, a long-time client, has come into the practice with Taco, a Pomeranian. Upon walking to the counter to check out, Mr. Yazzi trips on the weight scale, which has recently been moved to the hallway between the examination rooms. He is able to catch himself and not fall; however, he twists his back, sending it into muscle spasms. He states that he is fine; it was his fault for not looking down and seeing the scale on the floor. Ashleigh, the receptionist who saw the incident, offers him a chair to sit on to rest until his back relaxes. He declines to sit down, stating he just needs to get home and lie down in bed. Ashleigh is afraid that the client may sue the practice.

What Should Ashleigh Do?

Ashleigh should first notify the owner and practice manager of the incident and write down the entire incident before details are forgotten. Pictures should be taken of the scale and how the client tripped. If the client calls and threatens to sue the practice, the professional liability company should be called and informed of the incident.

Second, the practice should invest in some large protective barriers that clients can see to prevent them from tripping on the low-lying scale. Pictures of the barriers should also be taken, indicating the corrective action the practice has taken to prevent incidents such as this from occurring again.

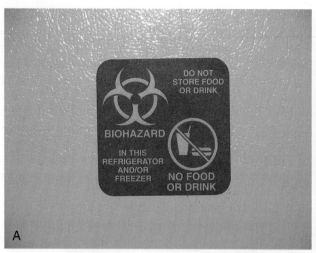

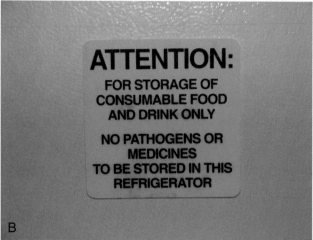

FIGURE 21-8 A, Biohazard materials, including vaccinations and tests, should never be stored with human food intended for consumption. **B,** Consumable food should never be stored with biohazard materials. Magnets can be placed on refrigerators to indicate contents.

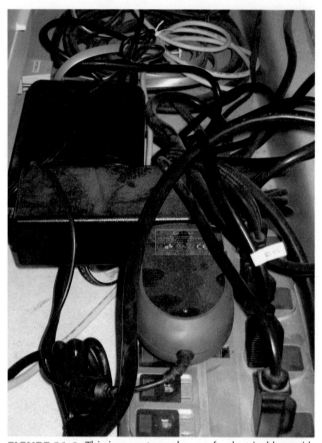

FIGURE 21-9 This is an extremely unsafe electrical box with six electrical plugs.

be overweighed with products, causing them to fall on team members. If product on an upper shelf is needed, a stepstool should be used; never climb on countertops or shelves to get products.

Autoclaves produce intense heat and should always be properly vented before opening the door. Steam should

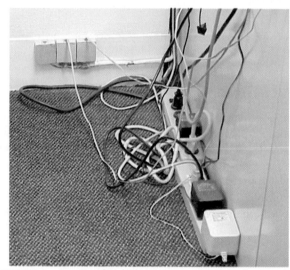

FIGURE 21-10 Overloaded surge suppressors of extension cords can start a fire. (From Bassert JM, McCurnin DM: *McCurnin's clinical textbook for veterinary technicians*, ed 7, St Louis, 2010, Saunders Elsevier.)

be allowed to dissipate slowly and completely before fully opening the door. The face and hands should be kept away from both the vent and door when venting and opening the autoclave.

> **PRACTICE POINT** Autoclaves can cause severe burns when the steam is released from the chamber; the arms, hands, and face should be kept away from the vent area.

Team members must always use caution when working with large animals and chutes. A team member's body must never be placed in a chute with an animal. The animal can be led into the chute with a rope from the outside; large animals can injure team members when there

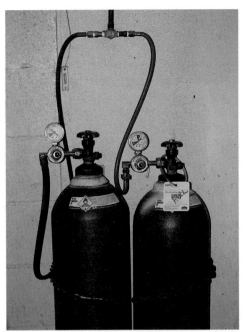

FIGURE 21-11 Oxygen tanks must be secured to a wall at all times.

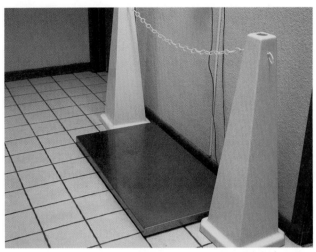

FIGURE 21-12 Barriers can prevent severe injuries.

is nowhere to escape. Large animal stalls may also need to be locked, preventing the theft of patients. Large, durable locks must be used that cannot be cut off.

Bathing and dipping patients can create a hazard; eye protection should be worn each time a bath or dip is performed. Pets tend to shake when they get wet; chemicals still present on the pet when it shakes could splash into someone's eyes, causing damage. If this happens it is imperative not to rub the eyes. Team members must find the nearest eyewash station and rinse the eyes for the suggested amount of time the appropriate MSDS suggests. Dipping areas should also be well ventilated because the fumes from many dips can be caustic.

Compressed oxygen tanks must be secured in an upright position with a chain. Unsecured tanks can get bumped into as team members are walking by, causing them to fall on a team member or to the floor (Figure 21-11). Tanks may explode on impact; therefore securing tanks is essential. All tanks should be kept away from heat sources such as furnaces, water heaters, and direct sunlight.

Team members must dress appropriately for the job, as outlined in employee manuals. For safety purposes, open-toed shoes are not allowed; if team members will be working with large animals, steel-toed boots may be required. Jewelry should be kept to a minimum because long earrings and bracelets could get tangled up in pets, causing injury to both team members and patients.

Noise levels can reach 110 dB in some practices, especially those that board a large number of dogs. If team members will be exposed to loud noises for extended periods, they are advised to wear earplugs rated for

20 dB and higher. According to OSHA, 85 dB is the maximum noise level that can be safely withstood.

Restraint is always a safety concern in every practice. Each team member must be trained in the proper procedures for restraining patients to prevent doctors, fellow team members, and clients from being bitten. Muzzles must be used when indicated regardless of how the client feels. Team member protection is the top priority.

> **PRACTICE POINT**   A muzzle must be used when a fractious dog is presented to the team members for evaluation.

If weight scales are placed on the floor, barriers may be placed at each corner preventing team members and clients from tripping over the scale (Figure 21-12). This is a common hazard in the veterinary practice, and all precautions must be taken to prevent injury.

IMPLEMENTING SAFETY PLANS AND PROTOCOLS

Four easy steps will help implement any safety plan within a practice. Gathering information is the first step, followed by delegation and preparation, training, and finally implementation.

When gathering information for the safety plan, a safety officer must be designated. This individual must be highly motivated and task oriented. The safety officer is in charge of several administrative duties, including ensuring that the radiograph machines are registered with the correct state department, that the Drug Enforcement Agency registration is current for the practice and for all doctors, that the job safety poster is visible to all team members, and that a log of employee injuries is kept and a summary provided every February. The safety officer should evaluate the entire facility monthly and list any item that is a hazard or could be one in the future.

Hazards include slippery floors, sharp corners, damaged radiology shielding, chemicals, and biohazard containers. Many more topics can be added to the lists of both administrative duties and hazards to inspect for; these are only examples (Box 21-3).

The safety officer should have a meeting with the entire team to discuss the importance of the safety plan, go over the "Right to Know" rule (see text that follows), and review the rights of the practice as well as those of the employees. Information should be gathered from team members of hazards they have recognized in

> **PRACTICE POINT**   Team members can help develop a hazard plan and initiate its use.

Box 21-3   Safety Topics
• Anesthetic gas safety • Bite injuries • Diamond labels listing hazards associated with chemicals • Emergency prevention plans • Employees' rights and responsibilities • Ethylene oxide • Evacuating animals • Formaldehyde • Handling chemical spills • Handling human blood • How to use a fire extinguisher • MSDSs; location of and how to use • Occupational noise exposure • Personal protective equipment; use and location • Proper lifting techniques • Proper restraint • Radiation safety • Rendering first aid to humans

the practice that may have been overlooked during the safety officer's walk-though inspection.

During the delegation and preparation phase, hazards can be placed in different sections. Each hazard can then be analyzed for ways to correct and stabilize the hazard, determine what PPE would be needed for the hazard, and order PPE and other materials.

The third phase includes training on each hazard within each section and the use of PPE for those hazards. Implementing the program is now easy to accomplish because sections of the practice have been evaluated, the practice has the proper materials needed, and the staff has been trained. When an emergency occurs, the staff will know the proper response to accommodate that emergency. It is important to review different sections regularly to remind the staff that hazards exist but so do the proper methods of handling the emergency (Table 21-2).

HAZARD COMMUNICATION: THE RIGHT TO KNOW

OSHA's Hazards Communication Standard requires that all team members who come in contact with hazards in the practice be aware of those hazards and instructed on how to protect themselves from those hazards. This applies to all chemicals, including anesthetic gases, radiology chemicals, alcohol, and formalin. To establish compliance, a practice must have:

- A designated safety manager. This employee is responsible for training all team members and ensuring the safety program meets standard requirements.
- A written plan.
- A summary of all hazardous chemicals available, including injectable medications, pesticides, antiseptics/disinfectants, and laboratory agents, as well as those listed above.

Table 21-2 Occupational Hazards		
Hazard	Associated Problems	Common Solutions
Animal handling	Animal bites, zoonotic disease transmission	Proper restraint devices
Ethylene oxide	Spills, improper use	Proper safety training
Ergonomics	Back injuries	Proper lifting techniques
Facility hazards	Old lead paint, slippery tile	Update facility; nonskid shoes
Fire	Exiting facility promptly and safely	Fire evacuation plan, accessible extinguishers, emergency lighting
Food	Ingestion of toxic chemicals and organisms	Separate refrigerator; no food in working areas
Housekeeping	Chemical mixing and toxicities	Do not mix cleaning products
Medical waste	Poking or cutting self with needles, glass, or blades	Appropriate use of biohazard containers
Radiology	Radiation exposure, toxic chemicals	Safety training, use of personal protective equipment; ventilate room; do not mix chemicals
Violence	Disgruntled clients or employees, angry family members, robberies	Listen

- MSDSs available at all times. If any chemicals are transferred to another container, the new container must be accurately labeled with descriptions and potential hazards. This includes disinfectants that are transferred to a spray bottle to clean exam room tables.
- An explanation of the labeling system.
- A protocol for emergency evacuation.
- A training program implementing the use of PPE and monitoring devices as well as the hazards of the practice. This is required for all practices with 11 or more employees.

Written Plan

The introduction of the communication plan should stress the commitment the practice has to workplace safety and employee heath. The safety officer can be named in the introduction, and a brief explanation of the system used to indentify chemicals and their hazards can be provided. An overview of the MSDS filing system may follow, along with the training objectives and how those objectives will be accomplished.

Material Safety Data Sheets

MSDSs are fact lists for chemicals and provide important information related to hazards (Figure 21-13) (also see the Evolve site that accompanies this text). Information included on sheets is as follows:
- The identity of the chemical
- Physical and chemical characteristics
- Health hazards
- Permissible exposure limits
- Whether the product is a carcinogen (cancer producing)
- Emergency first-aid procedures
- Specific hazards

MSDSs must be maintained for every hazardous chemical kept in the practice. Sheets must be kept current within 3 years of the date printed on the sheet. Manufacturers and distributors have MSDSs on hand; many are available on CD for easy referencing and printing.

OSHA allows a few MSDS exemptions (meaning an MSDS is not required). This includes many articles used by the practice; tape, hematocrit sealer, pens, and so forth are all exempt from MSDSs. Food and nutritional products, common household cleaning items, and drugs sold in tablet form are also exempt. Cleaning items must be used in the same format that a household would use them to be exempt. If tablets can be directed to be crushed or made into a dissolving solution, then an MSDS must exist. Capsules, gels, and solutions are not exempt from MSDSs.

Protocol for Emergency Evacuation

Emergency evacuation plans should include team members, clients, and patients. Patients are the last to be evacuated, and only after the situation has been evaluated and deemed safe for the rescue. This is an especially difficult topic for employees to accept and enforce; however, team member safety is of utmost importance. The protocol should also include how emergency personnel will be contacted, designate a central meeting place outside the facility, and include practice drills to improve the efficiency of the staff. The more physically and mentally prepared by role playing the staff is, the more effective the plan will be in case it is ever needed.

Training Program

A training program must include the description of the hazard, the correct PPE needed in case of emergency, how to use the PPE, and the location of the PPE.

Each hazard within the practice must be listed individually with the correct response procedures. Meetings should be held for team members to ask questions and practice using the PPE. Role playing is also suggested because employees who use PPE under stressful situations sometimes forget the basics of the equipment. The more familiar they are with the equipment, the better success team members will have in case of emergency. Videotaping the meetings for future team members to watch is suggested; they should then also have the ability to use the equipment hands-on.

Diamond Labeling System

The National Fire Protection Association uses colored diamond labels to indicate the risks associated with health, fire, reactivity, and special hazards of specific chemicals. These diamond stickers are placed at the entry point of the practice, along with the room the hazard is located in (Figure 21-14). These are not only important for team members, but also for emergency personnel if they need to enter the practice; the stickers allow them to quickly determine what hazards are in the practice and their location. These labels must also be placed on chemicals that are transferred from their original bottle (disinfectants placed in spray bottles for cleaning).

2006-July-05

003845
ACEPROJECT 50ML
ACEPROMAZINE MAL PVL

MATERIAL SAFETY DATA SHEET

1	PRODUCT AND COMPANY IDENTIFICATION

Product Name: Acepromazine Maleate Injection
Product No.: NADA 117-531
GHS Product Identifier: Not applicable

Synonyms: Not available
Molecular Formula: Mixture, not appplicable
Molecular Weight: Not applicable
CAS Number: Mixture, not applicable
Chemical Family: Phenothiazine Tranquilizer/Sedative

Manufacturer:
Boehringer Ingelheim Vetmedica, Inc.
2621 North Belt Hwy
St. Joseph, MO 64506-2002

Emergency Telephone:
Transportation Emergency: (800) 424-9300

Medical Emergency (24HR): (800) 530-5432

Intended Use:
Tranquilization aid and preanesthetic agent in
dogs, cats and horses

Non-emergency Telephone: (800) 821-7467

2	HAZARDS IDENTIFICATION

Emergency Overview

Physical State: 50 mL multidose vial of 10 mg/mL sterile liquid
Color: Yellow
Oder: Odorless

WARNING!
Harmful if swallowed-For dog, cat and horse injection only.
Not for human use.
May cause drowsiness or dizziness.
Causes eye irritation.

FIGURE 21-13 Example of an MSDS.

Chemical Spills

Spills can occur in any situation; accidents happen. A preparedness plan will help facilitate easy cleanup and prevent unnecessary exposure. A spill kit should be developed and maintained, and each team member must know where the kit is located. A safety program should instill role playing so each member knows how to use the kit in case of emergency.

When developing a spill kit, hazardous chemicals that are kept inside the practice need to be identified. MSDSs indicate the best cleanup method if a spill occurs. The information should be consolidated into an information sheet that is easy to understand. The sheet can then be laminated for protection.

> **PRACTICE POINT** Chemical spill kits are easy to assemble and do not require a large amount of space.

A spill kit should include a large plastic container to keep contents together. Inside there should be cat litter, a dustpan and broom, a pair of nitrate gloves, eye protection, and a laminated copy of cleanup procedures. The spill kit should be centrally located and easy to access.

Chemical Spill Cleanup Procedures

• Remove unnecessary people and pets from area to prevent spreading and exposure to chemical.
• Increase ventilation to area. Open windows and turn on exhaust fans and vents.

Acepromazine Maleate   2006-July-05
Injection

Precautionary Statements:
Accidental human injection can cause serious local reactions or anaphylactic reaction and
systemic effects.
Not for use in animals intended for food.
Keep only in original container.
Keep at a temperature not exceeding 30° C.
Fire-fighting: Use foam, carbon dioxide, dry powder and water fog or material appropriate for
surrounding fire.
Avoid contact with eyes, skin and clothing.
Wash thoroughly with soap and water after handling.
Wear suitable gloves and eye/face protection.
Spills: Cover with absorbent or contain. Collect and dispose.
In case of accident or if you feel unwell, seek medical advice immediately (show the label where possible).
Have the product container or label with you when calling a poison control center or doctor, or
going for treatment.
If swallowed, seek medical advice immediately and show this container or label.
In case of contact with eyes, rinse immediately with plenty of water for at least 15 minutes. Get
medical attention.
This material and its container must be disposed of in a safe way.
Keep out of reach of children.
Keep away from food, drink, and animal feedstuffs.

Acute effect:
Hypotension can occur after rapid intravenous injection causing cardiovascular collapse.
Tranquilizers are potent central nervous system depressants and they can cause marked sedation
with suppression of the sympathetic nervous system.
May produce an additive action when given in conjunction with other depressants.
Will potentiate general anesthesia.
In horses, paralysis of the retractor penis muscle has been associated with the use of phenothiazine
derivative tranquilizers. The risk should be duly considered prior to administration to male horses
(castrated and uncastrated).
Accidental Intracarotid injection in horses can produce clinical signs ranging from disorientation
to seizures to death.

Precautions/Contraindictions:
Should be avoided in pregnant or lactating animals. Should be used with caution in older animals,
animals with liver disease, heart disease, injury, or debilitation. Should not be used in animals
with a history of epilepsy, those prone to seizures or those receiving a myelogram (lowers the
seizure threshold). Should not be used in animals with tetanus or strychnine poisoning. Use with
caution in giant dog breeds and greyhounds due to their increased sensitivity to acepromazine.

Overdosage:
Overdose can cause excessive sedation, slow respiratory and heart rate, pale gums unsteady gait, poor
coordination, and inability to stand. May cause sudden collapse, unconsciousness, seizures and death.
Phenylephrine and norepinephrine are the drugs of choice to treat acepromazine-induced hypotension.
Barbiturates or diazepam may be used for the treatment of seizures associated with overdose.

FIGURE 21-13, cont'd

- Put on protective gloves. Put on gown if needed.
- Cover spill with absorbable material, either cat litter or paper towels.
- Clean up saturated absorbent material.
- Place chemical in trash bag and dispose of it properly.
- Wash area with plain water. Allow to dry.
- Wash hands.
- Replace materials used in spill kit.

DEVELOPING A HOSPITAL SAFETY MANUAL

A hospital safety manual (HSM) should include an overview of all materials covered above. It should include the hazardous communication plan, the MSDS filing system, and an explanation of secondary container labeling systems. An HSM can be created for each individual clinic or ordered. Tabs can be used to separate topics and allow easy identification. Topics included in an HSM can include, but are not limited to:

- General rules
- Accident prevention
- Anesthesia
- Chemicals
- Chemical spills
- Fire prevention and response
- Infection control
- Laboratory
- Radiation
- Restraint

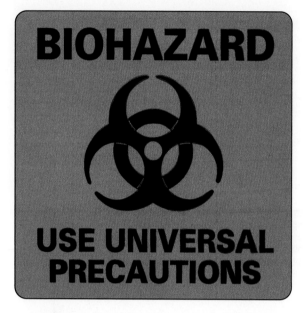

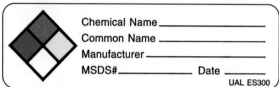

FIGURE 21-14 Biohazard sign and diamond labeling system.

> **PRACTICE POINT** Hospital safety manuals should be easy to navigate and placed in a convenient, centralized location.

ACCIDENT REPORTING AND INVESTIGATION

Every accident that occurs in the practice must be reported to the safety manager and/or practice manager and owner. If medical treatment is needed, appropriate paperwork should be available for the employee to take to the doctor or hospital (Figures 21-15 and 21-16). Paperwork may include the First Notice of Accident or Injury and Illness Incident Report (Figure 21-17) and/or a Workers' Compensation Insurance Claim Form. This will ensure that the employer's insurance is charged for the visit, not the team member's. When the employee returns from the medical visit, paperwork should be sent to the appropriate companies, state, or local authorities. Since workers' compensation varies by state, each practice must have a full understanding of the required filing procedures. Practices with 11 or more employees must record all accidents on an OSHA Form 300. Only injuries resulting in death or the hospitalization of five or more employees must be reported to OSHA. OSHA Form 300 must be kept for 5 years.

> **PRACTICE POINT** Every accident must be reported to the owner or practice manager and recorded on OSHA Form 300.

DOCUMENTATION

Documentation of the safety program must exist. Outlines of training programs, attendees, dates, and signatures should be kept on file. A summary of all hazardous chemicals, a workplace safety manual, and any workplace injuries and illnesses must be kept together. Injuries for the previous year must be posted on the staff bulletin board from February 1 through April 30 on OSHA Form 300A. OSHA Form 300A is a summary form of OSHA 300.

FIRE PREVENTION

The two most common causes of fire in the veterinary practice are overloaded electrical circuits and items stored too close to heat sources. Too many pieces of equipment plugged into one circuit can cause an instant electrical fire. If more circuits are needed, a certified electrician should be contacted to add more circuits for the practice. Newspapers, blankets, files, and supplies must not be stored near a furnace, water heater, or heat source, and portable heaters should never be left unattended.

> **PRACTICE POINT** Practices with 10 or more employees must have a written OSHA plan that includes fire prevention and response.

Practices with 10 or more employees must have a fire prevention and response plan. This should be included in the HSM and reviewed at safety training meetings. Fire prevention measures include a monthly walk-through of the facility. Fire extinguishers should be checked for damage or any evidence of tampering. Smoke and fire alarms should be tested; if the building is equipped with a sprinkler system, that should be evaluated as well. Fire extinguishers must be checked by a safety company at least yearly to ensure the efficacy of the extinguisher. Walk-through inspections and inspections of equipment should be documented. The response portion of the plan should include the evacuation of employees and clients, escape routes and procedures, a procedure to account for all team members, and a method to report the fire. The name of the safety officer should be included as well. A fire could happen to any practice at any time. It could occur with no one in the building or during the busiest time of the day.

FIRE CODES AND INSPECTIONS

Fire codes vary by location, so each practice should become familiar with codes in its geographic area. In general, the fire department is responsible for inspections of businesses and for ensuring that they are compliant with regulations established. Requirements may

How to Fill Out the Log

The *Log of Work-Related Injuries and Illnesses* is used to classify work-related injuries and illnesses and to note the extent and severity of each case. When an incident occurs, use the *Log* to record specific details about what happened and how it happened.

If your company has more than one establishment or site, you must keep separate records for each physical location that is expected to remain in operation for one year or longer.

We have given you several copies of the *Log* in this package. If you need more than we provided, you may photocopy and use as many as you need.

The *Summary* — a separate form — shows the work-related injury and illness totals for the year in each category. At the end of the year, count the number of incidents in each category and transfer the totals from the *Log* to the *Summary*. Then post the *Summary* in a visible location so that your employees are aware of the injuries and illnesses occurring in their workplace.

You don't post the *Log*. You post only the *Summary* at the end of the year.

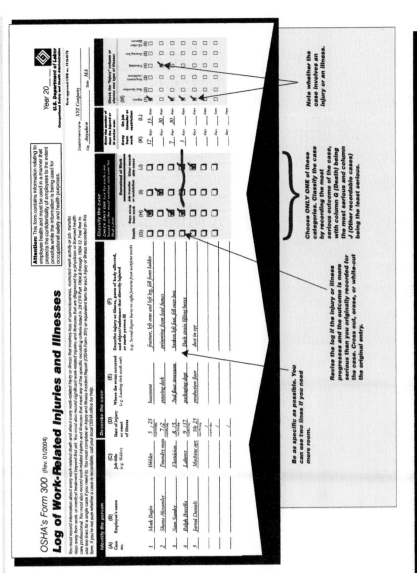

FIGURE 21-15 OSHA Form 300. (Courtesy Occupational Safety and Health Administration, Department of Labor, Washington, DC.)

OSHA's Form 300 (Rev. 01/2004)

Log of Work-Related Injuries and Illnesses

You must record information about every work-related death and about every work-related injury or illness that involves loss of consciousness, restricted work activity or job transfer, days away from work, or medical treatment beyond first aid. You must also record significant work-related injuries and illnesses that are diagnosed by a physician or licensed health care professional. You must also record work-related injuries and illnesses that meet any of the specific recording criteria listed in 29 CFR Part 1904.8 through 1904.12. Feel free to use two lines for a single case if you need to. You must complete an Injury and Illness Incident Report (OSHA Form 301) or equivalent form for each injury or illness recorded on this form. If you're not sure whether a case is recordable, call your local OSHA office for help.

Attention: This form contains information relating to employee health and must be used in a manner that protects the confidentiality of employees to the extent possible while the information is being used for occupational safety and health purposes.

Year 20____

U.S. Department of Labor
Occupational Safety and Health Administration

Form approved OMB no. 1218-0176

Establishment name _____

City _____ State _____

Identify the person

(A) Case no.	(B) Employee's name	(C) Job title (e.g., Welder)

Describe the case

(D) Date of injury or onset of illness	(E) Where the event occurred (e.g., Loading dock north end)	(F) Describe injury or illness, parts of body affected, and object/substance that directly injured or made person ill (e.g., Second degree burns on right forearm from acetylene torch)
month/day		
month/day		
month/day		
month/day		
month/day		
month/day		
month/day		
month/day		
month/day		
month/day		
month/day		
month/day		
month/day		

Classify the case

CHECK ONLY ONE box for each case based on the most serious outcome for that case:

(G) Death	Remained at Work (H) Days away from work	(I) Job transfer or restriction	(J) Other recordable cases

Enter the number of days the injured or ill worker was:

(K) Away from work	(L) On job transfer or restriction
___ days	___ days
___ days	___ days
___ days	___ days
___ days	___ days
___ days	___ days
___ days	___ days
___ days	___ days
___ days	___ days
___ days	___ days
___ days	___ days
___ days	___ days
___ days	___ days
___ days	___ days

Check the "Injury" column or choose one type of illness:

(M)

(1) Injury	(2) Skin disorder	(3) Respiratory condition	(4) Poisoning	(5) Hearing loss	(6) All other illnesses

Page totals ▶

Be sure to transfer these totals to the Summary page (Form 300A) before you post it.

Public reporting burden for this collection of information is estimated to average 14 minutes per response, including time to review the instructions, search and gather the data needed, and complete and review the collection of information. Persons are not required to respond to the collection of information unless it displays a currently valid OMB control number. If you have any comments about these estimates or any other aspects of this data collection, contact: US Department of Labor, OSHA Office of Statistical Analysis, Room N-3644, 200 Constitution Avenue, NW, Washington, DC 20210. Do not send the completed forms to this office.

Page ___ of ___

FIGURE 21-15, cont'd

OSHA's Form 300A (Rev. 01/2004)

Summary of Work-Related Injuries and Illnesses

Year 20____

U.S. Department of Labor
Occupational Safety and Health Administration

Form approved OMB no. 1218-0176

All establishments covered by Part 1904 must complete this Summary page, even if no work-related injuries or illnesses occurred during the year. Remember to review the Log to verify that the entries are complete and accurate before completing this summary.

Using the Log, count the individual entries you made for each category. Then write the totals below, making sure you've added the entries from every page of the Log. If you had no cases, write "0."

Employees, former employees, and their representatives have the right to review the OSHA Form 300 in its entirety. They also have limited access to the OSHA Form 301 or its equivalent. See 29 CFR Part 1904.35, in OSHA's recordkeeping rule, for further details on the access provisions for these forms.

Number of Cases

Total number of deaths	Total number of cases with days away from work	Total number of cases with job transfer or restriction	Total number of other recordable cases
(G)	(H)	(I)	(J)

Number of Days

Total number of days away from work	Total number of days of job transfer or restriction
(K)	(L)

Injury and Illness Types

Total number of . . .
(M)

(1) Injuries _____

(2) Skin disorders _____

(3) Respiratory conditions _____

(4) Poisonings _____

(5) Hearing loss _____

(6) All other illnesses _____

Establishment information

Your establishment name _____

Street _____

City _____ State _____ ZIP _____

Industry description *(e.g., Manufacture of motor truck trailers)*
_____

Standard Industrial Classification (SIC), if known *(e.g., 3715)*
_ _ _ _

OR

North American Industrial Classification (NAICS), if known *(e.g., 336212)*
_ _ _ _ _ _

Employment information *(If you don't have these figures, see the Worksheet on the back of this page to estimate.)*

Annual average number of employees _____

Total hours worked by all employees last year _____

Sign here

Knowingly falsifying this document may result in a fine.

I certify that I have examined this document and that to the best of my knowledge the entries are true, accurate, and complete.

_____ *Company executive*   _____ Title

(____) ____ - ____ *Phone*   __/__/__ Date

Post this Summary page from February 1 to April 30 of the year following the year covered by the form.

Public reporting burden for this collection of information is estimated to average 58 minutes per response, including time to review the instructions, search and gather the data needed, and complete and review the collection of information. Persons are not required to respond to the collection of information unless it displays a currently valid OMB control number. If you have any comments about these estimates or any other aspects of this data collection, contact: US Department of Labor, OSHA Office of Statistical Analysis, Room N-3644, 200 Constitution Avenue, NW, Washington, DC 20210. Do not send the completed forms to this office.

FIGURE 21-16 OSHA Form 300A. (Courtesy Occupational Safety and Health Administration, Department of Labor, Washington, DC.)

OSHA's Form 301
Injury and Illness Incident Report

U.S. Department of Labor
Occupational Safety and Health Administration

Form approved OMB no. 1218-0176

Attention: This form contains information relating to employee health and must be used in a manner that protects the confidentiality of employees to the extent possible while the information is being used for occupational safety and health purposes.

This *Injury and Illness Incident Report* is one of the first forms you must fill out when a recordable work-related injury or illness has occurred. Together with the *Log of Work-Related Injuries and Illnesses* and the accompanying *Summary*, these forms help the employer and OSHA develop a picture of the extent and severity of work-related incidents.

Within 7 calendar days after you receive information that a recordable work-related injury or illness has occurred, you must fill out this form or an equivalent. Some state workers' compensation, insurance, or other reports may be acceptable substitutes. To be considered an equivalent form, any substitute must contain all the information asked for on this form.

According to Public Law 91-596 and 29 CFR 1904, OSHA's recordkeeping rule, you must keep this form on file for 5 years following the year to which it pertains.

If you need additional copies of this form, you may photocopy and use as many as you need.

Completed by _____

Title _____

Phone (_____) _____ – _____   Date ___/___/___

Information about the employee

1) Full name _____

2) Street _____

City _____ State _____ ZIP _____

3) Date of birth ___/___/___

4) Date hired ___/___/___

5) ☐ Male ☐ Female

Information about the physician or other health care professional

6) Name of physician or other health care professional

_____

7) If treatment was given away from the worksite, where was it given?

Facility _____

Street _____

City _____ State _____ ZIP _____

8) Was employee treated in an emergency room?
   ☐ Yes
   ☐ No

9) Was employee hospitalized overnight as an in-patient?
   ☐ Yes
   ☐ No

Information about the case

10) Case number from the Log _____   *(Transfer the case number from the Log after you record the case.)*

11) Date of injury or illness ___/___/___

12) Time employee began work _____ AM / PM

13) Time of event _____ AM / PM   ☐ Check if time cannot be determined

14) **What was the employee doing just before the incident occurred?** Describe the activity, as well as the tools, equipment, or material the employee was using. Be specific. *Examples:* "climbing a ladder while carrying roofing materials"; "spraying chlorine from hand sprayer"; "daily computer key-entry."

15) **What happened?** Tell us how the injury occurred. *Examples:* "When ladder slipped on wet floor, worker fell 20 feet"; "Worker was sprayed with chlorine when gasket broke during replacement"; "Worker developed soreness in wrist over time."

16) **What was the injury or illness?** Tell us the part of the body that was affected and how it was affected; be more specific than "hurt," "pain," or sore." *Examples:* "strained back"; "chemical burn, hand"; "carpal tunnel syndrome."

17) **What object or substance directly harmed the employee?** *Examples:* "concrete floor"; "chlorine"; "radial arm saw." *If this question does not apply to the incident, leave it blank.*

18) *If the employee died, when did death occur?* Date of death ___/___/___

Public reporting burden for this collection of information is estimated to average 22 minutes per response, including time for reviewing instructions, searching existing data sources, gathering and maintaining the data needed, and completing and reviewing the collection of information. Persons are not required to respond to the collection of information unless it displays a current valid OMB control number. If you have any comments about this estimate or any other aspects of this data collection, including suggestions for reducing this burden, contact: US Department of Labor, OSHA Office of Statistical Analysis, Room N-3644, 200 Constitution Avenue, NW, Washington, DC 20210. Do not send the completed forms to this office.

FIGURE 21-17 OSHA Log 301. (Courtesy Occupational Safety and Health Administration, Department of Labor, Washington, DC.)

exist regarding exit signs and emergency lighting. Fire extinguishers are required, as are smoke detectors.

Exit Signs and Lighting

Signs must indicate where the exit is located (Figure 21-18). If a door looks like an exit but is not, it must be labeled "Not an Exit."

Emergency lights are required and must be tested on a yearly basis to ensure that they are working properly. Lights should be installed in locations that light the pathway to the exit, as well as in locations where team members might be performing duties that could result in injury if the lighting system fails (Figure 21-19).

> **PRACTICE POINT**   Emergency lighting is required by law.

Fire Extinguishers

Fire extinguishers must be located no more than 75 feet from any distance within the practice and placed 32 to 48 inches above the ground surface. Along with being placed in a central location of the clinic, extinguishers should be placed near the exit doors of the practice (Figure 21-20).

All employees must be trained in the use of a fire extinguisher. If a training facility is available, team members should practice using extinguishers because common sense often disappears during an emergency. Practicing will help instill automatic reactions. Team

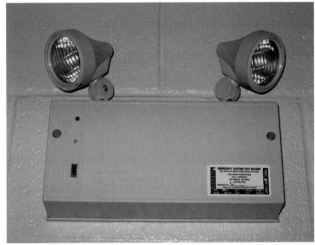

FIGURE 21-19 Emergency lighting is required and must be tested on a yearly basis.

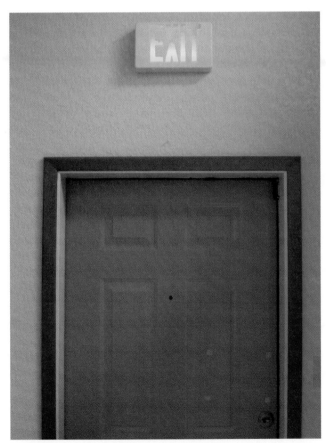

FIGURE 21-18 All exits must be indicated as such by an exit sign.

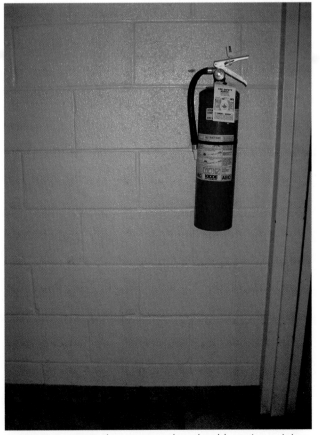

FIGURE 21-20 Each team member should receive training in the use of a fire extinguisher.

members can remember the word "pass" to help initiate the use of an extinguisher when needed:

P = **P**ull the pin.

A = **A**im low. Point the extinguisher to the bottom of the fire.

S = **S**queeze the handle.

S = **S**weep from side to side at the base of the fire until it appears to be out.

Before fire extinguishers are used, employees should make sure that the fire alarm has been sounded. Team members should never attempt to fight a fire that is larger than the immediate area and, if it is spreading, they must exit the building.

Fire extinguishers are made of carbon dioxide, dry chemicals, halon, or water. Carbon dioxide is most effective on class B and C fires (liquid and electrical) but is only effective for 3 to 8 feet because the carbon dioxide disperses quickly. Dry chemical fire extinguishers are used for a variety of fires and contain an extinguishing agent and compressed gas as a propellant. Halon extinguishers contain a gas that interrupts the chemical reaction taking place when fuel burns. Halon is used to protect electrical equipment because it does not leave any residue to clean up. Water fire extinguishers contain water and compressed gas and are used for class A fires (combustible) only.

Smoke Detectors

Batteries should be replaced on a yearly basis whether a change is needed or not. Monthly testing will ensure the product is in working condition.

> **PRACTICE POINT** Replace smoke alarm batteries yearly!

Fire Sprinklers

Many older buildings do not have fire sprinkler systems and have been grandfathered in. New buildings are required to have sprinkler systems, which must be evaluated frequently to ensure they are in proper working condition.

Blocked Entries/Exits

Entries and exits must not be blocked with anything, not even for a few minutes. In the event of a fire, anything that might prevent emergency exiting could have devastating effects.

Eyewash Station

Eyewash stations are required of every safety program and must be available if a team member or client gets a chemical or foreign object in the eye. A variety of eyewash stations are available, ranging from handheld bottles to stations connected to a consistent water supply. The most common are the eyewash stations that simply

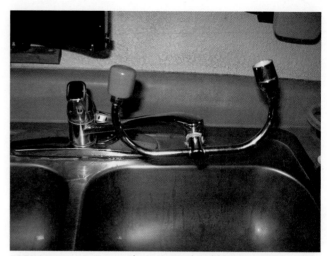

FIGURE 21-21 Eyewash stations should be centrally located.

attach to the top of a water faucet spout and are capped until needed. If the station is needed, a lever on the station is turned to allow water pressure to dispense; water is squirted in an upwards direction, allowing the employee to place his or her eyes in direct contact with pressurized water (Figure 21-21). This allows the flushing of any chemical that entered the eye. Most chemicals recommend flushing for 5 to 10 minutes; this information can be obtained from the MSDS. Water feels uncomfortable when flushing first begins because it is not the same pH as the eye and does not have the same salt content; however, team members must understand flushing is essential to remove potentially harmful substances and objects.

> **PRACTICE POINT** Eyewash stations are easy to install and should be centrally located in the practice.

Eyewash stations that connected to a consistent water supply are ideal because they apply the same amount of pressure to the eye for a period of time. Handheld bottles run out of water and do not supply constant pressure. If a faucet-mounted station is used, the hot water should be disconnected to prevent further injury to the eye. Each team member should practice using the eyewash station so that all are familiar with it in the event of an emergency. Eyewash stations should be marked with a sticker or sign indicating equipment location.

ESCAPING ANIMALS

Every preventive measure must be taken to prevent the escape of an animal. Many reasons exist for a patient to become scared and try to escape, and the practice can be held liable for the escape of an animal. Windows should never be left open, regardless of whether there is a screen on the window or not. Cats can claw through screens. Doors should never be left open; dogs may escape from restraint or slip a leash. Dogs are also great at being able to escape from kennels without the knowledge of team members. Any dog that is being removed from a cage or kennel should have a slip leash applied, not the owner's collar and leash. Many times, the owner's collar and leash are very loose and the animal can pull right out. A slip leash tightens around the neck, preventing the dog from slipping away.

Feral animals should be handled with caution at all times. If an examination is necessary, they should be placed in a quiet room that does not have any other animals in it. The desired room should have minimal shelving and breakable items if the animal escapes from restraint. Some feral animals can be examined with mild restraint; slow and cautious movements should be used to prevent startling the animal. If the animal escapes, it should be given some time to calm down. If this cannot occur, then capture techniques will need to be used. A fish net may help capture a feral cat; a rabies pole may be needed for an aggressive dog. All caution must be taken to prevent being bitten. Feral animals may need sedation before any exam for the safety of the staff.

All caution must be used when walking dogs outdoors. Ideally, practices should have a fenced-in area to walk dogs to help prevent an escape. Again, slip leashes should be used at all times; specific dogs may be denied walks based on the likelihood of them becoming scared and trying to escape while outside. In situations such as this, the owner may be asked to come and walk the dog during the day.

VETERINARY PRACTICE and the LAW

Clients who are injured while on the premises of the veterinary hospital may be tempted to sue the practice for injuries that occurred, along with pain and suffering. All attempts must be made to prevent a situation in which an injury can occur.

Team members who are injured on the job must report injuries immediately and seek medical help if warranted. Workers' Compensation must pay for the injury; however, an inspection and an increase in rates may result from the claim. Inspections are deemed necessary to ensure that practice is using safe working policies.

Team members must be alert as to all hazards that can occur on the premises at all times. Hazards can harm team members, clients, and patients. Wet floors must be identified and labeled for staff and clients. Wet floors should be towel dried to prevent someone from slipping. Barrier signs should be posted around an object on the floor to prevent people from tripping on it. Oxygen tanks should be secured to a wall to prevent team members from accidently bumping into them and knocking them over.

Self-Evaluation Questions

1. What is a zoonotic disease?
2. How should an animal heavier than 40 lb be lifted onto a table?
3. What is OSHA?
4. What is the Right-to-Know poster?
5. What is an MSDS?
6. What is the purpose of PPE?
7. When does OSHA Form 300A have to be posted?
8. What is an eyewash station?
9. What is a biohazard material?
10. What are some hazardous chemicals used in veterinary practice?

Recommended Reading

Lappin M: General concepts in zoonotic disease control, *Vet Clin North Am* 35:1, 2005.

McKelvey D: *Safety handbook for veterinary hospital staff*, Lakewood, CO, 1999, AAHA Press.

OSHA: employee workplace rights, Washington, DC, 1994, OSHA Publications Office.

Seibert P: *The complete veterinary practice regulatory manual*, ed 5, Calhoun, TN, 1996, Safety Vet.

Stowe JD, Ackerman LJ: *The effective veterinary practice*, Guelph, Ont, Canada, 2004, *Lifelearn, Inc.*

Veterinary safety: workplace topics for your veterinary practice, Schaumburg, IL, 2003, American Veterinary Medical Association Professional Liability Trust.

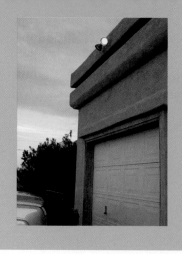

Security

Chapter Outline

Computer System
Theft
Security System
Cameras and Recording Devices
Perimeter Lighting

Emergency Calls
Mobile Practices
Methods of Defense
    Personal Protection Devices
Safety of Hospitalized Patients

Learning Objectives

Mastery of the content in this chapter will enable the reader to:
- Define the importance of one-way door locks.
- Describe methods used to protect a computer system against embezzlement and hackers.
- Describe methods used to protect the practice against theft from both employees and thieves.

- Identify an effective security system for the practice.
- Define perimeter lighting.
- Define personal protection devices.

Key Terms

Computer Hacker
One-Way Door Locks
Perimeter Lighting

Personal Protection Device
Security System

Security for team members and the practice must be considered a top priority. Practices have an ethical obligation to provide a safe and secure working environment for employees as well as a safe and secure hospital for clients and their pets. Safety goes beyond the standard preventions for slips and falls; security must be included and viewed from several aspects. Computer systems must be protected from employees, clients, the general public, and especially hackers. The practice must be protected from robbers and thieves, and clients and patients must be protected from harm and danger.

Practices should use deadbolts on all doors and one-way locks on all doors except the client entrance. When the business is open, the deadbolts must remain unlocked. The one-way door lock only allows access into the building with a key, but clients and employees can exit anytime. The client entrance door must let clients enter and exit as needed; therefore a standard door lock can be installed. All doors must be locked before the last team member leaves the premises to ensure the safety of the practice.

Entrances must be protected and monitored for those who enter. Any door other than the one clients enter must be locked at all times. A person could enter through any unlocked door in the rear of the practice and hide until the practice closes. He or she could harm employees quickly and force them into inconceivable actions. It is imperative to secure doors, and they must remain locked from the outside at all times. One-way door locks allow employees and clients to escape if an emergency occurs.

COMPUTER SYSTEM

The computer system is a valuable asset to the practice and must be protected from hackers, employees, and clients. A computer hacker is an individual or group or individuals who attempt to break into programs or networks that are restricted. Once they gain access to the restricted program, the hackers can cause damage to the program or network. This damage can range from changing prices to deleting transactions as well as installing viruses that can cripple the system. Chapter 8 describes several products that can be used to protect a system from hackers. Antivirus software, firewalls, and antispyware should be installed on each computer that is linked to the system to aid in the protection.

> ◎ **PRACTICE POINT** Computers must be backed up daily at the end of each shift.

Practices should ensure that the system is backed up on a nightly basis, either to an off-premises location or onto a CD that is removed from the system. If a thief breaks into the practice at night and steals the computer or causes severe damage to it, information can be fully reinstalled onto a new computer.

It is terrible to assume that computers must be protected from employees; however, employees will, on occasion, steal client mailing lists and sell them, either to a competing veterinarian or to a mail order company that is willing to pay for the names and addresses.

> ◎ **PRACTICE POINT** Veterinary computer software should be password protected for specified procedures.

Passwords should be put in place on a computer system, allowing only certain individuals access to financial reports, mailing lists, and deletion codes. Office managers should be the only employees allowed to delete transactions, and practice managers and owners should be the only team members allowed to change or delete product and service codes. Managers should also be the only authority to change and/or override prices of products and services. Managers should review the audit trail daily looking for any signs of embezzlement or theft.

If computers are located in exam rooms, a password-protected screen saver should be enabled. Clients waiting to be seen may try to access the Internet or their record. Confidential information may be obtained by these clients if they access the practice management system.

THEFT

Theft can occur at any time, either by an employee or by a person who enters the building with the intent to commit a crime. Employee theft can range from embezzling cash to stealing products and/or food. Procedures must be implemented to prevent either situation from occurring. Cash transactions must be recorded immediately, both in the computer and in the client's record. Receipts must be produced for clients indicating their account has been paid with cash. End-of-day totals must match the cash in the drawer, along with all credit card and check transactions. The deposit must then be double checked by the practice manager, ensuring that the deposit made to the bank at the end of the day matches the end-of-day deposit in the computer. If any discrepancy exists, it must be investigated immediately. Review Chapter 2 for more information on end-of-day reconciliation security features.

Team members purchasing products should always have the designated office manager enter the products or services into the computer. This ensures consistency in entering codes and allows someone other than the team member purchasing the product to determine the total. If owners, associates, or practice managers see an employee taking product that has not been charged for out of the building, the employee should be questioned immediately, not days later.

Practices must always be prepared for criminal intent. Practices are the target for theft of both drugs and cash. Many practices do not keep a large amount of cash on hand, especially since the payment trend has shifted to debit cards instead of cash for payment of

---

What Would You Do/Not Do?

Chade, a new veterinary assistant, observed a long-term associate place a box of Heartgard in her purse and leave the practice. She does not yet know what the procedures are for charging employees for products and assumes that the associate has been charged for the product. Two months later, she sees the same associate place cephalexin capsules in a pill vial without creating a label for the medication. Chade has learned that labels are created once a product is entered into the computer, which then charges appropriately. Chade is unsure about the process but feels that the associate may be taking product from the clinic. She is unsure whether she should talk to the owner about the associate. She feels that because she is the new employee, that the owner or practice manager may not believe her.

What Should Chade Do?

The practice should have an open-door policy regarding communication, making it easy for Chade to talk with her superiors about the possible employee theft. She should talk with the owner or practice manager when other employees are not around and address her concerns. She should detail both incidents and explain that she is not trying to get anyone in trouble, but rather to protect the practice from loss associated with shrinkage. She may suggest the installation of a video camera system to help deter employee theft, and offer to find a variety of systems for the practice to consider.

services. However, thieves continue to believe that veterinary practices hold a large amount of cash on premises. Individuals also want ketamine, which has a large dollar value on the streets. It is imperative that all drugs be locked in a safe that cannot be moved. Review Chapter 16 for information on safes approved by the Drug Enforcement Agency.

If a person with criminal intent enters the practice, all money should be given to him or her from the cash drawer. Team members should not risk injury or death to themselves, clients, or other team members to protect the small amount of money that the practice has on premises. If the thieves request drugs, give them whatever they want; the sooner they leave the practice, the safer the team members and clients will be. All doors should be locked and police should be called immediately.

> **PRACTICE POINT**   Remaining calm during a robbery is essential to help prevent team members from being injured by the thieves.

If the team is able to get a description of the thieves, it will be helpful to police, along with a description of the vehicle used to get away. Details can be hard to obtain in stressful situations such as this.

SECURITY SYSTEM

Security systems should be installed to protect the premises while the practice is closed. Sensory devices should be placed on all windows and doors; if any window or door is broken or opened after the system as been activated, an alarm will sound. Systems may also have a motion detector; once the alarm has been activated, any motion that is detected inside the building will trigger the alarm (Figure 22-1). Many security systems are connected to a monitoring system, which will automatically place a call to police if the alarm is triggered. Many practices have keypads at the employee entrance, allowing the alarm to be set or deactivated. Others have a badge reader; employees must swipe their badges to gain access to the building. This also allows employee monitoring during closed hours. Both devices can prevent entry if an employee is terminated and tries to reenter the building after the practice has closed.

> **PRACTICE POINT**   Security systems are mandatory to protect the practice after hours.

Many security devices have the ability to send pages, text messages, or alerts to owners and practice managers regarding who has activated and deactivated the system and when. This allows the monitoring of the practice over the weekend, if and when employees are on the premises when they should not be. Unfortunately, some robberies are the result of an inside job or tipoff; all perimeters must be monitored closely to protect the business in all fashions.

Some security systems have the option of installing panic buttons. These buttons are excellent in the event of a robbery or assault and should be placed in the front office in a convenient, yet hidden, location. If an emergency occurs, team members can hit the panic button to automatically call 911.

Emergency and specialty clinics often install buzzers at their front doors, adding a second level of protection for team members. When clients arrive, they push a buzzer; the receptionist can verify the clients and allow access.

Emergency clinics must take special precautions for safety because they are open throughout the night and weekend. This is a particularly easy time for criminals to target the business. Many emergency clinics have fewer employees at night, and there are fewer witnesses to observe unlawful actions.

Some practices may also install security devices on pharmacy doors, allowing the monitoring of team members who enter and exit the pharmacy room. This can decrease shrinkage (i.e., employee theft).

CAMERAS AND RECORDING DEVICES

Cameras can be placed at all entrances and exits, allowing recording of all employees and clients as they enter and leave the premises (Figure 22-2). Cameras and monitoring systems should be of high quality, allowing replication of images if needed. Action can be recorded on DVD-R, which allows more information to be stored than a CD, and can be written over with the permission of the operator. Cameras can be linked through the server, allowing an owner to view actions occurring

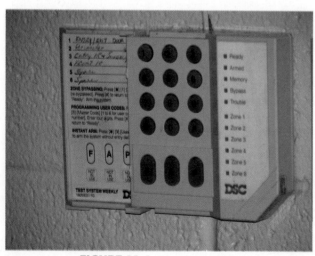

FIGURE 22-1 Security system.

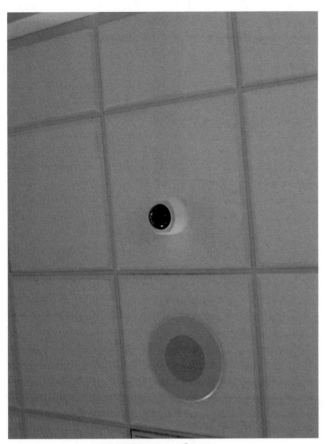

FIGURE 22-2 Camera.

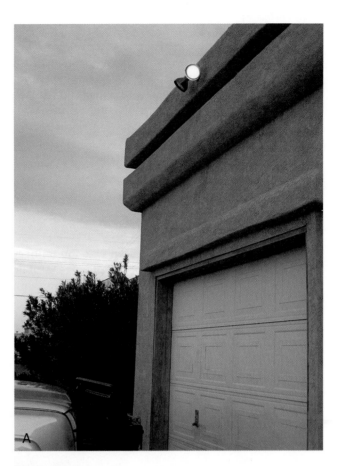

A

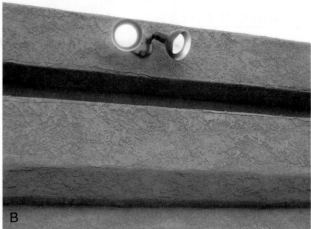

B

FIGURE 22-3 A and **B,** Perimeter lighting.

through a home computer. If the alarm was triggered due to a loose animal, the police can be notified of the false alarm.

Cameras can also be placed over cash drawers, near controlled substance locations, and within the pharmacy location to thwart potential employee embezzlement.

PERIMETER LIGHTING

The practice must have excellent lighting on the outside of the building and parking lot for the protection of clients and employees (Figure 22-3). Potential criminals may find a dark corner and wait for an employee to leave the building alone at night. They may either attack the employee in the parking lot or follow the person to another location. The same can occur for clients, who are less observant when leaving practices; they are generally preoccupied with their pets and loading them safely into the vehicle. Bright lights act as a deterrent to criminals and provide a safer environment.

> **PRACTICE POINT**   Parking lots and the perimeter of the building must be lit well for the protection of both team members and clients.

When team members are leaving a practice, they should use the buddy system, with a minimum of two employees leaving together. If only one employee needs to leave, two others should walk the team member to his or her car, then return to the practice as the car is leaving. If team members must be at a practice alone (weekend treatments, etc.) they should be instructed never to answer the door. Thieves are creative at being able to get into a business after hours, especially if they see a lone employee inside. Team members should always inspect the outside premises before leaving to ensure no one is lingering in the parking lot.

EMERGENCY CALLS

Many practices in small communities are on call for emergencies. In such situations, veterinarians are at an increased risk for attempted assaults, and all precautions should be taken when meeting clients. Calls should not be taken alone; a technician should arrive with the doctor, regardless of the time or day. Clients should be viewed through the "peephole" in the door to visualize the pet and ensure that the client has an actual emergency.

MOBILE PRACTICES

Mobile practices are at an increased risk for robbery and assault due to the mobility of the practice. Mobile veterinarians may carry drugs with them, along with cash, making them excellent targets for assailants. Veterinarians should always carry cell phones with emergency numbers programmed for quick access. Carrying some type of device for personal protection is recommended.

> **PRACTICE POINT**   Mobile veterinary units are especially vulnerable to thieves, and every safety precaution must be taken.

METHODS OF DEFENSE

A recommendation for a monthly meeting topic is methods of defense in case any violent crime or assault occurs. It is also advisable to have a local defense expert provide valuable training for the staff. Experts can locate areas of weakness in safety in and around the practice and can create scenarios for team members to role play. The more aware team members are of a possible assault, the better they are able to respond.

> **PRACTICE POINT**   Personal defense courses should be recommended for all team members.

Personal Protection Devices

The ASP Tactical Baton is the most tactically sophisticated impact weapon currently available (Figure 22-4). Easily carried and readily available, ASP batons have an incredible psychological deterrence and control potential. ASP batons are small to carry, but once swung to open the baton extends immediately, providing excellent protection for an individual. ASP batons can be kept in the front office with the receptionist for defense against would-be attackers. The receptionist would be able to swing the baton open in the event of an attack. ASP batons are also ideal for mobile veterinarians.

Mace is a brand of tear gas that is often used by police to deter potential attackers. Mace must be sprayed directly at the attacker and creates an intense burning sensation in the eyes and lungs. Mace can be extremely effective when used correctly.

Tasers are often thought of as weapons used by law enforcement to subdue those who are apprehended. Fortunately, models are also available for personal protection. A taser is an electroshock weapon that uses electrical current to disrupt voluntary control of muscles. Someone struck by a taser experiences stimulation of his or her sensory nerves and motor nerves, resulting in strong involuntary muscle contractions. Tasers do not rely on pain compliance and are thus preferred by some law enforcement over non-taser stun guns and other electronic control weapons.

Both ASP batons and tasers may require training in some states. Practices and mobile veterinarians should inquire with the local police department about the use and regulations of such devices. The manufacturers of both products offer courses with certified trainers to

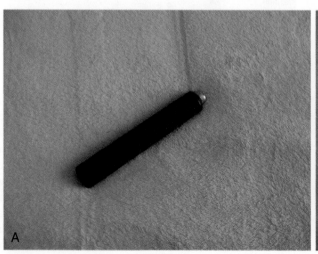

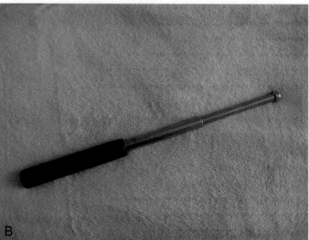

FIGURE 22-4 **A,** ASP Baton unextended. **B,** ASP Baton extended.

allow individuals to become comfortable with the use of such items. Both personal protection devices can cause great harm to another individual and should never be used carelessly.

SAFETY OF HOSPITALIZED PATIENTS

Patients that are hospitalized must be protected at all times. It has been reported that criminals sometimes break into a practice, steal a few items, and release all the animals that are hospitalized or being boarded. If it is possible to lock doorways between the practice and cages, patients are at less of a risk of being targeted. However, if a fire occurs in the building after hours, this may hamper rescue efforts.

VETERINARY PRACTICE and the LAW

One function of the veterinary practice that has been affected by the Patient Privacy Act is patient check-in. Clients who sign in may sign in on a sheet with adhesive pull off strips for each line so that clients cannot read names of those who have signed in before them. The privacy rule does permit incidental disclosures as long as the practice has reasonable guards against disclosure of personal information. Clients may be called to the examination room by their pet's name, protecting the privacy of their last names. Silent pagers can also be used, paging clients as a room becomes available.

It is also important to protect the computer screen from clients; personal information should not be viewable to clients as they check in or out. Screen privacy protectors can be applied to monitors, preventing the viewing of documents from an angle. A shredder should also be available to shred documents as needed, protecting clients' personal information.

Self-Evaluation Questions

1. Why should computer systems be backed up at the end of every shift?
2. Why should computer software be password protected?
3. What is the purpose of one-way door locks?
4. What should team members do if an armed individual enters the practice and demands money or drugs?
5. How can security systems provide practice protection?
6. Why is exterior perimeter lighting so critical?
7. What is an ASP baton?

Clinical Assisting in the Veterinary Practice

Veterinary assistants and technicians play a vital role in the success of the practice, especially when it comes to clinical assisting. The veterinarian(s) must be able to depend on the assistants to obtain accurate histories of the patient, restrain animals properly for examination, and perform diagnostic procedures efficiently and correctly. Procedures completed incorrectly or by cutting corners can yield unreliable and false results, resulting in poor patient care. Procedures completed incorrectly also contribute to the loss of money for the practice because tests must be repeated at no charge to the client.

It is imperative for veterinary assistants and technicians to understand the risks associated with anesthesia and surgery and relay that information to clients. Many clients do not understand that such risks are present and may become extremely upset if a tragic event occurs while their pet is in the hospital. Not only do the medications present a risk for surgery, but the surgical packs, equipment, and room must be prepared correctly to prevent nosocomial infections, which can also present risk for the patient. Correct instrument cleaning procedures, autoclaving techniques, and pack preparation must be initiated and enforced.

Anesthesia machine maintenance and administration of gases fall in the hands of assistants and technicians, who must be able to troubleshoot and correct problems within minutes. A machine working at optimal levels and a machine that is barely functioning can mean life or death of a patient, and the assistant and technician must be able to prevent death from machine error. Autoclaves must also be maintained, allowing packs to be sterilized correctly, killing all infectious agents.

All equipment must be maintained in some fashion within the practice; properly maintained equipment lasts longer and provides optimal results for the life of the equipment. Properly maintained equipment increases efficiency of the team and provides superior service to clients and less stress to patients.

Pharmacology is another important topic for veterinary assistants and technicians. Team members must become familiar with products that are carried in the practice, drug dosages, and routes of administration. This lessens the chance of a mistake from occurring if

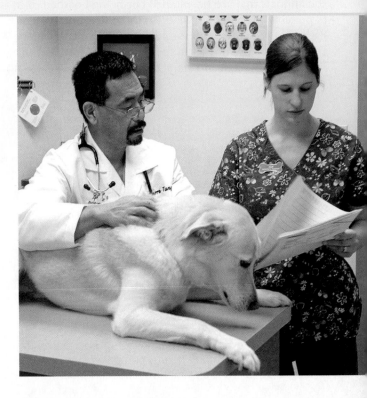

a direction is misinterpreted. Many times, unintentional mistakes occur on behalf of the veterinarian or credentialed technician, and assistants or other technicians may catch the mistake. This is why teamwork is so important: helping each other while providing exceptional patient care. Knowledge of drugs is also important so that clients can be educated on the side effects of products as well as interaction with other drugs. Client education is essential.

Practices see many puppies and kittens and provide care through a pet's senior years. Often clients ask nutritional advice of the team. Assistants must be familiar with the nutritional needs of patients and be able to recommend appropriate diets. Many therapeutic diets are available, and team members should be familiar with those carried by the practice. Parasite prevention and education are essential for puppy and kitten owners as well adult animals that live in highly endemic areas. Warm and humid climates attract a variety of parasites; it is the responsibility of the practice to educate the clients of the risks associated with those parasites. Programs should be implemented to control and prevent diseases associated with these parasites.

Emergencies may come at any time during open office hours. Team members must be familiar with common emergencies and have supplies prepared in case the emergency is real and severe. Many conditions occur to animals that may not be an emergency; however, being prepared for the worst case is best. The same applies to common disorders seen by the practice; the more informed the team members are about diseases or conditions, the more information can be relayed to owners.

With all the knowledge that is gained through practice, school, and life experiences, professional development occurs on a daily basis. It is important to every team member to continue developing skills. Many self-assessment tests can be completed indicating strengths and weaknesses of an individual, allowing continuous improvement of the weaknesses. Employment opportunities go far beyond a veterinary practice, allowing the skills obtained in practice to be used in other areas of the industry. Team members must be prepared to market themselves in a professional and diligent manner; the first impression is a lasting impression. At some point, everyone must consider retirement. It is never too early or too late for retirement planning; as the cost of living increases, so does the cost of retirement. Saving money for the future is essential because Social Security may not be around forever.

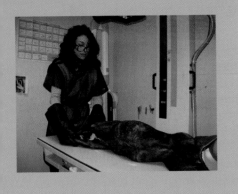

Clinical Assisting

Chapter Outline

Learning Objectives

Mastery of the content in this chapter will enable the reader to:

- Identify common diseases and vaccinations.
- Define diagnostic equipment and procedures.
- Explain the importance of preanesthetic procedures.
- Calculate medication doses.
- Explain the importance of labeling medications.

- Explain to owners how to administer medications.
- Define the nutritional needs of puppies and kittens.
- Differentiate therapeutic diets based on characteristics.
- Define common emergencies.
- Explain the most common diseases of animals.

Key Terms

Adjuvant
Anesthesia
Anorexia
Carnivore
Electrocardiogram
Enucleated

Fomites
General Anesthesia
Gingivitis
Hypothyroidism
Injection Site Sarcoma
Killed Vaccine

Kilocalorie
Lethargy
Local Anesthesia
Modified Live Vaccine
Omnivore
Recombinant Vaccine

There are many facets involved with assisting veterinarians and veterinary technicians. There are excellent books (referenced at the end of the chapter) available that give greater detail for the topics listed below. This chapter is intended to provide brief information for the new student and team member. Once these basis skills have been mastered, a review of the books referenced will help develop more advanced skills.

EXAMINATIONS

Taking a History

It is the responsibility of all team members, but especially veterinary assistants and technicians, to check the patient into a room and obtain a complete history from the client. Chapter 14 provides detailed instructions on how to take an accurate history. It is very important to know if a pet has been vomiting or has diarrhea, how long it has had the presenting symptoms, and whether the owner can correlate any symptoms with abnormal events. The history taker must write down all the information provided by the owner; the details may provide a valuable tool for the doctor as an attempt is made to make a diagnosis. A good history taker is a valuable asset to the practice.

Restraint

It is the duty of the team to prevent the veterinarian or veterinary technician from being bitten by the patient. Restraint is one of the most important tasks that must be learned and mastered. Patients can be wiggly and excited. All patients have their own emotions and deal with stress differently. They may be scared and may bite out of fear; others will bite because of pain or because they are aggressive. Every animal should be treated as if it could bite, puppies and kittens included. When doctors look into the patients' eyes and ears, they may become scared and bite out of fear. Dogs and cats can bite the tip of the doctor's nose when they are looking in a patient's eyes. Cats are quick with their forefeet and will strike with no warning.

> **PRACTICE POINT** It is the responsibility of the team member restraining the pet to prevent the doctor from being bitten.

Time and experience will teach new team members the best way to restrain animals and how much restraint is needed for each individual. Some cats may react best with little restraint; when the scruff is grabbed for restraint, they begin to object.

All animals should be observed while being restrained. The patients should remain pink and able to breathe well. If the patient's mucous membranes become blue (cyanotic) at any time, the animal should be given a break.

If a muzzle is needed at any time, team members should not hesitate to use it (Figure 23-1). Muzzles are made to protect team members from being bitten! Some owners may argue that their pet does not need a muzzle; however, for everyone's safety, including the owner's, muzzles should be used. Both dog and cat muzzles are available and come in a variety of sizes. Muzzles should fit snugly on a dog's nose. If the dog can open its mouth, the muzzle is too large, and the purpose of the muzzle is defeated. Cat muzzles should fit snugly over the entire head. Cat bags and towels may also be helpful to prevent team members from becoming scratched (Figure 23-2). The full cat body is placed inside the bag with only the head exposed. Most bags have two small openings that will allow front legs to be pulled through if needed.

> **PRACTICE POINT** A muzzle should never be left on an unattended pet because it may vomit and aspirate stomach contents.

What Would You Do/Not Do?

Sami Yung has brought Spot into the practice for her annual examination. Because there is a large Asian population in the area, the veterinary practice has learned two things about the Asian culture; people are brought up to respect elders, and they have a great respect for harmony. If they do not understand something, they may not admit it so as to avoid disrupting harmony. Mrs. Yung speaks a moderate amount of English, but in the past has not administered medications to her pet as directed. The team feels that it may due to a misunderstanding. Spot is 7 years old now and is advised to have a senior wellness exam, including bloodwork, urinalysis, and an ECG. Mrs. Yung approves the estimate for the senior wellness exam, which reveals a urinary tract infection (UTI). Teresa, the veterinary technician working with Mrs. Yung, believes that Mrs. Yung may not understand the recommendations, although she signed the estimate. Dr. Dreamer examines Spot and explains to Mrs. Yung that a urinary tract infection has been diagnosed, and a further workup is recommended to determine the cause. Mrs. Yung only nods her head, but never asks any questions or states yes or no when asked specific questions.

What Should Teresa Do?

Because Teresa is always concerned about clients and their level of understanding, she has determined that Mrs. Yung may not understand everything that is being stated to her. Teresa should create another estimate for a further workup. She should be able to find printed information regarding UTI workups, including radiographs to rule out stones and a culture for bacteria. Teresa should be able to advise Mrs. Yung to find a family member or friend to review the information with her, and schedule a follow-up visit in 2 days to determine what the next step will be or if conservative treatment will be the only option. It is imperative to understand the cultural diversity and actions of clients, how language and cultural barriers may affect their understanding of veterinary procedures, and whether or not they communicate this to team members. Team members must take these factors into consideration and do their best to help clients understand the treatments recommended for their pets.

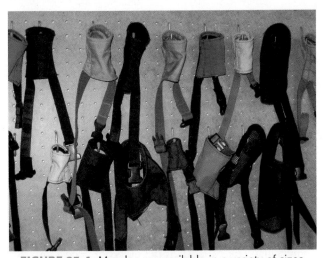

FIGURE 23-1 Muzzles are available in a variety of sizes.

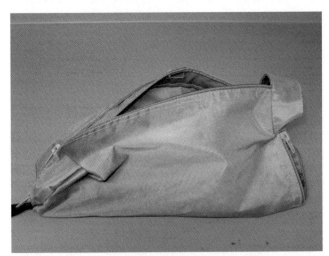

FIGURE 23-2 Cat bags are efficient for restraining aggressive cats.

VACCINATIONS AND DISEASES

Pets are exposed to a variety of diseases throughout their lifetime and should receive vaccinations to protect against potential disease or infection. Vaccination protocols can vary due to the age of the animal, location within the United States, colostral antibodies, vaccine type and route, nutritional status of the patient, and whether any other medications are being administered. Vaccine manufacturers print protocol guidelines on the product information insert to help veterinarians develop protocols for each species.

Vaccines are available in three types: modified live, killed, or recombinant. Modified live vaccines use a

> **PRACTICE POINT** Vaccination reactions can occur at any time, and every client must be advised of the risks associated with the administration of vaccines.

virus or bacteria that has been passed through a culture to reduce its virulence, whereas a killed vaccine introduces an inactivated virus into the body. Recombinant vaccines are available in two types. The first is the subunit vaccine, produced by a microorganism that has been engineered to make a protein, which then elicits an immune response in a target host. Another is the recombinant vector type, in which harmless genetic material from a disease-causing organism is inserted

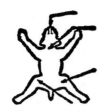

FIGURE 23-3 Stamp.

into a weakened virus or bacterium (the vector). When the vector organism replicates, the genetic material that was inserted elicits the desired immune response.

The animal generates an immune response to antigens in the vaccine, thus providing protection from disease. Killed vaccines use an adjuvant to enhance an immune response to the vaccine; vaccines made with modified live viruses do not need an adjuvant because viral antigens alone can induce a strong enough response to provide protection. Recombinant vaccines provide superior, faster, and safer protection than modified live or killed vaccines. However, at present only a few vaccines use recombinant technology.

Most vaccinations are given subcutaneously (under the skin) and take several weeks to reach optimal immunity levels. Vaccines must be shipped on ice and kept cool until the pet receives them. Warm temperatures will deactivate vaccines; it is therefore imperative that they remain refrigerated until used. Some vaccines are only in liquid form; others require reconstitution with a sterile diluent before use. For those that require reconstitution, a sterile syringe and needle are aseptically inserted into the bottle of sterile diluent and the entire milliliter of diluent is removed. The needle is then inserted into the powder vial and the diluent is injected. The syringe and needle can be removed and kept clean. The vial can be mixed by rotating it back and forth. Once all the powder has dissolved, the needle can be reinserted into the vial and the vaccine removed. It is important to remember that the needle should not touch anything except the rubber stopper; fingers must stay away from the needle! Sterile syringes should always be used. Never use resterilized syringes for vaccines; the process from the autoclave will deactivate the vaccination.

A variety of combinations of vaccinations are available on the market; the preference rests with the veterinarian as to which combination to order. It is highly recommended to indicate in the medical record where the vaccine was given. Some vaccines may cause localized reactions, and if the location of administration has been documented in the record, vaccine reaction can be ruled in or ruled out. Stamps are available to chart the location easily (Figure 23-3).

Common Diseases

Boxes 23-1 through 23-3 are not a complete list of diseases, but rather a summary of diseases for which there are vaccines. A brief description of the disease and

Box 23-1	Common Canine Infectious Diseases

CORONAVIRUS

A contagious viral infection of the gastrointestinal tract that causes vomiting and diarrhea. Symptoms are similar to those of parvo, but the virus is not as hardy as the parvovirus, nor is the disease as life threatening.

DISTEMPER (CDV)

A widespread and often fatal disease that can cause vomiting, diarrhea, pneumonia, and neurologic problems. The disease is transmitted by aerosol droplets from all body excretions of infected animals. Death is common with distemper, and recovery is rare.

HEPATITIS

A viral disease that targets the liver. When infected, adult dogs may recover; however, it is often fatal in puppies.

KENNEL COUGH

An extremely contagious infection of the upper respiratory tract that is characterized by a persistent dry, hacking cough. The infection is transmitted by aerosol droplets. Contributing infections include adenovirus (CAV-2), CDV, and the bacteria *Bordetella bronchiseptica,* as well as the parainfluenza virus.

LEPTOSPIROSIS

A bacterial infection that may lead to permanent kidney and liver damage. It is contagious to humans and is spread through contact with infected urine or contaminated soil or water.

LYME DISEASE

A disease transmitted by ticks that infects both humans and animals. The disease can affect the joints, kidneys, and other tissues. This disease is common in the southern and eastern United States.

PARVOVIRUS (CPV)

A highly contagious and potentially fatal disease that causes severe vomiting and bloody diarrhea. It is especially dangerous in young dogs, but all unvaccinated dogs are at risk of contracting this severe disease. This disease attacks all rapidly dividing cells, including those of the intestinal tract and the bone marrow. The disease is transmitted by contact with contaminated feces and vomit. This virus can stay in the ground for 2 years; therefore contaminated areas should be disinfected well. The best treatment available is to hospitalize the pet and keep it on intravenous fluids and antibiotics.

RABIES

A fatal viral infection of the central nervous system that can affect all mammals, including humans. The virus is transmitted through the bite of an infected animal, contact with saliva of an infected animal, or through fomites of an infected animal. Routine vaccination is the key to controlling this deadly disease.

Box 23-2	Common Feline Infectious Diseases

CALICIVIRUS (FCV)

An upper respiratory infection of cats with signs similar to those of feline rhinotracheitis. In addition, ulcers may be seen on the tongue and in the mouth. FCV also has a carrier state, in which healthy-looking cats are carriers of the virus. Infection is acquired by ingestion or inhalation of infectious virus present in saliva, secretions, or excretions from infected cats.

FELINE INFECTIOUS PERITONITIS (FIP)

This viral disease is most often seen in young adult cats. Once clinical signs are exhibited, the disease is progressive and leads to death. There are two types of clinical disease: the wet form and the dry form. In the wet form, large amounts of fluid build up in the body cavities, especially the abdominal cavity. In the dry form, the clinical signs are variable depending on the organ systems that are affected, such as the intestines, kidneys, liver, lungs, nervous system, or eyes. The dry form usually has a longer clinical course and death may not occur for a year or more. The virus may be contracted by ingesting infected feces.

FELINE IMMUNODEFICIENCY VIRUS (FIV)

This is a retrovirus that causes immunodeficiency in cats. It is in the same subfamily as human immunodeficiency virus, the causative agent of human AIDS. Stomatitis, upper respiratory infection, recurrent infections, persistent diarrhea, fever, and wasting are common signs of FIV. Transmission occurs through saliva.

FELINE LEUKEMIA VIRUS (FeLV)

Infection with this virus can cause serious disease and death in cats. The virus decreases the ability of the immune system to respond to infection and may lead to the development of different types of cancer. FeLV is passed from cat to cat by direct contact (saliva). It is not contagious to people. FeLV is the leading cause of death in cats.

PANLEUKOPENIA (FPV)

A widespread and potentially fatal disease that may cause a sudden onset of severe vomiting and diarrhea, fever, and loss of appetite. It is extremely dangerous in kittens but can also be fatal in adults. Even when recovery occurs, a normal-looking kitten may shed the virus for up to 6 weeks. The virus is shed in secretions and excretions from infected animals.

FELINE PNEUMONITIS CHLAMYDIA (FPN)

This is another common respiratory infection in cats producing sneezing, fever, and a thick discharge from the eyes. Chlamydial infection may be associated with the development of more serious bacterial complications.

RABIES

A fatal viral infection of the central nervous system that can affect all mammals, including humans. The virus is transmitted through the bite of an infected animal, contact with saliva of an infected animal, or through fomites of an infected animal. Routine vaccination is the key to controlling this deadly disease.

FELINE VIRAL RHINOTRACHEITIS (FVR)

A common respiratory infection of cats, which can be fatal in kittens. Sneezing, decreased appetite, and fever, followed by a thick discharge from the eyes and nose are often observed. FVR also has a chronic state, in which recovered cats become carriers for life. These carriers may or may not experience signs of the disease and will shed the virus intermittently. Transmission of the virus requires direct contact with infectious secretions or excretions.

---

symptoms is also included. Some tests are available for in-house diagnostics to determine if a pet has a disease, whereas other tests need to be submitted to an outside laboratory for diagnostics. Table 23-1 summarizes tests available for diagnostics.

DIAGNOSTICS

Many factors are considered when determining a diagnosis. History, physical exam, and laboratory results all provide information to the veterinarian. Diagnostic testing can take hours to accomplish and can depend on the client's financial situation. Clients should be provided with estimates before starting any diagnostics, so that they may elect to proceed with one test at a time.

Laboratory tests may include in-house bloodwork or panels sent to an outside laboratory (see Chapter 9). In-house lab work may consist of complete blood count (CBC) and chemistries (both abbreviated and complete panels are available), heartworm tests, fecals, urinalyses, cytologies, FeLV/FIV tests, and parvovirus tests. A variety of companies produce a number of tests that are available for use in practice; the product insert should be used as a guide to completing each test correctly. Directions that are not followed correctly can yield inconclusive results, producing a false-positive or –negative result. Not only does this provide substandard medicine, it decreases the profits of the veterinary practice. Any failed tests should be repeated and reported to the practice manager in case the tests are tracked.

> **PRACTICE POINT** In-house tests and testing equipment can increase the bottom line of the practice when used on a routine basis.

Bloodwork

It is imperative for the veterinary assistant and technician to become familiar with general tests that are run in-house. Clients will ask what test correlates with what bodily system, and these questions must be answered clearly and confidently. Table 23-2 lists the names of common tests and the system with which the test correlates.

| Box 23-3 | Common Large Animal Diseases |

The following infectious viruses have vaccinations available for protection.

EQUINE
Encephalomyelitis (Eastern, Western, and Venezuelan Equine Encephalomyelitis)
The virus is commonly carried by mosquitoes, birds, and rodents and can result in moderate to high mortality rates (within 2 to 3 days after signs begin). Symptoms include fever (106° F), hypersensitivity to sound, excitement, and restlessness. Shortly thereafter, the signs associated with brain lesions appear: drowsiness, drooping ears, and abnormal gait. The last stage is paralysis, and then death. Venezuelan equine encephalitis is a foreign animal disease and is reportable.

Influenza
This is the most common respiratory virus, and outbreaks spread rapidly (incubation of 1 to 3 days). Symptoms include fever, cough, and upper respiratory signs.

Potomac Horse Fever (Ehrlichiosis)
Unknown transmission, but multiple vectors are suspected, including the American dog tick. Symptoms include depression, high fever (107° F), profuse watery diarrhea, and colic. Concurrent laminitis may also occur.

Rhinopneumonitis (EHV-1)
Caused by several herpes viruses; can induce a fever of 106° F for several days. Presenting symptoms include clear nasal discharge and coughing that may last for several weeks. Mares may abort fetuses 3 to 4 months after infection. Antibiotics are used to treat secondary infections.

"Strangles" or Distemper (*Streptococcus Equi* Infection)
Submandibular and retropharyngeal lymph node swelling and fever are often seen, often accompanied by coughing and nasal discharge. Lymph nodes often rupture, and the contents are extremely contagious.

Tetanus
A clostridial disease also known as *lockjaw.* Spores are introduced through a break in the skin and are often associated with lacerations from fence wounds. Symptoms of tetanus include muscle rigidity and spasms; if left untreated, it will result in death. Success of treatment depends on how far the disease has progressed.

Rabies
A fatal viral infection of the central nervous system that can affect all mammals, including humans. The virus is transmitted through the bite of an infected animal, contact with saliva of an infected animal, or through fomites of an infected animal. Routine vaccination is the key to controlling this deadly disease.

CATTLE
Bovine Viral Diarrhea (BVD)
BVD is a multisystemic viral disease. Classic symptoms of BVD include diarrhea, depression, anorexia, dehydration, and oral erosions. Chronic BVD is known as *mucosal disease* and is 100% fatal. Persistent infections may occur.

Brucellosis (Bang's Disease)
Brucellosis is caused by *Brucella abortus*, which is a coccobacillus. Transmission occurs via ingestion of organisms that are shed in milk and uterine discharges. Symptoms include abortions in healthy cows. *Brucella* is a zoonotic disease and is therefore reportable.

Clostridial Infection
Clostridia spores live in the soil and may be ingested while eating or enter the body through an open wound. Various *Clostridia* forms exist, which can cause severe enteritis and dysentery (with high mortality rates) in young calves, lambs, and pigs. *Clostridia* can cause sudden death.

Infectious Bovine Rhinotracheitis (IBR)
Contagious; carriers can be seen. IBR causes upper respiratory signs, especially during times of stress (shipping); therefore also known as *shipping fever.* Symptoms may also include secondary bronchopneumonia, diarrhea (enteric form), abortion, and severe hyperemia of the muzzle (commonly referred to as *red nose*).

Moraxella Bovis Infection (Pink Eye)
Contagious pink eye is especially common in Herefords. Symptoms include conjunctivitis, corneal edema, and blindness.

Rabies
A fatal viral infection of the central nervous system that can affect all mammals, including humans. The virus is transmitted through the bite of an infected animal, contact with saliva of an infected animal, or through fomites of an infected animal. Routine vaccination is the key to controlling this deadly disease.

SHEEP AND GOATS
Clostridial Infection (Especially Type D)
Clostridia is a bacterium that grows best under anaerobic conditions and often comes from contaminated soil. Enterotoxemia is most likely to occur and is easily preventable with vaccination.

Tetanus
Same as in the horse.

Cytology

Cytologies are prepared for a number of reasons; the most common of which is to look at cells under the microscope. Cytology preparation can depend on the sample, the doctor, and the stain that will be used.

Different cells take up stain differently, which helps in diagnosis. Many veterinarians and technicians become proficient at reading cytologies; however, a histopathologist that is employed by a laboratory can provide a more definitive diagnosis.

Urinalysis

Urine samples can provide a wealth of information for the veterinarian, and several tests can be performed on one sample. Most urine samples are obtained by free catch; either the owner has obtained a sample or an assistant has walked the dog and caught a midstream

Table 23-1	Tests Available for Common Diseases	
Disease	In-House	Laboratory
FELINE		
Calici		PCR
FIP		PCR, antibody
FIV	X	ELISA, Western blot
FeLV	X	ELISA, IFA
Panleukopenia		PCR
Pneumonitis, chlamydia		PCR
Herpesvirus		PCR
Rhinotracheitis		
Heartworm	X	ELISA
CANINE		
Coronavirus		PCR
Distemper		PCR, conjunctival scrape
Adenovirus		PCR
Bordetella infection		PCR
Leptospira infection		PCR, antibody
Lyme disease	X	IFA, ELISA
Parvovirus	X	PCR, fecal antigen
Heartworm	X	ELISA
Herpesvirus		PCR
EQUINE		
Herpesvirus		PCR
Equine infectious anemia		AGID, cELISA
Equine influenza virus		PCR

PCR, Polymerase chain reaction; *FIP,* feline infectious peritonitis; *FIV,* feline immunodeficiency virus; *ELISA,* enzyme-linked immunosorbent assay; *FeLV,* feline leukemia virus; *IFA,* immunofluorescent assay; *AGID,* agar gel immunodiffusion; *ELISA,* enzyme-linked immunosorbent assay.

Table 23-2	Common Bloodwork Tests
Test	Associated With
AST	Liver
ALT	Liver
Total bili	Liver
Alk phos	Liver
GGT	Liver
Total protein	Protein
Albumin	Protein
Globulin	Protein
A/G ratio	Protein
Cholesterol	Lipids
BUN	Kidney
Creatinine	Kidney
BUN/crea ratio	Kidney
Phosphorus	Mineral
Calcium	Mineral
Glucose	Diabetes
Amylase	Pancreas
Lipase	Pancreas
Sodium	Electrolytes
Phosphorus	Electrolytes
Na/K ratio	Electrolytes
Chloride	Electrolytes
Triglycerides	Lipids
Magnesium	Mineral
WBC	White blood cell count
RBC	Red blood cell count
HGB	Hemoglobin concentration
HCT	Hematocrit
MCV	Mean corpuscular volume
MCH	Mean cell hemoglobin
MCHC	Mean cell hemoglobin concentration
Total T-4	Thyroid
T-4 equil. dialysis	Thyroid
TSH	Thyroid
Bile acids	Liver

AST, Aspartate aminotransferase; *ALT,* alanine aminotransferase; *bili,* bilirubin; *Alk phos,* alkaline phosphatase; *GGT,* gamma-glutamyl transferase; *A/G,* albumin/globulin; *BUN,* blood urea nitrogen; *crea,* creatinine; *Na/K,* sodium/potassium; *equil.,* equilibrium; *TSH,* thyroid-stimulating hormone.

urine sample (Figures 23-4). Other methods of collection include cystocentesis or catheterization (Figure 23-5). If a urine sample will be sent to the laboratory for culture, a sample acquired by cystocentesis is highly recommended because it is a sterile sample that is obtained without any contamination. Cystocentesis is the process of inserting a needle into the bladder and withdrawing a sample.

The tests that can be completed on urine are numerous; the most common tests completed in the hospital include specific gravity, stick urinalysis, and sediment (Boxes 23-4 and 23-5). The specific gravity provides the concentration of the urine and is a key indicator of how well the kidneys can concentrate the urine. Certain disease processes can affect the concentration, including renal disease and diabetes.

A stick urinalysis is performed by dipping a urinalysis stick into the sample itself (if it is a sterile sample, the urine should be dropped onto each testing block) (Figure 23-6).

The sediment is essential to verify the information provided by the stick.

Fecal Analysis

Fecal analysis is extremely important in puppies and kittens and in pets with diarrhea. A fecal analysis can diagnose internal parasites such as *Giardia*, *Coccidia*, roundworms, hookworms, whipworms, or tapeworms.

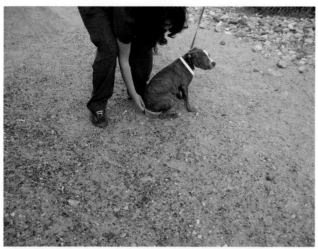

FIGURE 23-4 Urine may be caught by free catch when walking dogs.

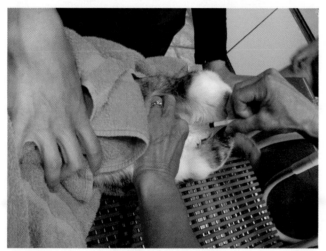

FIGURE 23-5 Urine can be obtained from dogs and cats by cystocentesis.

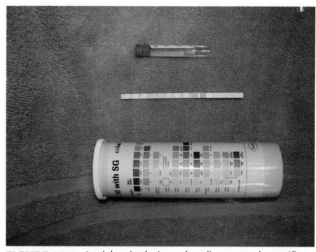

FIGURE 23-6 A stick urinalysis and sediment and specific gravity measurements should be performed on every urine sample.

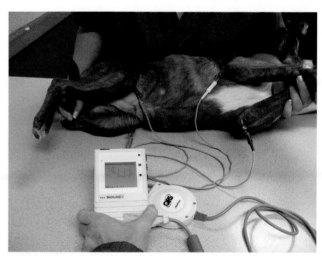

FIGURE 23-7 Electrocardiograms are effective diagnostic aids.

Box 23-4	Urine Dipstick Tests

- Leukocytes
- Blood
- pH
- Ketones
- Glucose
- Bilirubin
- Nitrates

Box 23-5	Urine Sediment Evaluations

- White blood cells
- Red blood cells
- Epithelial cells
- Bacteria
- Casts
- Crystals

It can also indicate severe bacterial overgrowth and determine if a sample should be sent to the laboratory for further diagnosis.

Electrocardiogram

Electrocardiograms, often referred to as EKGs or ECGs, are recordings of the heart's electrical activity. The recording traces the entire heartbeat process, through both the systolic and diastolic phases. Arrhythmias and conduction disturbances of the heart can be detected on ECGs, and an ECG is highly recommended before administering anesthesia to patients (Figure 23-7).

Blood Pressure

Measurement of blood pressure is an underutilized tool in veterinary medicine. Variations in blood pressure are characteristic of a number of diseases. By definition, blood pressure is the pressure exerted by the blood on the wall of the vessel. The systolic pressure is the maximal force caused by the contraction of the left ventricle of the heart. The diastolic pressure is the minimal force during the relaxation phrase, when the aortic and pulmonic valves are closed. The mean arterial pressure is the average pressure of both.

DIAGNOSTIC IMAGING

Most practices use a radiograph machine to produce high-quality x-rays. A radiograph is a visible record produced by x-rays penetrating an object. Radiographs can provide a great amount of detail in a short amount of time.

Safety

Care must be taken when taking radiographs. Safety cannot be emphasized enough. Studies indicate that excess radiation causes cancer, birth defects, a decreased life span, and fertility issues. Protection must be worn at all times while taking radiographs (Box 23-6 and Figure 23-8). Lead thyroid collars, gowns, and gloves are the absolute minimum that should be provided to all team members allowed to take radiographs. Eye goggles are also a good idea (eyes cannot be replaced!) to provide ultimate protection. Team members who are exposed to radiation on a daily basis have a higher incidence of reproductive, thyroid, and eye cancers.

Lead aprons, collars, and gloves should never be folded; any fold can crack the lead and allow radiation to penetrate the team member, decreasing safety (Figure 23-9). All apparel should be hung on a wall or laid flat on a table surface to prevent cracking. Aprons, collars, and gloves should be radiographed yearly to check for any cracks that may have appeared (Figure 23-10). Radiographs should be compared year to year, and safety equipment should be replaced as soon as visible cracks appear. Team member safety cannot be compromised.

Guidelines

Several regulations must be followed to comply with guidelines set for employee safety. All team members in the room during the radiograph process must be older than 18 years. Dosimetry badges must be worn at all times, and pregnant team members should especially avoid exposure to radiation. Personal protective equipment (PPE) must be worn. Employers must enforce the use of PPE, and employees must wear PPE. According to the Occupational Safety and Health Administration (OSHA), employers can be fined for not providing or enforcing the use of PPE, and employees can be fired for not wearing PPE. Excess radiation can have detrimental effects, and all protection must be used.

A dosimeter measures radiation exposure and should be worn on the collar at the thyroid gland level.

Box 23-6	Radiology PPE

- Lead thyroid collar
- Lead gown
- Goggles
- Lead gloves
- Dosimetry badge

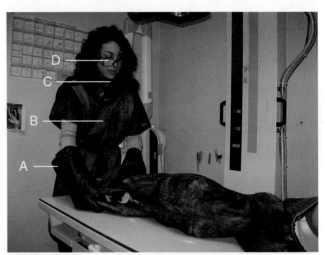

FIGURE 23-8 Personal protective equipment must be worn at all times when radiographing a pet. *A,* Lead gloves. *B,* Lead gown. *C,* Lead collar. *D,* Protective goggles.

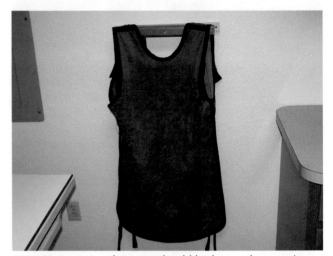

FIGURE 23-9 Lead aprons should be hung when not in use to prevent the lead from cracking.

The maximum permissible dose (MPD) is 5000 millirems per year (a millirem is 1/1000 rem), and should be monitored closely. The average exposure is 5 rem per year for a small or mixed practice. The United States Nuclear Regulatory Commission has determined that the MPD is a dose that is unlikely to harm a person over a lifetime of taking radiographs. Every precaution should be taken to keep radiation exposure low by wearing all protective gear. If a practice manager notices high levels

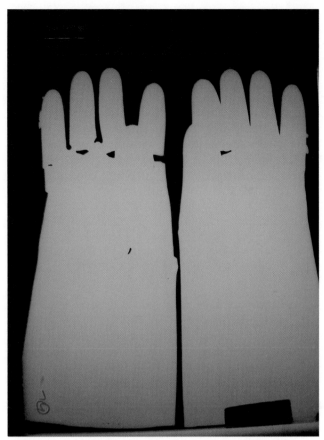

FIGURE 23-10 Personal protective equipment should be x-rayed yearly for cracked lead. This pair of gloves has several areas of damage and must be replaced.

of exposure on a dosimetry report, an investigation should be launched to determine the source of radiation. Machines may malfunction, and this may be the only way to detect the excess radiation being emitted.

All radiograph machines must be monitored and inspected by an Environmental Protection Agency (EPA) official yearly. The EPA certificate must be posted in the radiology room.

A radiology log can be helpful to team members when a digital system is not used. Figure 17-1 shows an example, listing the date, client and patient name, area being studied, position, and machine settings. This type of log allows team members to retrieve settings used in previous radiographs in case repeat or follow-up radiographs are required. To compare radiographs, the same setting should be used on both. Different settings may produce slight differences in quality of images, thereby making comparison difficult. Digital radiographs have setting information stored with the image, allowing exact settings to be used.

Films must be stored in a system that allows quick and easy retrieval. Digital radiographs are stored in the patient's file, allowing quick access at all times. Regular films may be alphabetized by the client's last name

or patient name, or numerically by client ID number. Whichever system is used, it must be simple and prevent lost films. Lost films are the biggest hassle of film storage. Many clinics now use a scanner or digitizer to enter radiographs onto a CD for easy retrieval, freeing up storage space once taken by radiographs. This also eliminates lost radiographs.

Radiograph checkout logs should also be implemented when owners take x-rays for second opinions or when films are sent to a specialist. Figure 17-2 shows a log that allows radiographs to be traced if they have not been returned.

Digital Radiographs

With the technology available today, digital x-rays have begun to replace the standard x-ray system. With digital x-rays, the tube is coupled with a specialized receiver that changes x-rays into electrical signals. The image is digitized and displayed on a computer screen, then stored on a DVD, CD, or magnetic optical disk (MOD). The advantages of a digital system are numerous. The processing time is reduced to seconds because film does not have to be processed. Images can be viewed immediately and can be manipulated with software to lighten, darken, or magnify the image. If a film needs to be repeated for positioning only, it can be done in a shorter amount of time. Views are stored within the computer system and/or disk, so images are never lost. Images can also be sent to a specialist for a second opinion by phone, DSL, or T1 cable line.

Fluoroscopy

Fluoroscopy involves projecting a continuous x-ray beam onto an image intensifier. Fluoroscopic units are suited for the study of moving structures and can provide the maximum information regarding the processes of the moving structures. Fluoroscopic studies are usually limited to gastrointestinal studies, myelography, and heart and vascular studies. They are rarely used in veterinary medicine for economic reasons.

Ultrasound

The use of ultrasound is becoming popular within veterinary practices, especially as the price of units decreases. Ultrasound is noninvasive and well tolerated by patients. A major disadvantage is the learning curve associated with using the unit. It takes practice and patience to master ultrasound imaging; the diagnosis is only as good as the diagnostician.

Ultrasound uses sound technology. The frequency of sound is computed into an image with an equation that involves wavelength and frequency. Sound reflection forms the basis of an ultrasound image. The thicker the tissue, the less sound is reflected, creating a darker image on the screen. The thinner the tissue, the more sound is reflected, creating a lighter image of the organ.

Ultrasound can be useful in diagnosing and evaluating tendon injuries, tendon sheath infections, adhesions, or foreign bodies. Joints can be evaluated for injury, neoplasia, or osteomyelitis. Abdominal cavities can be evaluated for fluid, cancer, or congenital defects. The list of uses for ultrasound is endless, making it a useful diagnostic tool when evaluating pets for disease.

Computed Tomographic Scanning

Computed tomographic (CT) scanning is performed by passing a thin x-ray beam through the patient and measuring the x-ray attenuation at multiple sites within a thin slice of a patient's anatomy. A computer then configures the data and provides a cross-sectional image on a video monitor. In veterinary medicine, a CT scan is generally used to diagnose neurologic disorders within the spinal column or brain. It can also be helpful to identify musculoskeletal, thoracic, and abdominal disorders.

Patients must be fully anesthetized to prevent movement within the machine. The patient is placed in a ventrodorsal position on a table that moves through the machine. As the table moves, the CT scanner obtains cross-sectional data. Two studies are generally performed: the first without any contrast media, the second after an intravenous injection of iodinated contrast. Contrast allows visualization of vascular structures.

Magnetic Resonance Imaging

Magnetic resonance imaging (MRI) is the newest imaging modality for veterinary medicine. MRI is similar to CT scanning in that it takes thin slices in cross-section and transfers the images to a video screen. MRI differs in that it does not use radiation to create the image; it uses radiowave signals in which hydrogen nuclei have been disturbed by a radiofrequency pulse. MRI produces superior results; clearer images and sensitivity to the composition of tissues are just two qualities worth mentioning. These qualities are excellent for diagnostics involving the brain and spinal cord.

Some veterinary teaching hospitals and veterinary specialty practices use MRIs; most animals are referred to a human hospital, imaging center, or a truck-based mobile MRI unit. Patients must be anesthetized for these centers; therefore the veterinarian must provide everything that would be needed for anesthesia, resuscitation (if needed), and recovery. The animal's bowels and bladder should be empty, and it should be parasite free.

Because MRIs use a strong magnetic field, anything metal must be removed from the room. The magnetic field will forcefully pull any metal object into the magnet, injuring anything in its path. Therefore animals must be anesthetized with injectable anesthesia. This can be a disadvantage because it can be difficult to monitor patients while they are undergoing the procedure. MRIs generally take 45 to 60 minutes to complete. They can be done with and/or without contrast media.

SURGERY

Surgery entails a wide variety of topics. Team members should familiarize themselves with the following summaries, then seek further training. A surgical procedure does not start in the operating room; it begins with client education. Clients must fully understand the procedure their pet will be receiving and understand the risks associated with anesthesia. With the appropriate drug choice, monitoring, and recovery, the anesthetic risk is decreased. Client communication and education is the No. 1 preoperative procedure.

> **PRACTICE POINT** Clients must be fully informed of the risks and benefits of procedures being performed on their pets, especially vaccinations and surgeries.

After clients have received all appropriate education regarding the procedure and the risk of anesthesia, they must sign an anesthetic release. Examples of anesthetic release forms are provided in Chapter 2. It is imperative that the client's phone number, cell phone, and/or pager be listed in case an emergency occurs and the client must be contacted during the procedure.

Clients must be informed of the risks and benefits the pet is subject to before the procedure is performed. Informed consent ensures that the client has been advised, understands the risks, and agrees to the procedures elected. Chapter 4 defines informed consent in more detail.

Preanesthetic Documentation

Preanesthetic questions MUST be addressed and documented. It should be confirmed that patients have been held off food and water (NPO) per practice instructions. Owners must be given the option (if it is not hospital policy) to have preoperative tests performed on their pet before anesthesia.

> **PRACTICE POINT** All communications with clients must be documented in the record.

- **Bloodwork:** The very minimum that should be offered is bloodwork that evaluates the kidney and liver function, as well as red blood cells, white blood cells, and platelet function. Most manufacturers offer preoperative panels that include blood urea nitrogen, creatinine, alanine aminotransferase, alkaline phosphatase, glucose, total protein, and a complete blood count. Anesthesia is metabolized by the liver and kidneys; it is imperative to know if they are functioning correctly. If a patient is deficient in platelets, it is helpful to know this before surgery; a patient with low platelets could bleed to death.

- **ECG:** An ECG is an excellent indicator of heart disease. An ECG will detect premature ventricular contractions or other abnormalities that may necessitate postponement of surgery.
- **IV catheter and fluids:** If IV fluids are not a requirement of the practice, the owner should be strongly advised to permit them. IV fluids help maintain the patient's blood pressure while under anesthesia, help support the kidneys, and allow an access port to the vein in case of emergency. If a patient goes into cardiac arrest while under anesthesia, drugs can be administered much faster through an existing line versus placing a catheter in an emergency.
- **Histopathology:** If a patient is having a mass or growth removed, clients should be advised to send the growth to a pathologist to determine the correct pathology. Many cancerous tumors look benign but are not. A pathologist who reviews cytologies as a profession can make an informed diagnosis of masses submitted.

If a patient is going to be spayed or neutered, it should be checked for testicles. Owners cannot always tell the correct gender of an animal; therefore it must be verified before surgery (it is frustrating and wasted time when a veterinarian cuts into the abdomen of a patient looking for a uterus to find out it is a male!). If a mass will be removed from the patient, the hair should be clipped (before the owner leaves) to verify the mass or masses that the owner has agreed to remove. If any other masses are found on physical exam, the owner should be called for permission to remove the additional masses.

Each patient should receive a physical exam at least 12 hours before anesthesia. The heart and lungs should be evaluated with both heart rate and respiratory rate noted. The mucous membranes should be pink, and the capillary refill time should be within 2 seconds. The pulse should be strong; any pulse deficits should be noted. The abdomen should feel normal to palpation, as should the lymph nodes. The pet should be well hydrated and have a normal temperature, and a weight should be taken for the current visit.

Anesthesia

Once all the parameters are evaluated and the patient is deemed healthy enough for surgery, an anesthetic protocol will be developed. Each patient is unique, and consideration should be given to each patient regarding the anesthesia protocol.

Anesthesia is the loss of sensation that can be induced by a number of drugs. Local anesthesia deadens sensory nerves; an injection of lidocaine is given at the site of the procedure. General anesthesia influences and desensitizes the central nervous system; it produces unconsciousness. Spinal anesthesia interrupts the function of nerves.

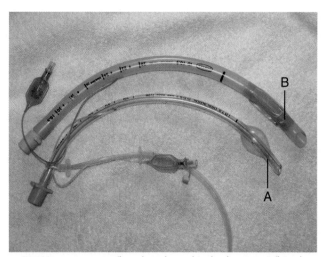

FIGURE 23-11 A, Inflated endotracheal tube. **B**, Deflated endotracheal tube.

Endotracheal Tubes

Patients that are undergoing anesthesia should always be intubated. Intubation prevents the patient from aspirating contents from the stomach if it vomits while under anesthesia. Intubation also prevents mucous and salivary secretions from entering the lung field. Intubation is extremely important during dental procedures. Excess water from the scaling instruments can pool in the lungs, causing severe complications for the patient. Along with these precautions, endotracheal tubes deliver anesthetic gases to the patient (Figure 23-11).

> **PRACTICE POINT** Endotracheal tubes deliver gas to the patient and prevent contents from the stomach from being aspirated.

PHARMACOLOGY

Pharmacology is a very important topic, and one with which assistants and technicians must be familiar. Pharmacology not only deals with drugs that are dispensed, it also involves knowledge about the administration of drugs, drug interactions, and the amount of a drug that is to be given with each dose.

> **PRACTICE POINT** Team members must become familiar with the products and with the classification of drugs the practice carries.

Chemical, Nonproprietary, and Proprietary Names

Drugs are also commonly referred to by three different names. The chemical name describes the chemical composition of the product. The nonproprietary name, also referred to as the *generic name,* is a more concise name given to the chemical compound. Examples of

ABC Veterinary Clinic
1000 Anyroad, Anytown, PA 19874
555-555-5555

Client name________ Patient _______ Species ______ Date ______

Address ________________________

Rx

Refills 0 1 2 3 4 ________________ DVM

FIGURE 23-12 Sample prescription order form.

nonproprietary names include aspirin, acetaminophen, or amoxicillin. The proprietary name, or trade name, is the name of the drug given by the manufacturer. Examples of proprietary names include Baytril, Tylenol, and Amoxi-Tabs. Because many manufacturers produce similar products, a single generic drug can be sold under several trade names. Amoxicillin is sold under Amoxi-Tabs, Robamox-V, and Amoxil (among others).

Dosage forms include tablets, capsules, solutions, injectables, topicals, ointments, creams, pastes, and implants. Tablets or capsules can be given orally. Some suppositories are packaged in caplet form but are given rectally. Solutions can be given orally in a suspension or syrup; they can also be applied to the eye and/or ears. Injectables can be given under the skin, in the muscles, or in the vein. Topicals are generally applied to the skin and can be manufactured in a solution, ointment, or cream base. Ointments can be applied topically or in the eye. Paste is generally administered orally, and implants are placed under the skin for release of a drug over an extended period of time.

Prescriptions

A prescription is an order from a licensed veterinarian directing a pharmacist to prepare a drug for use by a client's animal (Figure 23-12). A valid veterinarian/patient/client relationship must exist for a veterinarian to write a prescription, and the drug must be meet proper requirements for labeling. Documentation must be kept in the pet's record regarding the prescription. Valid prescriptions must contain the following information: date, client's name, pet's name, and species; the drug name, concentration, and number of units to dispense; directions for the client treating the animal; the doctor's name, address, and phone number; the abbreviation "Rx"; and the veterinarian's signature.

Dispensing Medications

Medications that are dispensed must be in childproof containers. If a child accesses a medication container and becomes poisoned, the veterinarian can be found liable. Many clients may request containers that are not childproof; pill vials and lids can be specially ordered that can be reversed, allowing the flip side of the lid to close the container without the use of the child-proof side. It must be verified with the owner, however, that no children reside in the premises.

Calculations and Conversions

Calculating the dose of medication is easy, but calculations must be verified with the veterinarian before administration to ensure correct dosing. The following information is needed before the calculation procedure:

- Pet's weight
- Recommended dose of medication (milligrams per kilogram of body weight)
- Strength or concentration of medication supplied (e.g., milligrams of drug per milliliter or milligrams per tablet)

Chapter 24 covers the topics of conversions, equations, and examples of medication calculation in depth. Every team member must be familiar with common drugs and doses and double-check medications for errors. Mistakes are less likely to occur if more team members double-check medications before dispensing.

Administration of Medications

Medications can be given in a variety of methods. PO means per os, or by mouth. SQ means under the skin, or subcutaneous. IM is intramuscular, or in the muscle, whereas IV means in the vein, or intravenously.

Medications given by mouth can be difficult to administer because many patients do not cooperate. If the pet is allowed to eat, the medication can be offered in food; the pet must be monitored to ensure it ingests the tablet. Many pets are creative and eat around the pill. If the pill is not taken in food form, the jaw must be opened and the pill must be placed in the rear of the mouth. It must be placed as far back on the tongue as possible because the animal can spit the pill out. Once it has been placed on the back of the tongue, the mouth should be closed and held shut immediately. The throat should be rubbed to induce swallowing. Water should then be given with a syringe, helping the pill slide into the stomach. Without water, many pills can lodge in the esophagus, causing ulcers and lesions when the pill begins to break down. This can be an extremely painful condition that will prevent the pet from eating and drinking for days. Pill poppers are also available to aid in the medication of pills.

One must use caution and double-check that the medication is being administered by the correct route. Many drugs have different effects if administered the wrong route. Not only can the medications have an adverse affect, the patients may be overdosed or underdosed if the drug is given improperly. Every veterinary assistant and technician must become familiar with the drugs supplied in the practice and the common routes of administration for each one. Assistants and technicians should also be familiar with common doses and be able to determine incorrect dosing or administration procedures. Assistants and technicians are the second eyes and ears for veterinarians and will frequently detect unintentional mistakes. It is always better to double-check than to administer a potentially fatal dose of medication.

Controlled substances are covered in Chapter 16 and should be reviewed carefully. Controlled substances must be logged correctly and balanced. Any discrepancy over 3% at the end of the year must be reported to the local police department, the Drug Enforcement Agency (DEA), and the state board of veterinary medicine. If theft occurs, the missing product must be reported immediately.

Expired Medications

Medications often expire in the veterinary practice. This can present a large loss for the business; therefore preventing drugs from expiring is essential. Inventory and inventory management are critical; by controlling the inventory, losses can be cut (see Chapter 15).

If a product expires, the manufacturer or distributor that the practice ordered the product from should be determined, and the return policy reviewed. Some companies will replace expired medication with later dating, preventing the practice from taking a loss. If they do not return the product, it will need to be disposed of properly. Expired medication cannot be sold. Not only

is selling expired product against the law, the efficacy of the product has been determined to be less than what is deemed appropriate.

Expired tablets can be dissolved in water, poured over a small amount of cat litter, and then discarded. Injectables can be poured in cat litter as well. The Environmental Protection Agency (EPA) has advised against the practice of pouring expired medication down the drain or in the toilet because the possibility of contaminating water sources is high.

Controlled substances that expire must be sent to a return agency that certifies the destruction of drugs (see Chapter 9).

Over-the-Counter Pharmaceuticals

Over-the-counter (OTC) pharmaceuticals include products that are available at the pharmacy or grocery store without the need for a prescription. OTC drugs include Robitussin (dextromethorphan), Benadryl (diphenhydramine), Dramamine (dimenhydrinate), Chlor-Trimeton (chlorpheniramine), Tagamet (cimetidine), and Imodium (loperamide). The list is extensive because many products can be purchased OTC.

Labels

Every medication that is dispensed from a veterinary practice must have a label on it. Each label must state the client's name, pet's name, and date; the name, address, and phone number of the practice; the veterinarian prescribing the drug; the name of the drug, its strength, and expiration date; and the directions for the client. Each label must also read "Keep out of the reach of children."

Warning labels can be affixed to medication vials to catch the client's attention (Figure 23-13). ("Refrigerate and mix well before using," and "This prescription cannot be refilled without an examination," are examples of labels that can be generated.) Box 23-7 gives examples of common abbreviations used in making labels.

> **PRACTICE POINT** Clients must be warned of the side effects of all medication.

Drugs

Drugs are placed into categories according to their function and the properties of the active ingredient. The active ingredient is defined as the main chemical that provides the desired result. Other chemicals may also be added to carry the drug, provide synergistic features, or provide a flavor.

Antiinflammatories

Drugs that reduce inflammation are called *antiinflammatories.* They often reduce pain, and some reduce fever as well. There are two types of antiinflammatories: steroidal and nonsteroidal. Steroidal antiinflammatories are

Box 23-7	**Common Abbreviations**
A complete list of abbreviations is available in the appendices.	
SID	once daily
BID	twice daily
TID	three times daily
QID	four times daily
QOD	every other day
cc	cubic centimeter
g or gm	gram
hr	hour
s or sec	second
m or min	minute
lb or #	pound
mg	milligram
mL	milliliter
od	right eye
os	left eye
ou	both eyes
au	both ears
ad	right ear
as	left ear
PO	by mouth
prn	as needed
q	every
stat	immediately
t or tsp	teaspoon
T or tbl	tablespoon

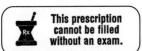

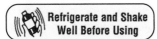

CAUTION:
Failure to use and refill this medication may lead to fatal heartworm disease.

FIGURE 23-13 Example of labels.

known as *glucocorticoids* and can be classified as short acting, intermediate, or long acting. Short-acting glucocorticoids generally relieve pain for less than 12 hours, whereas intermediate glucocorticoids relieve pain for 12 to 36 hours. Intermediate glucocorticoid examples include prednisone, prednisolone, triamcinolone, methylprednisolone, and isoflupredone. Long-acting glucocorticoids include dexamethasone, betamethasone, and flumethasone, which provide relief for more than 48 hours. Overuse of steroidal antiinflammatories can result in Cushing syndrome; physical symptoms may not appear for weeks.

Nonsteroidal antiinflammatories (NSAIDs) are regarded as a safer class of drug for pain relief because their side effects are generally fewer and less severe than those of glucocorticoids. Aspirin, ibuprofen, ketoprofen, and naproxen are NSAIDs available OTC. Flunixin meglumine (Banamine), carprofen (Rimadyl), deracoxib (Deramaxx), and firocoxib (Previcox) are some NSAIDs commonly used in veterinary medicine. Dimethyl sulfoxide (DMSO) is applied topically, primarily in horses.

Antimicrobials

Antimicrobials are drugs used to kill or inhibit bacteria, protozoa, viruses, or fungi. Antibiotics include penicillins, cephalosporins, bacitracins, aminoglycosides, fluoroquinolones, tetracyclines, sulfonamides, lincosamides, macrolides, metronidazole, nitrofurans, chloramphenicols, and rifampin. Amphotericin, ketoconazole, itraconazole, and griseofulvin are antifungal drugs. Each type of antibiotic or fungal agent is chosen based on the particular type of bacteria or fungus for which the patient is being treated. Each class of antibiotics has a variety of drugs available within its class, each of which may also have different properties based on its chemical composition.

Antiparasitics

Antihelmintics are used to treat various types of internal parasites. Fenbendazole, thiabendazole, oxibendazole, and albendazole are examples of antihelmintics used in practice. Organophosphates are used for external parasites such as fleas, ticks, and flies. Pyrethrins and pyrethroids are the largest group of insecticides marketed in the United States. Insect growth regulators and sterilizers are also becoming popular and are very safe to use on pets.

Cardiac Drugs

Many drugs have effects on the cardiovascular system but are not classified as cardiac medications. Medications must be analyzed for interactions or enhancement with other drugs. Antiarrhythmic drugs are used to produce a normal conduction sequence. Lidocaine, procainamide, and quinidine reverse arrhythmias.

PRACTICE POINT Different medications may have enhancing effects when administered together; drug interaction should be investigated before dispensing new medication.

Vasodilators open constricted valves, making it easier for the heart to pump blood to the vessels. Hydralazine, nitroglycerine, enalapril, and captopril are examples of vasodilators available.

Diuretics increase urine formation and promote water loss. Patients in cardiac failure tend to retain water and sodium, causing edema and ascites. Examples of diuretics include furosemide and spironolactone.

Disinfectants and Antiseptics

Disinfection is the destruction of pathogenic microorganisms or their toxins. Antiseptics are chemical agents that kill or prevent the growth of microorganisms on living tissues. Disinfectants are chemical agents that kill or prevent the growth of microorganisms on objects (surgical equipment, tables, floors, etc.). Alcohols are commonly used as antiseptics, but they are ineffective against bacterial spores and must remain in contact for several seconds to be effective against bacteria. Quaternary ammonium compounds are used to disinfect objects. They are generally safe and nonirritating to the skin and noncorrosive to objects but are ineffective against parvovirus. Clorox is an example of a chlorine compound; it is effective on fungi, algae, parvovirus, and vegetative forms of bacteria. It is not effective against bacterial spores. Betadine is an example of an iodophor and is used to disinfect tissue. Biguanides are commonly used to clean cages, surgical sites, and minor wounds. Chlorhexidine is the most common example; it may have residual activity when left in contact with the surface of the skin.

Endocrine Drugs

Hyperthyroidism, an increase in the production of the thyroid hormone, is common in cats. Methimazole is the most common treatment and can be supplied in tablet or topical form.

Hypothyroidism, a decrease in the production of the thyroid hormone, is more common in dogs. Levothyroxine is usually the drug of choice for this condition.

Insulin is responsible for the movement of glucose from the blood into the tissue cells. In diabetes mellitus, insufficient insulin is produced resulting in high blood glucose levels. The treatment of choice is the administration of insulin, which is supplied in a variety of trade names, all of which are developed by different methods. Types of insulin currently available include NPH, glargine, Vetsulin, and PZI.

Gastric Drugs

Drugs that affect the gastrointestinal tract are called *gastric drugs*. They can be further described by their function within the gastrointestinal tract. Emetics are drugs that induce vomiting, whereas antiemetics prevent or decrease vomiting. Examples of emetics include apomorphine and ipecac, whereas examples of antiemetics include acepromazine, chlorpromazine, metoclopramide, and maropitant (Cerenia). Diphenhydramine, dimenhydrinate, and maropitant can also reduce vomiting associated with motion sickness.

Antidiarrheals combat diarrhea, whereas adsorbents and protectants prevent toxins from attaching to, or coming in contact with, the gastrointestinal wall. Examples of antidiarrheals include diphenoxylate (Lomotil), loperamide, aminopentamide (Centrine), and bismuth subsalicylate (Pepto-Bismol). Activated charcoal is an example of an adsorbent.

Laxatives and stool softeners facilitate evacuation of the bowels. Metamucil is an excellent source of indigestible fiber, which helps retain water in the feces. Milk of Magnesia and phosphate salts create a strong osmotic force and attract water into the bowel of the lumen. Lubricants include mineral oil or cod liver oil and make the stool more slippery.

Antacids and antiulcer drugs reduce acidity of the stomach or reduce acid production. Examples of drugs that reduce acidity include calcium carbonate (Tums, Maalox), Rolaids, and aluminum hydroxide gel (Amphojel). Drugs that reduce acid production include cimetidine (Tagamet), ranitidine hydrochloride (Zantac), and famotidine (Pepcid). Sucralfate (Carafate) treats ulcers by adhering to the ulcer site.

Nervous System

Anesthetics are a class of drug that affects the nervous system. Examples of injectable anesthetics include propofol, ketamine, and tiletamine with zolazepam (Telazol). Gas anesthetics include nitrous oxide, methoxyflurane, halothane, isoflurane, and sevoflurane.

Tranquilizers and sedatives reduce anxiety and produce a relaxed state. Acepromazine can be used alone to produce the desired effect. Diazepam, midazolam (Versed), and clonazepam are used in conjunction with other drugs as part of a preanesthetic plan. Xylazine and medetomidine (Domitor) produce a calming effect and decrease the ability to respond to stimuli.

Analgesics are drugs that reduce the perception to pain without affecting other sensations. Butorphanol (Torbugesic), oxymorphone (Numorphan), meperidine (Demerol), and buprenorphine (Buprenex) are examples of analgesics.

Anticonvulsants are drugs used to control seizures. Phenobarbital and diazepam are the most common choices of drugs used in veterinary medicine.

Stimulants are drugs used to stimulate the central nervous system. Doxapram (Dopram) is a stimulant used to increase respiration in animals with apnea.

Respiratory

Antitussives block the cough reflex, whereas mucolytics, expectorants, and decongestants are designed to break up mucus in the respiratory tract. Butorphanol, hydrocodone, codeine, and dextromethorphan are commonly used antitussives. Mucomyst is an example of a mucolytic, whereas guaifenesin is an expectorant.

Bronchodilators inhibit constriction of the smooth muscle surrounding the deep bronchioles. Terbutaline, albuterol, theophylline, and aminophylline are examples of bronchodilators used in veterinary medicine.

THERAPEUTIC DIETS

Often, the term *prescription diet* is thought of as requiring a prescription for the product to be sold. This is not true. Therapeutic diets, as they should be called, require a valid doctor/client/patient relationship as recommended by the manufacturer (Figure 23-14). These diets are recommended for certain diseases or conditions and may aid in the treatment of such disease; they should be fed at the recommendation of a veterinarian. For example, a diet high in protein to treat obesity should not be fed to a cat with renal failure, who would most benefit from a low-protein diet. Assistants and technicians should be familiar with diets available, the conditions they treat, and the benefits and risks of each. The following section on nutrition covers a wide range of therapeutic diets available, along with a description of diseases or conditions that they aid in the treatment of.

> **PRACTICE POINT**   Therapeutic diets do not require a prescription; however, they must be sold by a veterinarian.

Therapeutic diets have been developed to aid in the treatment of or maintenance plan for disease but do not cure the disease. Clients must understand that foods cannot cure diseases or conditions.

AAFCO

The Association of American Feed Control Officials (AAFCO) was established in response to the increasing number of diets available on the market, some of which did not meet the specific nutritional needs of animals. AAFCO is made up of a variety of individuals and is not regulated or managed by any pet food manufacturer. Any foods that are recommended should meet the expectations and testing of AAFCO.

A label that reads "complete and balanced" must either meet a nutrient profile or pass a feeding trial. The food must meet all nutrient minimum and maximum ranges that have been established by AAFCO as being safe.

> **PRACTICE POINT**   Not all pet foods are tested; they simply state that they meet AAFCO requirements.

Minimum level requirements were established for protein, fat, carbohydrate, and essential amino acids as diseases associated with nutrient deficiencies have become more prominent. Maximum level requirements were established for calcium, phosphorus, magnesium, fat, water-soluble vitamins, and trace minerals to prevent nutrient excess, which has become a larger problem with the pet foods available in today's market.

Maximum levels for methionine, zinc, and vitamins A and D have been established for adult cat foods,

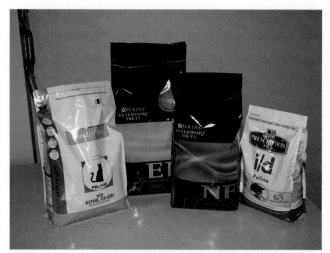

FIGURE 23-14 Examples of therapeutic diets.

reflecting current studies available on the toxic effect of these nutrients. Taurine levels have been established for both canned and dry cat food because the bioavailability of taurine is decreased in canned food.

All foods must either be categorized as growth and lactation or maintenance. Foods can state "for all life stages," which indicates the food has been able to meet stringent requirements for both categories. Canine growth and lactation nutrient requirements have higher levels of zinc, iron, and fat and decreased levels of calcium, phosphorus, and sodium.

To compare diets, food must be looked at on a "dry matter basis." AAFCO's definition of dry matter basis (DM) is the level of nutrients contained in a food. A "guaranteed analysis," or "as fed basis" must be converted to DM to effectively compare diets. For example, a canned diet contains approximately 75% moisture, whereas a dry diet contains approximately 10% moisture. To effectively compare the two products, the moisture content must be removed.

Ingredients are listed on the label by weight and can include moisture. Therefore some products may list chicken as the main ingredient, but the chicken may only weigh more than the corn or wheat products that follow because of its moisture content. Moisture is burned off during the cooking process; therefore it is important to look at the entire ingredient and nutrient profile when determining the appropriate diet for a patient.

The most commonly used unit of measurement is the kilocalorie (kcal), defined as the amount of heat necessary to raise the temperature of one kilogram (kg) of water by one degree Celsius. Calories are used to maintain physical activity, digestion, growth, and basal metabolism. Most foods are recommended in kcal/8 oz cup or kcal/can. Puppies and kittens require a larger amount of energy early in life and a lesser amount as they age. It is important to follow the feeding recommendations established by the pet food manufacturer because diets vary by company as well as within a specific product line. Tables 23-3 and 23-4 list the AAFCO nutrient requirements for both puppies and kittens, respectively.

Nutrients are required for basic bodily function, including acting as structural components, enhancing chemical reactions, transporting substances throughout the body, maintaining temperature, and providing energy. Nutrients are divided into six categories:

1. **Water:** Water is the most important nutrient and has several functions. It helps regulate temperature, provides shape and resilience to the body, enhances chemical reactions, and transports substances through the body.
2. **Carbohydrates:** Carbohydrates include sugars, starches, and fiber and function primarily to provide energy.
3. **Protein:** Protein is composed of various amino acids and provides energy. Protein is the principle structural component of body tissues and organs.
4. **Fats:** Fats supply energy and essential fatty acids that the body cannot produce.
5. **Minerals:** Minerals comprise all inorganic elements in food. Minerals play a large role in enzyme and hormone systems.
6. **Vitamins:** Both water-soluble and fat-soluble vitamins are cofactors in enzyme reactions and play a role in DNA synthesis.

Homemade diets are generally incomplete and therefore are not recommended. When preparing meals, owners may omit ingredients because of a lack of money or inability to find a product or may change a product because of personal preference. Many homemade canine diets contain excessive protein but are deficient in calories, calcium, vitamins, and microminerals. Many diets have an inverse calcium/potassium ratio. Feline diets tend to be deficient in fat, energy, and micronutrients. Uncooked recipes contain high levels of pathogenic bacteria that not only risk harm to the pet receiving the diet, but to the owner preparing the meal as well.

> **PRACTICE POINT**   Most homemade diets do not meet dietary guidelines for pets and therefore are not recommended.

Choosing the correct diet for a puppy or kitten requires evaluation of the breed, age, activity level, and environmental conditions. Some breeds are less active than others, and a house-bound dog will likely use less energy than a farm dog. Large-breed dogs need a slower growth rate to help decrease skeletal abnormalities. Many breeds are predisposed to obesity. Puppies and kittens that develop a large number of adipose cells during growth may also be predisposed to obesity as adults. Clients should be educated well on preventing obesity by learning to score their pets' body condition to prevent a number of diseases related to obesity in the senior years.

Puppies

A healthy mother that is well nourished should be able to provide complete nutrition for a puppy for the first 3 to 4 weeks.

A healthy puppy will nurse actively and vigorously. A malnourished puppy will constantly cry, become inactive, and fail to gain weight. Pregnant and nursing mothers should be fed a high-quality puppy food; they use the extra protein, calories, and fats to nourish the puppies.

More neonates die from a lack of knowledge of husbandry and nutrition than from disease. Birth weight is the single most important predictor of neonate survival. Those that are less than 25% of the average birth weight are at a higher risk of hypoglycemia, hypothermia, and pneumonia. Hypothermia decreases the motility of the gastrointestinal tract, thereby slowing the digestion of nutrients. Body weight should be monitored daily to ensure normal weight gain.

Average birth weight for toy-breed puppies is 100 g to 200 g; large-breed puppies average 400 g to 500 g, and giant-breed puppies average 700 g. Low birth weight produces poor performance and increased morbidity and mortality rates; it can be caused by congenital cardiac and pulmonary defects. Inadequate nutrition leads to dehydration and muscular weakness. Puppies not gaining weight may not be receiving enough calories and therefore require supplementation. In general, growing puppies need twice as much energy as adults for growth, activity, and body maintenance.

If one puppy is not gaining weight while the rest of the litter is, an exam should be performed to check for a cleft palate or any other oral abnormalities. If the exam appears normal, giving the underfed puppy time alone with the mother may be beneficial. The litter may be pulled away from the mother for approximately 5 to 10 minutes, giving the underweight puppy time with the mother. This process should be repeated three or four times daily, allowing the puppy to increase its milk intake.

Mother's milk is the gold standard. Occasionally, milk replacer may be needed due to the mother's refusal to care for the young, the death of the mother, or her inability to produce enough milk for the litter. Neonates that weigh less than 30% of their littermates or those losing weight after 48 hours may also need extra supplementation. Neonates that die after 48 hours of birth most likely have died from starvation.

Successful hand-rearing of orphans can depend on several factors, including appropriate feeding schedule, selection of milk replacer, meeting the caloric needs of the neonate, and proper feeding methods.

Newborns should be fed every 3 hours for the first week. Once the puppy has doubled the birth weight, feeding can be decreased to every 4 hours. This can take 7 to 10 days for a normal healthy puppy and 14 days for a puppy receiving milk replacer.

Table 23-3　AAFCO Recommendations for Puppies

Nutrient	Units DM Basis	Growth and Reproduction Minimum	Adult Maintenance Minimum	Maximum
DOG FOOD NUTRIENT PROFILES*				
Protein	%	22.0	18.0	
Arginine	%	0.62	0.51	
Histidine	%	0.22	0.18	
Isoleucine	%	0.45	0.37	
Leucine	%	0.72	0.59	
Lysine	%	0.77	0.63	
Methionine-cystine	%	0.53	0.43	
Phenylalanine-tyrosine	%	0.89	0.73	
Threonine	%	0.58	0.48	
Tryptophan	%	0.20	0.16	
Valine	%	0.48	0.39	
Fat†	%	8.0	5.0	
Linoleic acid	%	1.0	1.0	
MINERALS				
Calcium	%	1.0	0.6	2.5
Phosphorus	%	0.8	0.5	1.6
Calcium/phosphorus ratio		1:1	1:1	2:1
Potassium	%	0.6	0.6	
Sodium	%	0.3	0.06	
Chloride	%	0.45	0.09	
Magnesium	%	0.04	0.04	0.3
Iron‡	mg/kg	80.0	80.0	3000.0
Copper§	mg/kg	7.3	7.3	250.0
Manganese	mg/kg	5.0	5.0	
Zinc	mg/kg	120.0	120.0	1000.0
Iodine	mg/kg	1.5	1.5	50.0
Selenium	mg/kg	0.11	0.11	2.0
VITAMINS				
A	IU/kg	5000.0	5000.0	250000.0
D	IU/kg	500.0	500.0	5000.0
E	IU/kg	50.0	50.0	1000.0
Thiamine¶	mg/kg	1.0	1.0	
Riboflavin	mg/kg	2.2	2.2	
Pantothenic acid	mg/kg	10.0	10.0	
Niacin	mg/kg	11.4	11.4	
Pyridoxine	mg/kg	1.0	1.0	
Folic acid	mg/kg	0.18	0.18	
B_{12}	mg/kg	0.022	0.022	
Choline	mg/kg	1200.0	1200.0	

*Presumes an energy density of 3.5 kcal ME/g DM, based on the modified Atwater values of 3.5, 8.5, and 3.5 kcal/g for protein, fat, and carbohydrate (nitrogen-free extract), respectively. Rations greater than 4.0 kcal/g should be corrected for energy density; rations less than 3.5 kcal/g should *not* be corrected for energy.

†Although a true requirement for fat per se has not been established, the minimum level was based on recognition of fat as a source of essential fatty acids, as a carrier of fat-soluble vitamins, to enhance palatability, and to supply an adequate caloric density.

‡Because of very poor bioavailability, iron from carbonate or oxide sources that is added to the diet should not be considered as a component in meeting the minimum nutrient level.

§Because of very poor bioavailability, copper from oxide sources that is added to the diet should not be considered as a component in meeting the minimum nutrient level.

¶Because processing may destroy up to 90% of the thiamine in the diet, allowance in formulation should be made to ensure the minimum nutrient level is met after processing.

DM, Dry matter; *ME*, metabolized energy.

Table 23-4   AAFCO Recommendations for Kittens

Nutrient	Units DM Basis	Growth and Reproduction Minimum	Adult Maintenance Minimum	Maximum
CAT FOOD NUTRIENT PROFILES*				
Protein	%	30.0	26.0	
Arginine	%	1.25	1.04	
Histidine	%	0.31	0.31	
Isoleucine	%	0.52	0.52	
Leucine	%	1.25	1.25	
Lysine	%	1.20	0.83	
Methionine-cystine	%	1.10	1.10	
Methionine	%	0.62	0.62	1.50
Phenylalanine-tyrosine	%	0.88	0.88	
Phenylalanine	%	0.42	0.42	
Threonine	%	0.73	0.73	
Tryptophan	%	0.25	0.16	
Valine	%	0.62	0.62	
Fat†	%	9.0	9.0	
Linoleic acid	%	0.5	0.5	
Arachidonic acid	%	0.02	0.02	
MINERALS				
Calcium	%	1.0	0.6	
Phosphorus	%	0.8	0.5	
Potassium	%	0.6	0.6	
Sodium	%	0.2	0.2	
Chloride	%	0.3	0.3	
Magnesium‡	%	0.08	0.04	
Iron§	mg/kg	80.0	80.0	
Copper (extruded)¶	mg/kg	15.0	5.0	
Copper (canned)¶	mg/kg	5.0	5.0	
Manganese	mg/kg	7.5	7.5	
Zinc	mg/kg	75.0	75.0	2000.0
Iodine	mg/kg	0.35	0.35	
Selenium	mg/kg	0.1	0.1	

Continued

Formulated puppy milk replacer is available from veterinary distributors. Both powder and liquid forms are available. Powder formula lasts longer, and the unused powder can be frozen for 6 months. Once formula has been reconstituted, it should be used within 48 hours; the unused portion should be refrigerated in a glass container. Liquid milk replacer should also be used within 48 hours once the can has been opened, refrigerating the unused portion. Formulated milk replacer is superior to homemade versions because it generally provides the correct balance of protein, fat, carbohydrates, vitamins, and minerals needed for growing puppies. Reconstituted milk replacer should be warmed to 95° to 100° F in a warm-water bath. Milk should never be placed in the microwave because it can become too hot, causing severe burns to the patient.

If puppy milk replacer is temporarily unavailable, an emergency formula may be used. This formula provides approximately 1.2 kcal/mL. A 1-lb puppy would receive approximately 60 mL/day, divided over eight feedings. This

PRACTICE POINT Small-breed puppies commonly suffer from hypoglycemia; frequent feedings may need to be instituted until 6 months of age.

emergency formula is strictly that, and should be replaced with an appropriate puppy milk replacer as soon as possible.

The ingredients and caloric density of the puppy milk replacer can change with the manufacturer. Always review the label recommendations for the product being administered. The total feeding per day should be divided into eight feedings per 24 hours the first week and then decreased to five feedings per 24 hours thereafter. Smaller and toy breeds require more frequent feedings to prevent hypoglycemia. The frequency of feedings can slowly be decreased as the amount being fed slowly increases, along with the age of the puppy.

The urogenital area should be stimulated after every feeding to encourage urination and bowel movements. A

Table 23-4   AAFCO Recommendations for Kittens—cont'd

Nutrient	Units DM Basis	Growth and Reproduction Minimum	Adult Maintenance Minimum	Maximum
VITAMINS				
A	IU/kg	9000.0	5000.0	750000.0
D	IU/kg	750.0	500.0	10000.0
E‖	IU/kg	30.0	30.0	
K**	mg/kg	0.1	0.1	
Thiamine††	mg/kg	5.0	5.0	
Riboflavin	mg/kg	4.0	4.0	
Pantothenic acid	mg/kg	5.0	5.0	
Niacin	mg/kg	60.0	60.0	
Pyridoxine	mg/kg	4.0	4.0	
Folic acid	mg/kg	0.8	0.8	
Biotin‡‡	mg/kg	0.07	0.07	
B_{12}	mg/kg	0.02	0.02	
Choline§§	mg/kg	2400.0	2400.0	
Taurine (extruded)	%	0.10	0.10	
Taurine (canned)	%	0.20	0.20	

*Presumes an energy density of 4.0 kcal/g ME, based on the modified Atwater values of 3.5, 8.5, and 3.5 kcal/g for protein, fat, and carbohydrate (nitrogen-free extract), respectively. Rations greater than 4.5 kcal/g should be corrected for energy density; rations less than 4.0 kcal/g should *not* be corrected for energy.

†Although a true requirement for fat per se has not been established, the minimum level was based on recognition of fat as a source of essential fatty acids, as a carrier of fat-soluble vitamins, to enhance palatability, and to supply an adequate caloric density.

‡If the mean urine pH of cats fed ad libitum is not below 6.4, the risk of struvite urolithiasis increases as the magnesium content of the diet increases.

§Because of very poor bioavailability, iron from carbonate or oxide sources that is added to the diet should not be considered as a component in meeting the minimum nutrient level.

¶Because of very poor bioavailability, copper from oxide sources that is added to the diet should not be considered as a component in meeting the minimum nutrient level.

‖Add 10 IU vitamin E above minimum level per gram of fish oil per kilogram of diet.

**Vitamin K does not need to be added unless diet contains greater than 25% fish on a DM basis.

††Because processing may destroy up to 90% of the thiamine in the diet, allowance in formulation should be made to ensure the minimum nutrient level is met after processing.

‡‡Biotin does not need to be added unless diet contains antimicrobial or antivitamin compounds.

§§Methionine may substitute choline as methyl donor at a rate of 3.75 parts for 1 part choline by weight when methionine exceeds 0.62%.

DM, Dry matter; *ME,* metabolized energy.

moist, warm cotton ball can be used to stimulate movement. Once puppies are about 3 to 4 weeks of age, they will urinate and defecate without stimulation.

At 3 or 4 weeks of age, dry puppy food can be mixed with water and/or formula in a 1:3 ratio to form a gruel. If canned food is preferred, a 2:1 ratio can be made (canned food/formula and/or water). By 6 weeks of age, 50% of the puppies' diet should be from unmixed puppy food.

Water should be offered starting at 5 weeks of age. Puppies should still be receiving hydration from either their mother or the milk replacer, but water intake will increase once offered. Puppies should be allowed to play in the water at first; once they are acquainted with it, they will begin to drink it.

Puppies can be weaned at approximately 6 to 8 weeks. Early weaning is discouraged because it can lead to malnutrition, stress-related disease, and behavioral problems. It is important to watch the overall caloric intake because puppies can become obese, leading to a variety of diseases later in life. From the time of weaning until 6 months of age (9 months in large breeds), it is advised to feed puppies three times a day (more frequently for smaller and toy breeds). Thereafter, dogs should be fed twice daily on a regular schedule.

Large-Breed Puppies

Nutrition plays an important role in large-breed puppies and can lead to skeletal disease from an increased growth rate. Genetics and environmental components also play a role in disease development, but designing an adequate nutrition program can decrease the potential for a disease process.

Large-breed puppies require fewer calories per unit of body weight and mature more slowly than small-breed puppies. Rapid growth occurs in the first few months in all breeds but occurs over a longer period in large breeds. It is important to take into consideration the age, breed, gender, body condition, genetics, and environment. It is also important to understand how nutrients contribute to the expression of skeletal disease.

Excess dietary energy and caloric intake may support a growth rate that is too fast for appropriate skeletal development and that results in a higher number of skeletal abnormalities. Fat has a higher caloric density than protein or carbohydrates; therefore increased fat may be a primary contributor to excess energy intake. Extra energy is stored as fat once the maximum growth rate has been achieved. Excess energy leads to increased growth rate; increased growth rate leads to increased skeletal abnormalities. Abundant caloric intake contributes to accelerated growth rate and excess weight gain.

Excess protein has not been shown to affect large-breed puppies. Decreased protein has been shown to affect the skeletal system; therefore a diet should contain more than 25% protein on a DM basis. Excess calcium affects the skeletal system by increasing the severity of osteochondrosis. The absolute value of calcium appears to be more significant than the calcium/potassium ratio. Therefore it is contraindicated to supplement large-breed puppies with calcium when they are fed a complete and balanced commercial diet. AAFCO has demonstrated the safety and efficacy of a 1.1% calcium (on a DM basis) diet for large-breed puppies.

> **PRACTICE POINT** Large-breed puppies should not receive supplements of any kind; supplements may increase the risk of skeletal abnormalities.

Vitamins A, C, and D and trace minerals (copper and zinc) are all involved in skeletal development. There is a lack of studies evaluating excess amounts of vitamins A and C, copper, and zinc in the diet and their relationship to skeletal abnormalities. Vitamin D metabolites regulate the uptake of calcium and phosphorus from the gastrointestinal tract. Commercial diets contain between 2 and 10 times the amount of vitamin D recommended by AAFCO; therefore supplementation is absolutely discouraged. However, a proper balance of vitamins A, C, and D and minerals is very important to skeletal development.

Osteochondrosis desiccans (OCD) is a disruption in bone ossification that results in focal lesions. OCD occurs in the growth cartilage. Factors affecting OCD include age, gender, breed, rapid growth rate, and excess nutrients. Great Danes, Labrador Retrievers, Newfoundlands, and Rottweilers are at an increased risk. Overnutrition and/or excess caloric intake results in abnormal weight gain for the skeletal structure, disrupting the chondrocytes and leading to OCD.

Canine hip dysplasia is a genetic disorder of large and giant breeds but can be influenced by nutrition. Evidence suggests that rapid growth and weight gain in early development increase the risk for this condition.

Feeding methods can help control excess nutrient intake. Three methods of feeding include free-choice feeding, time-restricted feeding, and food-restricted feeding. Free-choice feeding allows the pet to eat ad libitum, thereby increasing the risk for excess nutrient intake. Time-restricted feeding allows the owner to feed two or three times per day for a set period. This may encourage the pet to eat ravenously, passing the normal satiety mechanism. Food-restricted feedings allow the owner to control caloric intake, maintaining optimal growth rate and body condition.

The body condition should be evaluated every 2 weeks. Food can be adjusted as needed to decrease excess fat, thereby decreasing the growth rate. Puppies should be scored on a 9-point scale as to how easy it is to palpate the ribs and spine. The ideal body condition score is an hourglass shape when viewed from above, with a definitive waist behind the ribs. Figure 23-15 demonstrates the appropriate technique for determining the body score of a canine.

Environment, genetics, and nutrient composition play key roles in skeletal development. The effects of skeletal disease in large-breed puppies can be minimized by regulating nutrient and caloric intake. The goal should be to regulate growth rate, not maximize it. Feeding an AAFCO-approved commercial diet is recommended to help achieve this goal.

Kittens

Normal, healthy kittens should be able to nurse vigorously. Healthy mothers can provide complete nutrition for kittens for the first 4 weeks of life. Signs of kittens receiving inadequate nutrition include constant crying, inactivity, and no weight gain.

The normal birth weight of healthy kittens is between 90 and 110 g. Kittens should gain 10 to 15 g per day and double their birth weight by day 10. Thereafter, kittens should weigh an average of 1 lb per month of age until 4 months. Formula-fed kittens grow more slowly, only doubling their body weight at 14 days, rather than 10, regardless of appropriate caloric intake.

Kittens require the most energy during their first 2 weeks of life, or 20 kcal/100 g/day. Kittens can begin to consume gruel at about 3 to 4 weeks of age. Gruel can be made of a dry kitten food mixed with formula and/or water (2:1) and fed in a saucer. They will increase consumption over the next 2 weeks, during which time the amount of water and/or formula added to the kitten food can be decreased, eventually weaning them onto kitten food.

Orphan kittens or kittens failing to gain weight can be fed a kitten milk replacer. Veterinary distributors carry a variety of replacers, as described in the canine section.

If kitten milk replacer is temporarily unavailable, the emergency formula established above may be used. A 100-g kitten would receive approximately 24 mL per day, divided over eight feedings. This emergency formula is strictly that and should be replaced with an appropriate kitten milk replacer as soon as possible.

Vigorous orphans with a good suck reflex may be bottle fed in a sternal recumbency, with the head elevated, simulating a nursing position. Weaker kittens may need to be tube fed. Kittens that do not receive colostrum may be more susceptible to infection at about 35 days postnatal.

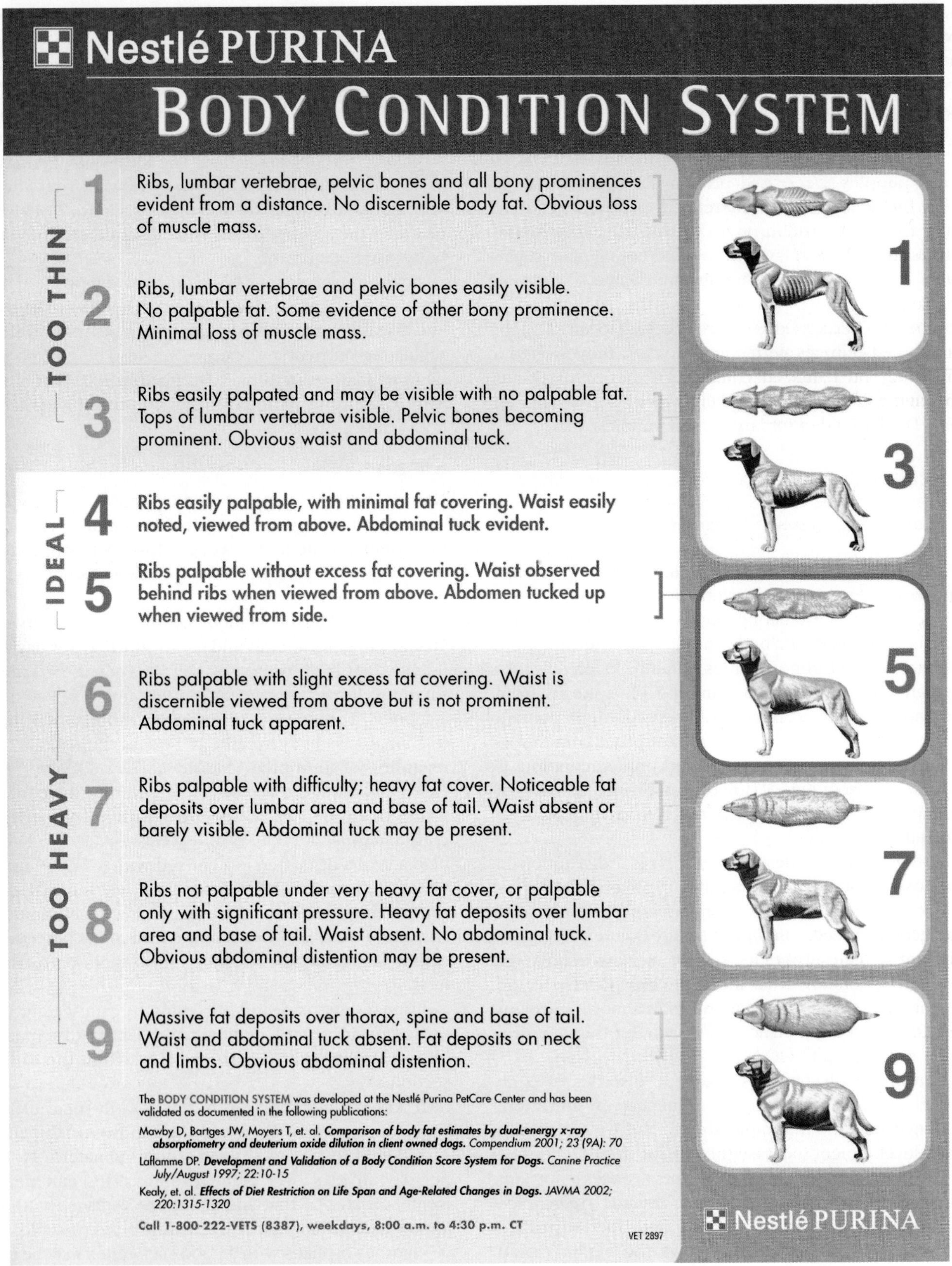

Nestlé PURINA
BODY CONDITION SYSTEM

TOO THIN

1 Ribs, lumbar vertebrae, pelvic bones and all bony prominences evident from a distance. No discernible body fat. Obvious loss of muscle mass.

2 Ribs, lumbar vertebrae and pelvic bones easily visible. No palpable fat. Some evidence of other bony prominence. Minimal loss of muscle mass.

3 Ribs easily palpated and may be visible with no palpable fat. Tops of lumbar vertebrae visible. Pelvic bones becoming prominent. Obvious waist and abdominal tuck.

IDEAL

4 Ribs easily palpable, with minimal fat covering. Waist easily noted, viewed from above. Abdominal tuck evident.

5 Ribs palpable without excess fat covering. Waist observed behind ribs when viewed from above. Abdomen tucked up when viewed from side.

TOO HEAVY

6 Ribs palpable with slight excess fat covering. Waist is discernible viewed from above but is not prominent. Abdominal tuck apparent.

7 Ribs palpable with difficulty; heavy fat cover. Noticeable fat deposits over lumbar area and base of tail. Waist absent or barely visible. Abdominal tuck may be present.

8 Ribs not palpable under very heavy fat cover, or palpable only with significant pressure. Heavy fat deposits over lumbar area and base of tail. Waist absent. No abdominal tuck. Obvious abdominal distention may be present.

9 Massive fat deposits over thorax, spine and base of tail. Waist and abdominal tuck absent. Fat deposits on neck and limbs. Obvious abdominal distention.

The BODY CONDITION SYSTEM was developed at the Nestlé Purina PetCare Center and has been validated as documented in the following publications:

Mawby D, Bartges JW, Moyers T, et. al. *Comparison of body fat estimates by dual-energy x-ray absorptiometry and deuterium oxide dilution in client owned dogs.* Compendium 2001; 23 (9A): 70

Laflamme DP. *Development and Validation of a Body Condition Score System for Dogs.* Canine Practice July/August 1997; 22:10-15

Kealy, et. al. *Effects of Diet Restriction on Life Span and Age-Related Changes in Dogs.* JAVMA 2002; 220:1315-1320

Call 1-800-222-VETS (8387), weekdays, 8:00 a.m. to 4:30 p.m. CT

VET 2897

Nestlé PURINA

FIGURE 23-15 Determining body condition score in dogs. (Courtesy Nestle Purina, St. Louis, Mo.)

Neonates may need help to learn how to bottle feed. Some take to bottle feeding well, whereas others need assistance. The nipple should be proportionate to the kitten's size and fill its mouth. A drop of milk should readily form when the bottle is inverted. If not, enlarge the nipple opening with a hot 22-g needle. Kittens nursing from a too-small nipple may generate negative suction. Increasing the size of the nipple and/or the size of the hole helps weaker patients nurse more effectively.

The gag reflex does not develop until approximately day 10; therefore kittens should not be forced to bottle feed. Aspiration and/or pneumonia can be a fatal consequence.

It is important to prevent overfeeding or feeding too fast. Gastric overdistention can cause delayed gastric emptying, bloat, and diarrhea. Regurgitation can occur through the nose. Excess air intake while nursing can also cause bloat and make the kitten uncomfortable. It is strongly advised to ensure proper body temperature because hypothermia can also cause delayed gastric emptying. The maximum stomach capacity for a neonate kitten is approximately 4 mL per 100 g of body weight.

Kittens should be fed every 2 to 4 hours for the first week, decreasing to every 4 to 6 hours the second week. Frequency can be decreased over the next 4 weeks while the amount being fed increases.

The urogenital area should be stimulated after every feeding to encourage urination and bowel movements. A moist, warm cotton ball can be used to stimulate movement. Kittens will begin to defecate and urinate without stimulation at about 3 to 4 weeks of age.

Kittens can be weaned at 6 to 8 weeks. Early weaning is not advised because separation from littermates can result in behavioral changes and a decline in social skills.

Kittens should be fed three times daily for 6 months, then twice daily for life. The label should be read on each food the kitten is eating to determine the correct amount to feed. If the kitten is eating both canned and dry food, the total caloric intake needs to be considered. As kittens mature, their energy requirements become less. At 10 weeks of age, the average daily energy requirement (DER) is 200 kcal/kg. By 10 months of age, the DER decreases to 80 kcal/day.

> **PRACTICE POINT** Kittens can easily become overweight, becoming obese adults as they mature.

Kittens can become obese, leading to a variety of diseases later in life. Some cats will limit themselves and simply "graze" all day, whereas others will eat until they have a distended abdomen. The same rules apply for kittens and cats that apply to puppies and dogs; owners should be educated well on body scoring their pets for obesity. The ribs and spine should easily be palpable, with an hourglass shape from above and a trim waistline behind the ribs. Figure 23-16 demonstrates the appropriate technique to determine the body score of cats.

Adults

The same body condition score applies to dogs and cats as they mature to adults and seniors. In general, adult foods should be lower in calorie content because the adult pet does not have the same energy requirements as puppies and kittens. Research has shown that adults can benefit from higher protein diets with less carbohydrates and fat. This is especially true for cats. Cats are strictly carnivores, meaning meat is their main source of protein. Carbohydrates are not required by cats and significantly contribute to the obesity problem seen in adults. Dogs are not strictly carnivores, but rather omnivores; they use both meat and vegetables for their sources of protein, carbohydrates, minerals, and fat.

> **PRACTICE POINT** Adult dogs and cats that have been altered have a decreased rate of metabolism; therefore fewer calories are needed to maintain body functions.

Seniors

Traditionally, senior patients were thought to need lower levels of protein because high levels of protein were thought to contribute to renal disease. Newer research has shown, however, that senior patients need higher levels of protein to help maintain muscle mass with low to moderate levels of fat to help maintain body mass.

Conditions That Can Be Treated or Maintained by Diet

Many conditions are diet responsive, whereas others must have medical management as well. Many diets can treat multiple diseases; the characteristics of a particular diet are vital to the treatment or maintenance of a disease or condition.

Allergies

Food allergies can be difficult to diagnose in patients because many different ingredients may contribute to the offending allergen. The goal, when determining what type of protein the pet may be sensitive to, is to eliminate all protein and carbohydrate sources for 8 weeks. A food trial of a hypoallergenic diet must be initiated with no other treats, trash, or snacks. A truly hypoallergenic diet is one that hydrolyzes (reduces the size of) the proteins to less than 18,000 Daltons (the size of the proteins). Once the pet's allergenic symptoms have subsided, the introduction of proteins can begin, one by one. Because hydrolyzed diets have been modified, the resulting protein is a medium-chain triglyceride, enabling the body to digest a higher amount

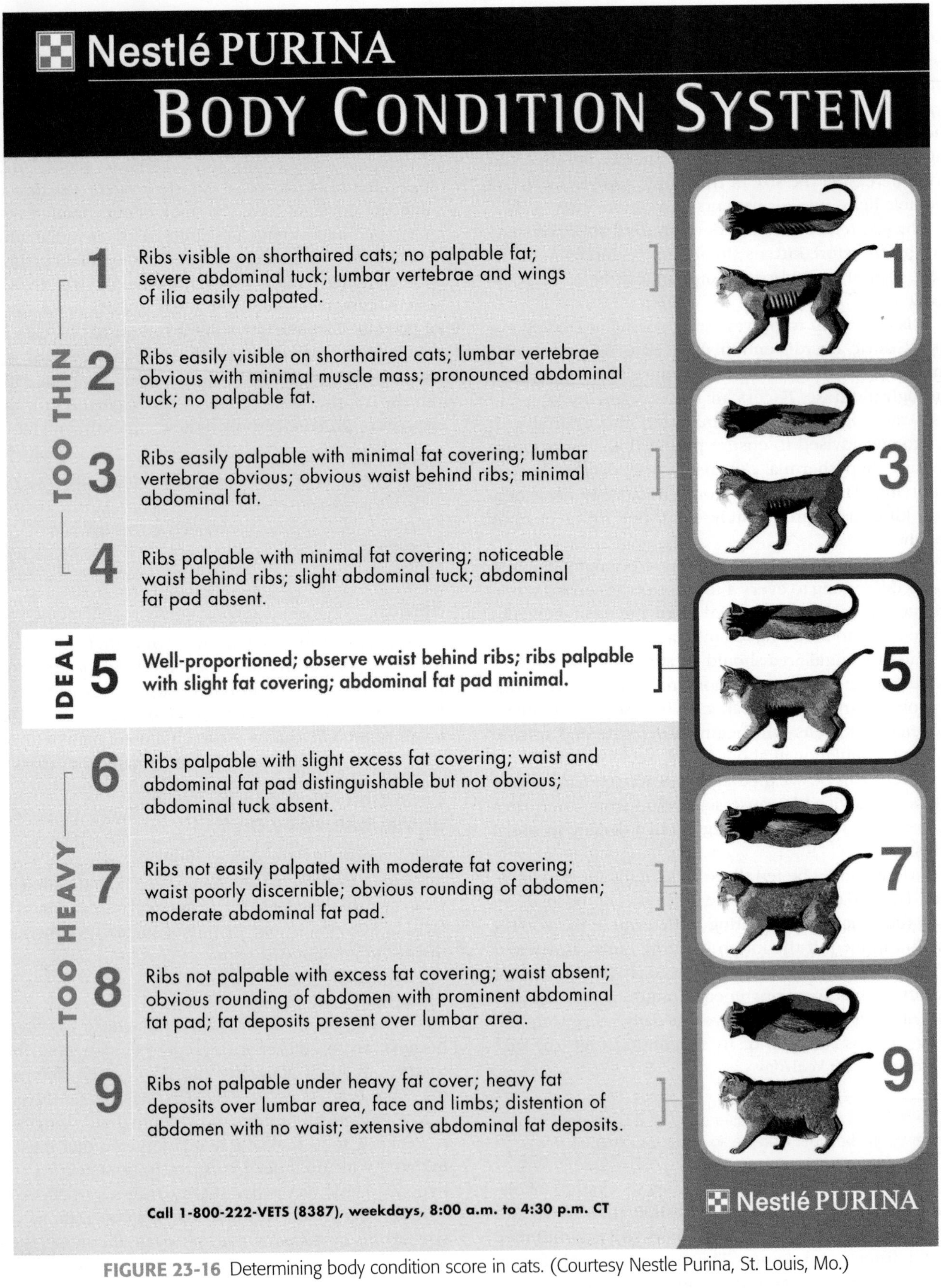

Nestlé PURINA
BODY CONDITION SYSTEM

TOO THIN

1 Ribs visible on shorthaired cats; no palpable fat; severe abdominal tuck; lumbar vertebrae and wings of ilia easily palpated.

2 Ribs easily visible on shorthaired cats; lumbar vertebrae obvious with minimal muscle mass; pronounced abdominal tuck; no palpable fat.

3 Ribs easily palpable with minimal fat covering; lumbar vertebrae obvious; obvious waist behind ribs; minimal abdominal fat.

4 Ribs palpable with minimal fat covering; noticeable waist behind ribs; slight abdominal tuck; abdominal fat pad absent.

IDEAL

5 Well-proportioned; observe waist behind ribs; ribs palpable with slight fat covering; abdominal fat pad minimal.

TOO HEAVY

6 Ribs palpable with slight excess fat covering; waist and abdominal fat pad distinguishable but not obvious; abdominal tuck absent.

7 Ribs not easily palpated with moderate fat covering; waist poorly discernible; obvious rounding of abdomen; moderate abdominal fat pad.

8 Ribs not palpable with excess fat covering; waist absent; obvious rounding of abdomen with prominent abdominal fat pad; fat deposits present over lumbar area.

9 Ribs not palpable under heavy fat cover; heavy fat deposits over lumbar area, face and limbs; distension of abdomen with no waist; extensive abdominal fat deposits.

Call 1-800-222-VETS (8387), weekdays, 8:00 a.m. to 4:30 p.m. CT

Nestlé PURINA

FIGURE 23-16 Determining body condition score in cats. (Courtesy Nestle Purina, St. Louis, Mo.)

of the nutrients. Diets with these protein modifications can also be used for dogs with dermatitis, pancreatitis, gastroenteritis, exocrine pancreatic insufficiency, protein-losing enteropathy, inflammatory bowel disease, lymphangiectasia, and hyperlipidemia.

"Allergy diets" made of proteins the pet has never been exposed to before may also provide relief for food allergies. Trout, duck, venison, and rabbit are a few proteins available for both dogs and cats.

Diabetes

Dogs and cats with diabetes mellitus respond differently to diets. Cats, being strictly carnivores, respond to diabetic treatments better with a high-protein diet. Carbohydrates are not needed by cats; therefore low levels of carbohydrate in the diet help regulate the cat more efficiently. In fact, some cats regulate well with a high-protein diet alone and do not need daily injections of insulin.

Dogs must have a diet high in fiber, with moderate levels of protein and fat for diabetes regulation. Canines use carbohydrates for energy more than cats do; therefore the two species must have two different diets.

Gastroenteritis
Canine
Gastroenteritis is complex and can be a difficult disease to treat. A diet that is composed of medium-chain triglycerides is ideal because dietary fats from long-chain triglycerides (LCT) can be among the most complex nutrients to digest. The fermentation of undigested fats contributes to diarrhea. Medium-chain triglycerides (MCT) can provide a readily digested and easily utilized energy source because they have already been broken down for the animal. Because fewer steps are required to break down the chains, the dog can absorb a higher volume of nutrients more efficiently. Therefore a diet composed of MCTs, with moderate levels of fat and low fiber, will help promote intestinal hemostasis, preventing diarrhea. A diet with these characteristics can also treat dogs for pancreatitis, exocrine pancreatic efficiency, hyperlipidemia, inflammatory bowel disease, lymphangiectasia, or hepatic disease not associated with encephalopathy.

> **PRACTICE POINT** Recently, research has shown that the addition of beef colostrum to canine dry foods increases gastrointestinal stability, thereby reducing the risk of diarrhea.

Feline
Because cats tend to respond to fat and carbohydrates differently than dogs do, a diet composed of moderate levels of fat and low carbohydrates is ideal for cats with gastrointestinal issues. High protein is required by cats; therefore a diet that is high in protein, low in

carbohydrates, and moderate levels of fat is ideal. These characteristics will also provide a diet for those with hepatic lipidosis. Contraindications for this diet include cats with renal failure or hepatic encephalopathy.

Heart Disease
Patients with heart disease must consume a diet low in sodium to decrease the workload of the heart.

Joints and Arthritis
New research has shown that omega-3 fatty acids play a large role in decreasing inflammation associated with arthritis. Eicosapentaenoic acids compete with arachidonic acid for the cyclooxygenase enzymes, ultimately reducing the proinflammatory mediators produced. Diets should be high in fish sources to allow dogs to maximally benefit from the omega-3 fatty acids. Foods that contain added chondroitin may be ineffective because the manufacturing process breaks down the product, rendering it unusable by the pet's body.

Liver Disease
Because liver disease can be due to several different factors, different diets may be required for such diseases. See other sections in this chapter for characteristics of diets for hyperlipidemia, hepatic lipidosis, and hepatic encephalopathy.

Obesity
Animals respond to "light" or reduced-caloric foods in different ways. Some may need a therapeutic diet to help remove excess weight. A diet that is high in protein and crude fiber will help the pet feel full, inducing satiety. High protein may also increase the metabolism of the pet. In addition, a high protein/calorie ratio promotes the loss of body fat while helping minimize the loss of lean body mass during weight loss. Therefore an ideal obesity diet should be low in fat and high in protein and fiber. This diet would be contraindicated for animals that require a low-protein diet because of renal disease. The characteristics of this diet would also be ideal for those that have fiber-responsive colitis, constipation, hyperlipidemia, or feline overweight diabetes mellitus or for those with hairballs.

> **PRACTICE POINT** Diets high in protein promote healthy weight loss in pets.

Renal Disease
The role of dietary management in renal disease is to provide a diet low in phosphorus to help protect against hyperphosphatemia and associated renal damage. Restricted but high-quality protein in the diet minimizes the intake of nonessential amino acids, resulting in decreased amounts of nitrogenous waste products. Reduced levels of sodium help compensate for the

kidney's inability to regulate this mineral, whereas omega-3 fatty acids may reduce glomerular hypertension. Therefore an ideal renal failure diet should be restricted in protein, with decreased levels of phosphorus and sodium. This diet would be contraindicated in animals that require a high-protein diet. The characteristics of this diet would also be ideal for those with heart failure or with hepatic disease associated with encephalopathy.

Urinary Stone Formation

A diet that effectively reduces the stone formation of both struvite and calcium oxalate uroliths will minimize the risk of recurrence while maintaining urinary tract health. An ideal diet should produce urine with a pH of 6.2, with moderate levels of salt to promote water intake. High levels of protein satisfy the protein needs of cats. Cats with heart disease or renal failure should not consume diets with these characteristics. Dogs may need a urine acidifier depending on the type of stones diagnosed.

PARASITES

Parasites may be internal or external and occur in small and large animals. Internal parasites in small animals include roundworms, hookworms, threadworms, whipworms, tapeworms, and heartworms. Internal protozoan parasites of small animals include *Coccidia* and *Giardia*. Parasites of horses include roundworms, pinworms, strongyles, threadworms, and tapeworms. Ruminants are commonly infected by strongyles, lungworms, tapeworms, *Coccidia,* and *Trichomonas*. Pigs are often infected with stomach worms, ascarids, *Strongyloides, Oesophagostomum,* whipworms, lungworms, and kidney worms. External parasites include fleas, ticks, lice, and mites.

Parasite prevention programs should be implemented where possible because many parasites are zoonotic. Controlling parasites in large animals can be difficult; however, a program should be established to provide the most protection possible.

COMMON SMALL ANIMAL EMERGENCIES

Emergencies come in all sizes. Everyone needs to be prepared to handle an emergency at any time. Once the receptionist accepts the call, the owner's name, pet's name, and a phone number should be noted. The receptionist should ask as many questions as possible: what the emergency is, when it happened, and the current condition of the pet. Many clients will not be able to answer all the questions and may be in too much of a hurry to talk. The receptionist can then provide the information to the assistants, technicians, and doctors.

Anaphylactic Reaction

This is an immediate type of hypersensitivity reaction in which death may occur rapidly from respiratory and circulatory collapse. Causes of anaphylactic reactions include (but are not limited to) vaccines, bee or wasp stings, and medications.

Antifreeze Ingestion

Unfortunately, once a pet has ingested antifreeze, it may be too late to save its life. Unless the ingestion has occurred very recently, there is no effective treatment. Many people do not know when their pets have ingested antifreeze. Pets will not show symptoms for up to 12 hours after ingestion. They may be lethargic. A urine sediment sample can be checked to determine if any monohydrate crystals are present (this is a definitive diagnostic tool), or an ethylene glycol test can be run. The patient can be supported with IV fluids while monitoring the blood urea nitrogen and creatinine values. Antifreeze basically shuts down the kidneys and does not allow the pet to produce urine.

> **PRACTICE POINT**   Antifreeze is a sweet-tasting liquid that attracts pets.

Bleeding

Frequently, the location of an active bleed can be difficult to determine, especially in patients that are active or in pain. In general, application of pressure directly to the site can induce clot formation, which will slow the bleeding. Once the bleeding has slowed, identification and a treatment plan can be initiated.

Blocked Cat

Many owners do not realize that a blocked cat is an emergency. Once a cat is blocked and cannot urinate, the blood urea nitrogen and creatinine levels increase dramatically. The cat may present with a distended abdomen, lethargy, and lack of appetite. These cats need to have a urinary catheter put in immediately. They may need to be sedated for the procedure, but if lethargic enough, it may be possible to advance a catheter without sedation. Vinegar may help the advancing of the catheter. Once a catheter has been placed, a urine sample needs to be collected and a urinalysis performed. The cat needs to be put on IV fluids to help flush the system out, and the urinary catheter needs to be left in place for 12 to 24 hours. An Elizabethan collar must be applied to the cat so it cannot pull the catheter out. A closed urinary tract system (an empty IV line and bag) can be put on the catheter to collect the urine. The amount of urine produced by the cat can then be measured and recorded. After the urinary catheter has been pulled, the cat should be observed for appropriate urination (straining, blood in the urine, etc.). Blood values of urea nitrogen and creatinine must be rechecked in 48 hours to make sure they have come down. The cat will need to be placed on a special diet and remain on the diet for the rest of its life because blockage can recur at any time.

> **PRACTICE POINT** Blocked cats that go undiagnosed may suffer permanent kidney damage.

Cardiopulmonary Resuscitation

When an animal is in cardiorespiratory arrest, **everyone must be available to assist.** When performing cardiopulmonary resuscitation (CPR), one person performs chest compressions, one person must breathe for the pet, another technician maintains the ECG machine, and someone needs to be available to get medications as needed.

Dyspneic Animal

An animal having difficulty breathing should be put into the oxygen cage (or have an oxygen mask put on) immediately. The gums will generally be a purple or blue color in this situation.

Dystocia

Difficult labor occurs in both the dog and cat but is far more common in the dog. Several conditions result in the diagnosis of dystocia:

- No fetus present within 4 to 6 hours from the onset of labor or from when the last time a fetus was born.
- No attempt to deliver a fetus despite the presence of fetuses in the uterus.
- Weak or infrequent contractions.
- Depression, weakness, and signs of toxemia.
- No puppies born by 72 days of gestation.
- No puppies born after 2 to 3 hours of active labor.

Gastric Torsion

Several factors may predispose dogs to gastric torsion. Older, large, and giant purebred dogs with a deep and narrow thorax are at a higher risk. Some studies indicate dogs that eat fast, are fed one meal a day, and have a nervous temperament may also be at a higher risk. It is associated with pain and stress and swallowing large amounts of air. The stomach distends with air and often twists 180 degrees on its axis. Signs include nonproductive retching and a distended abdomen that sounds air filled when thumped. The animal can die quickly from blood not being returned to the heart. The first priority is to relive the air-filled stomach, then surgery to correct the torsion.

Car Accident

Having a pet be hit by a car is a very traumatic experience for the owner. Often, the best option for the veterinary practice is to take the animal to the treatment area and place the client in an exam room. This allows the team to evaluate the patient without the client in the way. Once the pet has been evaluated, the veterinarian can provide information to the owner. It is important to try to determine where the pet has been hit by the car; the chest, abdomen, extremities only, or the whole body. If the pet is severely injured, it will most likely go into shock; the temperature will drop, oxygen circulation will decrease, and the system will try to compensate for the damage. A pet in shock should be warmed immediately and started on IV fluids. Caution should be used when moving the pet until the extent of its injuries can be determined. The veterinarian can then make recommendations for therapy and treatment of existing wounds.

Heat Stroke

Heat stroke can be caused by a pet being left outside in extreme heat with no shade or water or by being left in a car with closed windows. Heat stroke patients often suffer irreversible damage that may go undetected for several days. Heat stroke patients present with temperatures in excess of 104° F, panting, and usually laterally recumbent. Although the goal when treating these patients is to decrease the temperature, it should be done slowly to prevent sudden hypothermia.

Proptosed Eye

A proptosed eye is when the globe of the eye has popped out of the socket. This is also a very traumatic experience for owners who can hardly look at the pet's face. Proptosed eyes are usually the result of trauma and commonly occur in small breeds with short noses. Pekingese, Pugs, and Boston terriers are the most common breeds to experience this trauma, although other breeds are susceptible. If the eye has just proptosed, and there is minimal damage to the muscles and tendons around the globe, it can occasionally be replaced into the socket and sutured shut. The majority of the time, the eye will have to be enucleated (removed) and the socket sutured closed.

Seizure

A seizure can have many different etiologies. Toxicity, head trauma, tumors, and epilepsy are only a few causes. Many breeds are predisposed to seizures. Some seizures only last for a few seconds; others may last for minutes. A seizure is characterized by the pet lying in a lateral recumbent position with the legs and body stiffening and shaking uncontrollably. The pet may lose control of its bowels during the seizure. Once it has finished shaking, it may be disoriented for several hours. Seizures can be controlled with medication.

> **PRACTICE POINT** A seizing pet can be extremely traumatic for owners; they may not be able to recall details of the onset of the seizure.

Toxicities

Toxicities can result from a variety of different things, including plants, chemicals, and medications. Animals may present with shaking, disorientation, impairment of balance, seizures, or lethargy. If the owner knows what product the pet ingested, Animal Poison Control can be called. Be sure to have the correct product name and, if possible, the package or container. Animal Poison Control charges a fee; however, it has information relating to animal toxicities, treatments, and protocols. If a pet has *just* ingested a toxin, vomiting should be induced immediately. Apomorphine, as directed by the veterinarian, can be administered into the corner of the eye to induce vomiting. After most of the stomach contents have been emptied, the apomorphine should be rinsed from the conjunctival area and charcoal should be given. This will help absorb any toxins left in the stomach.

Rodenticides

Different rodenticides are composed of different chemicals. Each product should be reported to Poison Control to get the specific details. The most common product is Decon, which causes an animal to become anemic. These animals are treated with an injection of vitamin K and released with a minimum 30-day supply of oral vitamin K.

Tylenol

Tylenol (acetaminophen) is toxic to both dogs and cats. The animal's body cannot break down the active ingredient in Tylenol, which therefore causes toxicity. If the pet has just ingested Tylenol, vomiting should be induced with apomorphine. The pet should be started on intravenous fluids and continue treatment at the discretion of the veterinarian.

COMMON EQUINE EMERGENCIES

Colic

Colic is a general term that encompasses abdominal pain and is most commonly associated with gastrointestinal pain. Colic can be due to gas distension, torsion of the intestines, or nephrosplenic entrapment (the intestine can become obstructed in the space between the kidney and spleen). Symptoms can range from mild (kicking at belly) to severe discomfort (rolling and unable or unwilling to walk). Treatment can be either medical or surgical. Medical treatment consists of sedation to help control pain, nasogastric intubation to check for reflux, and the administration of mineral oil and fluids. The veterinarian may or may not recommend IV fluids. If the horse does not respond, surgery is advised. Uncontrollable pain is one of the most important signals for surgery. Surgery consists of an exploratory laparotomy to determine the cause of the pain and should be performed in an appropriate facility where sterility can be maintained.

Laceration

Lacerations can be caused by a number of things, including wire fencing, stalls, or loading accidents.

COMMON BOVINE EMERGENCIES

Down Cow

A "down cow" is one that is unable or unwilling to stand. Down cows may be suffering from hypocalcemia, also known as *milk fever* (especially likely in high-producing cows that have just begun lactation) or *obturator nerve paralysis*. Hypocalcemia is treated with intravenous calcium gluconate. Nerve paralysis is treated with dexamethasone (if a cow is pregnant, dexamethasone can lead to abortion; therefore caution should be used in its administration).

Dystocia

Cows may have difficulty in calving due to the size or malpresentation of the calf. Dystocia can sometimes be easily corrected by a veterinarian repositioning the calf; obstetric chains may be needed to help pull the calf out. Dystocia can lead to a cesarean section if the calf cannot be removed. If the calf is dead or too large to be pulled, a fetotomy (cutting the calf and delivering in pieces) may be performed.

Uterine Prolapse

A prolapse of the uterus often occurs shortly after calving. A cow may present with a large, red, and bloody body of tissue protruding from the vagina. The cow rarely appears in distress but may be straining (unable to urinate). Treatment consists of trying to put the uterus in its proper location.

COMMON OVINE AND CAPRINE EMERGENCIES

Sheep commonly suffer from both dystocia and hypocalcemia, similar to cows. The treatment is the same.

Pregnancy Toxemia

Pregnancy toxemia is seen in late-term ewes. The ewes may appear depressed or staggering or may be down. Pregnancy toxemia is caused by a nutritional deficiency leading to ketosis, ketoacidosis, and fatty liver. It is often associated with a sweet smell (ketones) on the breath. Ketones can be observed in the urine, and glucose levels in the blood may be low. Ewes can be treated with propylene glycol via stomach tube and with intravenous fluids with added dextrose. If the lambs are dead or the ewe is valuable, a cesarean section can be performed.

COMMON CANINE DISORDERS

Dogs can present with a variety of ailments; some are breed specific and others are species specific. It is imperative that the receptionist, assistant, and technician team be well informed on the most common diseases to provide clients with information about and be able to answer their basic questions.

Allergies

Allergies are a common problem among dogs and can be related to food or environment. Food allergies are a response to certain proteins in the diet; allergies to beef, chicken, or salmon are common. Pets with food allergies may suffer from vomiting, diarrhea, sensitive skin, and/or anal gland infections. To rule out suspected proteins as the source of allergic symptoms, pets must be placed on a food trial and fed a truly hypoallergenic diet. A hypoallergenic diet is one in which the proteins have been hydrolyzed (reduced in size), which prevents the pet's immune system from recognizing the protein and mounting an allergic response to it. A food trial must last for a minimum of 8 weeks; the pet cannot receive treats of any kind (this includes heartworm preventive if it is in the form of a flavored tablet). If the symptoms clear, then the pet has a true food allergy. If the symptoms do not completely clear, then the pet may have some existing environmental allergies as well. If the pet responded to the food trial, then individual proteins may be reintroduced to the diet one at a time to determine which protein the pet is allergic to. Once the symptoms return, a diagnosis can be made. The pet should not eat any food with that type of protein on the ingredient list.

Pets can have environmental allergies to grass, pollens, or molds and can be treated with antihistamines to relieve the symptoms. Just as with humans, some antihistamines may not work with an individual pet; therefore other antihistamines should be tried. Blood tests can also determine which environmental conditions a pet may be allergic to. Allergy injections can be formulated to help alleviate the symptoms. A variety of companies can compound allergy injections.

Anal Gland Impaction and/or Infection

Anal glands are located near the rectal area at approximately the 4 o'clock and 8 o'clock positions. These glands are used for scenting the pets' stool and frequently become impacted or infected. Smaller breeds tend to have more difficulty with these glands and often need assistance to express them. Many dogs will scoot on the carpet, expressing them and infuriating the owner with the horrible smell left behind. It is a common myth that

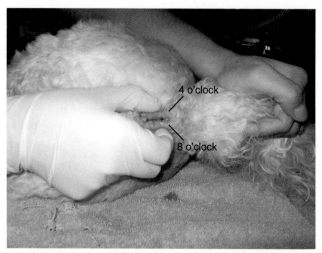

FIGURE 23-17 Anal glands are located at approximately the 4 o'clock and 8 o'clock positions around the anus.

dogs that scoot have worms; in fact, a majority of the time the anal glands are full or impacted (Figure 23-17).

Normal material from the anal glands should have a liquid consistency, with a slight brown color. Dark, thick material is not normal and may indicate that the pet needs to have its glands expressed more regularly. White liquid debris can indicate infection. Often, infected anal glands will rupture, becoming an anal gland abscess. At this point, the pet may need antibiotics and regular flushing of the draining tract.

Fiber can be added to the diet of some pets; by increasing the bulk in the stool, natural expression of the glands will occur. Others may need to have the glands expressed on a regular basis, either by the groomer, veterinary assistant, or veterinary technician.

Ear Infection

Ear infections are common in all breeds of dogs, especially those with ears that flop over. The warm, dark, and moist environment attracts yeast and bacteria. Pets may present with symptoms of scratching their ear or head tilt, or the ear may be tender to the touch or have debris emanating from it.

It is advised to perform a cytology study of the ear to determine what type of bacteria or yeast may be residing in the ear canal. This can determine the appropriate treatment that will be recommended by the veterinarian. Cytology must be completed before the ear is cleaned; therefore technicians and assistants may want to gather the appropriate equipment to complete it. Once the appropriate medication has been dispensed, owners should be advised of the appropriate way to clean ears (described later in this chapter).

Ear infections may start as a result of allergies and are also more frequent in pets that swim in pools and lakes and in dogs that are hypothyroid. Cocker Spaniels are the most common breed to have both allergies and hypothyroidism, predisposing them to recurring ear infections.

Gingivitis

Gingivitis is inflammation of the gum line around both the inside and outside of teeth. Gingivitis can create a terrible odor, as bacteria live in and around the plaque buildup. Gingivitis can be prevented by regular teeth brushing. Many pets learn to enjoy their teeth being brushed, but it takes time and patience from the owner. Educating owners to brush their pets' teeth is an excellent puppy and kitten education topic. Animals learn to accept it when they are young; starting young prevents the disease later in life.

Gingivitis and dental disease are very common in smaller breeds of dogs because they do not chew on toys, bones, or sticks as they age. Larger breeds of dogs always find something to chew on. The actual mechanism to help keep teeth clean is similar to flossing; the simple scraping of an object against the teeth scrapes off plaque and bacteria. Once plaque builds up and calcifies, it turns to tartar, which requires a dental prophylaxis to remove. Without a dental treatment, gingivitis leads to periodontal disease, which ultimately leads to tooth loss. As bacteria build in the mouth, they begin to circulate in the bloodstream and can affect such organs as the kidneys and heart. Gum and dental disease prevention is key to maintaining a healthy body for the pet's life.

Hypothyroidism

Hypothyroidism is underproduction of thyroid hormone and most often occurs in dogs older than 2 years. Presenting symptoms include lethargy; obesity; dull, dry hair coat; and ear infections. A blood test is performed to diagnose the disease. Hypothyroid dogs are then started on a thyroid supplement, which is generally given twice daily. The thyroid levels are then checked 4 to 6 weeks later and 4 to 6 hours after the pill is given. A pet's activity level generally improves, along with the hair coat, once supplementation has started.

Kennel Cough

Kennel cough, usually caused by *Bordetella*, is a common bacterial or viral infection that is extremely contagious to other dogs. It is very common in boarding facilities, pet shops, and animal shelters. Symptoms include a dry, hacking cough that can be induced upon palpation of the trachea. Dogs usually feel normal otherwise and continue to eat, drink, and play as normal. An antitussive agent (anticough) can be prescribed to relax the muscles of the trachea if needed. Antibiotics may be needed if the veterinarian feels that a secondary infection is starting or that the cough is due to a bacterial infection. Viral kennel cough must run its course because antibiotics will not kill a virus.

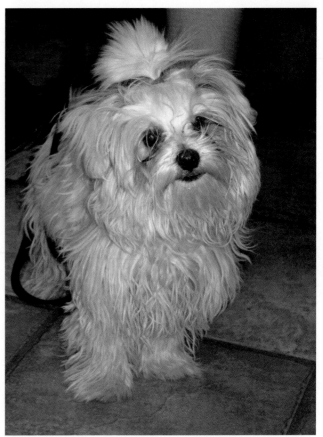

FIGURE 23-18 Ocular discharge can be abnormal. The patient should be examined by a veterinarian.

Owners of pets with kennel cough should be advised to confine their pets to a restricted area to prevent contact with other dogs until the symptoms have subsided. If pets are presented to the practice with symptoms of kennel cough, they should be placed into an exam room immediately, offered an isolation room, or asked to wait outside. This will prevent the further spread of this contagious disease.

Ocular Discharge

Ocular discharge is important to treat. Allowing eyes to drain excessively may increase the chance of permanent damage. Clear discharge may be normal for some smaller breeds and may be due to a blocked tear duct. Colored discharge, such as green or yellow discharge, can indicate an eye infection or damage to the surface of the eye (Figure 23-18). When clients call and are concerned about possible drainage from their pet's eye, they should be advised to come in to be seen as soon as possible.

Skin Diseases

Skin diseases can be due to a variety of ailments. The most common skin diseases seen are caused by allergies, infections, or mites. Allergies may cause a "hot spot," an area that has become irritated as the pet continues to lick and chew at it. Hot spots are localized, red lesions and are generally larger than the owner anticipates. Skin infections are characterized by scabby areas, with a small amount of purulent discharge oozing from the area. Both hot spots and infected lesions should be clipped and cleaned with a broad-spectrum cleaner. Antibiotics may be started, as well as shampoo or antihistamines to relieve skin irritation.

Mites can be difficult to diagnose, depending on the type of mite. *Demodex*, the common mite of mange, can be easily diagnosed with a skin scrape. Mites can be seen under the microscope and are easily treated. Dogs with mange usually present with patches of missing hair. Sarcoptic mange can be more difficult to diagnose because this mite resides in the hair follicles. Deep skin scrapes must be taken, which rarely yield *Sarcoptes*. Pets present with hair loss and intense pruritus (itching). A diagnosis is usually made when the pet's symptoms begin to remit with treatment.

Ringworm is a fungal skin disease that is zoonotic to people and other pets. The most common characteristics of ringworm include red, raised lesions on the face, nose, and ears, with hair loss on the rest of the body. Dermatophyte test media (DTM), or fungal cultures, must be performed to rule out ringworm. If the DTM is positive, the client must be educated on proper eradication methods because ringworm can be difficult to eliminate.

Obesity

Obesity is a common disease that is on the rise. Many owners feel that they need to give their pets extra attention and love and do so by feeding too many treats. Obesity decreases a pet's life span and increases diseases such as osteoarthritis, heart disease, and hip dysplasia.

> **PRACTICE POINT** Leaner pets live an average of 1.8 years longer than those that are overweight.

Clients must be educated that leaner pets live longer lives, cost less to maintain, and are happier pets. Obesity programs may need to be instituted in the practice to decrease the number of obese patients. More importantly, if the owner is obese, instilling an activity program for the pet may increase the activity of the owner, ultimately increasing the health level of the client. Obesity must be tackled in America for both pets and clients.

Tumors

Tumors can be benign or malignant and must be removed to confirm the diagnosis. Fine-needle aspiration may be performed to attempt to view the cells that make up the tumor; however, trained pathologists that read such samples on a daily basis should make the diagnosis. A tumor may look benign or feel like a lipoma (fatty tumor) when, in reality, a smaller malignant mass may lie within.

Benign tumors are localized and do not metastasize to other regions of the body. Malignant tumors can metastasize to other parts of the body. Mast cell tumors, round cell tumors, and transitional cell carcinomas are just a few malignant tumors. Benign tumors do not generally require any treatment other than complete excision; malignant tumors require excision, along with chemotherapy or radiation treatment. A pathologist can recommend the best treatment when a mass has been submitted to the lab. Further consultation can occur with an oncology specialist in the area.

COMMON FELINE DISORDERS

Cats present with a variety of diseases or problems, many of which can be difficult to diagnose and manage.

Abscesses

An abscess is a large pocket of pus and debris that has sealed over, retaining the bacteria inside. Many abscesses start from a cat bite wound or puncture that immediately seals over. The bacteria are left inside and replicate, causing an infection. Many cats present with fever, lethargy, and tenderness to touch in a specific area. Others may present with a ruptured abscess; the wound has opened, draining its contents. An abscess, if not already ruptured, will need to be opened and drained. The wound will then need to be flushed and the cat placed on antibiotics.

Asthma

Cats with asthma present with upper respiratory distress; they cannot breathe normally and are gasping for air. Most cats can only sit on their chests during an asthma attack because this is the only position that is comfortable. Cats may also "open mouth breathe"; they are trying to obtain more air by breathing through their mouths instead of their noses.

Cats with asthma generally need a radiograph to rule out other diseases. Asthma can be treated with a combination of several drugs, and cats can live long lives with asthma.

Feline Lower Urinary Tract Disease

Feline lower urinary tract disease (FLUTD) is common in male cats from 2 to 10 years of age. FLUTD is the blockage of the urinary tract between the bladder and the penis; the cause is unknown but is thought to be genetic or food related. Cats present with a painful abdomen, straining to urinate and meowing in discomfort. This is an emergency because the cat is unable to urinate. Most cats must be sedated immediately, have a urinary catheter placed that must remain in place for 12 to 24 hours, and be started on intravenous fluids. Many cats suffer kidney damage; therefore blood urea nitrogen and creatinine values must be evaluated and monitored.

FLUTD can be severe and life threatening. Once cats have become unblocked, the owner must be aware that the condition can recur at any time. Many cats are difficult to unblock and may reblock within a short period. Cats should be observed for normal urination for the rest of their lives. A special diet should be recommended that will maintain the urine pH within a neutral zone.

Hyperthyroidism

Hyperthyroidism is common in cats. Affected pets present with weight loss and vomiting. Cats look anorexic but have a vigorous appetite. The thyroid gland overproduces thyroid hormone, resulting in an excessive metabolism. Bloodwork determines if a cat is hyperthyroid. Medication is usually an effective treatment. Methimazole is the most common drug given and can be given once or twice a day, depending on the cat. If the cat does not easily take a pill, then a transdermal gel is available that can be applied to the ear pinnae.

> **PRACTICE POINT** Radioactive iodine treatment is also available to treat cats with hyperthyroidism.

Once a cat has been on the medication for 4 to 6 weeks, the thyroid level can be tested again to ensure the cat is receiving the correct dose.

Thyroid disease unfortunately can mask other diseases. Often, once the thyroid disorder has been treated, other diseases, such as renal and cardiac disease, will manifest.

Megacolon

Megacolon in cats is just as it sounds; it is an enlarged colon that often constipates cats. Many cats present with a distended and painful abdomen. Radiographs can be taken to diagnose megacolon. Enemas are often given to relieve the constipation. Medications must be given to the affected cat for life, and they must eat a special diet. Cats not receiving medication will reblock with feces and will need to have future enemas. Some cats block severely and must be anesthetized to perform a warm-water enema to release the contents.

Ringworm

Ringworm is a common disease of cats, who can be symptomatic or asymptomatic carriers. Symptomatic is defined as showing lesions or hair loss, allowing areas to be cultured on a DTM. Asymptomatic carriers do not have any symptoms and are simply carriers of the fungus.

If one household has a cat positive for ringworm, it is recommended to test other cats in the house as well to determine if all must be treated. Cats can be orally medicated and bathed to treat the fungus.

Ringworm can be especially difficult to eradicate in the household setting. Strict cleaning procedures must be initiated and involve the carpet, upholstery, vents, and vacuum.

HOUSEKEEPING

It is imperative that the practice stay in immaculate condition at all times. Odors travel quickly through the practice; therefore urine, feces, anal gland secretions, and other unpleasant odors must be removed immediately. Odors are also absorbed into the walls, baseboards, and tile grout; once the odors have permeated, they may be impossible to remove.

Chemicals used to clean floors should never be mixed. The label on bleach products reads to dilute to a 10% or 20% solution and not to mix with other products. Caustic vapors may result, causing harm to patients and team members. Labels must be read clearly to dilute the product to the correct strength to have a solution that kills viruses, fungi, or bacteria, whichever the product is designed to eradicate.

Trash should be emptied several times a day. Trash cans absorb odors that can also travel through the practice. Rooms must be cleaned after every patient, preventing the transmission of odors and diseases.

Walls should be cleaned weekly, if not more often; blood, hair, and dirt collect on walls and cabinets and must be cleaned off as soon as they are spotted.

Potted plants that sit on the floor must be cleaned frequently because animals often urinate on them. The entire pot must be cleaned. It should be moved each night while cleaning the practice, removing hair and dirt that has collected under the plant.

Blinds, fans, vents, baseboards, and door frames must be dusted weekly. Dirt collects in these locations quickly, and clients notice the dirt as they are waiting in the examination rooms.

The outside of the practice must remain clean as well. Feces must be removed daily, and common urination areas must be scrubbed with a dilute Clorox solution. Urine stains walls and sidewalks and produces a terrible smell. Trash must be removed from the parking lot, including cigarette butts and cans. Windows should be washed weekly and dirt swept away from the entrance and exit areas. The outside of the building must be as presentable as the inside of the practice.

BOARDING

Some practices allow their clients to leave their pets at the hospital when they leave town. Other practices may have a boarding facility that is separate from the practice. It is ideal to have separate facilities to allow hospitalized patients to recover in a quieter, cleaner environment. It also prevents boarding patients from being exposed to diseases or pathogens that hospitalized patients may be harboring.

Admitting

Admitting procedures for boarding animals are critical. The goal of any facility is to provide a safe, well-monitored, and caring environment. Every animal that is admitted must be reviewed for medications, feeding schedules, special diet, exercise requirements, and any other special needs. See Chapter 5 for examples of boarding admission forms. Release forms should include the above-mentioned information, and the owner should sign the bottom of the release. Release forms are absolutely critical when accepting patients for boarding. The release form must include the client's name, pet's name, and all available emergency contact information. If anything happens to the pet while the client is away, the practice must be able to contact the owner. The practice should also have established guidelines and the owner's consent that emergency procedures will be administered if and when an event should happen.

Release forms should also ask specific questions regarding the pet: What food does the pet eat and how often? What medications does the pet receive and how often? Has the pet had any vaccine or drug reactions in the past?

All patient blankets, collars, leashes, toys, and food must be clearly marked with the patient's name and owner's last name. All products left with the animal should be indicated on the release sheet. If a patient soils a blanket during the stay, it must be returned to the cage once washed. Kennels and cages may have a plastic holder on each to accommodate all personal items, preventing misplacement during the pets stay.

Facilities cannot be overcrowded, unsanitary, or loud; these factors can produce a stressful atmosphere for animals and team members. Boarding facilities or practices should have a boarding reservation software management system that allows the control of patient intake. Reservation management systems are similar to hotel reservations; they allow the team member to review available cages for a specific length of time.

The boarding center must be staffed by a kennel assistant as much as possible, allowing for the cleaning of cages as soon as patients defecate or urinate. Animals cannot be allowed to lie in their urine or feces for long periods. Animals boarded should always receive a bath before returning home because the odor of the facility will be present on the pet when it is discharged. This can be an unpleasant odor that makes clients wonder if their pets were cared for or left alone.

Every consideration should be given to the patient's dietary needs. If the practice does not carry a patient's food, clients should be advised to bring their own food. Changing the diet can cause a pet to have diarrhea; adding a stressful situation increases the chances of the pet experiencing stress colitis, a condition that also causes diarrhea. Medications should be administered as close to the normal times as possible, especially if insulin is being administered to a diabetic patient. Once the release sheet has been completed by the owner and team member, a treatment sheet should be filled out for the patient, indicating specific instructions for the kennel attendant. This allows each patient to receive individual care in a kenneled situation.

Isolation should be available for those patients with diseases that can be contagious to other patients in the boarding facility. Every precaution should be taken for patients to prevent the cross-contamination of disease; however, it can still occur. Kennel cough, or infectious tracheobronchitis, and feline upper respiratory diseases are spread though respiratory secretions and fomites. A fomite, or fome, is any object or material on which disease-producing agents can be conveyed. It is imperative that all bowls, litter pans, and blankets be washed in a warm, diluted bleach formula to prevent the spread of disease. If a dog is observed coughing or a cat is observed sneezing, it should be moved to an isolation area immediately.

> **PRACTICE POINT**   Pets that are boarding commonly experience stress colitis, a condition that results in diarrhea.

Patients that are boarding may have options to receive treatments and special care while they are at the facility. It is important to always ask the client for permission before performing any service. Spa days are becoming very popular. Pets are pampered with a day of bathing, grooming, nail trims, ear cleaning, and anal sac expression; some may receive a massage!

Nail Trims

Nail trims should be offered to all patients because clients often cannot trim them at home. Long nails can have detrimental effects on the patient; altered gait, potential lameness, and ingrown nails are just a few. Resco-type nail trimmers work great. On white or clear nails, the quick can be visualized. The quick is the vein that runs midway through the nail; it is generally pink. If the quick is trimmed, it is extremely uncomfortable to the pet and causes the nail to bleed. Kwik Stop powder can be applied to the nail or a silver nitrate stick can be used. The quick should be dabbed to absorb excess blood, and then the stick can be rolled in the quick bed. This can also be painful to pets. Short, quick actions can minimize the discomfort. Black nails can be hard to trim without cutting the quick because it cannot be visualized as easily as in white nails. It is advised to only trim the hook of the nail on black toenails. The quick will recede with each nail trim the pet receives. If a pet has excessively long nails, they can be trimmed a small amount every 2 to 3 weeks until the desired length is achieved. Owners with sensitive skin should be warned that freshly trimmed nails are sharp and can scratch their skin easily. For elderly clients, patients' nails may be rounded off with a Dremel tool to decrease the sharpness of the nails.

CONDO FACILITIES

Many facilities offer condominium-like housing for patients. Cat condos have several tiers available so that cats can move around. Toys may be available, or owners can bring their own. All toys and condos must be disinfected before exposure of the next patient. Canine condos may have themes associated with them (e.g., a cowboy room). This room may have painted walls, a step-up cot with a blanket, and a horse trough for water. Others may have water fountains or stereos to play music for the pets. Televisions may loop dog or cat videos to entertain patients.

Blankets and/or cots should be provided for pets to rest on; this can add comfort to the pets' stay, especially older and arthritic patients. Raised cots lift patients off the floor during colder times of the year. Blankets need to be watched; some patients love to chew on them. If a patient is known as a chewer, discretion should be used when allowing blankets to remain in the cage. All blankets should be washed in hot water with a dilute bleach solution. Blankets should be changed every day, regardless of whether or not they appear clean. Blankets can harbor odors, which penetrate the pet's hair coat. Blankets may also still look clean when patients have urinated on them, leaving patients to lie in their own urine.

With the newest updated technology, web cameras can be installed in kennels, allowing owners to see their pets anytime on the computer. This is an added benefit for owners, and they love the ability to check in. Practices and facilities must be diligent about cleaning and ensure that the facility appears clean and friendly at all times.

Owners seek veterinary practices to board their patients for security and a guarantee that their pets will receive the treatment required while they are gone. This is especially true for patients that are unhealthy. Diabetics, senior patients, or those that receive any special medications must be monitored and medicated daily. All boarding patients must be monitored for urination, defecation, appetite, and activity. Increased water intake and urination must be noted, as well as any diarrhea, anorexia (lack of appetite), or lethargy (lack of energy). All the above should be noted on the treatment sheet, and a doctor should be notified. If patients are seen limping, an exam by the veterinarian may be warranted; with the owner's consent, an NSAID may be administered.

Clients may elect to have procedures completed on the patient while boarding. Dentals, ovariohysterectomies, and castrations can be completed early in the boarding time, and the incision can be observed throughout the pet's stay. If a pet becomes too active in the kennel, drugs may be administered to calm the pet.

When releasing patients to owners, they should smell clean, look clean, and have all their personal items. If any procedures were performed during the stay, a release sheet should be provided to the owners with follow-up instructions, including permitted activity and when to give the next dose of medication. A report should also be generated regarding the pet's stay in the facility. Clients love to receive "report cards" of their pets; this is an excellent marketing tool and allows clients to feel that their pet is special.

VETERINARY PRACTICE and the LAW

Laboratory procedures must be performed with precision to obtain accurate test results. Each step must be performed according to directions; proper timing and the correct number of drops of conjugate to sample are essential for accurate results. Incorrect results could result in euthanasia or the incorrect treatment of a disease. Ultimately, a malpractice lawsuit could be filed.

Vital signs must be taken and recorded every time a patient is seen for an examination and on a daily basis for hospitalized patients. Because vital signs are measured so frequently, team members often minimize the importance of these results. Changes in vital signs may be the first indicator of disease or illness, so meticulous attention must be paid and comparisons should be made between current and past values.

Self-Evaluation Questions

1. Why are informed consent forms so critical in veterinary medicine?
2. What is a carnivore?
3. What are the characteristics of an effective allergy diet?
4. Why is the admitting procedure for patients that are boarding so important?
5. What information is required on a medication label?
6. Interpret the following prescription: Diphenhydramine; 1 cap PO EOD × 21d.
7. Give an example of a nonsteroidal antiinflammatory drug.
8. Why should all communication with the client be documented in the record?
9. Why should a receptionist double-check medication that is dispensed to clients?
10. What is a vasodilator?

Recommended Reading

AAFCO guidelines. Available at http://www.fda.gov/Animal Veterinary/Products/AnimalFoodFeeds/PetFood/default.htm, 2010.

Han CM, Hurd CD: *Practical diagnostic imaging for the veterinary technician*, ed 3, West Lafayette, IN, 2004, Mosby Elsevier.

Hand M, Thatcher C, Remillard R, et al: *Small animal clinical nutrition*, ed 4, Orinda, CA, 2000, Mark Morris.

Kirk R: *Current veterinary therapy XIII*, Philadelphia, 2000, WB Saunders.

McCurnin D, Bassert JA: *Clinical textbook for veterinary technicians*, ed 7, St Louis, 2010, Saunders Elsevier.

Sirosis M: *Principles and practices of veterinary technology*, ed 2, St Louis, 2004, Mosby Elsevier.

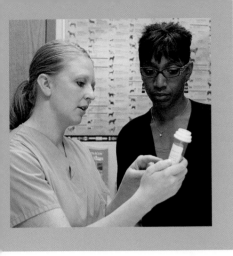

Calculations and Conversions

Chapter Outline

Monthly Finance Charges
Accounts Receivable Percentages
Inventory Turns per Year
Developing an Effective Product Markup
   Dispensing Fees
Developing an Effective Service Markup
Cost/Benefit Ratio

Break-Even Analysis
Payroll Calculations
Drug Calculations
   Percentage Solutions
   Teaspoons and Tablespoons
Intravenous Fluid Calculations

Learning Objectives

Mastery of the content in this chapter will enable the reader to:
- Calculate monthly finance charges.
- Calculate accounts receivable percentages.
- Calculate inventory turns per year.
- Develop an effective product markup.
- Develop an effective service markup.

- Calculate cost/benefit ratio.
- Calculate a break-even analysis.
- Calculate payroll.
- Calculate drug doses.
- Calculate intravenous fluid doses.

Every team member should be familiar with the common calculations that are used in veterinary practice. Receptionists and office managers are generally responsible for determining finance and statement charges for client account receivables. They may also be responsible for product markup when products are special ordered for a client. Office managers may be responsible for payroll and for determining the cost/benefit ratio of special promotions or the purchase of equipment. Each team member must be familiar with drug calculations and equations because every team member must double-check medications before they leave the premises; this can prevent a fatal mistake.

Most of the following equations have been covered in previous chapters. The purpose of this chapter is to allow the reader to become comfortable with equations used in everyday practice. The reader should practice the examples given because practice results in improved skills. Math can be a difficult task, but with a little practice anyone can become proficient at conversions and calculations (Box 24-1).

Many of the conversions should be memorized by team members; this will allow tasks to be completed more easily. A copy of the conversion table can be hung in a central location in the veterinary practice so that all team members can benefit. Conversion tables also provide a way to double-check work.

MONTHLY FINANCE CHARGES

Monthly statement fees must cover the cost of the statement being produced. This includes team member time, paper, ink, stamps, and envelopes. It may also be encouraged to add a finance fee; credit cards charge finance fees, why shouldn't a veterinary practice? State regulations must be verified as to what percentage of a bill is allowed as a finance charge.

Items to consider when determining the cost of a statement fee:
- Number of statements to run
- Cost of invoice (paper, ink, envelopes, and stamps)
- Labor (pay rate of team member preparing statements, including taxes)
- Finance rate (if applicable)

Example A: What minimum dollar amount should be added in order to recover costs associate with monthly statements?

Box 24-1 Common Conversions

1 kg = 1000 g = 10,000 mg
1 kg = 2.2 lb
 • kg to lb: multiply by 2.2
 • lb to kg: divide by 2.2
1 g = 1000 mg = 0.001 kg
1 grain = 64.8 mg
1 lb = 0.454 kg = 16 oz
1 lb = 454 g
1 mg = 0.001 g = 1000 mcg
1 L = 1000 mL = 10 dL
 • L to mL: multiply by 1000
 • mL to L: divide by 1000
1 mL = 1 cc = 1000 mcL
1 mL = 15 gtt
1 T = 3 t
1 t = 5 mL
1 T = 15 mL
1 oz = 30 mL
1 gal = 3.786 L
1 gal = 4 qt = 8 pt = 128 fl oz
1 pt = 2 c = 16 oz = 473 mL
1 km = 1000 m
1 m = 100 cm = 1000 mm

kg, Kilogram; *g*, gram; *mg*, milligram; *mcg*, microgram; *lb*, pound; *L*, liter; *dL*, deciliter; *mL*, milliliter; *mcL*, microliter; *cc*, cubic centimeter; *gtt*, drop; *T*, tablespoon; *t*, teaspoon; *gal*, gallon; *qt*, quart; *pt*, pint; *oz*, ounce; *fl oz*, fluid ounce; *c*, cup; *m*, meter; *cm*, centimeter; *mm*, millimeter.

• 100 statements to run
• Cost per invoice is determined to be $0.99
• Labor: The team member's hourly salary is $12, and it takes 6 hours to complete the task. Taxes are approximately 20% of the pay rate.

$$\text{Labor: } \$12 \times 6 \text{ hours} = \$72 \times 20\% = \$14.40$$

$$\text{Total labor: } \$86.40 \, (\$72.00 + \$14.40)$$

$$\text{Labor per invoice: } 0.86 \, (\$86.40 / 100)$$

$$\text{Labor + Set costs: } \$1.85/\text{invoice}$$

A statement fee of at least $1.85 must be applied to each invoice to recover costs. If the practice chooses to use a finance fee instead, the following would apply:
• An invoice has a balance of $98.45. The interest rate is 6.25%.

$$\$98.45 \times 6.25\% = \$6.15$$

$$\$98.45 + \$6.15 = \text{New balance of } \$104.60$$

If a practice wishes to use both a monthly statement fee and finance charge:

$$\$98.45 + \$6.15 + \$1.85 = \$106.45$$

Example B: *What is the client's new balance after monthly statement fees have been printed?*

• 55 statements to run
• Cost per invoice is determined to be $0.99
• Labor: The team member's hourly salary is $9, and it takes 3 hours to complete the task. Taxes are approximately 20% of the pay rate.

$$\text{Labor: } \$9 \times 3 \text{ hours} = \$27 \times 20\% = \$5.40$$

$$\text{Total labor: } \$32.40 \, (\$27.00 + \$5.40)$$

$$\text{Labor per invoice: } 0.32 \, (\$32.40/100)$$

$$\text{Labor + Set costs: } \$1.31$$

The practice chooses to have a set monthly fee of $5 per invoice and no monthly finance charge.
• An invoice has a balance of $354.08.

$$\$354.08 + \$5 = \text{New balance} = \$359.08$$

Practice Set: Monthly Statement Fees

Determine the minimum monthly statement fee and the new balance based on the following scenarios. Answers appear on the Evolve site accompanying this text.
1. 250 statements
 • Set costs per invoice of $1.05
 • Labor: 2.5 hours; hourly pay rate = $8.50/hr; 20% for taxes
 • Set monthly statement fee of $6.50
 • Finance charge of 10%
 • Balance: $563.09
2. 39 statements
 • Set costs per invoice of $0.85
 • Labor: 2.0 hours; hourly pay rate = $12.50/hr; 20% for taxes
 • No monthly statement fee
 • Finance charge of 14.25%
 • Balance: $54.09
3. 50 statements
 • Set costs per invoice of $1.85
 • Labor: 4 hours; hourly pay rate = $19.50/hr; 20% for taxes
 • Set monthly statement fee of $8.50
 • Finance charge 0%
 • Balance: $201.98

ACCOUNTS RECEIVABLE PERCENTAGES

What percentage of the gross revenue is tied up in accounts receivable?

Less than 0.5% of gross revenue should be tied up in accounts receivable. A practice that produces $895,000 per year should have a total of only $4475 in accounts receivable each month! If the amount were 3%, it would total $26,850 per month. It should be the goal of every clinic to have the lowest accounts receivable possible!

$$\$895,000 \times 0.5\% = \$4475$$

$$\$895,000 \times 3\% = \$26,850$$

Example A:
Gross revenue (GR) for a veterinary practice is $595,000; accounts receivable (AR) total is $14,950. What is the percentage tied up in AR?

$$\$14,950/\$595,000 = 0.025 \times 100 = 2.5\%$$

The AR total is divided by the total GR to obtain a numerical amount (don't forget, to obtain a percentage the numerical answer must be multiplied by 100).

Example B:
GR for a practice is $1,902,798.98. AR is 3%. What is the total dollar amount tied up in AR?

$$\$1,902,798.98 \times 3\% = \$57,083.97 \text{ total AR}$$

Example C:
The predicted GR for a practice is $800,000 and the practice's goal is to keep accounts receivable less than 1%. What amount can the AR total to meet this goal?

$$\$800,000 \times 1\% = \$8000$$

Practice Sets: Accounts Receivable Percentages

Answers appear on the Evolve site accompanying this text.
1. GR is $495,958.02; AR totals 14%. What amount is tied up in AR?
2. GR is $2,891,098.04; AR totals $109,004.09. What percentage is tied up in AR?
3. GR is $355,758.72; AR totals 5%. What amount is tied up in AR?
4. GR is $1,564,642.98; AR totals $19,104.09. What percentage is tied up in AR?

INVENTORY TURNS PER YEAR

Turns per year is defined as the number of times an inventoried product turns over in a practice. This helps determine correct reorder quantities and points. Each practice should set a goal of eight to 12 turns per year. To determine the inventory turns per year, the beginning inventory is added to the ending inventory and the result is divided by two. This results in the average inventory per year. The total amount of product purchased during that period divided by the average yields the number of turns per year for that product. Taking the equation one step further, dividing the number of days in the year (365) by the number of turns per year produces the average shelf life of the item.

Example A:
• 35 bottles of Keflex 500 mg were purchased between January 1, 2007, and December 31, 2007.

• Beginning inventory = 4
• Ending inventory = 1

$$4 + 1 = 5$$
$$5/2 = 2.5$$
$$35/2.5 = 14$$

Keflex turned over 14 times during 2007.

Example B:
• 36 bottles of eye drops were purchased in 2007.
• Beginning inventory = 2
• Ending inventory = 2

$$2 + 2 = 4$$
$$4/2 = 2$$
$$36/2 = 18$$

The product turned 18 times. This is an excellent value!

Example C:
• Convenia was purchased eight times during 2007.
• Beginning inventory = 1
• Ending inventory = 1

$$1 + 1 = 2$$
$$2/2 = 1$$
$$8/1 = 8$$

The product turned eight times during 2007.

DEVELOPING AN EFFECTIVE PRODUCT MARKUP

The markup of a product is defined as the cost (of the product) multiplied by a percentage calculated to recover hidden costs associated with inventory management. Many practices will mark products up 100% to 200%. A product markup must be at least 40% to break even. Shopped items, such as vaccines and routine surgeries, should be kept competitive with the local or regional veterinary practices. Nonshopped items must be increased to accommodate the lower priced shopped items. Special services and supplies must be marked up appropriately to cover the extra charges that generally accommodate the special service.

Example A:
A tablet of acepromazine costs the practice $0.10 per tablet.
• A markup of 100% = $0.10 × 100% = $0.10
  Therefore $0.10 (initial cost) + $0.10 (100% markup) = $0.20.
• A markup of 200% = $0.10 × 200% = $0.20
  Therefore $0.10 + $0.20 (200% markup) = $0.30.

Example B:
A bottle of Rimadyl costs the practice $86.
• A markup of 100% = $86 × 100% = $86

Therefore, $86 (initial cost) + $86 (100% markup) = $172.

- A markup of 200% = $86 × 200% = $172
  Therefore $86 + $172 (200% markup) = $258.

Dispensing Fees

Practices may also add a product dispensing fee as well as a minimum prescription charge. The average dispensing fee ranges from $8 to $14 to cover the cost of the label, the pill vial, and the time used to count the medication. If a bottle of shampoo or a full bottle of medication is dispensed, the average dispensing fee ranges from $3 to $5. Many practices initiate a minimum prescription fee of $14 to $18 to help recover hidden pharmacy costs.

Hidden pharmacy costs include costs associated with expired medications, ordering and shipping costs, and insurance and taxes on products and supplies. These costs can increase rapidly and must be covered.

Example A:

- Product cost: $1.06 per tablet
- 100% markup
- 20 tablets dispensed
- Dispensing fee of $11.95
- Minimum prescription fee of $12.95
- What is the client's total cost?

$$\$1.06 \times 100\% = \$1.06$$

$$\$1.06 + \$1.06 = \$2.12 \times 20 \text{ tablets} = \$21.20$$

$$\$21.20 + \$11.95 = \$33.15 \text{ total cost}$$

(The prescription met the minimum prescription charge; therefore the additional charge was not needed.)

Example B:

- A bottle of shampoo costs $11.95 per bottle
- 100% markup
- One bottle dispensed
- Dispensing fee of $5.95
- Minimum prescription fee of $16.95
- What is the client's total cost?

$$\$11.95 \times 100\% = \$11.95$$

$$\$11.95 + \$11.95 = \$23.90$$

$$\$23.90 + \$5.95 = \$29.85 \text{ total cost}$$

(The prescription met the minimum prescription charge; therefore the additional charge was not needed.)

Example C:

- Product cost: $0.06 per tablet
- 200% markup
- 60 tablets dispensed
- Dispensing fee of $11.95
- Minimum prescription fee of $14.95
- What is the client's total cost?

$$\$0.06 \times 200\% = \$0.12$$

$$\$0.06 + \$0.12 = \$0.18 \times 10 \text{ tablets} = \$1.80$$

$1.80 + $11.95 = $13.75 *would be* the client's total cost; however, the charge has not met the minimum prescription fee. Therefore the client cost is $14.95.

Practice Set: Developing Effective Product Markup

Answers appear on the Evolve site accompanying this text.
1. Dermazole shampoo: $10.50 per bottle
   - 200% markup
   - Doctor dispenses two bottles
   - Dispensing fee of $5.95
   - Minimum prescription fee of $14.95
   - What is the client's total cost?
2. Product cost: $3.06 per tablet
   - 100% markup
   - One tablet dispensed
   - Dispensing fee of $11.95
   - Minimum prescription fee of $14.95
   - What is the client's total cost?
3. Product cost: $0.72 per tablet
   - 200% markup
   - 15 tablets dispensed
   - Dispensing fee of $11.95
   - Minimum prescription fee of $14.95
   - What is the client's total cost?
4. Pet vitamins: $3.50 per bottle
   - 100% markup
   - One bottle dispensed
   - Dispensing fee of $5.95
   - Minimum prescription fee of $14.95
   - What is the client's total cost?

DEVELOPING AN EFFECTIVE SERVICE MARKUP

- **Overhead costs per minute + Direct costs + Return on time to the doctor**

Overhead costs can be determined from the previous year's financial statements and include every cost except veterinarian compensation and drug and supply costs. Most overhead costs range from $1.50 to $2 per minute.

- **Overhead costs** = Total cost of utilities + Mortgage + Staff salary + Building maintenance, etc., divided by the number of business days per year. These costs can then be broken down by minute.

Direct costs include all materials used for any given procedure. Once all direct costs have been calculated, double it to include the costs of ordering, shipping, and unpacking the products. If a practice only charges the true direct costs, income will be lost.

- Total cost of products to provide service × 2

Return on doctor time is calculated according to the average base salary of the veterinarians of the practice. Per-minute charge is then determined from the average salary.
- Average salary of veterinarians in practice: $90,000
- Average number of hours worked per year: 2080
- $90,000/2080 = $43.26 per hour
- $43.26/hour = $0.72 per minute

Example A:
Costs associated with the application of a splint on a broken leg:
- Time to complete a procedure: 15 minutes
- Overhead costs: $2 × 15 minutes = $30
- Direct cost of product: $12.50 × 2 = $25
- Veterinarian time: $0.72 × 15 = $10.80

The client's cost to apply the splint and products used: $30 + $25 + $10.80 = $65.80. (Additional costs should be added for exam, radiographs, etc.)

Example B:
Costs associated with a physical examination:
- Time to complete a procedure: 15 minutes
- Overhead costs: $2 × 15 minutes = $30
- Direct cost of product: $0
- Veterinarian time: $0.72 × 15 = $10.80

The client's cost for a physical examination: $30 + $10.80 = $40.80.

Example C:
Costs associated with ear canal flushing:
- Time to complete a procedure: 15 minutes
- Overhead costs: $2 × 15 minutes = $30
- Direct cost of product: $32.50 × 2 = $64
- Veterinarian time: $0.72 × 15 = $10.80

The client's cost for an ear canal flushing: $30 + $64 + $10.80 = $104.80.

Practice Set: Calculate an Effective Service Markup

Use the following information for the scenarios below. Answers appear on the Evolve site accompanying this text.
- Average salary of veterinarians in practice: $135,000
- Average number of hours worked per year: 2000
- Overhead costs: $2.10 per minute

1. Exam for ear infection = 20 minutes
   - Direct cost of supplies = $3.25

2. Laceration repair = 35 minutes
   - Direct cost of supplies = $25.97

3. Examination/fine-needle aspiration of a growth = 45 minutes
   - Direct cost of supplies: $1.98

4. Behavioral consultation = 65 minutes
   - Direct cost of supplies: $0

COST/BENEFIT RATIO

Before promotions can be developed, a cost/benefit analysis should be completed. This will allow the team to determine whether the promotion will be profitable.

Example A:
- Target: Increase the number of dentals by 100 for a 1-month period
- Client cost of a basic dental procedure: $157
- Cost associated with promotion of target: labor estimated at 3 hours at $15/hour, with 20% overhead for taxes

3 × $15 × 20% = $54	**$54**
Postage: $0.42 × 100 =	**$42**
Paper: $0.40/paper (four cards per paper)	
$0.40/4 = $0.10/card: $0.10 × 100 =	**$10**
Ink: $19.99/cartridge; one cartridge produces 200 postcards	
$19.99/200 = $0.10/card: $0.10 × 100 =	**$10**
Labels: $19.99/500 labels = $0.04/card: 0.04 ×	
100 =	**$4**
Total cost to target clients:	**$120**

- Cost associated with producing a basic dental: labor estimated at 1 hour; $12/hr with 20% overhead for taxes

$12 × 20% = $14.40	**$14.40**
Drugs:	**$5.50**
Equipment use:	**$54**
Overhead (10%):	**$15.70**
Total cost associated with a dental:	**$89.60**
Profit associated with one dental =	
$157 − $89.60	**$67.40**

Adding 100 dentals for the month will increase gross revenue by $15,700 ($157 × 100). Profit will increase by $6620: $6740 (profit of a dental: $67.40 × 100) − $120 (cost of target promo).

It will benefit the practice to promote this goal.

Example B:
- Target: Increase heartworm preventive sales by 100 boxes.
- Cost associated with promotion of target: labor estimated at 3 hours at $15/hour, with 20% overhead for taxes

3 × $15 × 20% = $54	**$54**
Postage: $0.42 × 100 =	**$42**
Paper: $0.40/paper (four cards per paper)	
$0.40/4 = $0.10/card: $0.10 × 100 =	**$10**
Ink: $19.99/cartridge; one cartridge produces 200 postcards	
$19.99/200 = $0.10/card: $0.10 × 100 =	**$10**
Labels: $19.99/500 labels = $0.04/card:	
$0.04 × 100 =	**$4**
Total cost to target clients:	**$120**
Cost of heartworm preventive (average):	**$24/box**
Cost to client:	**$48/box**
Average profit:	**$24/box**

Increasing sales of heartworm preventive by 100 for the month will increase gross revenue by $4800. Profit will increase by $2280 ($2400 − $120).

It will benefit the practice to promote this goal.

BREAK-EVEN ANALYSIS

A break-even analysis should be completed before purchasing equipment. The break-even point is the point at which the sales of a service will cover all costs related to the equipment, including maintenance, supplies, and the capital itself. A break-even point can be determined by dividing the total cost of the equipment by the cost to the client. The resulting number gives the number of times the service must be performed to break even.

Example A:
A practice wishes to purchase a digital dental radiograph unit. The unit costs $11,000.
- What should the practice charge the client for a set of radiographs?
- How many radiographs must be taken to break even?
- Will the equipment be profitable for the practice?

The practice has determined that the average charge for a set of dental radiographs is $88; therefore it will charge the client $88.

The cost associated with taking the radiographs has been determined to be $22; this includes the technician's time to take the views and the veterinarian's time to interpret the views.
- Overhead costs are $1 per minute; 15-minute procedure

$$15 \, \text{minutes} \times \$1 = \$15$$

- One technician at $15 per hour; 15 minute procedure

$$\$15 \times 1 = \$15/60 \, \text{minutes}$$
$$= \$0.25 \, \text{per minute} \times 15 \, \text{minutes} = \$3.75$$
$$\$3.75 \times 20\% \, (\text{taxes}) = \$0.75$$
$$\$3.75 + \$0.75 = \$4.50$$

- One veterinarian to interpret view: 3 minutes
  - Average salary of veterinarians in practice: $90,000
  - Average number of hours worked per year: 2080
  - $90,000/2080 = $43.26 per hour
  - $43.26/hour = $0.72 per minute

$$\$0.72 \times 3 \, \text{minutes}: \$2.16$$

$$\$15 + \$4.50 + \$2.16 = \$21.66; \text{round up to} \$22$$

$$\text{Client cost} - \text{Practice cost} = \text{Profit}$$

$$\$88 - \$22 = \$66$$

$11,000/$66 = 166.67 views; therefore 167 views must be taken to break even.

If two dentals are completed on a daily basis and both dentals have radiographs completed, it will take 83 business days to recover the cost of the equipment.

$$167/2 = 83$$

After 83 business days, $66 profit will be made on each radiograph charge.

Example B:
The practice wishes to purchase a Tono-Pen.
- Unit cost: $3000
- Average national client charge: $29.99 (per company representative)
- What is the estimated number of pets that will receive eye pressure checks?
- How long until the equipment will be paid for?
- Will the equipment be profitable?
- Overhead costs $1 per minute; 15-minute procedure

$$15 \, \text{minutes} \times \$1 = \$15$$

- One technician at $15 per hour; 15-minute procedure

$$\$15 \times 1 = \$15/60 \, \text{minutes}$$
$$= \$0.25 \, \text{per minute} \times 15 \, \text{minutes} = \$3.75$$
$$\$3.75 \times 20\% \, (\text{taxes}) = \$0.75$$
$$\$3.75 + \$0.75 = \$4.50$$

- One veterinarian to examine and perform procedure: 15 minutes

$$0.72 \times 16 \, \text{minutes} = \$11.52$$

$$\$15 + \$4.50 + \$11.52 = \$31.02; \text{round down to} \$31$$

This example reveals that charging $29.99 for a pressure check does not cover the costs associated with the pressure check ($31). Team members must decide to increase the cost to the client or add an additional charge for the examination.

Practice Set: Break-Even Analysis

Answers appear on the Evolve site accompanying this text.
1. The practice will purchase a LaserSite to evaluate CBCs in-house.
- Procedure time: 5 minutes
- Cost: $22,000
- Average CBC charge: $33
- Average number of CBCs completed per day: 8
- Overhead costs: $2.10/minute
- Costs associated with running a CBC (tech time, supplies): $12
- How long until the equipment will be paid for?
- Will the equipment be profitable?

2. The practice will purchase a chemistry machine for in-house diagnostics.
- Procedure time: 5 minutes

- Cost: $5000
- Average chemistry charge: $66
- Average number of chemistries per day: 8
- Overhead costs: $2.10/min
- Costs associated with running a chemistry (tech time, supplies): $17
- How long until the equipment will be paid for?
- Will the equipment be profitable?

PAYROLL CALCULATIONS

Example A:
Salary formula: Team member is paid by salary only.
- A veterinarian receives $60,000 in salary per year
- Payday occurs on the first and the fifteenth of each month

$$\$60,000/24 = \$2,500 \text{ gross pay per pay period}$$

The definition of gross pay is the total amount earned before taxes or other withholdings.

Example B:
Pro-sal formula: A combination of salary and production-based pay.
- A veterinarian is paid $60,000 base salary per year
- 10% production bonus once production has reached $10,000 per month
- Bonuses are paid monthly for the previous month's production
- Payday occurs on the first and the fifteenth of each month (24 pay periods per year)

$$\text{Salary pay: } \$60,000/24 = \$2500 \text{ per check}$$

- The veterinarian produced $33,000 for the previous month

$$\$33,000 \times 10\% = \$3300$$

The gross pay for the first is $2500 + $3300 = $5800. The gross pay for the fifteenth is $2500.

Example C:
Production-based pay: An associate is paid by production only.
- A veterinarian is paid 20% production of all services and products.
- Payday occurs on the first and the fifteenth of each month.

The payroll manager should pull a report of production of that specific associate from the first to the fourteenth of the month.
- $15,000 was produced from March 1, 2009, to March 14, 2009

$$\$15,000 \times 20\% = \$3000 \text{ gross pay}$$

The second pay period report runs from the fifteenth to the thirtieth or thirty-first of the month.

- $16,236 was produced from March 15, 2009, to March 31, 2009

$$\$16236 \times 20\% = \$3247.20 \text{ gross pay}$$

Example D:
Hourly-based pay: Employees are paid by the hour at a regular rate for the first 40 hours; anything over 40 hours is paid overtime.
  Regular rate calculations:
- Wanda is paid $10 per hour and works 34 hours per week.
- Payroll is paid every other Monday; therefore the work week is Monday, 12 AM through Sunday, 12:59 PM.

$$34 \text{ hours per week} \times 2 = 68 \text{ hours per 2-week period}$$

$$68 \text{ hours} \times \$10 = \$680 \text{ gross pay}$$

Example E:
Overtime rate calculations:
- Ann has worked 44 hours during week 1
- She has worked 32 hours during week 2
- She is paid $10 per hour
- Overtime is paid at $15 (1½ times the regular rate)

$$\text{Week 1: } 40 \text{ hours} \times \$10 = \$400; 4 \text{ hours} \times \$15 = \$60$$

$$\text{Week 2: } 32 \text{ hours} \times \$10 = \$320$$

$$\$400 + \$6 + \$320 = \$780 \text{ gross pay}$$

Example F:
- Alex accrues 44 hours in week 1.
- He accrues 52 hours during week 2.

$$\text{Week 1: } 40 \text{ hours} \times \$10 = \$400, 4 \text{ hours} \times \$15 = \$60$$

$$\text{Week 2: } 40 \text{ hours} \times \$10 = \$400, 12 \text{ hours} \times \$15 = \$180$$

$$\$400 + \$60 + \$400 + \$180 = \$1,040 \text{ gross pay}$$

Practice Set: Determining Gross Pay per 2-Week Pay Period

Answers appear on the Evolve site accompanying this text.
1. Team member 1: $10 per hour; 12 hours week 1; 52 hours week 2
2. Veterinarian paid by production only, 35%: gross revenue first through fourteenth: $12,300.23; gross revenue fifteenth through thirtieth: $16,345.09
3. Team member 2: $15 per hour; 40 hours week 1; 40 hours week 2
4. Associate veterinarian paid salary only; $95,000 per year
5. Team member 3: $11.37 per hour; 52 hours week 1; 41 hours week 2
6. Veterinarian paid pro-sal: $50,000 base salary; 13% production bonus once production has reached $10,000 per month; bonus paid first of the month for the previous month's production. Production total: $26,524.67

Box 24-2 Drug Conversions

```
1 kg = 1000 g = 10,000 mg
1 kg = 2.2 lb
   • kg to lb: multiply by 2.2
   • lb to kg: divide by 2.2
1 g = 1000 mg = 0.001 kg
1 gr = 64.8 mg
1 lb = 0.454 kg = 16 oz
1 lb = 454 g
1 mg = 0.001 g = 1000 mcg
1 L = 1000 mL = 10 dL
   • L to mL: multiply by 1000
   • mL to L: divide by 1000
1 mL = 1 cc = 1000 mcL
1 mL = 15 gtt
1 T = 3 t
1 t = 5 mL
1 T = 15 mL
1 oz = 30 mL
1 gal = 3.786 L
1 gal = 4 qt = 8 pt = 128 fl oz
1 pt = 2 c = 16 oz = 473 mL
1 km = 1000 m
1 m = 100 cm = 1000 mm
```

kg, Kilogram; *g,* gram; *mg,* milligram; *gr,* grain; *lb,* pound; *L,* liter; *dL,* deciliter; *mL,* milliliter; *mcL,* microliter; *cc,* cubic centimeter; *gtt,* drop; *T,* tablespoon; *t,* teaspoon; *gal,* gallon; *qt,* quart; *pt,* pint; *oz,* ounce; *fl oz,* fluid ounce; *c,* cup; *m,* meter; *cm,* centimeter; *mm,* millimeter.

DRUG CALCULATIONS

Every team member should be able to easily calculate drug doses because double-checking dispensed drugs can prevent a potential fatal error (Boxes 24-2 and 24-3).

Explanation 1

Step 1

Convert the body weight in pounds (lb) to kilograms (kg). In the United States, the most common weight measurement is pounds. Medication doses are recommended in milligrams per kilogram (mg/kg). There is 1 kg per 2.2 lb; therefore the number of pounds the patient weighs divided by 2.2 will yield the kilograms of body weight.

Step 2

Calculate the drug dose. The recommended dose is generally given in milligrams per kilogram. Therefore if 22 mg of a drug is recommended for each kilogram of body weight, 22 mg multiplied by the body weight will give the total number of milligrams needed for the patient.

Step 3

Calculate the volume of drug needed per dose. The concentration of the product is generally given as 22 mg per tablet, or 25 mg per milliliter, and so forth. If the patient needs 22 mg, then one 22-mg tablet will be needed to

Box 24-3 Examples of Drug Calculations

What volume of a drug solution should be given to a 25-lb dog if the advised dose is 5 mg/kg and the concentration of the solution is 50 mg/mL?

Step 1. Convert pounds to kilograms:

$$25 \text{ lb}/2.2 = 11.36 \text{ kg}$$

Step 2. Calculate the drug dose:

$$X \text{ mg} = \frac{5 \text{ mg}}{\text{kg}} \times 11.36 \text{ kg} = 5 \times 11.36 = 56.8 \text{ mg}$$

Step 3. Calculate the volume of solution needed:

$$\frac{50 \text{ mg}}{\text{mL}} = \frac{56.8 \text{ mg}}{X \text{ mL}} = \frac{56.3 \text{ mg}}{50 \text{ mg/mL}} = 1.1 \text{ mL}$$

What volume of a drug solution should be given to a 7.9-lb cat if the advised dosage is 10 mg/kg and the concentration of the solution is 5 mg/mL?

Step 1. 7.9 lb/2.2 = 3.59 kg

Step 2. $X \text{ mg} = \dfrac{10 \text{ mg}}{\text{kg}} \times 3.59 \text{ kg} = 10 \times 3.59 \text{ kg} = 35.9 \text{ mg}$

Step 3. $\dfrac{5 \text{ mg}}{\text{mL}} = \dfrac{35.9 \text{ mg}}{X \text{ mL}} = \dfrac{35.9 \text{ mg}}{5 \text{ mg/mL}} = 7 \text{ mL}$

How many 25-mg tablets should be dispensed for a 10-lb cat if the recommended dose is 5 mg/lb twice daily for 7 days?

Step 1. 10 lb × 5 mg = 50 mg/dose
Step 2. 50 mg/25 mg = 2 tablets/dose
Step 3. 2 tablets twice daily = 4 tablets/day
Step 4. 4 tablets/day × 7 days = 28 tablets

How many 500-mg capsules should be dispensed for a dog that weighs 55 lb and needs 20 mg/kg every 8 hours for 14 days?

Step 1. 55 lb/2.2 = 25 kg
Step 2. 25 kg × 20 mg/kg = 500 mg
Step 3. 1 capsule every 8 hours = 3 capsules/day
Step 4. 3 capsules/day × 14 days = 42 capsules total

treat the patient per dose. If the patient needs 11 mg, then the concentration supplied divided by the amount needed will yield the volume to give the patient. In this example, if the patient needs 11 mg and a 22-mg tablet is supplied, then half a tablet will be administered.

Step 4

Determine the total amount of product needed to dispense for the client. If the patient needs half a tablet twice daily for 7 days, then multiply ½ by 2; this yields 1 tablet per day. One tablet per day × 7 days yield

7 tablets. Seven tablets must be dispensed to this client for treatment of the patient.

Explanation #2

$$\frac{Dose\,(D) \times Weight\,(W)}{Available\ concentration\,(C)}$$

D is the dose of the drug as recommended by the manufacturer, usually written in milligrams per pound or kilogram. The dose for a particular drug may vary by species or treatment. For instance, Torbugesic has one dose if used for pain and another if used for coughing.

W is the weight of the animal being treated; this value can be in pounds or kilograms.

D × *W* is the desired dose (how much drug should be given to the patient per dose).

C is the concentration of the available drug to be administered, usually written on the label in milligrams per milliliter for liquids or milligrams for tablets and capsules. Drugs may come in multiple concentrations. For instance, amoxicillin is supplied as 50-mg tablets, 100-mg tablets, and 50-mg/mL oral suspension.

(D × W)/C therefore represents how much of the available medication to give.

Example A:
A pet needs 320 mg (desired dose) of a drug with a concentration of 50 mg/mL (available). How many milliliters should be administered?

$$320\ mg/50\ mg/mL = 6.4\ mL$$

Example B:
A pet needs 114 mg (desired dose) of a drug with a concentration of 100 mg/tablet (available). How many tablets should be given?

$$114\ mg/100\ mg\ tablet = 1.14\ tablets$$

Because 0.14 of a tablet cannot be given, a team member would give one 100-mg tablet.

Percentage Solutions

Some injectable solution concentrations are written as a percentage instead of milligrams per milliliter. Atropine, for example, is a 2% solution. Therefore the solution in question contains 2 g of atropine for every 100 mL of solution. Because drugs are not typically administered in grams per 100 mL, this amount must be converted to something more familiar. First, it should be determined how many grams are in 1 mL. To accomplish this, divide 2 g by 100 mL to get 0.02 g/mL. In general, doses are given in milligrams per milliliter rather than grams per milliliter; therefore the next step is to convert 0.02 g to milligrams by multiplying by 1000 mg/g to get 20 mg. Therefore 2% = 20 mg/mL.

Shortcut: Unless you like doing all these calculations, you can simply multiply the percentage by 10 and change the units to milligrams per milliliter.

Example C:
- 3% solution = 3 × 10 = 30 mg/mL
- 0.2% solution = 0.2 × 10 = 2 mg/mL
- 1.5% solution = 1.5 × 10 = 15 mg/mL

Now, put it all together:
- How many milliliters would be required for 274 mg of a 0.75% solution?

  0.75% = 7.5 mg/mL; 274 mg (desired dose) divided by 7.5 mg/mL (available concentration) = 36.5 mL
- How many milliliters would be required for 485 mg of a 4% solution?

  4% = 40 mg/mL; 485 mg (desired dose) divided by 40 mg/mL (available concentration) = 12.1 mL

To determine how many milligrams are in the amount of milliliters of a solution that was administered:

$$\%\ Solution\,(in\ mg/mL) \times mL = mg$$

Example D:
- How many milligrams were administered if 3.5 mL of a 1% solution were given?

  $$1\% = 10\ mg/mL \times 3.5\ mL = 35\ mg$$
- How many milligrams were administered if 4.3 mL of a 10% solution were given?

  $$10\% = 100\ mg/mL \times 4.3\ mL = 430\ mg$$

Practice Set: Drug Calculations

Answers appear on the Evolve site accompanying this text.

1. A pet needs 50 mg of a tablet, and the medication is available as a 100-mg tablet. How many tablets will be needed?
2. A pet needs 35 mg of a solution, and the medication is available as a 100-mg/mL solution. How many milliliters will be needed?
3. A pet needs medication at a dose of 5 mg/kg, and the medication is available in 25-mg tablets. The pet weighs 10 lb. How many tablets will be administered?
4. A pet needs a medication at a dose of 100 mg/kg, and the medication is available in a 100-mg/mL solution. The pet weighs 25 lb. How many milliliters will be administered?
5. A pet needs 25 mg of a 2% solution. How many milliliters will be administered?
6. A pet needs butorphanol for pain at a dose of 0.04 mg/kg and the medication is available in a 10-mg/mL solution. The pet weighs 4 lb. How many milliliters will be administered?
7. A veterinarian writes a script for 25 mg of acepromazine to be given every 8 hours for 5 days, and the medication is available in 25-mg tablets. How many tablets will be dispensed?

Box 24-4 Examples of IV Fluid Calculations

DRIP SETS
- 15 gtt/mL for patients >20 lb
- 60 gtt/mL for patients <20 lb

FLUID RATES
- Surgical rate: 11 mL/kg/hr
- Maintenance rate: 66 mL/kg/24 hr
- Twice (doubled) maintenance rate: 132 mL/kg/24 hr

STEPS
1. Convert pounds to kilograms (2.2 lb per kilogram)
2. Calculate milliliters per hour
3. Calculate drops per minute

EXAMPLE 1
- 45-lb dog, 15 gtt/mL drip set
- Maintenance rate = 66 mL/kg/24 hr
1. 45 lb/2.2 = 20.45 kg
2. 20.45 kg × 66 mL/kg/24 hr = 20.45 kg × 66 mL/kg = 1350 mL/24 hr
3. 1350 mL/24 hr = 56.25 mL/hr

4. Place on IV pump; if no pump is present, continue:
5. 56.25 mL/hr = 56.25 mL/60 min = 0.9375 mL/min
6. 0.9375 mL/min = 0.9375 mL/60 sec = 0.156 mL/sec
7. 0.156 mL/sec × 15 gtt/mL (drip set) = 0.156 mL × 15 gtt = 0.234 mL/gtt
8. 0.234 mL/1 gtt = Reciprocate = 1/0.234 mL = 1 gtt/4 sec

EXAMPLE 2
- 25-lb dog, 15 gtt/mL drip set
- Surgical rate = 11 mL/kg/hr
1. 25 lb/2.2 = 11.36 kg
2. 11.36 kg × 11 mL/kg/hr = 11.36 kg × 11 mL = 125 mL/hr
3. Place on IV pump
4. 125 mL/hr = 125 mL/60 min = 2.08 mL/min
5. 2.08 mL/min = 2.08 mL/60 sec = 0.035 mL/sec
6. 0.035 mL/sec × 15 gtt/mL (drip set) = 0.035 mL × 15 gtt = 0.52 mL/gtt
7. 0.52 mL/gtt = Reciprocate = 1/0.52 = 1 gtt/2 sec

gtt, Drop.

8. Translate the following prescription so that a client would be able to understand it: Give 25 mg Benadryl PO TID × 2 weeks. Benadryl is available as 25-mg capsules. How many capsules would be dispensed?
9. A pet needs 5 mg/kg of Albon PO SID on day 1, then 2.5 mg/kg PO SID for 5 more days. The medication is available in 125-mg tablets and the pet weighs 25 lb. How many milligrams will the pet need? How many tablets will be dispensed for the owner?

Teaspoons and Tablespoons

Many over-the-counter products are labeled in teaspoons (t or tsp) and tablespoons (T or tbsp); the team must be able to give the client correct conversions.
- 1 t = 5 mL
- 1 T = 15 mL

Therefore if the label states that the concentration is 25 mg/t, then the product contains 25 mg/5 mL, or 5 mg/mL. If the label states that the product has 25 mg/T, then the product contains 25 mg/15 mL, or 1.67 mg/mL. Once the correct milligrams per kilogram has been verified with the veterinarian, the team can determine the number of milliliters to be administered.

INTRAVENOUS FLUID CALCULATIONS

Patients on intravenous (IV) fluids must be monitored throughout administration to ensure they are receiving the correct amount. Too much fluid could drown a patient; too little fluid might prevent the patient from improving.

Fluid administration sets are available in two sizes for small animals. Also called *drip sets,* these sets help control the amount of fluids delivered to the patient. A macrodrip is a 15 dr/mL (drops per milliliter) drip set; a microdrip is a 60 dr/mL drip set.

Fluids are administered at a rate determined by the veterinarian, which can depend on the patient's fluid loss (Box 24-4). Basic rates are as follows:
- Surgical rate: 11 mL/kg/hour
- Maintenance rate: 66 mL/kg/24 hours
- Two times maintenance rate: 132 mL/kg/24 hours

Practice Set: Intravenous Fluid Calculations

Answers appear on the Evolve site accompanying this text.
1. A 22-lb dog needs IV fluids at a maintenance rate. How many milliliters per hour will the patient receive?
2. A 7-lb cat will have a dental and needs IV fluids at the surgical rate. How many milliliters per hour will the patient receive?
3. A 120-lb dog is experiencing vomiting and diarrhea and must have IV fluids at two times maintenance. How many milliliters will he receive per hour?
4. A 32-lb dog needs IV fluids at a surgical rate. How many milliliters per hour will the patient receive?
5. A 50-lb dog needs IV fluids at two times maintenance. How many fluids will be administered in a 24-hour period?
6. A 4.5-lb cat requires maintenance fluids. How many milliliters per hour will the pet receive?

ACKNOWLEDGMENT

I would like to thank Laurie Rankin for her invaluable advice regarding the explanations for drug calculations and conversions in this chapter.

Professional Development

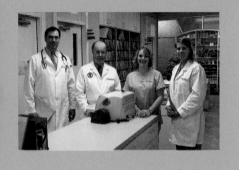

Learning Objectives

Mastery of the content in this chapter will enable the reader to:

- Identify the importance of professional development.
- Identify skills that one possesses.
- Discuss career fields that are available.
- Explain how to develop an effective cover letter.
- Explain how to develop an effective resume.
- Discuss how to email cover letters and resumes.

- List methods used to prepare for an interview.
- List questions to ask a potential employer.
- Discuss how to follow up after an interview.
- Differentiate offers of employment.
- Discuss retirement savings.

Key Terms

16 Personality Factors
Campbell Interest and Skill Survey
Career Planning

Cover Letter
Myers-Briggs Type Indicator
Personal Skills

Resume
Transferable Skills

Professional development is vital to every career. There are many aspects of career and professional development, and all are vital to an individual's success. The successful development of an individual can lead to the development of a successful team. Individuals must first assess themselves and determine their strengths and weaknesses; they can then work on the weaknesses while striving to improve the strengths. They must determine what successes they want in life, define what success is, and set professional and personal goals. Professional and motivated individuals will seek out experiences to improve themselves as well as opportunities to improve others.

On average, individuals will change jobs every 3.6 years and change careers three times before retiring. Training and development in areas other than veterinary medicine are essential. Training in leadership,

management, creativity, diversity, communications, and analytical skills will help even the most experienced individual. Many individuals change careers to veterinary medicine after being in another field for years, and the skills and knowledge they bring from other professions is essential for practice development. Each team member may possess a set of skills another does not; therefore everyone can benefit from one other.

Career planning is often intertwined with individual plans, goals, and successes. Career planning is the ongoing process of making career choices; these choices should be reviewed from time to time. Individuals may need to analyze themselves, their environment, and their occupation to determine if and when a change is needed.

When changes are needed, it is often overwhelming to start the process of looking for new employment. Self-confidence may falter, and suddenly the skills that once seemed so strong now seem useless. It is common to feel this way, but fortunately it is easy to turn that mindset around. The skills that one has acquired over the years are essential for survival. Skills such as interpersonal and verbal communication, critical thinking, writing, and leadership are all valuable resources for any employer. In addition to these essential skills, self-discipline, excellent morals, outstanding ethics, and creativity are skills that should be reflected on to help rebuild confidence.

> ◎ **PRACTICE POINT** Self-assessment tests help individuals determine their strengths and weaknesses, which will help guide them in choosing a career.

SELF-ASSESSMENT

Knowledge of oneself can enhance personal strengths while helping become aware of unknown weaknesses, tolerances, or risks (Figure 25-1). Personalities, styles, and accomplishments will help guide personal assessment. The Myers-Briggs Type Indicator, Campbell Interest and Skill Survey, 16 Personality Factors, and transferable skills assessments are just a few self-evaluation tests.

Myers-Briggs Type Indicator

The Myers-Briggs Type Indicator (MBTI) is widely applied in the career development field to help individuals make more informed career decisions. This is an assessment of individual preferences, not a test of right or wrong answers. The goal of the MBTI in career planning is to assist an individual in gaining and understanding personal preferences and to use that information to explore various careers that will be supportive, challenging, and interesting.

Campbell Interest and Skill Survey

The Campbell Interest and Skill Survey (CISS) measures self-reported vocational interests and skills. Similar to traditional interest inventories, the CISS interest scales reflect an individual's attraction for specific occupational areas. However, the CISS instrument goes beyond traditional inventories by adding parallel skill scales that provide estimates of an individual's confidence in his or her ability to perform various occupational activities. Together, the two types of scales provide more comprehensive, richer data than interest scores alone. The CISS instrument focuses on careers that require post–secondary education and is most appropriate for use with individuals who are college bound or college educated.

16 Personality Factors

Since its introduction more than 40 years ago, the 16 Personality Factors (16PF) instrument has been widely used for a variety of applications, providing support for vocational guidance, hiring, and promotion recommendations.

Transferable Skills

Transferable skills are the skills that have been gathered through various jobs, volunteer work, hobbies, sports, or other life experiences that can be used in the next job or new career. In addition to being useful to career changes, transferable skills are also important to those who are facing a layoff, new graduates looking for their first jobs, and those reentering the workforce after an extended absence.

> ◎ **PRACTICE POINT** Individuals who possess positive leadership skills are of great value to practices and manufacturing companies.

Personal Skills

Team players seem to excel both more and more quickly than those who choose to work as individuals. This does not mean that people must depend on a team to succeed, but it shows that they have been successful in adjusting to a team environment as well as sharing and delegating responsibilities effectively.

Positive attitudes are contagious, and those with positive attitudes excel faster than those with negative attitudes. People prefer to be around happy, energetic, and enthusiastic individuals; they tend to be creative problem solvers and contribute well to a team environment.

A strong work ethic is an excellent attribute to possess. A strong work ethic is defined as striving for the best and excelling at finding tasks to complete. These tasks are completed quickly and efficiently, with excellent and consistent results. A strong work ethic cannot be taught; it is a trait that one possesses. Team members exhibiting a good work ethic in theory (and ideally in practice) should be selected for better positions, more responsibility and, ultimately, promotion. Team members who fail to exhibit a good work ethic may be regarded as failing to provide fair value for the wage the employer is paying them and should not be promoted or placed in positions of greater responsibility.

Education is essential for professional development. College courses enhance current skills, develop new skills, and teach independence. Continuing education is required of credentialed veterinary technicians and veterinarians to help them maintain the skills they have obtained as well as learn new techniques. Science and medicine continually change, and it is imperative to stay current with the new, up-and-coming trends and treatments.

> ◎ **PRACTICE POINT** Family values may be ranked higher in importance than work and must be evaluated when choosing careers.

Self-Evaluation Form

Name _____ Position _____

Date of employment _____ Date of promotion(s) _____

How long in present position _____

Attendance Record:

Number of days absent this year: _____ Approved days: _____ Unapproved days: _____

Number of days absent last year: _____ Approved days: _____ Unapproved days: _____

Number of days late this year: _____ Number of days late last year: _____

Attendance is: _____ Excellent _____ Good _____ Poor

Work Performance:

Rate your job performance by circling the appropriate letter.

Quality of Work:

A. Consistently performs quality work; requires little supervision.

B. Work is neat and accurate; requires some supervision.

C. Quality of work is good; makes some mistakes.

D. Produces work that is passable; needs improvement.

E. Makes frequent errors.

Comments: _____

Quantity of Work:

A. Superior work production. Completes tasks ahead of schedule and completes more than required.

B. Good producer; meets task deadlines and completes more than required.

C. Volume of work is satisfactory.

D. Requires close supervision to complete tasks; needs improvement.

E. Very slow. Does not complete tasks on time.

Comments: _____

Job Knowledge:

A. Understands all aspects of veterinary medicine. Masters tasks and skills extremely well.

B. Has a good knowledge base and performs tasks well.

C. Understands most procedures, tasks, and skills.

D. Shows understanding of job but requires help and instruction.

E. Lacks sufficient understanding of tasks and performs duties ineffectively.

Comments: _____

Staff Relations:

A. Goes out of the way to cooperate and assist all team members. Works well with others.

B. Willing to provide assistance to most team members.

C. Cooperates and works with others.

D. Usually helpful; may occasionally exhibit poor assistance.

E. Poor attitude.

Comments: _____

FIGURE 25-1 A self-evaluation form helps identify strengths and weaknesses.

Evaluating the surrounding environment may also be essential when evaluating oneself. Personal issues, family, health, and finances have a heavy impact on decisions to change or advance careers. For many, family comes first, and it is important for those who feel this way to find an occupation that agrees with and allows this philosophy. Health can be of concern for many, as employment positions with a high level of stress can cause increased blood pressure and a higher risk for heart attacks. Finances may be the highest of

Patient and Client Relations:

A. Extremely good at client relations and education; excellent patient care.

B. Consistently good at client relations and education; good at patient care.

C. Deals effectively with clients and patients.

D. Attitude and behavior not consistent.

E. Frequently rude or blunt.

Comments: _____

List four essentials that you are doing well:

1. _____
2. _____
3. _____
4. _____

List four essentials that need improvement:

1. _____
2. _____
3. _____
4. _____

Signature _____ Date _____

FIGURE 25-1, cont'd

all concerns, especially in the veterinary community. Veterinarians and technicians are not paid very highly, which forces many out of the veterinary health care profession and into sales, marketing, or research.

Questions may be asked and researched every so often to determine if a career change or advancement is needed. Further questions can be asked of individuals in the field when examining the possibility of change (Box 25-1).

Individuals may reevaluate the positions they currently hold. A manager may look to become certified by the Veterinary Hospital Managers Association. A technician may become specialized within a field such as internal medicine or emergency and critical care. A veterinarian may become board certified in a specialty. The possibilities are endless; it takes a motivated leader to find a niche that is a perfect fit.

MARKETING SKILLS

All the above skills help individuals market themselves as they look for employment. Team environments are going to look for a team-motivated individual to join their staff. Potential employers want a positive, smart, and motivated individual to join their team; confidence and personality must be visible to the potential employer or a resume may be tossed aside.

Marketing starts with personal interactions within a profession or industry being investigated. Individuals must appear professional and confident as they explore

Box 25-1 Questions to Consider Before Applying for a New Job

- Can this job change with the economy?
- Do I believe in the science the company produces and the products it develops?
- Do I have the ability to learn new topics, subjects, and fields?
- Does this job have a career track?
- How will a change benefit my family?
- If the job is in research or sales, does the company have excellent products?
- Is a change consistent with my values?
- What is my work style?
- What is the company's potential for growth?
- What traits do I have?
- What unique characteristics can I bring to this job?
- Will my family support a change?

employment opportunities (Figure 25-2). Many benign conversations can quickly change to an unscheduled interview once managers and representatives begin discussing employment opportunities.

EMPLOYMENT OPPORTUNITIES

Team members must have personal goals as well as employment goals. It is important not to forget oneself and one's personal life, especially as dedicated and

What Would You Do/Not Do?

Julie has been a full-time employee at ABC Veterinary Clinic for 5 years and has reached a plateau. She feels that her skills are not being utilized as much as they could be, which has made her resent her position. She feels that it is time to look for a position at another practice. Upon submission of her resume to several other practices, one in particular has shown interest and has called for an interview. The interview seems to go well for both parties. The potential employer asks for a list of references, and asks permission to call her current employer. Julie is hesitant to give permission to call her current employer, as she feels he may be upset with her for looking for other employment.

What Should Julie Do?

First, it would have been wise for Julie to discuss her job dissatisfaction with the current employer before she decided to look for new employment. If Julie is a great employee, the current employer may simply need to make changes to utilize Julie's skills to their fullest potential. If a change does not occur, then the current employer has been made aware of Julie's dissatisfaction and knows that she will be applying elsewhere.

Second, Julie should state to the potential employer that she prefer that the current employer be called as the last reference because she feels the he will be upset with her and she may suffer retribution as a result. It is important to be fair and honest with both individuals to prevent a shock to the current employer while impressing the potential employer.

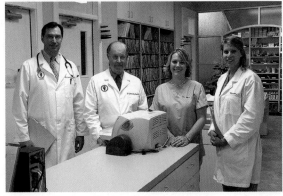

FIGURE 25-2 A professional appearance is a marketing tool that projects quality. (From Bassert JM, McCurnin DM: *McCurnin's clinical textbook for veterinary technicians*, ed 7, St Louis, 2010, Saunders Elsevier.)

PRACTICE POINT   Technicians can enjoy careers in general practice, specialty practice, sales, marketing, research, or management.

hardworking as many technicians are. They must make time for themselves; vacation, personal, or sick time, if awarded, should be used on a regular basis. It is imperative to take care of oneself to prevent burnout.

There are many different paths technicians can take in the field of veterinary medicine. Career opportunities include the many facets of clinical practice. General and specialty practice are very rewarding careers. General practice allows technicians to see a variety of animals, diseases, and treatments. Specialty practice limits the amount of diseases and species seen but allows specialization in specific areas such as internal medicine, surgery, dermatology, dentistry, or emergency and critical care.

Research and development can add challenges and rewards to any career by developing new products, foods, or treatments for a variety of species and diseases. Research has received negative attention in the past, and the media especially feels that research always involves harming animals. This is untrue and has been proven at excellent research facilities.

Veterinary manufacturers and distribution companies are always seeking the qualifications of credentialed and experienced technicians. Sales and marketing teams look for methods to target consumers, and technicians have the experience that these teams are looking for. Many companies require a bachelor's degree for employment; it is imperative to finish a bachelor's program in case a switch in careers is ever contemplated.

Management of a general or specialty practice takes time, patience, leadership, and independence. Technicians that have superseded expectations in practice are generally promoted to manage practices. While the technician portion is easy to manage, running an entire business is a whole new ballgame. Attending classes and learning from peers will help the most inexperienced businessperson succeed.

Excellent technicians are also excellent educators. They have experience teaching clients as well as other team members about veterinary medicine. Those who take time to help others will find a very rewarding career in teaching. There is nothing more gratifying than seeing a student progress and become a distinguished individual in the veterinary profession; since they had an excellent teacher, they become an excellent teacher to others (Figure 25-3).

Many sources exist for locating employment opportunities. Large manufacturing companies post research and sales positions on their Web sites. Word of mouth is also a valuable resource; many representatives know when their company is or will be hiring. Veterinary practices may advertise locally, nationally, in schools, and at veterinary conferences. National publications such as the *Journal of Veterinary Medicine*, *Veterinary Economics*, and *Vet Product News* list job announcements

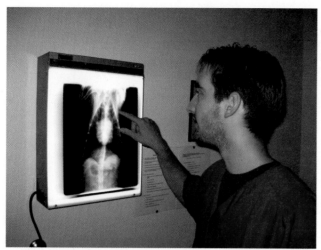

FIGURE 25-3 Many veterinary professionals choose teaching as a second career.

for all facets of veterinary medicine, including research, sales, and teaching opportunities.

PREPARING EMPLOYMENT DATA

Many times, the only impression a potential employer can make about an applicant is from the cover letter and resume that are submitted. Care must be taken to develop a professional, error-free cover letter and resume conveying positive attributes and work ethic.

Cover Letter

Cover letters are an introduction to the applicant, without repeating information contained in the resume. Three basic goals should be achieved with a cover letter: create interest, describe abilities, and request an interview. Cover letters may be needed when a resume is sent to the human resources department or to someone who is not the decision maker. They may also be used when a type of action is required by either the reader or the applicant. For example, an applicant may notify the reader that a follow-up phone call will be made in a specified number of days.

> **PRACTICE POINT** Cover letters and resumes are sometimes the only introduction the reader has about a potential employee.

A cover letter should be printed on the same type of paper the resume is printed on, with similar font type and size. Full contact information should be at the top of the page, similar to the resume, along with a date and the anticipated reader's name and address. If the applicant is unsure of the target reader's information, some research should be done to determine who it is; this adds a personal touch to the letter, identifying that the applicant has put extra effort into the cover letter.

A formal greeting is appropriate for the opening paragraph. A title such as Mr., Mrs., or Dr. should be used along with "Dear." Do not use "To whom it may concern," as this devalues the cover letter immediately. The first paragraph should let the reader know where the information was found to apply for the job; a newspaper article, a friend, or a co-worker can all be cited. The first paragraph should also stimulate interest about the candidate (Figure 25-4).

The second paragraph is the body of the letter. This section is used to promote and highlight the activities that qualify the applicant for the position. This may be the hardest paragraph to write, but it includes the most valuable information, information that may not be immediately visible on the resume. If the writer has difficulty writing this paragraph, a friend may be enlisted to state the positive attributes the candidate possesses. Those attributes can then be listed in this paragraph.

The final paragraph is an action paragraph; it states what the next step of either the applicant or the reader should be. If the applicant states that he or she will call and follow up, a specific date should be given. If the applicant is asking for an interview, a simple statement is appropriate such as, "Please give me the opportunity to discuss my qualifications with you. My contact number is _____."

It is important to be proactive when searching for employment, and it is essential to set one's resume apart from the rest. The applicant should call and follow up on the resume to ensure that it was received. If the target reader has not had a chance to review the resumes on file, the name of the applicant will be familiar once he or she does review the resumes, as the applicant's name has already been stated once, if not twice. If a call cannot be placed, an email or follow-up letter is appropriate. It is important not to be too aggressive, but it is imperative to be assertive and follow up.

The closing signature should be thoughtful: "Thank you for your time," or "Cordially," are appropriate, along with the applicant's name. Any degrees or titles should follow the name, along with the signature of the applicant.

Resume

A resume is a marketing tool that is tailored to the specific job the applicant has interest in. The goal of a resume is to be granted an interview; therefore as a general rule, resumes should be concise and limited to one or two pages in length. Abbreviations and acronyms should be avoided, and the font should be easy to read. Recommended fonts include Ariel, Times New Roman, or Tahoma and should not be smaller than 10 point or larger than 12 point size.

1000 Terrace View Apts.
Blackburg, VA 24060
987-654-3210
stevenmasonvt@fastwave.biz

Mr. John Wilson
Personnel Director
Anderson Veterinary Hospital
3507 Rockville Pike
Rockville, MD 20895

Dear Mr. Wilson:

I read in the most recent journal of Pet Product News of your need for an experienced veterinary technician in the Rockville area. I will be returning to the Rockville area immediately after graduation in May and believe I have the necessary credentials to fill your position.

I have worked at various veterinary hospitals prior to attending college. As you can see from my resume, I have also assisted graduate students with several research projects.

In addition to my practical experience, I will complete the requirements for my veterinary technician degree in May. As you know, Purdue is one of the leading universities in veterinary technology, specializing in business management. I am confident that my veterinary technician degree, along with years of experience, makes me an excellent candidate for your position.

I would welcome the opportunity to interview with you. I will be in the Rockville area during the week of April 12th and would be available to speak with you at that time. I will contact you in the next 10 days to answer any questions that you may have.

Thank you for your consideration,

Sincerely,

Steven Mason

Enclosure

FIGURE 25-4 A sample cover letter.

PRACTICE POINT   Resumes must not have errors!

As a resume is being created, the writer should keep a few things in mind. Potential employees should put themselves in the shoes of the potential employer. What is the potential employer looking for? What qualifications is the employer looking for? What attributes are needed? These qualifications and attributes can then be emphasized in the resume.

All resumes should have contact information listed first, centered at the top of the first page. This includes the applicant's name, address, telephone number, and email address. An objective statement follows, which is a brief description of the position that is being applied

for and how the applicant's unique skills can contribute to the position. Education is cited next, listing schools by full name and address. Education should be arranged in chronological order, listing the most current first. Degrees should be listed, along with any major or minors, and the graduation date (Box 25-2).

Resumes can have a variety of arrangements, including chronological (most common), skill, or mixed order. Chronological order lists items starting with the most current position held. Education is generally listed first, followed by employment history. Job descriptions are included in the employment portion. Skills resumes may be used when changing careers. Education and work history are minimized, while the skills used to accomplish tasks are embellished. This may be of benefit

Box 25-2   Resume Rules
• Avoid lengthy job descriptions or descriptions of non-transferable job duties. • Be consistent. Use the same format throughout the resume. • Construct a resume using action verbs, adjectives, and key words that describe skills. • Describe accomplishments quantitatively where appropriate. • Do not list unrelated personal information or photographs. • Do not make statements that cannot be backed up with examples or proof. • Do not use the word "I" or indefinite or personal pronouns or articles such as "my," "our," "an," or "the." • Do not include physical attributes such as age, weight, or height. • Do not include salary information unless requested. • Emphasize qualities and experience. • Limit graphics. • Limit the length. One page should be sufficient unless extensive professional experience is included. • Make sure that it is free of spelling, grammatical, and typographical errors. • Never hand write a resume. • Never print resumes double sided. • Print the resume using a laser printer or very clear ink jet printer. • Select resume paper that is light in color and has a fairly plain background so it can be copied, scanned, or faxed easily. • Since computers and scanners vary, save a copy of the resume in a text-only format so it can be emailed easily or copied and pasted to a job Web site. Many companies scan resumes, but scanners have difficulty with lines, graphics, and some fonts. • Use headings that allow the reader to find needed information quickly.

Box 25-3   Positive Words
• Accomplished • Achieved • Assisted • Completed • Conducted • Coordinated • Creative • Demonstrated • Dependable • Enthusiastic • Flexible • Generated • Have initiative • Honest • Implemented • Improved • Increased • Initiated • Instructed • Listener • Maintained • Managed • Motivated • Organized • Persuaded • Prepared • Produced • Prompt • Recruited • Self-motivated • Streamlined • Team player • Trained • Updated

when trying to match the target skills to the position available. Mixed resumes offer a combination of both chronological and skills-based resumes, allowing focus on individual skills.

Employment history includes the name and location of the employer along with employment dates and responsibilities. Descriptions of job duties and responsibilities should be short and to the point (Box 25-3).

PRACTICE POINT   Positive words contribute to the overall image of the cover letter and resume.

Volunteer experiences can be listed after employment history, especially if volunteering was a large part of a previous employment period. Previous volunteer experience may also be vital to the skills targeted for the open position. Just as for employment history, the

name and location of the organization should be listed along with volunteer dates in chronological order. A brief description of duties should be included as well (Figure 25-5).

Membership organizations can be listed after volunteer experiences, especially if a leadership position has been held. A brief description of roles, responsibilities, and highlights should be documented.

References should be listed on a separate sheet of paper in alphabetical order. The applicant's contact information should be on the top of the sheet in case it becomes separated from the original resume. Reference information should include a full name, address, telephone number, and email address of each person listed. References should be reminded that they have been listed on the resume, preventing a shock when a potential employer calls.

If several jobs have been held, some related to career goals and some not, one might try creating a "Related Experience" section near the top of the resume to

Steven Mason

Current Address:
1000 Terrace View Apts.
Blackburg, VA 24060
987-654-3210

Permanent Address:
1650 Home Road
Rockville, MD 20895
123-654-0987

stevenmasonvt@fastwave.biz

Career Objective

Veterinary Technician: Seeking a challenging position in a dynamic environment that focuses on building strategic relationships with clients and promotes customer service while promoting high-quality veterinary medicine.

Education

Purdue University, Veterinary Technology Program
Bachelor of Science in Veterinary Technology   Expected graduation 5/10

Activities and Honors

- Captain, Intramural Softball Team; organized tryouts, selected team and coached an eight-week season
- President, Veterinary Technology Club; organized fundraisers as well as career days with local elementary schools

Experience

Animal Science Reproduction and Physiology Lab, Purdue University
08/09-present
Lab Research Assistant
- Researched, updated, and selected and more than 500 Holstein cows for a reproductive trial utilizing Lutalyse
- Drew blood, performed laboratory analysis on selected cows
- Assisted in calving

Animal Science Nutrition Lab, Purdue University
08/08-05/09
Lab Research Assistant
- Developed feeding protocols for calves
- Performed nutritional analysis on feedstuffs and fecal content
- Analyzed data, providing summary to graduate students

Ark Veterinary Hospital
08/07-08/08
Veterinary Assistant
- Assisted the veterinarians and veterinary technicians with restraint, examinations, and surgery
- Placed IV catheters
- Obtained blood samples
- Performed basic laboratory analysis utilizing Idexx Lasercyte and chemistry machines
- Completed urinalyses, fecal and microscopic examinations

FIGURE 25-5 A sample resume.

highlight career-related jobs. Other jobs could be listed under the headings "Other Experience" or "Supportive Experience" and have much more concise descriptions.

Creating a "Summary of Skills" list at the top of the page can be an excellent way to demonstrate job-related skills immediately, especially if applying for a position for which there has been no formal training.

Every resume and cover letter should be meticulously read by a trusting friend or professional. The writer is bound to make typographical errors that will be overlooked; a fresh set of eyes will pick up the errors before the target reader does (who will then form a negative thought regarding the professionalism of the applicant). A good friend will also scrutinize the information and offer tips for improvement. If a good friend is not available for review, a local college is sure to have excellent resources and staff available for such tasks.

PRACTICE POINT Many companies only accept resumes online; correct submission is essential.

Email and Internet Resumes

Many companies now accept resumes online, either by the Internet or email. It is important to know that the Internet and email changes the configuration of resumes and cover letters. The resume can be saved as a PDF file; this will allow it to be viewed exactly as it was created. If a cover letter will be submitted via email, it may be easier to cut and paste the cover letter into the body of the email. An applicant does not want to submit a cover letter that is deformed and unreadable, especially when it is the first document the target reader will open.

PREPARING FOR AN INTERVIEW

Preparing for an interview is similar to completing homework for a college course. One must be prepared and present the homework in a professional, logical manner (Box 25-4). Questions can be asked of oneself in preparation for an interview, and many additional questions asked during the interview may come from these basic questions (Box 25-5).

"Where are you at this time in your life?" This helps review the past and explains why the person is where he or she is today. Experiences, past employment, and lifestyle affect the development of an individual, including skills and attitude. Applicants should expect to answer questions about previous employment, gaps in employment history, or frequent changes in jobs. Skills, aptitudes, and responsibilities should be thought about when completing this section of the homework. (Where am I now? What changes need to take place? Why?)

> **PRACTICE POINT** It is essential to prepare for interviews; questions must be answered confidently and appropriately.

"Where are you going?" A potential employer wants to know what the goals of the applicant will be. Where will this potential employee be in 1 year, 5 years, or 10 years? Will he or she benefit the company? Will the company waste money training a person for less than 1 year of employment? On a personal level, the individual must determine goals, understand that goals do change, and accept the challenges that come along the way.

"How are you going to achieve your goals?" Additional schooling, employment opportunities, or volunteering experiences may help achieve goals and dreams. A particular job may result in a dream or goal an applicant has; if so, it is important to take the right steps to obtain that goal.

"What are your strengths and weaknesses?" It is advantageous to determine one's strengths and weaknesses. These questions will certainly be asked in an interview, and the potential employer will want to know

Box 25-4	Interview Rules

- Ask questions.
- Do not chew gum.
- Do not discuss salary immediately.
- Do not lack enthusiasm.
- Do not talk excessively or appear too aggressive.
- Dress accordingly.
- Make eye contact.
- Use proper grammar.

Box 25-5	Common Interview Questions

- Are you currently employed?
- Describe yourself.
- How did you learn about this profession?
- What are your goals? 5 years from now? 10 years from now?
- What can you bring to our team?
- What formal education have you received?
- What is your ideal job?
- What is your strongest asset?
- What is your weakest asset?
- What responsibilities have you enjoyed the least at your previous jobs, and why?
- What responsibilities have you enjoyed the most at your previous jobs, and why?
- What salary do you expect?
- Why are you interested in this company?
- Why do you feel you are qualified for this position?
- Why do you wish to change jobs?
- Why should our company hire you?

why. Many veterinary technicians' greatest weakness is the inability to say no. They take on too many projects, become overwhelmed, and perhaps do not complete any of them on time or above the expected level. A great asset may be listening and talking. A great employee may talk a lot, but clients love team members who are social, listen, and reply with valuable knowledge.

"What type of benefits or salary would you be willing to accept?" Benefits and salary are generally a decisive factor when determining employment; therefore full thought and consideration should be given to this topic before an interview. The topic may or may not evolve during the interview process; it will, however, evolve by the time an offer of employment is made. Veterinarians, veterinary technicians, and practice managers can refer to the Veterinary Hospital Medical Association, American Animal Hospital Association, or National Commission on Veterinary and Economic Issues for standards of pay in the region in which they reside or will potentially reside. This can provide a guide of acceptable ranges of payment. Other considerations are benefits that are available to team members. Many times, benefits packages far outweigh salary; therefore consideration must

Box 25-6	Questions to Ask Potential Employers

- Do you have an open-door policy regarding communications, problem solving, and personnel issues?
- Do you value your employees as team members or individuals?
- How many team members are employed?
- What are short-term goals for this company?
- What are the long-term goals of this company?
- What benefits are generally offered with this position?
- What is the biggest strength of this company?
- What is the staff turnover rate?
- What is the weakest attribute of this company?

be given to both. See Chapter 5 for benefits that are generally offered.

Applicants should learn about the business to which they are applying. Mission statements, values, or goals can be gained from Web sites for larger corporations; smaller practices may also have information available on their Web sites. If the applicant knows current employees of the company, questions can be asked about company policies, benefits, and promotional opportunities and procedures.

◉ **PRACTICE POINT**   When asked by potential employers, applicants should be able to explain employment gaps and frequent changes in jobs.

Depending on the type of company and position, wearing a suit may be appropriate. A suit may be overdressed for a veterinary assistant position; business casual dress may be considered. Appearances make an impression and can last forever; it is imperative to dress appropriately. If there is any question, dress a step above what might be expected.

Prepare questions for a potential employer (Box 25-6). An interview is for both the applicant and the employer. Applicants should want to know if they are an appropriate match for the practice or company. There is no need to waste the applicant's and employer's time if the morals, ethics, and goals do not match. A small notebook can be taken into the interview to remind the applicant of questions. Ask for a day to work in or observe the practice (if applicable). Learning about the environment is extremely important.

Arrive early for an interview. Latecomers are automatically assessed a mental penalty; lateness may indicate that the interview is not important to the candidate.

FOLLOW-UP AFTER THE INTERVIEW

A follow-up letter should be written 1 or 2 days after the interview. This is an indicator that the applicant is interested in the position, which may help set the resume and interview apart from others. A letter may include a statement of thanks and once again highlight the qualifications of the candidate and how the applicant's assets will benefit the company. If, after the interview and observation of the practice, the applicant chooses not to pursue employment opportunities, a letter should be written stating so. This not only saves the employer time and money, but the applicant may need to return in the future for an interview with the practice.

◉ **PRACTICE POINT**   Follow-up letters can positively influence the potential employer.

RECEIVING OFFERS OF EMPLOYMENT

It is important to remember the value one possesses. If more than one interview has taken place and multiple offers have been made, all offers should be considered before making a final decision. Potential employers should be told that several offers exist for employment, and that a response will be available in a stated time. (Be careful not to extend this time too far out, as potential employers may hire someone else.) Individuals must remember what their goals are: "What kind of employer do I want?" "What kind of work environment do I want?" "What is my goal for hours and salary?" Once a majority of expectations have been met, a decision can be made.

◉ **PRACTICE POINT**   Evaluate all offers of employment, including benefits, before making a decision.

It is advisable to receive the offer in writing, including the agreed salary, the raise and evaluation structure, and any benefits that are offered at the time of employment. Some employees may be put on a trial period, which prevents benefits from immediately being offered; the rules of the trial period should also be clearly stated in the offer.

RETIREMENT

Retirement should not be ignored while developing one's career. Whether an individual is changing to the veterinary profession, leaving the field, or creating a whole new dynamic, retirement is important to consider. Previous generations have had Social Security to rely on; although it does not produce a wealthy income, it at least provided enough money for food and shelter. Future generations may not have Social Security to depend on; if any money is left to distribute, it will not be enough for survival. It is therefore imperative to start planning as soon as possible.

◉ **PRACTICE POINT**   Retirement income will be essential to survive once generations X and Y come to retirement age.

If companies do not offer a retirement fund as a benefit, it is up to the individual to start one for himself or herself. One can contact a financial planning professional to determine what type of account would be best; it is advised to find one who is willing to educate and spend time finding the correct investments for each client. Co-workers, friends, and professionals in the community can offer recommendations.

It takes discipline to save money now, but it will be worth it later. Many practices or companies allow funds to be deducted directly from the payroll check and deposited into a savings or retirement account before the employee ever sees the money. This is helpful for enforcing a savings plan for those who lack the discipline to do so.

 VETERINARY PRACTICE and the LAW

When preparing for an interview, be aware of questions that cannot be asked of the applicant. The Equal Employment Opportunity Laws are a collection of federal laws that prohibit job discrimination, both during the interview process and once the applicant has been hired. Questions regarding religious affiliation, citizenship or place of birth, pregnancy, family or marital status, race, military affiliation, age, political affiliation, or holidays that are observed are off-limits. Persons who believe they have been discriminated against in the application process can file a report with the Equal Employment Opportunity Commission.

Self-Evaluation Questions

1. What is the MBTI?
2. Why should one prepare for an interview?
3. What is the purpose of a cover letter?
4. When would one use a skills-based resume?
5. Why should one ask potential employers questions?
6. How should one dress for an interview?
7. Why is professional development important to maintain?
8. What is the purpose of a follow-up letter?
9. Prepare a cover letter.
10. Prepare a chronological resume.

Recommended Reading

Ackerman LJ: *Management basics for veterinarians*, New York, 2003, ASJA Press.

Bolles RN: *What color is your parachute? 2009: a practical manual for job hunters and career changers*, Berkeley, CA, 2008, Ten Speed Press.

Green B: *Get the interview every time: Fortune 500 hiring professionals' tips for writing winning resumes and cover letters*, Chicago, IL, 2004, Dearborn Trade.

Jackson A, Geckeis K: *How to prepare your curriculum vitae*, ed 2, New York, 2003, McGraw-Hill.

Stowe JD, Ackerman LJ: *The effective veterinary practice*, Guelph, Ont, Canada, 2004, Lifelearn.

Index

Page numbers followed by f, t, or b indicate figures, tables, or boxes, respectively.